the retinal circulation

D K Markstone

george n. wise, B.S., M.D., D.Med.Sci. (Ophth.)

Professor of Ophthalmology
Albert Einstein College of Medicine;
Montefiore Hospital and Medical Center
Bronx, New York

colin t. dollery, B.Sc., M.B., Ch.B., F.R.C.P.

Professor of Clinical Pharmacology
Royal Postgraduate Medical School
University of London

paul henkind, A.B., M.D., M.Sci. (Ophth.), Ph.D.

Professor of Ophthalmology
Albert Einstein College of Medicine;
Montefiore Hospital and Medical Center
Bronx, New York

the retinal circulation

MEDICAL DEPARTMENT
HARPER & ROW, PUBLISHERS
NEW YORK, EVANSTON, SAN FRANCISCO, LONDON

THE RETINAL CIRCULATION

Printed in the United States of America. For information address Medical Department, Harper & Row, Publishers, Inc., 49 East 33rd Street, New York, N.Y. 10016.

First Edition

Standard Book Number 06–142767–5

LIBRARY OF CONGRESS CATALOG CARD NUMBER: 79–156133

contents

preface

"What glories lie within the eye"

The retinal circulation is important in many different fields of medicine. To the ophthalmologist, retinal vascular disease is one of the most common causes of visual disturbance and blindness. To the internist, examination of the retinal vessels provides invaluable evidence concerning the impact of systemic diseases such as hypertension and diabetes upon the microcirculation of a deep organ. To the vascular physiologist, the retina provides a supremely accessible microcirculation fitted with a natural transparent window through which vascular responses may be observed.

Clinical observation with the ophthalmoscope, slit lamp, and contact lens has provided a large body of clinical data on the development and course of retinal lesions. Recent advances in clinical techniques, notably the retinal camera with electronic flash and fluorescein angiography, have added a new dimension to studies of the retinal circulation. The possibility of studying changes in vessel caliber, blood flow, vascular leakage, and the like have shed light upon the pathogenesis of many retinal lesions hitherto known only as inexplicable clinical syndromes. Advances in the clinical and experimental study of retinal vascular disease have been paralleled by advances in pathologic techniques, such as the use of retinal digests and studies with the electron microscope.

In this book we have utilized these newer techniques of clinical, experimental, and histologic study in reaching our conclusions regarding the various retinal vascular diseases and their clinicopathologic correlations. As these problems are diverse and cover several disciplines, we believe that an interdisciplinary approach is of special value. Together we have interests in clinical ophthalmology, internal medicine, ocular pathology, and experimental vascular disease united in the common ground of the retinal circulation.

Our approach to the clinical description and understanding of retinal vascular disease is somewhat different from that adopted by other authors and requires a word of explanation. Retinal vascular disease tends to have its chief impact on either the arterial side of the circulation, as in arteriosclerosis or hypertension, or on the capillaries and veins, as in the diseases associated with capillary or venous obstruction and diabetes. Grouping diseases in this manner is helpful in understanding the very similar pathologic responses that may occur in conditions of varied etiology.

The human retina has a dual blood supply, and although the retinal vessels are much easier to observe, it is essential not to forget the role of the choroidal circulation. Less is known about normal and pathologic responses of the choroidal circulation. Exploration here is just beginning. Study of the choroidal circulation by fluorescein angiography and knowledge of the effect of increased choroidal oxygen tension upon the inner retinal layers are but two of the recent developments advancing knowledge in this area.

Throughout this book we have used the terms *retinal artery* and *retinal vein* rather than *arteriole* or *venule*. This usage is purely arbitrary and was adopted for the sake of uniformity rather than anatomic correctness. A similar approach was recently taken by Pickering (*Trans. Ophthal. Soc. U.K. 89:*38, 1969). Since many of the photographs were taken with older carbon arc fundus cameras, some will contain central oval, white spots or black linear marks due to the camera reflex.

This book is intended for both the practitioner in his office and the research worker in his laboratory. We hope that it will help each one to understand the other's problems.

Production of a book involves many people besides the authors. We should like to express our thanks to our colleagues, research fellows, and technical and secretarial staff, all of whom contributed in no small measure to our work. Special mention should be made of Drs. C. J. Bulpitt, D. W. Hill, J. V. Hodge, E. M. Kohner, L. N. F. de Oliveira, J. W. Paterson, P. S. Ramalho, and M. Shakib who have been essential members of the research team that carried out much of the experimental work we describe. We are particularly indebted to our retinal photographic staff, Henrick Malpica and Michael Tudball, for their efforts in preparing the illustrations. Our secretaries, Gwen Cox, Doris Ortega, Joyce Rolls, and Annette Todaro carried an especially heavy burden; without them this book could not have been produced. We are also grateful to Professor Norman Ashton and Drs. C. J. Ball, J. L. Baum, C. J. Bulpitt, J. E. Kennedy, E. M. Kohner, A. Patz, C. W. Rucker, M. Shakib, and P. F. Wendler for permission to reproduce illustrative material.

Professor Russell Fraser and Sir John McMichael gave us great support and encouragement in England, and Dr. P. Rutkowski was especially helpful with work conducted in the Retinal Clinic at New York University. Much of the work contributed by Drs. Wise and Henkind was carried out during the period of their faculty appointments in the Eye Department of New York University.

This book contains a great deal of our personal research, and a special note of thanks is owed to those government and private agencies that have supported this work: The National Institutes of Health (Research Grants No. NB-05059, and EY-00613), and The Seeing Eye in the United States; and The Medical Research Council and The Wellcome Trust in the United Kingdom.

G.N.W.
C.T.D.
P.H.

the retinal circulation

chapter 1

Development of Retinal Vessels

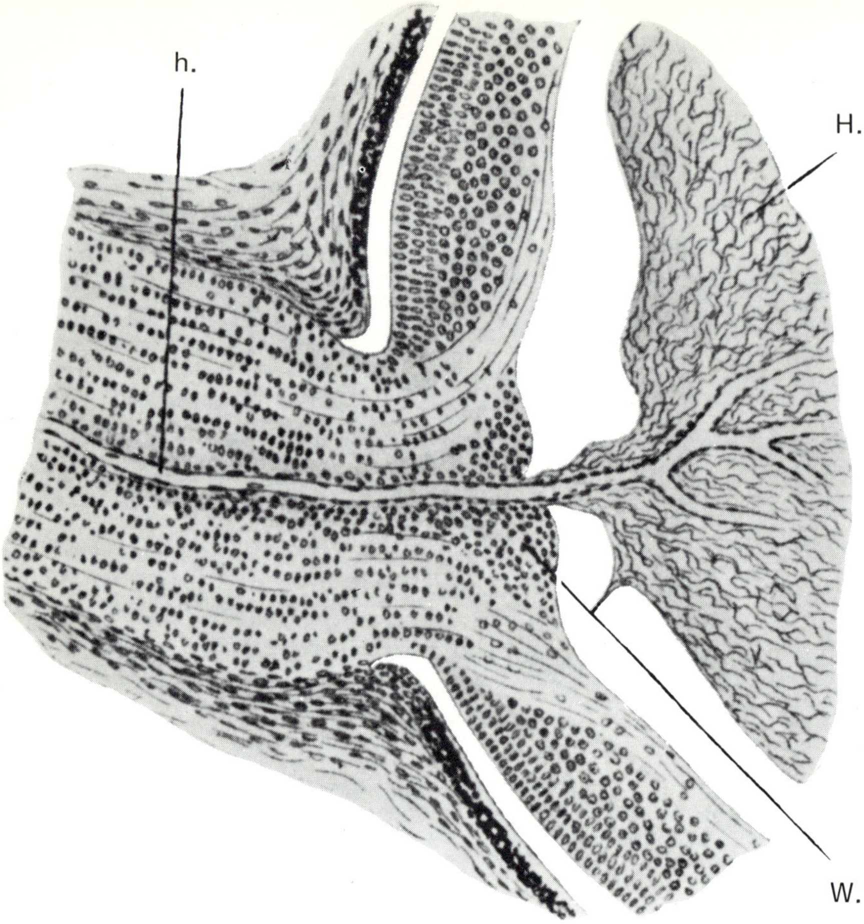

Fig. 1-1. Section through the point of entrance of the optic nerve in a 7-cm human fetus: **(h.)** hyaloid artery; **(H.)** vitreous body; **(W.)** cellular proliferation around hyaloid artery in which retinal vessels are forming. (From Versari.[21])

It is now accepted that the embryonic blood vessels arise from mesenchymal tissue at various sites within the body.[2,12] Once the embryonic circulation is fully established extension of the vascular system is solely by growth from preexistent vessels, and not from isolated mesenchyme. Where does the retinal vasculature fit into this scheme? It develops late in embryonic or even in postembryonic life, after most of the systemic vasculature has been laid down. The immature retina is composed strictly of nervous tissue elements and lacks mesenchyme. Therefore, vessels must develop from tissue entering the retina from without.

To date, the various stages in human retinal vessel development have not been fully studied, thus our discussion must rely, in part, on evidence gathered from lower species.

STUDIES IN MAN

Detailed study of the development of the human retinal vasculature dates back only to the early part of the twentieth century. Indeed, only in the past few years, by virtue of applying newer techniques, has it been possible to define the initial stages and pattern of such development. In the following section we provide an historical account of retinal circulatory development in man.

Versari[21,22] examined gelatin and Prussian blue-injected preparations as well as serial sections of more than 100 human fetal eyes, and he noted that retinal vessels de-

Fig. 1-2. Section through the point of entrance of the hyaloid artery into the eye of a 13-cm human fetus: **(H.)** vitreous body; **(a.l.)** hyaloid artery; **(h.)** hyaloid artery; **(a.r.)** retinal artery; **(v.r.)** retinal vein; **(W.)** cellular proliferation around the hyaloid artery from which the retinal vessels have formed. (From Versari.[21])

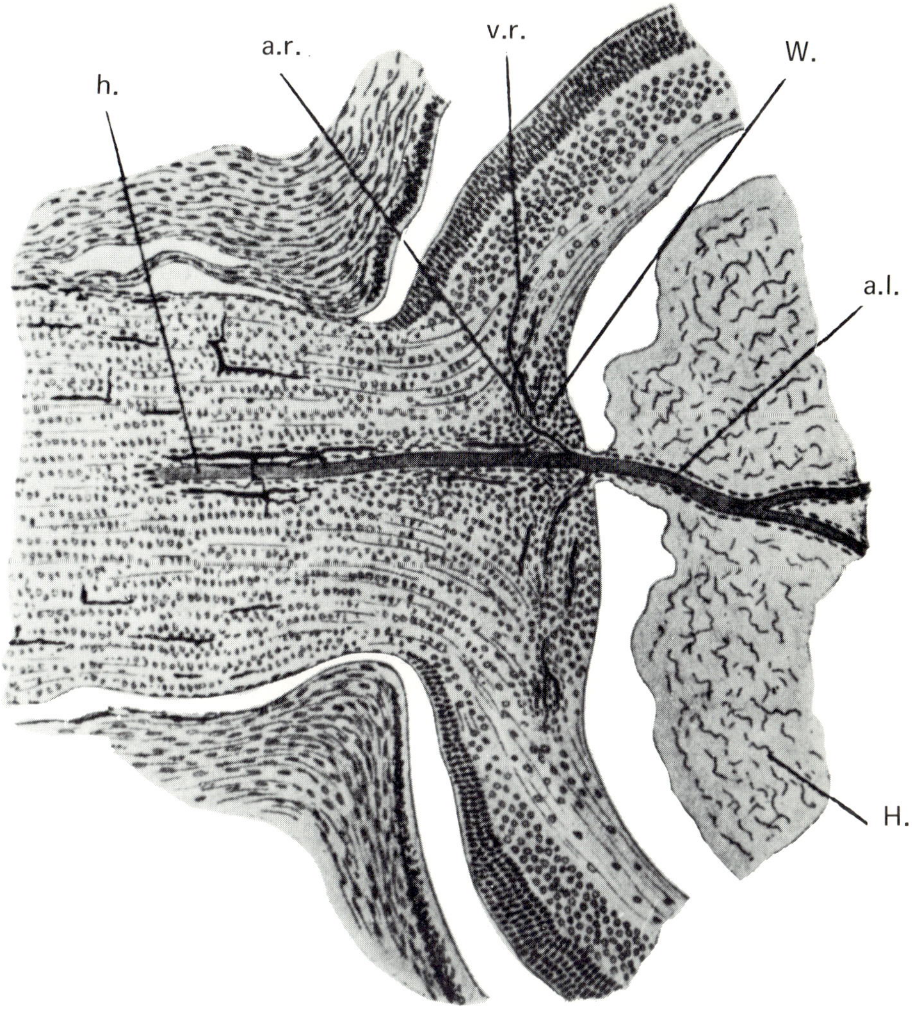

veloped from embryonic connective tissue around the hyaloid artery. In a fetus of 7-cm length he found cell cords in the substance of the cellular mass surrounding the hyaloid artery in the region of the papilla, and these were in continuity with the wall of the hyaloid artery (Fig. 1-1). Patent retinal vessels were observed in a fetus measuring 13 cm (Fig. 1-2). Versari also showed that the retinal vessels gradually penetrate from the superficial retina into the inner nuclear layer (Fig. 1-3).

Mann[11] noted that the central retinal artery is just recognizable at the 100-mm stage (fourth month) of gestation. At this time a bulbous swelling appears on the trunk of the hyaloid artery at its point of exit from the disc. From this enlargement, two small buds grow out to form the upper and lower main branches of the central retinal artery.

In 1948, Michaelson,[13] on the basis of studies conducted primarily on ink-injected fetuses, came to the following conclusions: (*1*) Vessel growth in the human retina is by a process of budding from preexistent vessels; (*2*) the formation of retinal capillaries is preeminently a function of the retinal veins, with only the arteriae afferentes (precapillary arterioles) originating from arteries; (*3*) if vein and artery are close to each other, vessel growth takes place predominantly from the side of the vein remote from the artery; and (*4*) the spread of capillary growth toward an artery extends only a certain distance, leaving finally, in the mature human eye, a well-marked, capillary-free zone around the arteries similar to that present in other mammalian retinas. He postulated that an extravascular tissue factor was responsible for the mode in which retinal capillaries developed, that the factor was possibly biochemical in nature, and that its action was essentially on retinal veins. His final conclusion was that the bulk of the capillary system in the retina of man can be considered part of the venous system. Michaelson's work has had a marked impact upon ophthalmology, however, the majority of his conclusions are no longer tenable. For example, retinal vessel growth does not start as budding from preexistent vessels, retinal capillary formation precedes and does not follow venous ingrowth, capillary growth is not predominantly from the venous side of the circulation, and the capillary-free zone is a secondary development occurring after the primitive retinal capillary bed is laid down.

The use of such techniques as retinal digestion, serial cross and flat sections, and electron microscopic studies in the rat have provided evidence that ink-injected preparations allow only a limited view of retinal vascular development (Fig. 1-4).

Ashton[3] has pointed out that undifferentiated spindle cells preceded either formed blood vessels or solid endothelial buds in the human fetal retina. His sections showed (Fig. 1-5) that the tip of the ingrowing vascular complex consists of spindle cells with associated polysaccharide granules which stain positively for periodic acid-Schiff reagent (PAS). Serpell[17] has identified the granules as glycogen. Ashton believes that the spindle cells are mesenchymal in nature and the normal precursors of retinal vascularization in the human fetus. Among other contributions, Ashton[4] also has noted that the developing vascular complex was accompanied by wandering macrophages which apparently act as scavengers, and seem to

Fig. 1-3. Sections through human fetal retina show the penetration of vessels from the inner retina (nerve fiber–ganglion cell layer) down into the inner nuclear layer. Diagrams are of injected retinas sectioned near the papilla. *A*, 19-cm fetus; *B*, 36-cm fetus; and *C*, 42-cm fetus. There are no deep vessels at the 19-cm stage. (From Versari.[21])

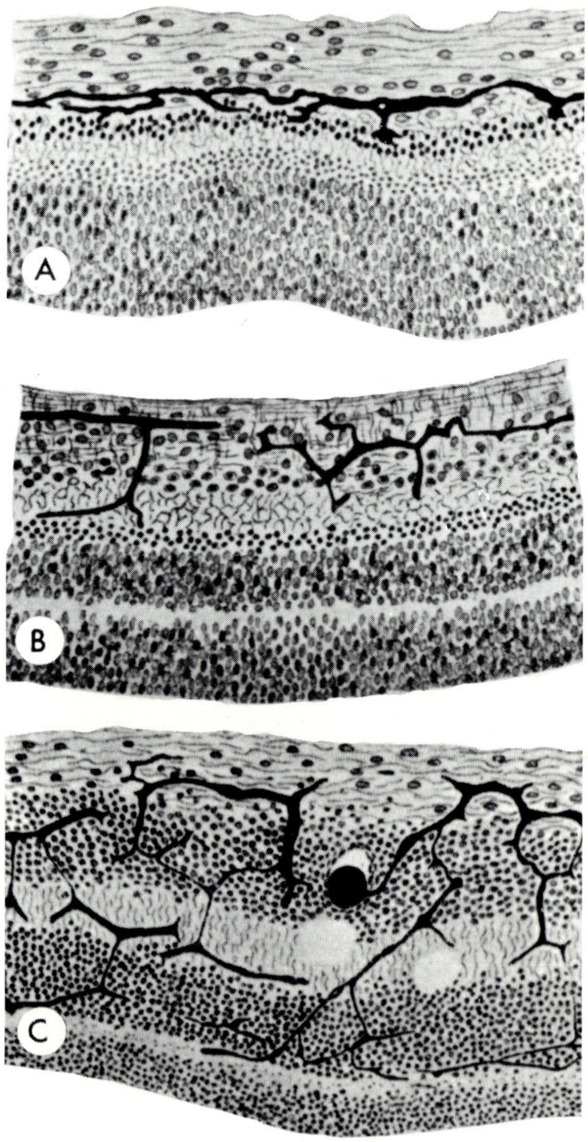

have some role in normal retinal vascularization in man. He also has demonstrated that the primitive immature network remodeled itself into the mature pattern by undergoing capillary retraction. In this process the redundant channels are obliterated and the endothelial cytoplasm and nuclei retract into adjacent patent capillaries leaving behind basement membrane bridges or strands. Ashton's statement, "It is clear that in the retina as elsewhere, vascular growth is remarkably labile, with proliferation, retraction, and cellular death constantly remodeling the developing network," is worth remembering.[4]

Nilhausen[14] has shown that the leading edge of the ingrowing retinal vascular system in the human fetus stains positively for alkaline phosphatase activity. This activity is lost in the mature retina.

Cogan,[7] primarily studying retinal digest preparations, has contributed greatly to our understanding of human retinal vessel development. He felt that solid endothelial cords, rather than undifferentiated cells, sprout from the nerve head, apparently from the same vessels that give rise to the hyaloid system. It should be pointed out, that in digest preparations the leading edge of cells, if not tightly bound to each other, could well be lost, leaving only the solid cords. Such a loss of the leading cells has been demonstrated in preparations of developing retinal vessels in the rat (Fig. 1-6). By the fifth fetal month the cords form a tight, uniform, chicken-wire pattern which is most prominent near the disc. The advancing vascular border is characterized by loops and free-ending sprouts (Fig. 1-7). Lumina containing occasional red blood cells are found at the fifth and sixth months. At the seventh and eighth months the primitive chicken-wire pattern extends almost to the ora serrata nasally and to the equator temporally. The advancing peripheral edge is characterized by a dense plexus of thin-walled vessels en-

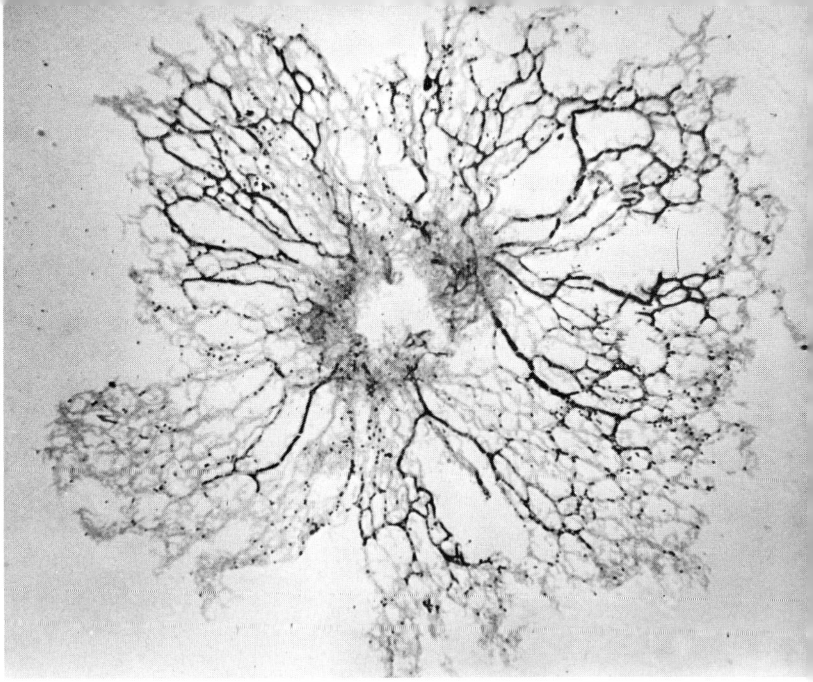

Fig. 1-4. Retinal digest preparation of a 24-hour-old rat. Initially the retina was inked and then was enzymatically digested. The vascular complex as seen in the digest is much more extensive than the portion which fills with ink. (From de Oliveira.[15])

Fig. 1-5. Flat section of retina of premature infant, shows ingrowing vascular complex. The peripheral tips are associated with PAS-positive granules. More posteriorly the vessels are developing and the granules have largely disappeared. PAS and hematoxylin, ×170. (From Ashton.[4])

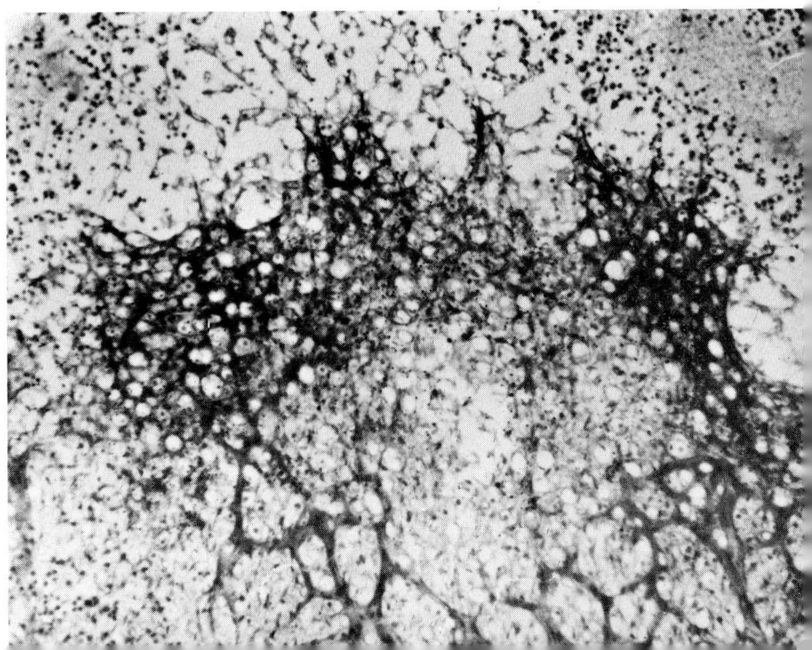

meshed in a mass of hyaline, PAS-positive material. Contrary to previous workers, Cogan has shown that retinal vessels were not completely differentiated by the eighth fetal month. Indeed, the adult pattern of retinal vascularization is not achieved until some months after birth, and the transition into mature vessels is gradual over the first few years of life. The immature vessels tend to be very cellular. Initially only endothelial cells are found, but at the third month after birth intramural pericytes can be seen on some capillaries. De Oliveira [15] has demonstrated intramural pericytes in the retinal vessels of newborn cats and human embryos (Fig. 1-8). By the fifth month of life intramural pericytes are present in all but the most peripheral capillaries. Another feature of the immature capillary is that its basement membrane takes only a weak stain with PAS, and that with maturity the basement membrane becomes more prominent.

The preceding paragraphs outline the work to-date. Ashton [5] has recently provided a useful summary of the state of our knowledge.

About the fifteenth or sixteenth week of human fetal life, spindle cells, presumably mesenchymal in nature, appear in the vicinity of the hyaloid artery at the disc. The cells seem to arise from the walls of the venous channels on either side of the hyaloid artery rather than from the artery itself. They proliferate into the nerve head and subsequently invade the nerve fiber layer of the retina. These cells, in active mitotic division, form the vanguard of the ingrowth and always precede the ingrowing patent channels until vascularization is completed at, or shortly after birth. The mesenchymal cells differentiate into endothelial cells, solid cords form, clefts develop between adjacent cells, intercellular junctions appear and they gradually canalize to form primitive capillaries in a polygonal network. No arteries or veins can be distinguished at this stage. Scattered capillaries begin to narrow, retract, and atrophy. Blood is shunted into remaining channels which enlarge to form major channels. At an early stage the arterial and venous channels can be recognized: The capillaries related to venous drainage form a smaller meshwork and are dilated and more cellular, while the capillaries near the arteries form a wider meshwork, and are narrower and less cellular. As the arterial and venous channels develop from the primitive capillary bed their side branches retract and atrophy and a perivascular capillary-free zone appears.

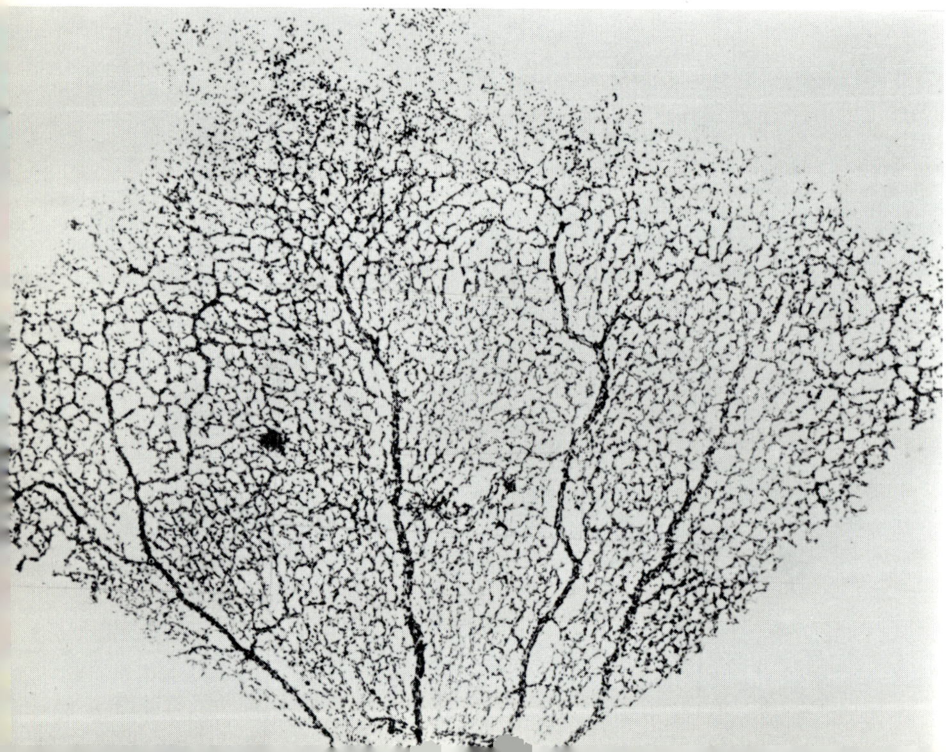

Fig. 1-6. Retinal digest preparation from a 4-day-old rat. Note loss of the mesenchymal meshwork at the upper left and upper right sides of the preparation. This gives the impression that the complex ends as cords in these areas, but the upper center portion of the figure shows that this is not so. PAS and hematoxylin, ×45. (From Henkind and de Oliveira.[9])

AGING OF RETINAL VESSELS IN MAN

Cogan has studied the senescence of human retinal vessels.[7] He found that the cells of the peripheral capillaries start to disappear about age 50. Sugi [20] has found that the cellular elements of peripheral capillaries tend to be lost at about age 40 in Japanese individuals. Cogan has noted that first the endothelial cells are lost leaving some capillaries only with intramural pericytes, but Sugi has found that both cell types diminish with about equal frequency. Capillaries which have lost endothelial cell nuclei appear to maintain their original caliber so long as intramural pericytes are intact. Eventually the latter also disappear leaving acellular channels devoid of blood. In those instances where the intramural pericytes are lost first one may find dilated capillaries, shunts, microaneurysms, and endothelial cell proliferation. Such a situation can apparently occur as a part of the normal aging process without concomitant diabetes or hypertension. For example, Sugi has found capillary microaneurysms in 35 of 63 eyes (55.5 per cent) of older patients without known hypertension or diabetes. Most of these aneurysms occurred at the retinal periphery. With increasing age there is a gradual diminution in the cellularity of most retinal capillaries. This affects the endothelial cells more than the intramural pericytes, and is more patchy than the generalized peripheral changes. The capillaries may also show basophilic stippling and sudanophilia. As the peripheral capillary arcades become acellular the internal limiting membrane becomes fused to the retinal vessels. As a result, many PAS-positive, spider-like processes develop on or about the vessels.

STUDIES IN ANIMALS

Observations on the development of the retinal vascular system date back to the nineteenth century. Kessler,[10] using osmium tetroxide for fixation (in 1877), studied the development of retinal vessels in the rat, and concluded that they arose independently of the hyaloid artery, presumably not by budding. Vessels developed from a cellular layer which grew into the retina. Schultze [16] and Voll,[23] studying the membrana vasculosa retinae in a number of species, noted that the retinal vessels arose independently

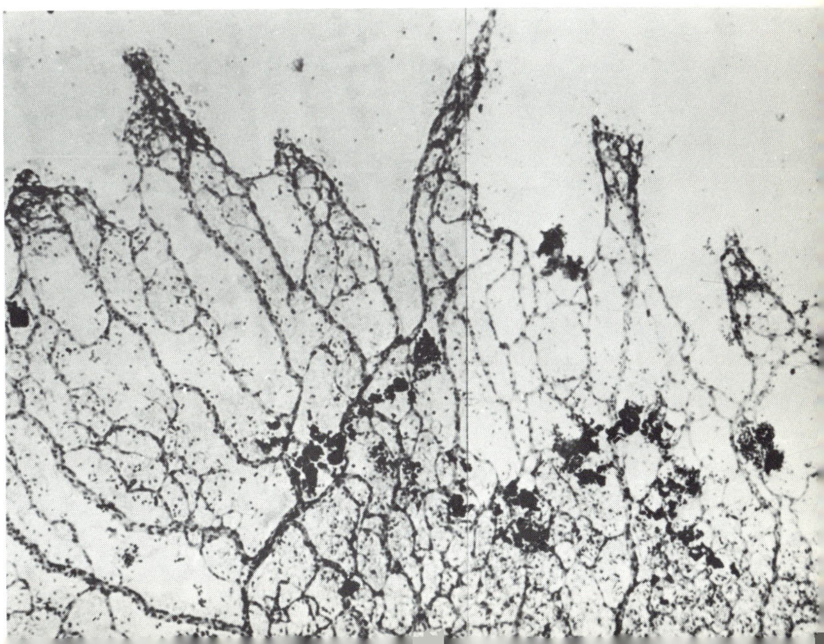

Fig. 1-7. Digest preparation of edge of the retinal vascular complex in a 22-week-old human fetus shows the loops and sprouts described by Cogan. (From de Oliveira.[15])

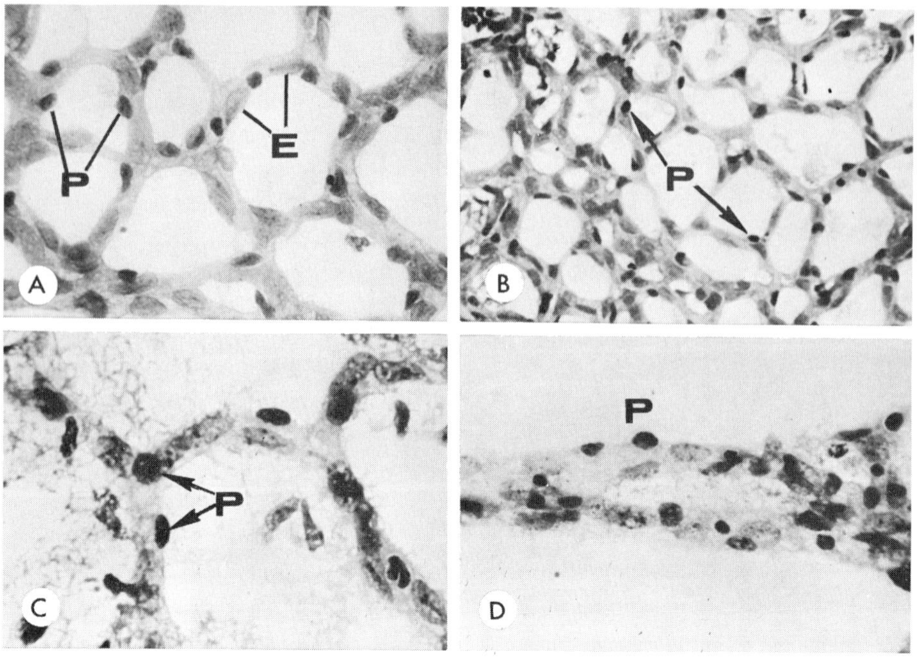

Fig. 1-8. Retinal digest preparations of a 24-hour-old kitten (*A* and *B*) and a 22-week-old human fetus (*C* and *D*) show the cellular morphology of the developing vessels. *A* is at the posterior pole, *B* is near the periphery, *C* is near the periphery, and *D* is at the periphery. **E,** endothelial cells; **P,** intramural pericytes. (From de Oliveira.[15])

Fig. 1-9. Section through the optic nerve and retina of a 2.5-cm sheep embryo; **mv** is the membrana vasculosa retinae developing from the mesenchymal cells which surround the hyaloid artery, **ah.** (From Voll.[23])

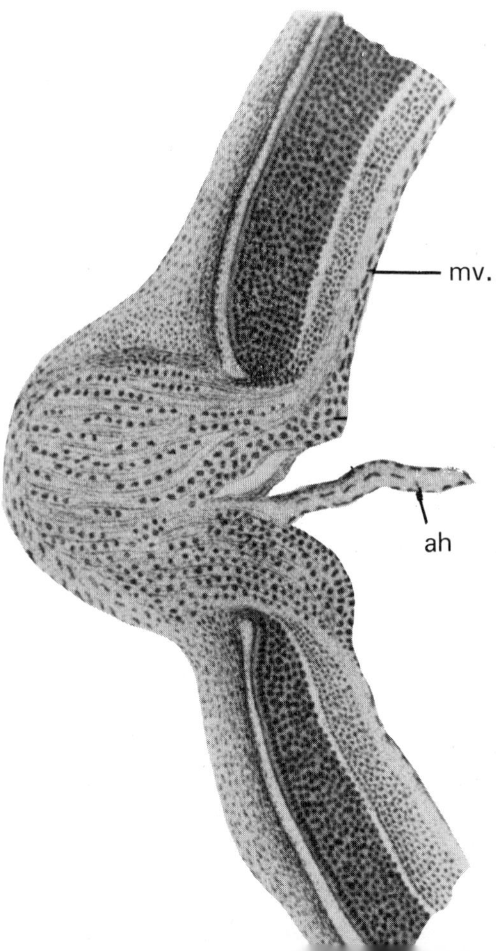

of the hyaloid artery and were preceded by a layer of mesenchymal cells which grew over the surface of the retina (Fig. 1-9). According to Schultze[16] this layer of mesenchymal cells develops late in embryonic life. These cells arrange themselves in a very distinct network and are hollowed out to form blood vessels.

The work of Michaelson[13] has been noted in the preceding section dealing with human vessel development. His conclusions were the same for animals and man and need not be repeated here. A number of his observations, however, have been confirmed by other workers. For example, Ashton,[4] utilizing retinal digest preparations, has confirmed that the developing retinal vessel network is composed of pentagonal spaces of varying size. The spaces tend to be larger on the arterial side of the capillary circulation and gradually diminish towards the venous side (Fig. 1-10). He also has noted that the number of endothelial cells is fewer in the capillaries on the arterial side as compared with those of the venous side of the system. Ashton has suggested that this difference in cellularity may be a direct or indirect result of oxygen tension upon endothelial growth.

Michaelson[13] has noted that the initial retinal vascular ingrowth lies in a two dimensional plane near the inner surface of the retina; only later does a deep capillary network develop from this superficially placed strata of vessels. Ashton and Blach,[6] Engerman and Meyer,[8] and Henkind and de Oliveira[9] have made similar observations.

Engerman and Meyer,[8] using a modified PAS-stain technique to study whole-mounted rat retinas, and Agrawal,[1] who examined rat retinal digests, were among the first mod ern workers to demonstrate that primitive cells preceded vessel ingrowth into animal retinae. Henkind and de Oliveira,[9] utilizing a variety of techniques including india-ink injections, retinal digestion, PAS-stained whole mounts, and combinations of these methods, described the various stages in the development of retinal vessels in ratlings. Initially, one sees only a cellular meshwork, perhaps a syncytium of primordial elements, without any hint of patent vascular channels (Fig. 1-11). This meshwork is also represented in the peripheral portion of the better-developed vascular system seen several days after birth. Just central to the undifferentiated mesh is a network of primitive capillaries, some patent, some apparently not, and little or no evidence of arteries or veins (Fig. 1-12). (While the terms "capillary," "artery," and "vein" are used to describe the early retinal vasculature, these vessels do not morphologically resemble those in adult life, but in time will evolve into the mature forms.) Extending centripetally back to the disc is a more-developed, though still immature, vascular pattern with a better-defined, patent capillary bed, and early arteries and veins (Figs. 1-10 and 1-13).

At this point it is pertinent to mention that it has been thought that a number of animal species, including rat, cat, and mouse, lack retinal vessels until after birth. This is unlike the human situation where the majority of the vascular bed is formed in utero. Shakib, de Oliveira, and Henkind,[19] have demonstrated that the rat starts to develop a retinal vessel complex at approximately 15 days of intrauterine development (beginning of third trimester), and a similar situation also seems to apply to the cat. However, the majority of patent vessels in these animal species do not appear until after birth. In this sense the first few days or weeks after birth in the animal resemble the situation of the human fetus in the early portion of the third trimester of pregnancy. For this reason newborn animals, the cat in particular, serve as excellent models for producing experimental retrolental fibroplasia.

ULTRASTRUCTURE

The ultrastructure of developing retinal vessels has been studied in the cat and rat.[18,19] The initial ingrowth consists of individual polygonal cells, derived either from the wall or immediately surrounding tissue of the hyaloid artery, which lie beneath the internal limiting membrane of the retina (Fig. 1-14). While similar to the cells found in the retinal capillaries of mature animals they contain more cytoplasmic organelles; these include membrane-bound vesicles, numerous ribosomal particles—free or in association with well-formed endoplasmic reticulum, abundant mitochondria, and a prominent Golgi system. Mitotic figures are common. Shakib and de Oliveira[18] have shown that the rough-surfaced endoplasmic reticulum contains a granular substance which is identical to the basement membrane which later develops around the vasculogenic cells. This, presumably, is the origin for the basement membrane material which appears to be secreted by developing endothelial cells and intramural pericytes. The cells of mature vessels have much less rough-surfaced endoplasmic reticulum.

Cords, disposed in hexagonal arrangement, develop as a collection of closely packed cells which do not show any junctional complexes between them, and their adjacent plasma membranes are separated from one another (Fig. 1-15). At times it is difficult to differentiate between cords and lumenized vessels. In this instance the presence of base-

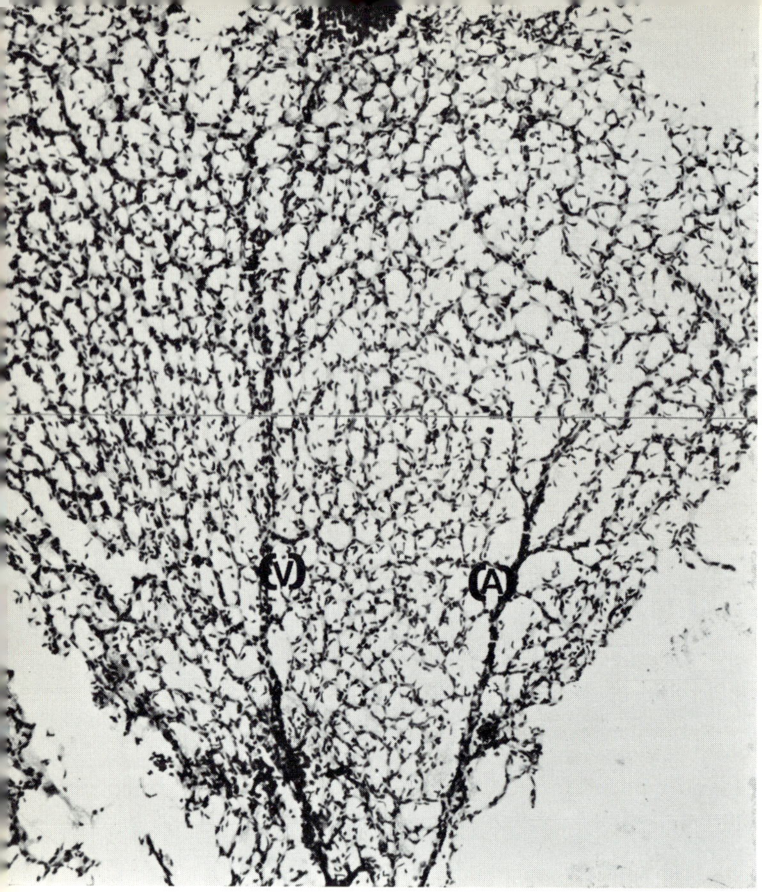

Fig. 1-10. Retinal digest preparation of a 5-day-old rat shows the pentagonal spaces between the developing capillaries. The spaces tend to be wider near the primitive artery **(A)** than near the vein **(V).**

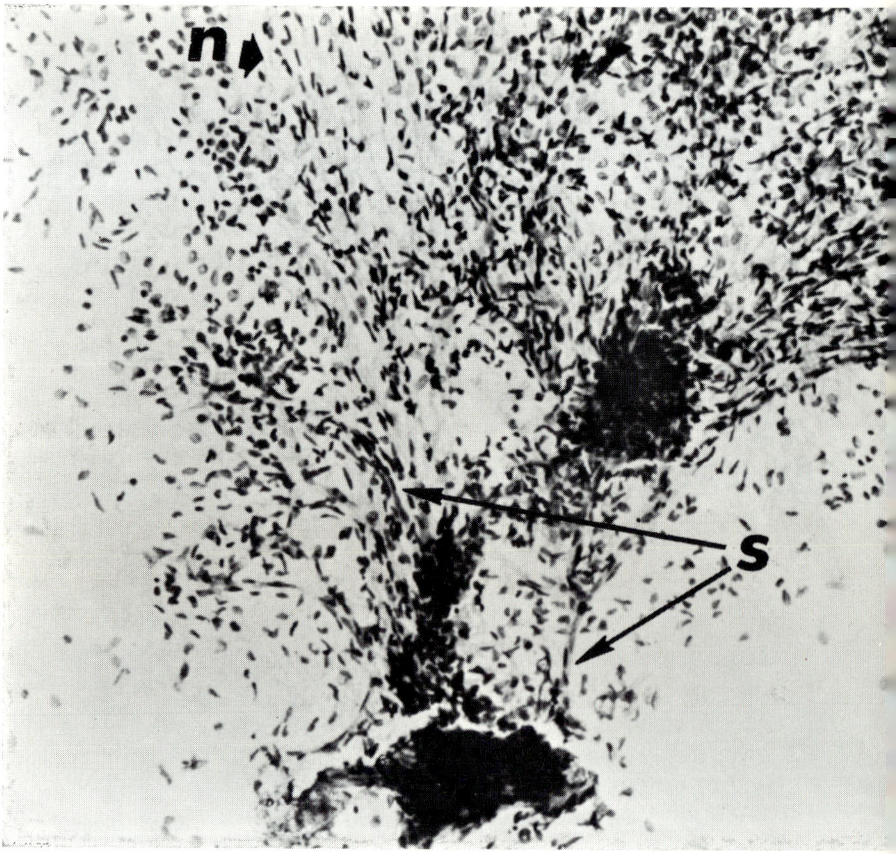

Fig. 1-11. Incomplete retinal digest preparation from a full-term fetal rat. Strands **(S)** of undifferentiated mesenchyme can be seen around the disc, and spindle-shaped nuclei **(N)** of the cells forming the vascular meshwork are present elsewhere. PAS and hematoxylin, ×250. (From Henkind and de Oliveira.[9])

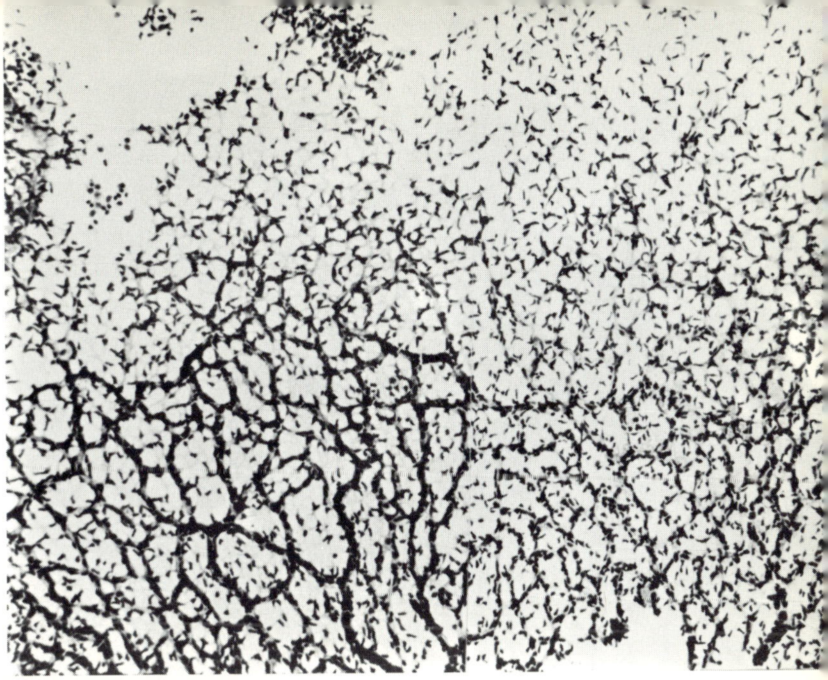

Fig. 1-12. Retinal digest preparation from a 5-day-old rat. Vascular cords and aligned cells are seen in the peripheral cellular meshwork. Most are continuous with patent vessels, but definite arteries and veins cannot be discerned. PAS and hematoxylin, ×100. (From Henkind and de Oliveira.[9])

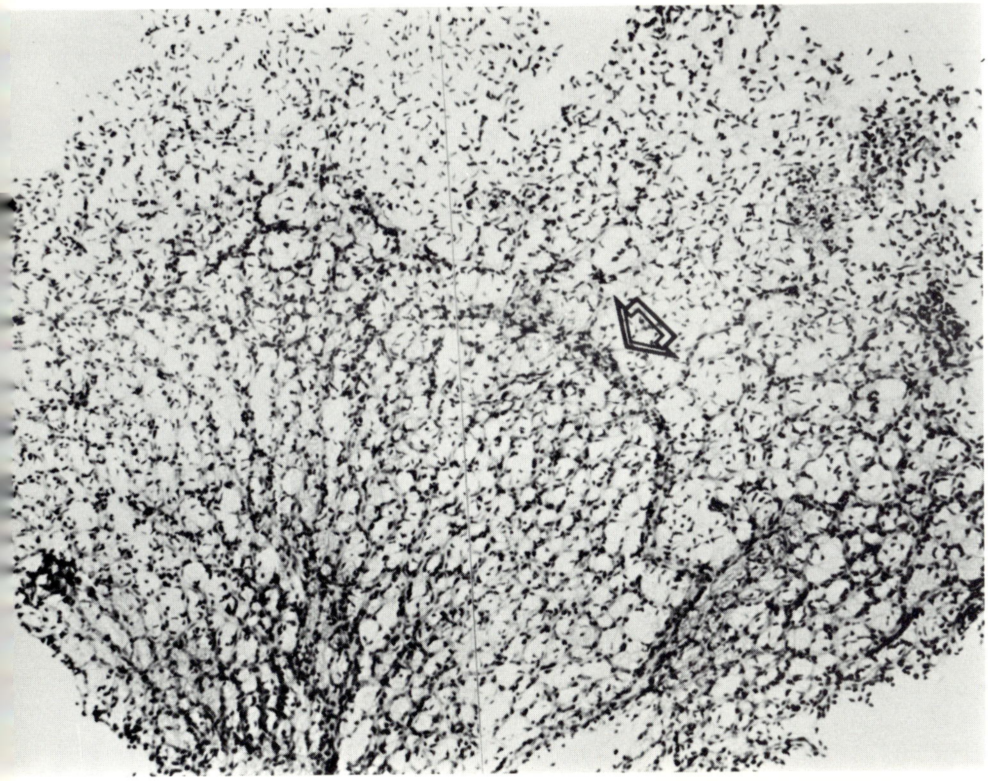

Fig. 1-13. Retinal digest preparation from a 3-day-old rat. The undifferentiated mesenchymal meshwork is at the periphery, while centrally there is the advancing zone of cords, primitive capillaries, and a larger vascular arcade **(arrow)** destined to develop into an artery or vein. PAS and hematoxylin, ×87. (From Henkind and de Oliveira.[9])

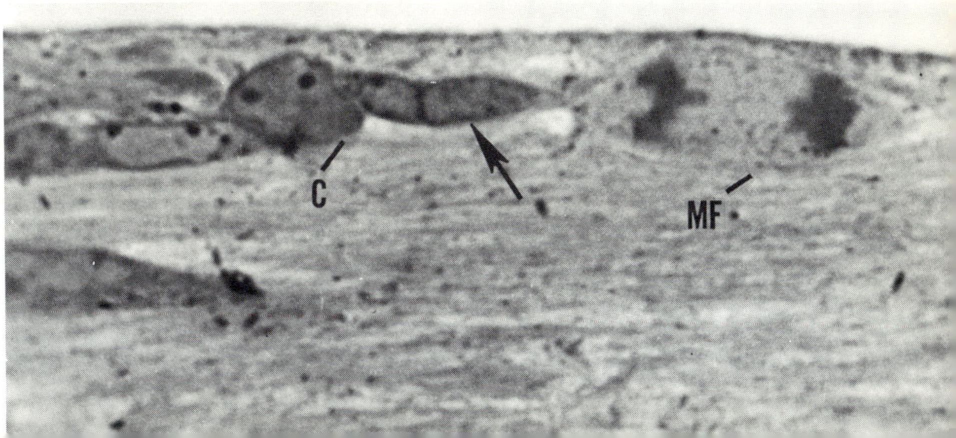

Fig. 1-14. Thick sections of a cord **(C)** show a cell at the distal end **(arrow). MF,** mitotic figure. Specimen from a 17-day-old rat fetus. ×1300. (From Shakib, de Oliveira, and Henkind.[19])

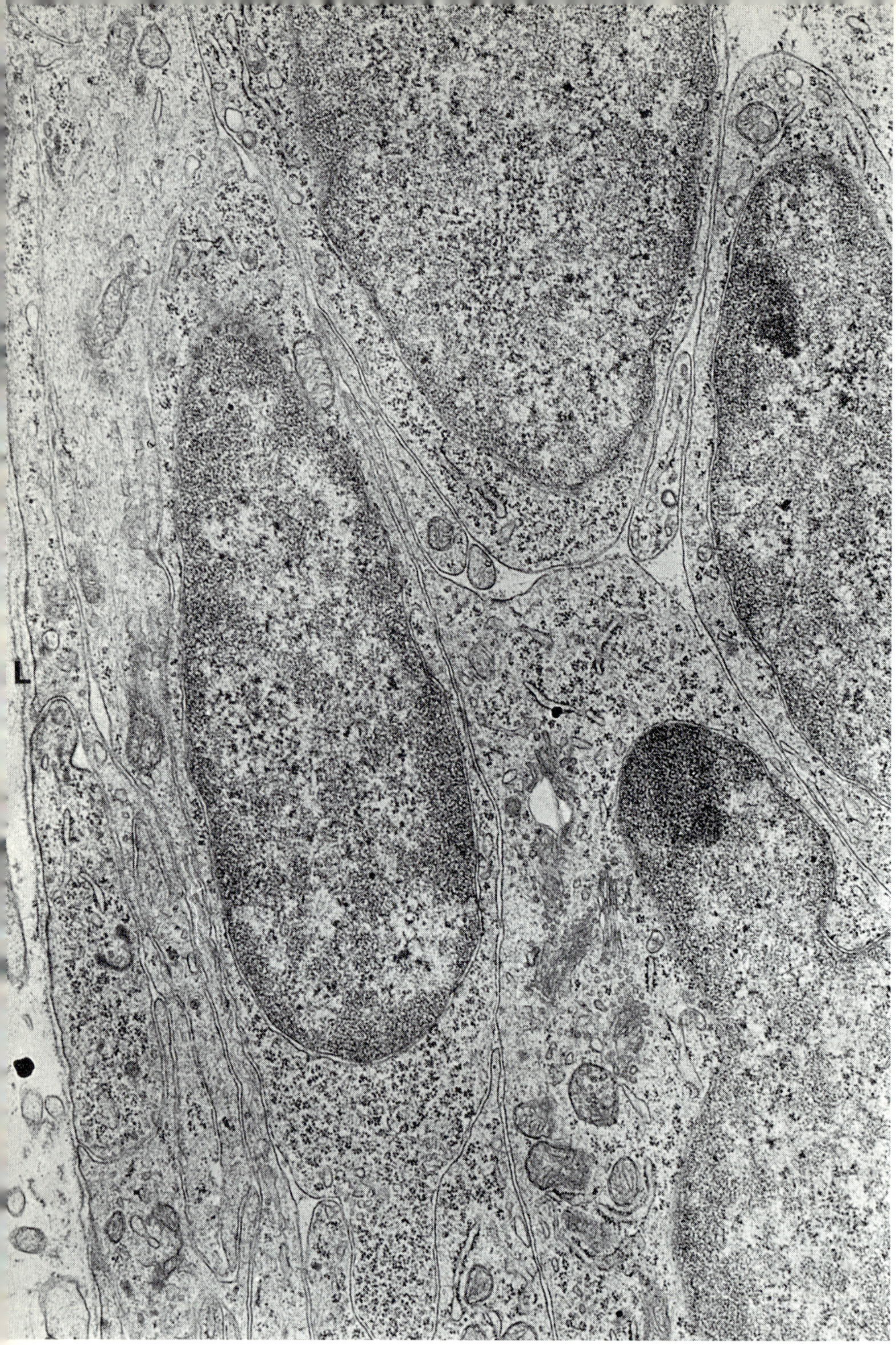

Fig. 1-15. Electron micrograph of a section of a cord of the retinal vascular system shows neither junctional complexes between the cells nor basement membrane material around them. Specimen from a 17-day-old rat fetus. **IL,** internal limiting membrane. ×20,000. (From Shakib, de Oliveira, and Henkind.[19])

Fig. 1-16. Electron micrograph of the wall of a blood vessel shows basement membrane **(BM)** between the cells and the neighboring tissue. Specimen from an 18-day-old rat fetus. ×19,000. (From Shakib, de Oliveira, and Henkind.[19])

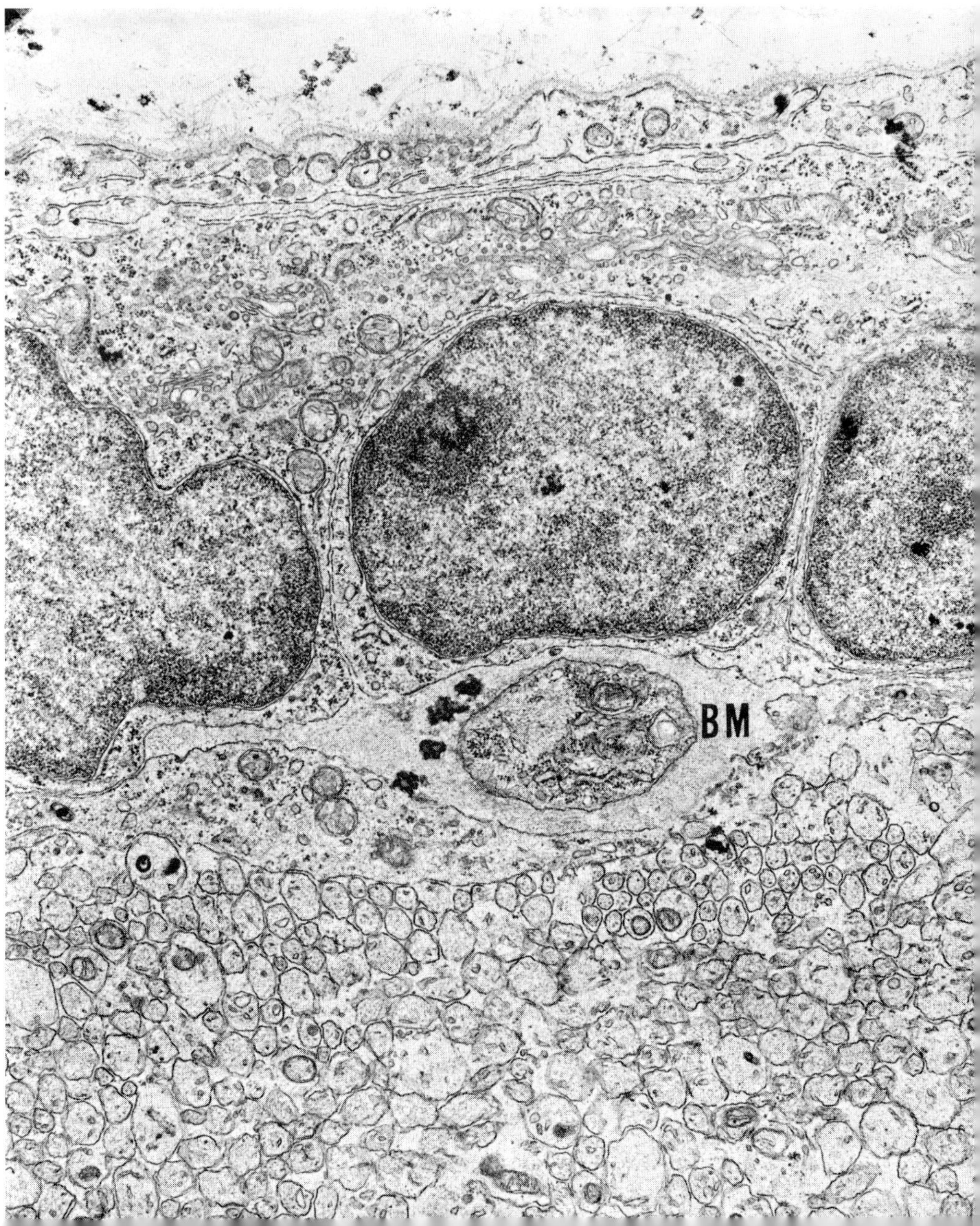

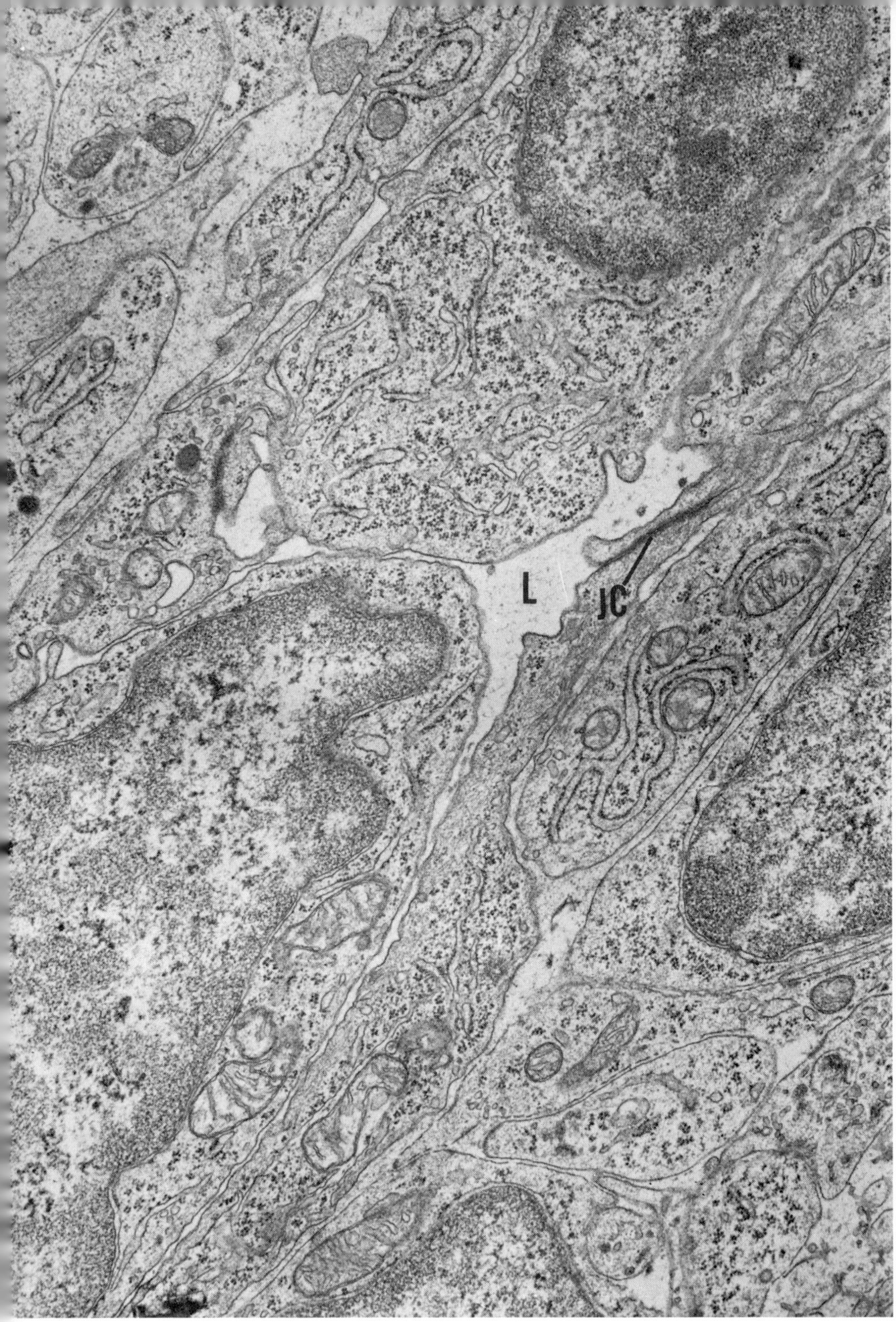

Fig. 1-17. Electron micrograph of an early retinal blood vessel shows a lumen **(L)** and well-formed junctional complexes **(JC)** between the endothelial cells. Specimen from a 17-day-old rat fetus. ×27,000. (From Shakib, de Oliveira, and Henkind.[19])

Fig. 1-18. *Opposite page.* Whole mount of an inked, PAS-stained, 5-day-old rat retina. *A*, A zone completely free of vascular components is seen around a retinal artery by transmitted light. *B*, Same area as *A*, but photographed with a Wratten No. 58 filter. Note the numerous vascular strands in the capillary-free zone. ×800. (From Henkind and de Oliveira.[9])

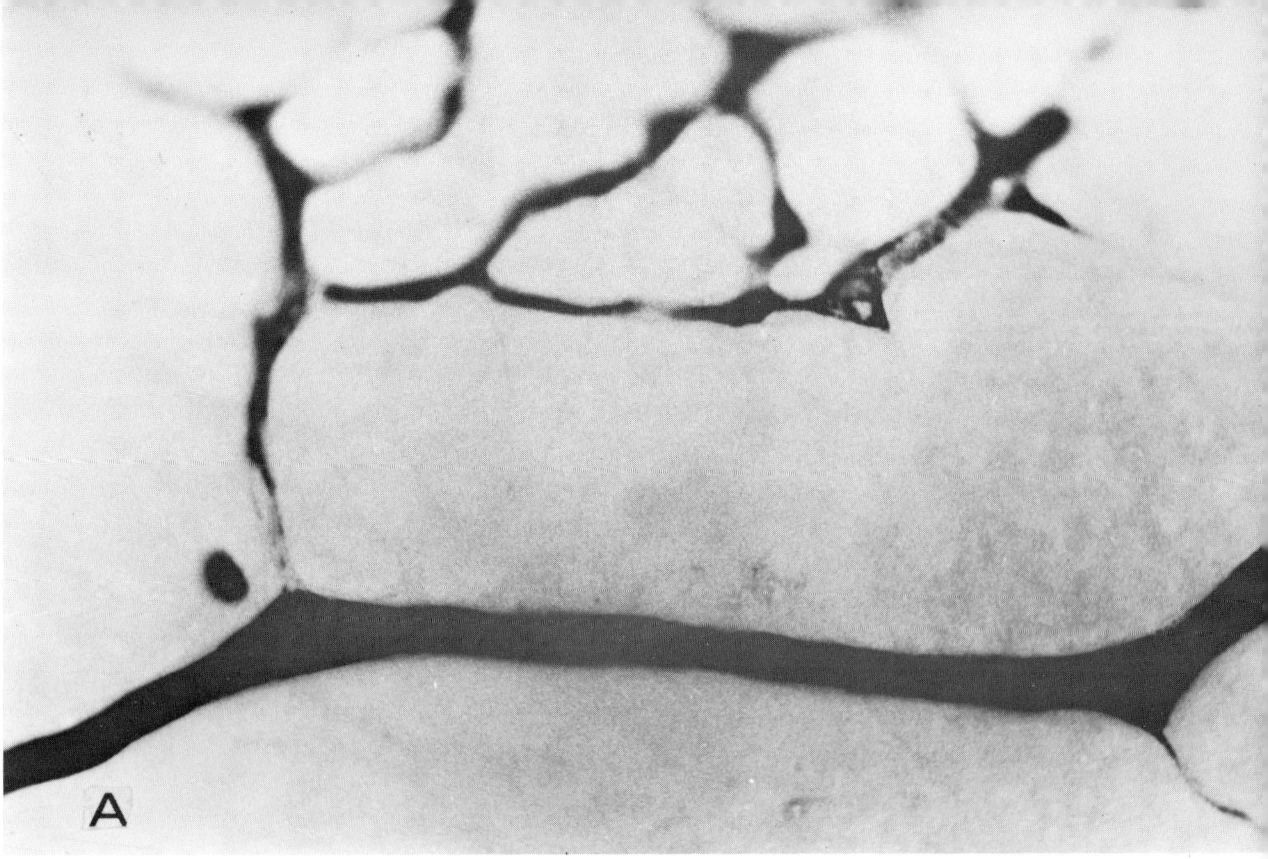

A

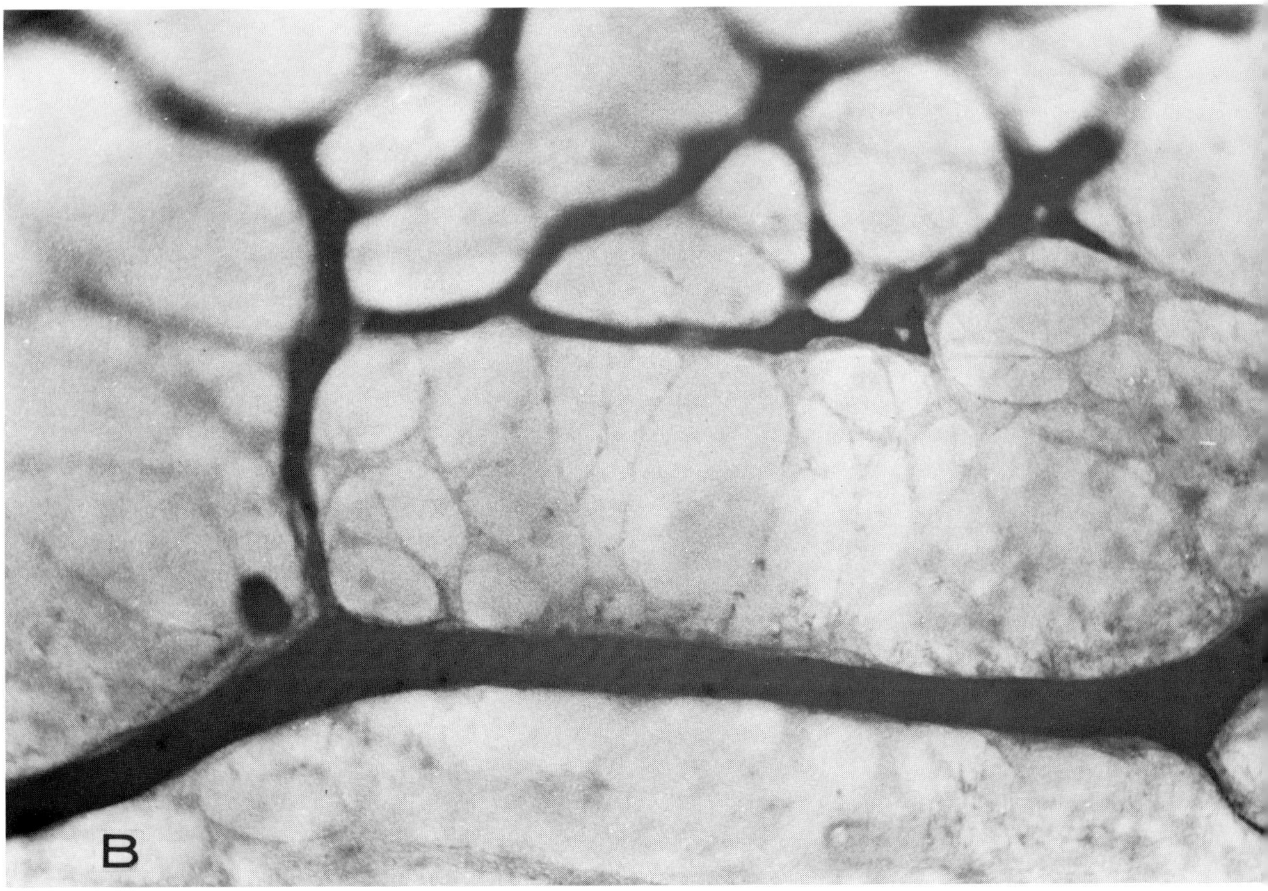

B

ment membrane around the cells is one criterion for the recognition of the vessel wall (Fig. 1-16).

The initial, newly formed blood vessels appear to be of capillary size, and they have a wall composed of one or two layers of cells surrounding a lumen which may contain red blood cells (Fig. 1-17). Abundant basement membrane material, less condensed than that seen in mature capillaries, is often found in the space between the cell wall of the blood vessel and the neighboring tissue (Fig. 1-16). Junctional complexes between cells are seen to be forming in the transition from the cords to the lumenized vessels. A distinctive finding is the presence of well-formed junctional complexes between the cells adjacent to the lumen (those destined to form the endothelium). There are no junctions between inner and outer cells nor between the outer cells (intramural pericyte precursors) themselves (Fig. 1-17). According to Shakib and de Oliveira,[18] with the appearance of basement membrane material

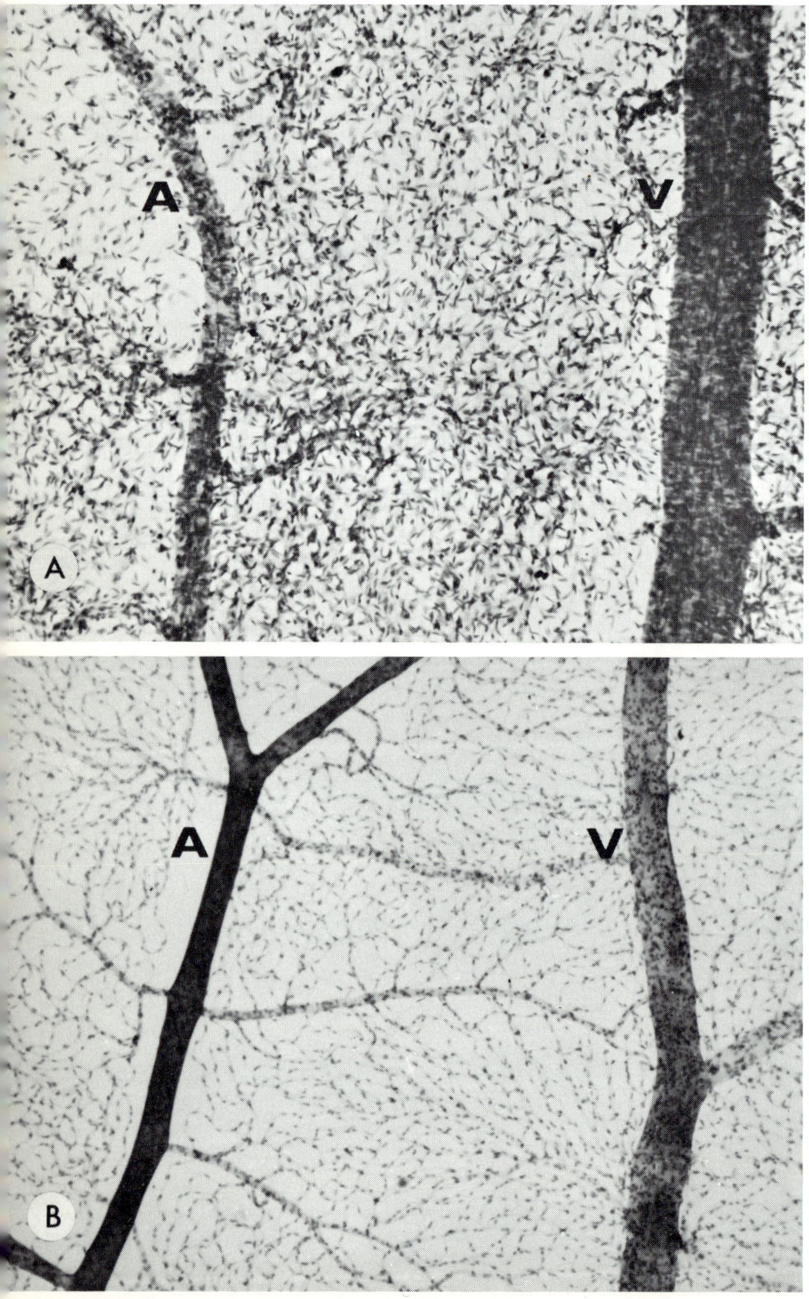

Fig. 1-19. *A*, Retinal digest preparation of a young pig. Note the dense capillary network and the absence of a capillary-free zone around the artery **(A). V,** vein. PAS and hematoxylin, ×87.

B, Retinal digest of a mature owl monkey (*Aotes trivirgatus*) showing the less dense capillary network and the well-defined capillary-free zone around the artery **(A). V,** vein. PAS and hematoxylin, ×50.

in the intracellular spaces, the outer cells are differentiated into intramural pericytes and the inner ones, directly in contact with the blood stream, evolve into endothelium. In their view the two cell types derive from the initial primitive mesenchymal cell which grows into the retina. Such a common origin has also been suggested by Agrawal.[1]

The cells of the deep capillary bed were found to arise from the superficial retinal vessels near the disc in the retina of the 1-day-old rat, and these cells appear to pierce the nerve fiber layer. They are morphologically similar to those forming the superficial vessels.[19]

DEVELOPMENT OF THE CAPILLARY-FREE ZONE

A capillary-free zone about arteries has been described for most species possessing retinal vessels. Michaelson,[13] from his interpretation of inked specimens, has postulated that the zone was a primary phenomenon, occurring because some factor prevented the new-growing capillaries from approaching the retinal arteries. Recent studies negate this point of view, and suggest that the capillary-free zone occurs secondarily in an early stage of vascular remodeling.[5,9]

In the rat, this zone is seen initially after vessels larger than primitive capillaries appear within the vascular complex. It develops as immature capillaries or primitive vascular mesenchyme retract or atrophy in the region surrounding newly formed arteries (Fig. 1-18). It is first seen 1 to several days after birth. To a lesser extent, there is capillary retraction around the developing veins. Ashton[5] has noted the surprising fact that a capillary-free zone fails to develop around the newly proliferating vessels in kittens whose initial retinal circulation was obliterated by excess oxygen.

While its significance is not completely understood, the occurrence of a capillary-free zone may merely reflect the normal process of retraction of primitive capillaries due to the need to maintain adequate pressure along the artery. If many capillaries drained the artery there would be a drop in pressure in the distal arterial segment. Furthermore, there appears to be a relationship between the width of the zone and the diameter of the capillary mesh. The capillary-free zone is broader in those species with a large capillary net diameter than in those with a close-set network (Fig. 1-19). In young pigs, which have a very dense, closely packed capillary network, we have been unable to demonstrate such a zone either in inked or digested retinal preparations. It has also been suggested that the development of the capillary-free zone may be related to oxygen or biochemical factors as yet unknown.

REFERENCES

1. Agrawal, P. K.: The cellular structure and development of the retinal vessels of the rat. *Orient Arch. Ophthal. 3:*23, 1965.

2. Arey, L. B.: "The Development of Peripheral Blood Vessels," In *The Peripheral Blood Vessels.* Ed. by Orbison, J. L., and Smith, D. E. Baltimore, Md., Williams & Wilkins, 1963, pp. 1–16.

3. Ashton, N.: Pathological basis of retrolental fibroplasia. *Brit. J. Ophthal. 38:*385, 1954.

4. Ashton, N.: Oxygen and the growth and development of retinal vessels. *In vivo* and *in vitro* studies. *Amer. J. Ophthal. 62:*412, 1966.

5. Ashton, N.: "The Mode of Development of the Retinal Vessels in Man." In *The William MacKenzie Centenary Symposium on the Ocular*

Circulation in Health and Disease. Ed. by Cant, J. S., St. Louis, Mo., Mosby, 1969, pp. 7–17.

6. Ashton, N., and Blach, R.: Studies on developing retinal vessels. 8. Effect of oxygen on the retinal vessels of the ratling. *Brit. J. Ophthal. 45:*321, 1961.
7. Cogan, D. G.: Development and senescence of the human retinal vasculature. *Trans. Ophthal. Soc. U.K. 83:*465, 1963.
8. Engerman, R. L., and Meyer, R. K.: Development of retinal vasculature in rats. *Amer. J. Ophthal. 60:*628, 1965.
9. Henkind, P., and de Oliveira, L. F.: Development of retinal vessels in the rat. *Invest. Ophthal. 6:*520, 1967.
10. Kessler, L.: *Zur Entwickelung des Auges der Wirbeltwiere.* Leipzig, Vogel, 1877.
11. Mann, I. C.: *The Development of the Human Eye.* Cambridge, England, University Press, 1928.
12. McClure, C. F. W.: The endothelial problem. *Anat. Res. 22:*219, 1921.
13. Michaelson, I. C.: The mode of development of the retinal vessels and some observations of its significance in certain retinal diseases. *Trans. Ophthal. Soc. U.K. 68:*137, 1948.
14. Nilhausen, K.: The vasoformative tissue in foetal retina with particular reference to the histochemical demonstration of its alkaline phosphatase activity. *Acta Ophthal. 36:*65, 1958.
15. de Oliveira, L. F.: *A Origem E O Desenvolvimento Dos Vasos Da Retina.* (Thesis, Lisboa, 1968.)
16. Schultze, O.: *Zur Entwickelungsgeschichte des Gefass-systems im Saugetier-auge.* Leipzig, Festschrift von Kolliker, 1892, p. 1.
17. Serpell, G.: Polysaccharide granules in association with developing retinal vessels and with retrolental fibroplasia. *Brit. J. Ophthal. 38:*460, 1954.
18. Shakib, M., and de Oliveira, L. F.: Studies on developing retinal vessels. 10. Formation of the basement membrane and differentiation of intramural pericytes. *Brit. J. Ophthal. 50:*124, 1966.
19. Shakib, M., de Oliveira, L. F., and Henkind, P.: Development of retinal vessels. 2. Earliest stages of vessel formation. *Invest. Ophthal. 7:*689, 1968.
20. Sugi, K.: Studies on the pathological changes in the retinal vessels of human eyes, using the trypsin digestion method. *Jap. J. Ophthal. 10:*252, 1966.
21. Versari, R.: Morfologia dei vasi sanguigni Arteriosi dell' Occhio dell' uomo et di altri mammiferi. *Ric. Labor. Anat. Norm.* (Rome) *5:*181, 1900.
22. Versari, R.: La morfogenesi dei vasi sanguigni della retina umana. *Ric. Labor. Anat. Norm.* (Rome) *10:*25, 1904.
23. Voll, A.: *Ueber die Entwickelung der Membrana Vasculosa Retinae.* Leipzig, Festschrift von Kolliker, 1892, p. 87.

chapter 2

Pattern and Location of Retinal Vessels

The earliest representations of the retinal vessels in the human eye were drawn shortly after the advent of the ophthalmoscope in 1850.[12] According to Keys and Rucker,[21] Adrian Van Trigt published the first illustration of the fundus of the human eye drawn from life in his thesis which appeared in 1853.[33] The following year, Ruete,[31] the inventor of the indirect ophthalmoscope, published a number of pictures of eyegrounds as seen by his method. While of historical interest, they scarcely compare with the skillfully drawn fundus illustrations of Jaeger[18] which were published in 1855. Jaeger spent upwards of 100 hours on a single illustration, and his plates reflect meticulous observation. In the past century more than 100 atlases have appeared which are devoted solely to the fundus of the eye.[21]

OPHTHALMOSCOPIC APPEARANCE

The optic nerve head, or disc, is the focus from which retinal arteries enter, and retinal veins leave the eye. It is the common practice to start an examination of the ocular fundus at the disc, and then to examine the retinal quadrants in turn, leaving the macular region for the end of the examination.

There are numerous variations of vascular pattern on the nerve head, these depend upon the level at which the major vessels divide (Fig. 2-1*A-D*). The central retinal artery and its primary branches lie nasally to the central retinal vein in the nerve head. It is usually easy to distinguish between arteries and veins; the former are narrower, brighter red, and run a straighter course than the corresponding veins. While the arrangement of the vessels is inconstant, and indeed is distinctive for each human being including identical twins, the general plan is for each quadrant of the retina to be supplied by a major artery and vein. These are termed supero- and inferotemporal, and supero- and inferonasal arteries and veins (Fig. 2-2). The nasal vessels run a shorter and more direct course than the temporal ones which tend to pursue an arcuate path above and below the macular region.

Retinal arteries and veins divide by dichotomous and side-arm branching (Fig. 2-3). The terminal arterioles come off at almost right angles from the main stem. It is possible to visualize, by direct ophthalmoscopy, the vessels down to their third or fourth divisions (15 to 20 μ), but the smallest channels, comprised of capillaries, precapillary arterioles, and postcapillary venules, are invisible.

Small arterioles and venules may run directly temporal from the disc to the nasal margin of the macula. In approximately 25 per cent of humans[11] a cilioretinal artery hooks around the temporal margin of the disc and provides the arterial supply for a portion of the macula (Fig. 2-4). Multiple cilioretinal arteries are an uncommon finding. Cilioretinal veins, where a retinal vein disappears at the disc margin presumably to enter the ciliary system, are rare.

At sites of arteriovenous crossings the arteries generally lie anteriorly (closer to the vitreous) to the veins. The majority of such crossings are in the superotemporal quadrant of the retina (Fig. 2-5). With bright illumination it is possible to see the venous blood column beneath an overlying arterial vessel. In man it is exceedingly rare to find arteries crossing arteries or veins crossing veins. Trifurcations of retinal vessels are also uncommon oddities.[5]

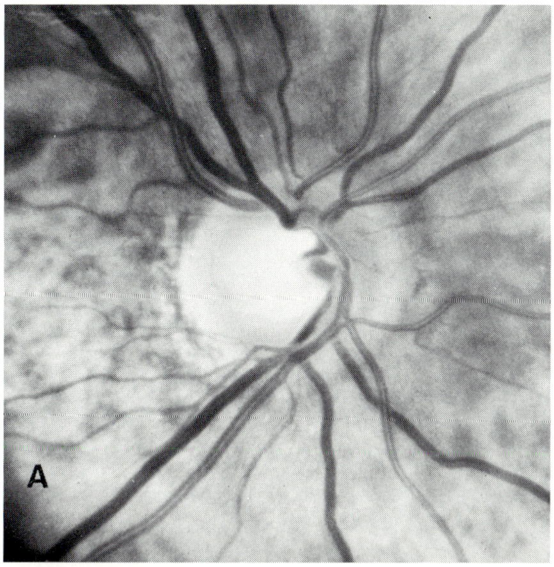

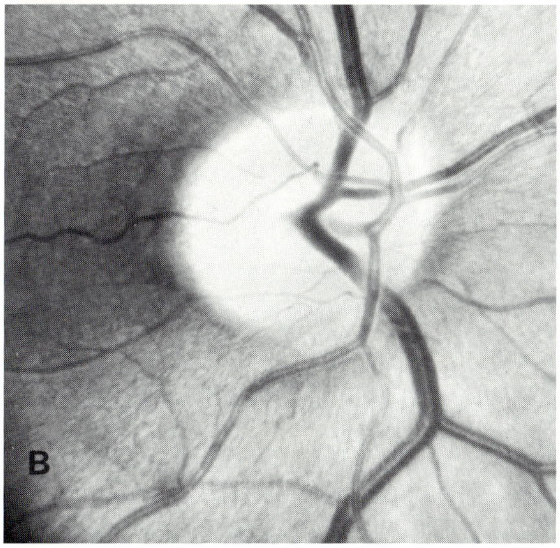

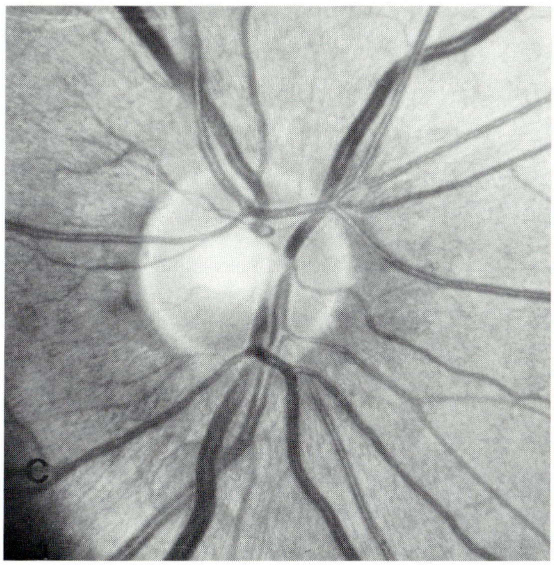

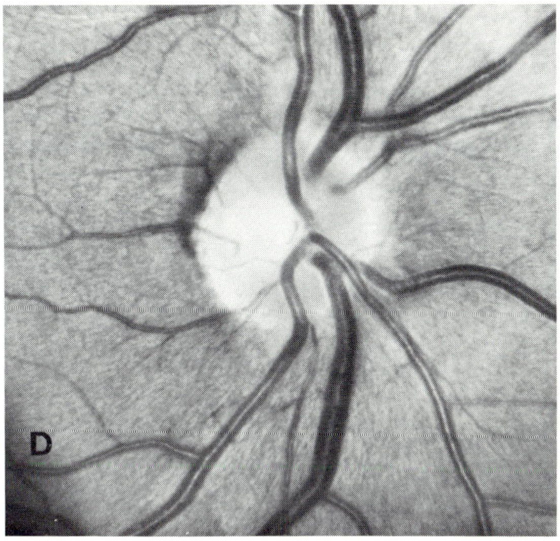

Fig. 2-1. *A–D*, Fundus photographs of the right discs of four humans. There is variation in the vessel pattern with each human possessing a distinctive appearance. The veins appear darker and broader than the arteries. In general, the central retinal artery lies nasally to the central retinal vein and this is most obvious in *B*. The branching of the retinal arteries is complex and unusual in *C*.

ANATOMIC STUDY

Ophthalmoscopy provides only a partial view of the retinal vasculature. To fully appreciate the various aspects of the retinal vascular pattern in detail a variety of techniques may be employed.[20] These include: vascular injection with material such as india ink,[3,29] latex,[19] or Berlin blue combined with retinal digestion—a technique that allows one to study both the intact vascular pattern and later the cellular detail of the vessels;[22] injection of red blood

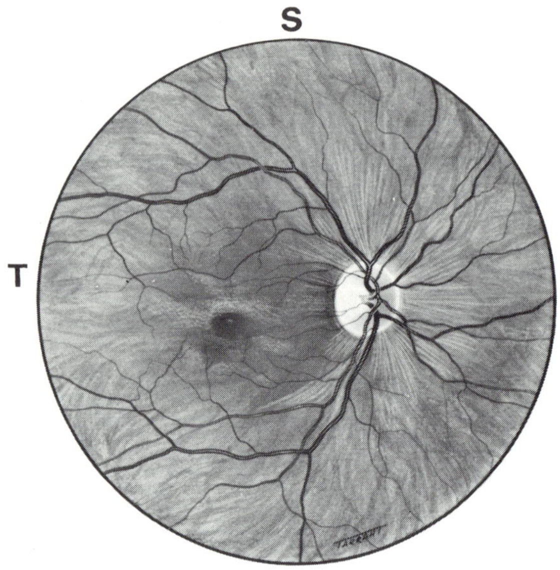

Fig. 2-2. Painting of a human fundus showing the pattern of the retinal vessels at the posterior pole of the right eye. The temporal vessels tend to curve around the macular region; **(S)** superior; **(T)** temporal.

Fig. 2-3. Fundus photograph of a human left eye, superotemporal to the disc. The **large arrows** point to dichotomous branchings of a vein (upper) and an artery (lower) and the **small arrow** points to a side-arm branch of the artery.

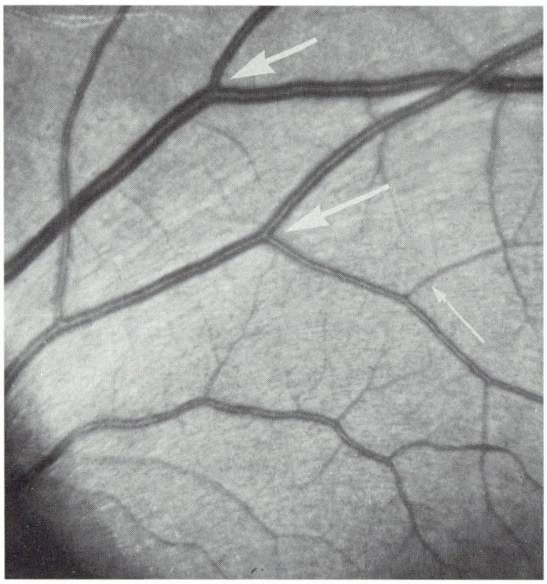

cells followed by benzidine staining,[28] colored gelatin;[30] intravascular silver staining;[10] retinal flat mounts or retinal digests stained with periodic acid-Schiff (PAS) reagent;[2,9,24] and, finally, routine histologic cross sections and flat sections stained with various agents.

EXTENT OF RETINAL VESSELS

In man the retinal vessels occupy the inner half of the neural retina. They extend outward from the disc in all directions spreading their network across the retina, but stopping short of the periphery and also sparing the fovea. Except for capillary-sized communications at the optic nerve head, which may link the retinal and ciliary vessel systems, there are no anastomoses with other vessels. The retinal circulation is end-arterial in nature; occlusion of the central retinal artery before it enters the eye leads to cessation of retinal blood flow and subsequent death of the inner retinal layers. Within the retina there are regional variations in capillary pattern and distribution and these will be discussed in the following paragraphs.

LOCATION OF RETINAL BLOOD VESSELS

The larger blood vessels lie in the innermost portion of the retina, and are usually separated from the internal limiting membrane by a thin coat of glial and neural elements. At the nerve head, which is not covered by the internal limiting membrane, the vessels are separated from the vitreous by a thin layer of glial tissue. Large vessels are found in the nerve fiber and ganglion cell layers except at arteriovenous crossing sites, in which case the deeper vessel may indent the retina down to the outer plexiform or outer nuclear layer (Fig. 2-6). Smaller vessels, the precapillary arterioles, postcapillary venules, and capillaries, are

Fig. 2-4. *Top right.* Fluorescein angiogram of a human left eye. A cilioretinal artery hooks around the inferotemporal margin of the disc. Note that it fills prior to other retinal arteries showing that it derives its blood from a ciliary artery rather than from the central retinal artery.

Fig. 2-5. *Middle right.* An arteriovenous crossing in the superotemporal portion of a human left eye. The artery crosses above the vein **(arrow)** before the venous bifurcation and lies beneath it after the bifurcation.

Fig. 2-6. *Bottom right.* Cross section through a human retina at a site of arteriovenous crossing. The vein **(V)** lies beneath the artery and indents the retina down to and including the outer nuclear layer. Epon-embedded section, toluidine blue, ×200.

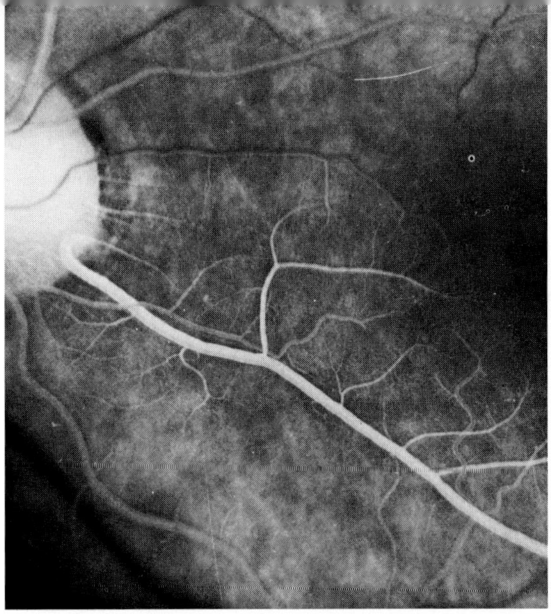

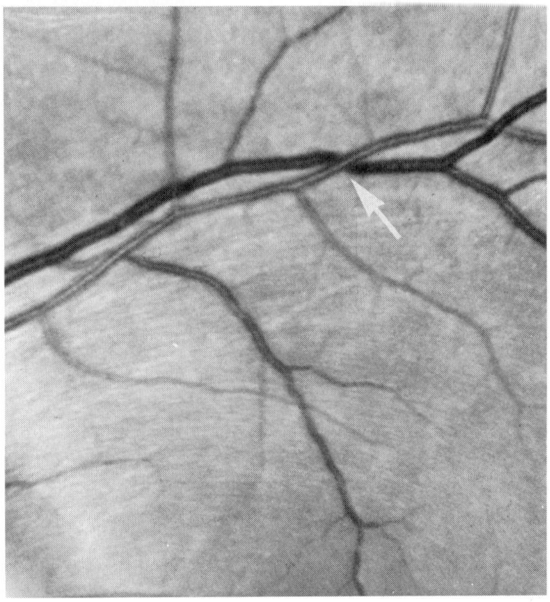

found between the nerve fiber and inner nuclear layers. In health they are never deeper than the boundary of the latter with the inner plexiform layer. The majority of retinal capillaries are present in the inner nuclear layer and the combined nerve fiber–ganglion cell layer. Lerche,[25] who has found the vascularity of the retina comparable to that of the central nervous system, provides the following figures for volume % of capillaries in the various retinal layers; inner nuclear layer 2.4 per cent, inner plexiform layer 0.5 per cent, ganglion cell and nerve fiber layer 1.3 per cent. No capillaries were present in either the outer plexiform or outer nuclear layers. Lerche noted that the choriocapillaris occupied 35 per cent of the volume of the inner choroid. This latter figure suggests the large role that the choriocapillaris plays in nourishing the outer layers of the retina.

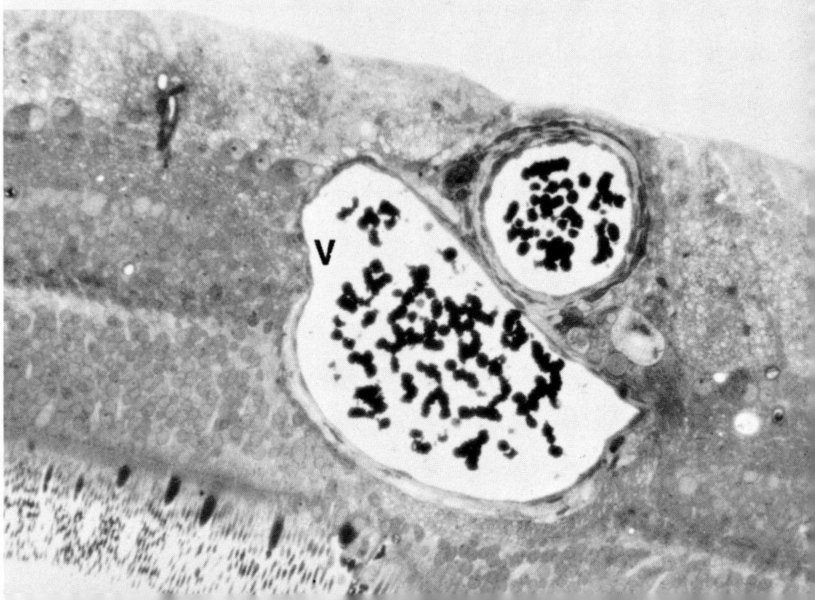

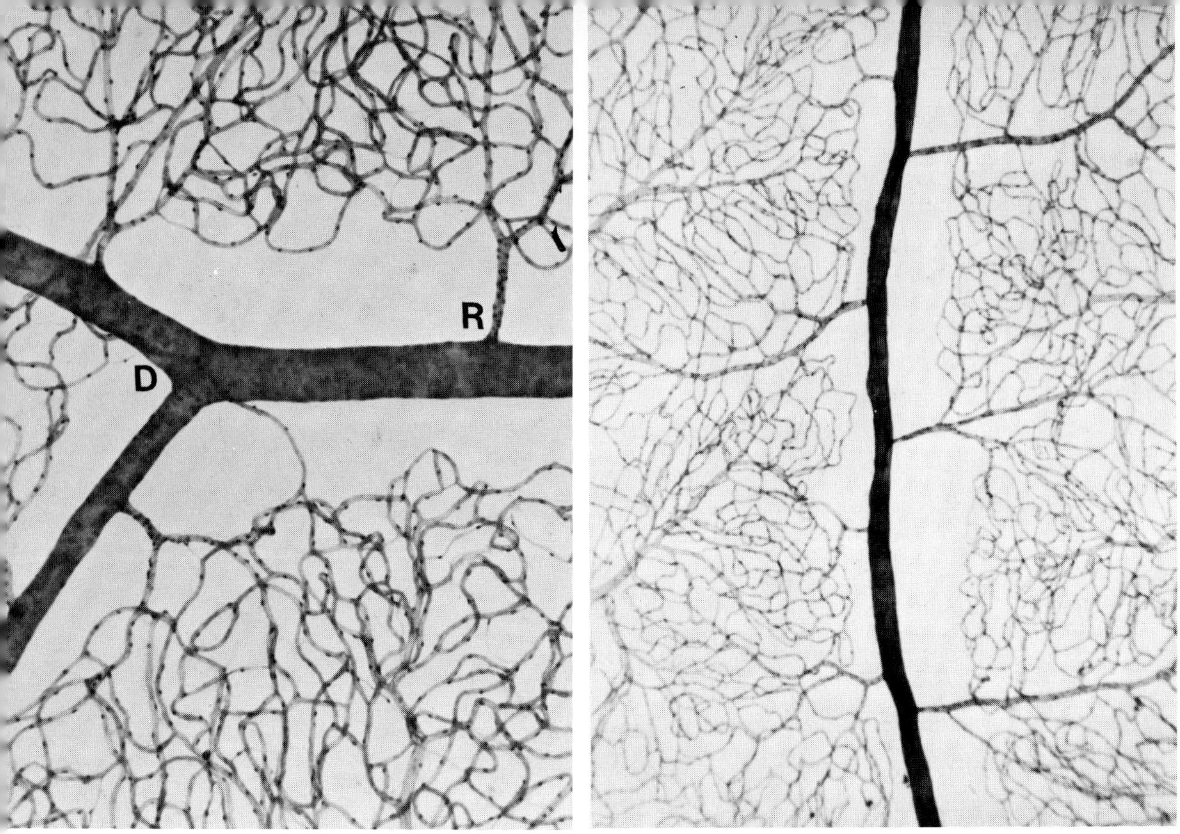

Fig. 2-7. *Left,* A dichotomous **(D)** and a side-arm or right-angle **(R)** branching of a human retinal artery. Digest preparation. PAS and Hematoxylin, ×75.

Right, Human retinal digest preparation shows terminal arterioles coming off at right angles from the parent stem. Note the capillary-free zone around the artery. PAS and hematoxylin, ×30.

Fig. 2-8. Pattern of vessels at the retinal periphery in man. The terminal artery **(A)** and vein **(V)** are linked by a broad capillary meshwork. Digest preparation. PAS and hematoxylin, ×50.

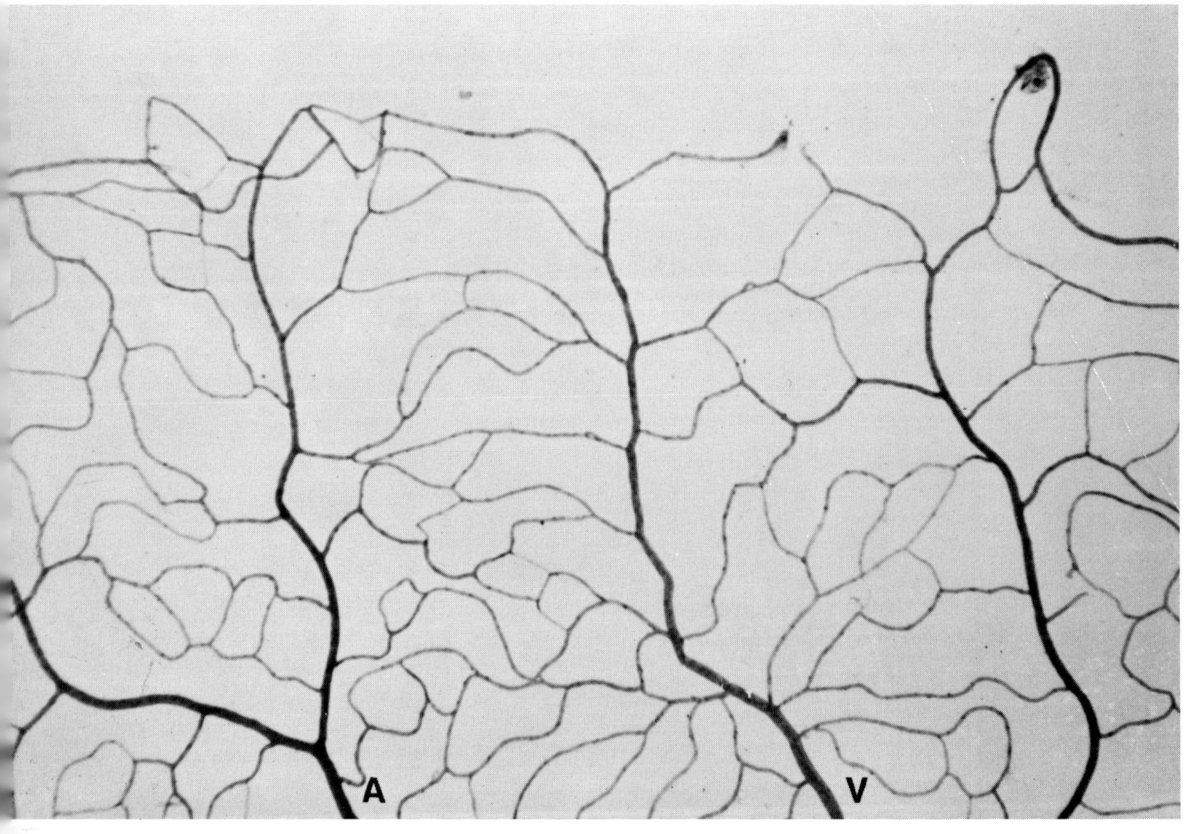

Fig. 2-9. Retinal digest showing the capillary-free zone of the human fovea. Note the long capillaries ringing the fovea which link the terminal arterioles and venules. ×26.

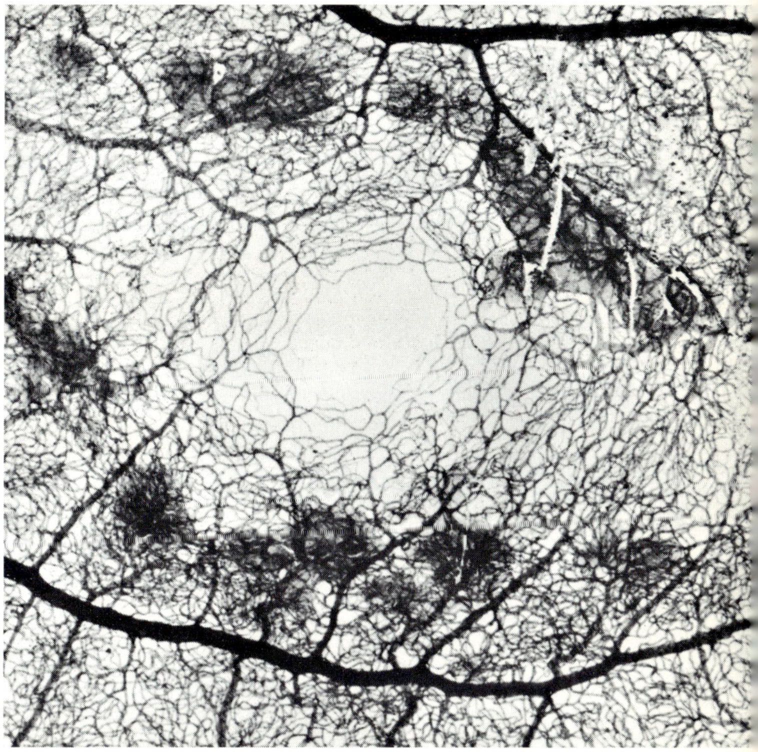

Vessels are absent from the fovea and retinal periphery. This is the result of retinal architecture. At the fovea itself there is a lack of the inner retinal layers in which the vessels normally reside. The slope of the fovea is such that only a single layer of capillaries is found in the perifoveal area, but as the surrounding retina thickens the capillary bed becomes multilayered. The thinness of the retinal periphery, which can receive nutrition from the underlying choroid, explains first the diminution, and finally the absence of capillaries in this region.

DISTRIBUTIONAL ARRANGEMENT OF RETINAL BLOOD VESSELS

Flat preparations, either inked or digested, best reveal the distribution of the retinal vessels.

The major arteries and veins share a common territorial distribution, but do not lie in the close juxtaposition often found in connective tissue structures.[7] The arteries subdivide by dichotomous branching, while the smaller terminal arterioles tend to come off at right angles from the parent stem (Fig. 2-7). The venous system has a somewhat similar arrangement, but occasional capillaries may join a major venous trunk directly. The terminal or precapillary arterioles, and the postcapillary venules form a regularly staggered or alternate arrangement and are linked by the interposed capillary bed. There are no arteriovenous shunts in the normal retina, however, at the retinal periphery the terminal arteries and veins are joined by rather large capillary communications (Fig. 2-8). Similar, but shorter and perhaps narrower channels link the terminal arterioles and venules which ring the perifoveal region of the macula, leaving a capillary-free zone some 400 to 500 μ in diameter (Fig. 2-9).

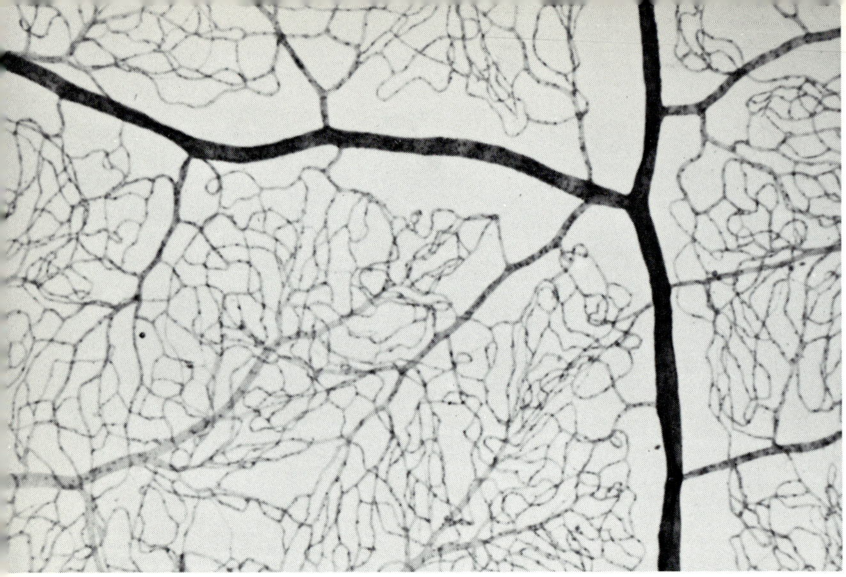

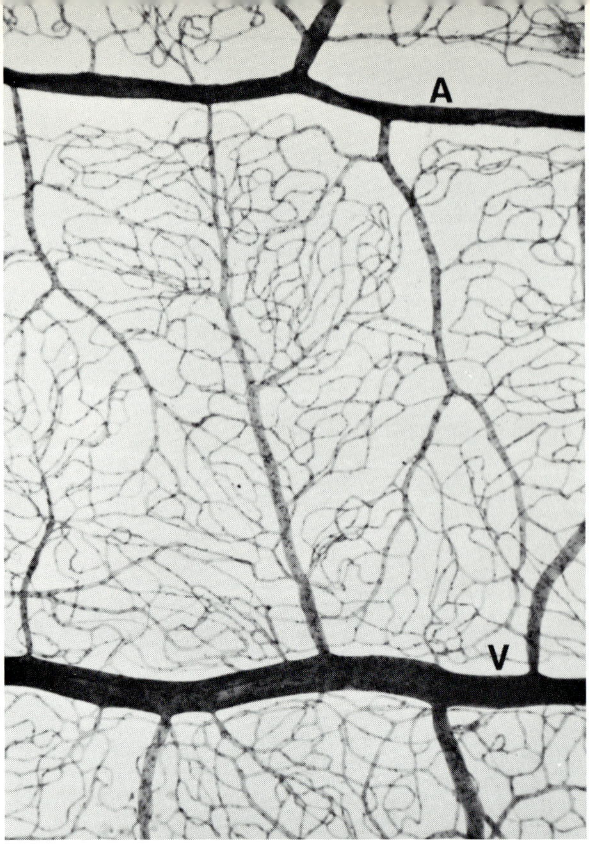

Fig. 2-10. *Above.* A human retinal digest preparation shows a capillary bed supplied by multiple arterial feedpoints. PAS and hematoxylin, ×30.

Fig. 2-11. *Top right.* Human retinal digest preparation. A broad capillary-free zone is present around the artery **(A)** and a much narrower zone is seen about the vein **(V).** PAS and hematoxylin, ×12.

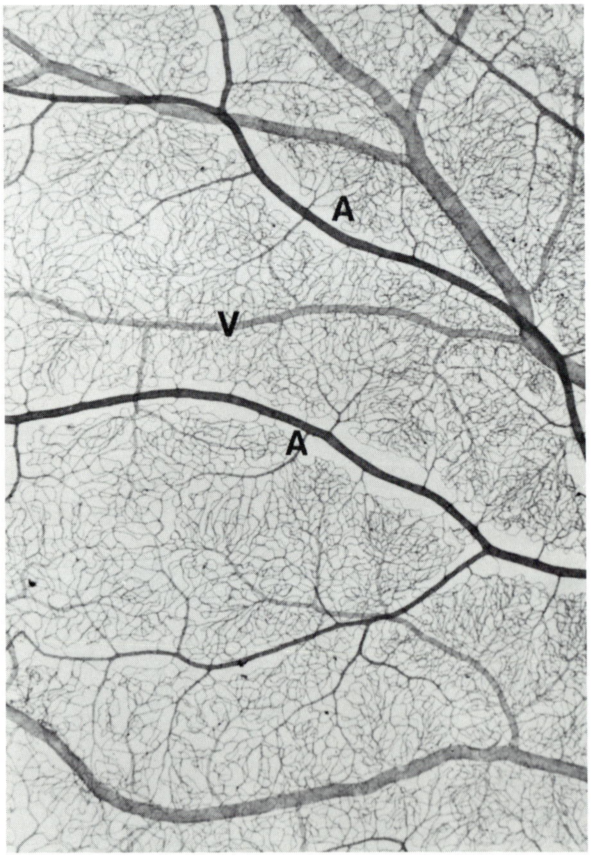

Fig. 2-12. *Bottom right.* Human retinal digest preparation in the region of the equator. Note the partially compartmentalized appearance of the capillary bed which appears to be "strung-out" between the adjacent arteries **(A)** and which is drained by an interposed vein **(V).** PAS and hematoxylin, ×12.

From a single terminal arteriole there arises a plexus of 10 to 20 interconnecting capillaries each approximately 5 μ in diameter. Cogan[6] has noted that the capillaries come off of a relatively large arteriole, and this suggests that the retinal capillary bed has a high-pressure head. The retinal capillary network has multiple arteriolar feedpoints,[16] a fact of considerable consequence when considering the effect of intraretinal vascular occlusion (Fig. 2-10). Blockage of a single terminal arteriole will not lead to total cessation of flow in the immediately surrounding capillary bed.

The retinal capillary bed is a complex meshwork of small-caliber channels which tend to be arranged in layers. According to Michaelson[27] there is a basic two-layered pattern: the deeper capillaries lying in the inner nuclear layer and forming a closer-set meshwork than the superficial capillaries which occupy the nerve fiber and ganglion cell layers. The mesh diameter varies in different parts of the retina with the deep or outer network averaging 50 μ with a range of 15 to 130 μ and the superficial or inner network averaging 65 μ with a range of 16 to 150 μ.[27] Terminal arterioles supply, capillary communications link, and postcapillary venules drain the networks. This basic two-layered pattern is modified at the posterior pole. In the peripapillary region, where the retina is thickest, there may be three layers plus a discrete capillary net in the superficial portion of the nerve fiber layer. At the central macular area the capillary bed thins out and in the perifoveal region there is only a single layer of capillaries (Fig. 2-9). Toward the periphery the deep net disappears leaving a single layer of wide-mesh, broad-caliber capillaries (Fig. 2-8).

Toussaint and his co-workers,[32] and Marquardt[26] do not feel that the retinal capillary bed can be considered to comprise separate lamina (with the exception of the superficial peripapillary capillaries which they consider to be discrete). Basing their observations on analyses of retinal digests they favor the view that the capillaries form a three-dimensional plexus with the capillaries suspended like a hammock between the arteriole and venule. However, injected whole mounts provide the definite impression of separate but interconnected capillary networks. Indeed, the concept of at least partially independent laminae of capillaries is consistent with the observation that some retinal vascular disorders affect predominantly the deeper capillaries, while others involve superficial ones. In this regard it is interesting that His[17] felt that the superficial capillary net was arterial and the deeper one venous. While this view has not been supported by other investigators[27] there is little question that postcapillary venules seem more prominent in the deeper layer, and that the precapillary arterioles are distinctly more allied to the superficial capillaries.

A broad zone, free of capillaries, is present around retinal arteries[27] (Fig. 2-11), see Chapter 1, Development of Retinal Vessels. According to Ashton[4] such a periarterial, capillary-free zone is unusual outside of the retina. We have noted, in various species, a relationship between the width of the capillary-free zone and the diameter of the retinal capillary mesh: the broader the mesh, the wider is the zone free of capillaries. A narrower and less prominent capillary-free zone around veins has been noted by Toussaint, Kuwabara, and Cogan.[32]

From the equator of the eye anteriorly it is possible to discern that the retinal capillary bed is somewhat compartmentalized (Fig. 2-12). A plexus of capillaries appears strung out between adjacent arteries. One or more veins drain the territory. A few capillaries cross under the arteries and link with the adjacent portions of the capillary bed. Whether this observation has clinical or physiologic significance is as yet unknown, but it bears further study.

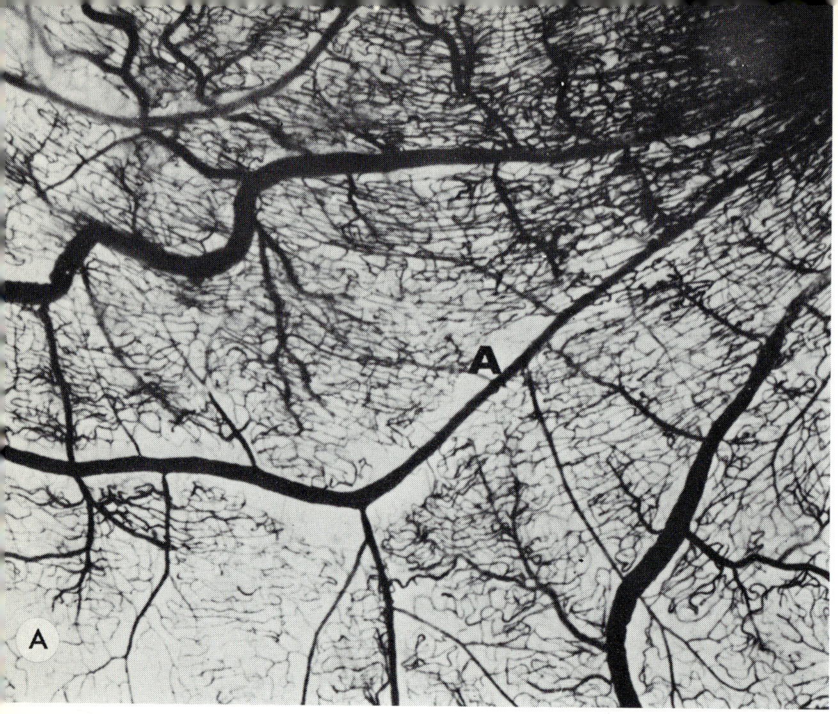

Fig. 2-13. *A*, India-inked human retina. Note the dense network of radial capillaries on either side of the inferotemporal artery **(A).** The radial peripapillary capillaries arise independently from intraretinal arteries but rarely cross a major arterial trunk.

B, Photomicrograph of a radial peripapillary capillary (between **arrows**) in the nerve fiber layer of a human without known retinal disease. Note the long length of the capillary. Near its center there is a suggestion of a connection with a capillary lying in the ganglion cell layer **(arrow head).** Weigert's resorcin-fuchsin, ×320.

(Both *A* and *B* from Henkind.[14])

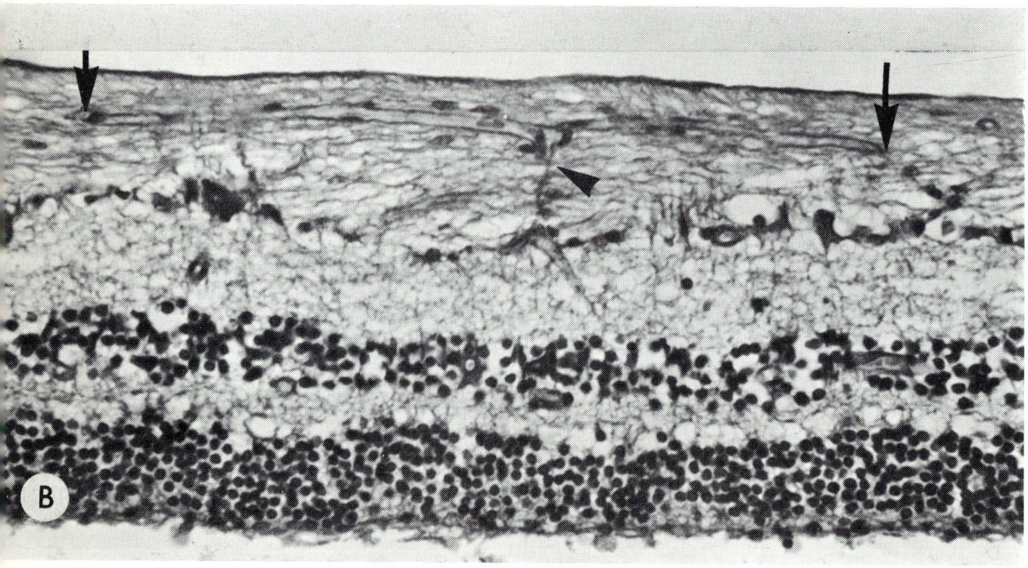

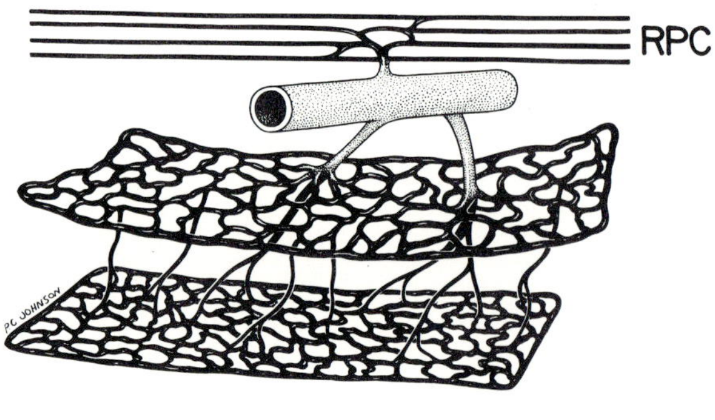

Fig. 2-14. Schema of the origin of radial peripapillary capillaries **(RPC).** They derive from the same retinal artery that supplies the deeper-lying capillaries. (From Henkind.[15])

RADIAL PERIPAPILLARY CAPILLARIES

Aside from the retinal capillaries discussed above there is a distinct strata of capillaries occupying the superficial portion of the nerve fiber layer in the peripapillary retina.[13–15, 28, 32]

Described initially by Michaelson and Campbell[28] in 1940, the radial peripapillary capillaries have received attention only in recent years. The most superficial of all retinal capillaries, they pursue relatively long, straight, or slightly curved paths, and have few communications with adjacent radial vessels or with the underlying capillaries (Fig. 2-13). Several such capillaries may run end to end as if in series. They originate from intraretinal precapillary arterioles, and drain into intraretinal venules or veins lying on the optic nerve head (Fig. 2-14). Separate arterioles are responsible for supplying various portions of the radial peripapillary capillary bed and these same arterioles also feed the deeper capillaries. Possibly the greater length of the radial capillaries with consequent higher resistance may cause blood to be deflected from the radial capillaries into the deeper capillaries when intraocular tension is increased.

In their distribution the radial capillaries resemble a double Bjerrum's scotoma[32] (Fig. 2-15). They are most prominent along the paths of the major superotemporal and inferotemporal vessels, and to a lesser extent are found in the nasal quadrants adjacent to the disc. The macular area lacks radial capillaries, thus one finds a deficiency in the radial capillary bed just temporally to the disc. A smaller indentation is present nasally. Radial capillaries cross underlying venules, but stop short of larger arterioles.[32]

By light microscopy the radial capillaries appear to have a comparable cellular structure and are of similar caliber to other retinal capillaries. The differences between these and other retinal capillaries can be summarized as follows: radial capillaries have a long path length measuring several hundred to several thousand micra while the other retinal capillaries are arranged in meshlike nets; radial capillaries have few arteriolar feedpoints while the other retinal capillaries have multiple arteriolar feedpoints; and the radial capillary bed has few anastomoses while the other retinal capillaries have multiple anastomoses.

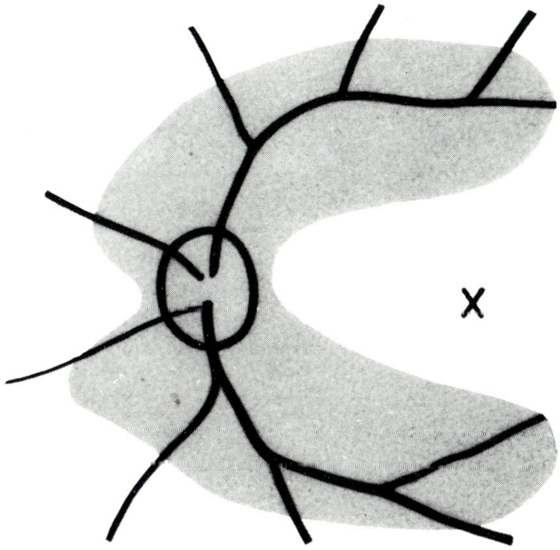

Fig. 2-15. The distribution of the radial capillaries resembles a double Bjerrum's scotoma. **X,** fovea. (From Henkind.[15])

The radial capillaries are responsible for nourishing the tissue surrounding them which consists mainly of the superficially placed nerve fibers. These neurons apparently originate from ganglion cells of the posterior pole of the eye and enter the center of the nerve head,[34] and they are the fibers presumably involved in early glaucoma field defects.

Several retinal lesions occur in the distribution of the radial capillaries and can probably be attributed to their derangement. Flame-shaped hemorrhages are most common at the posterior pole of the eye, and are most often seen in the supero- and inferotemporal quadrants, or just around the disc itself. Their linear pattern and superficial placement are indications that the bleeding is in the nerve fiber layer, most likely originating from the radial peripapillary capillaries. Michaelson and Campbell[28] have noted that the very superficial and linearly arranged hemorrhages seen in papilledema coincide in number and distribution with the radial capillaries. Cotton-wool spots are found mainly in the region of the radial capillaries in humans. In the pig, experimentally induced, cotton-wool spots have been noted to develop in areas of radial capillary obliteration.

Evidence is accumulating that the radial capillaries play a significant role in glaucomatous field defects. Their anatomic distribution coincides with the location of Bjerrum's scotomata. Elevation of the intraocular pressure in experimental animals, both in vitro and in vivo, caused selective underfilling or decreased flow in radial capillaries.[1,8] Kornzweig and his colleagues[23] have demonstrated the selective obliteration of radial capillaries in retinal digest preparations from 10 aged humans with glaucoma. In two individuals the disease process was unilateral as was the radial peripapillary capillary degeneration. Aging alone caused no significant change in these vessels.

REFERENCES

1. Alterman, M., and Henkind, P.: Radial peripapillary capillaries. 2. Possible role in Bjerrum scotoma. *Brit. J. Ophthal. 52:*26, 1968.
2. Ashton, N.: Vascular changes in diabetes with particular reference to retinal vessels. *Brit. J. Ophthal. 33:*407, 1949.
3. Ashton, N.: Injection of retinal vascular system in diabetic retinopathy. *Brit. J. Ophthal. 34:*38, 1950.
4. Ashton, N.: "The Mode of Development of the Retinal Vessels in Man." In *The William Mackenzie Centenary Symposium on the Ocular Circulation in Health and Disease.* Ed. by Cant, J. S., St. Louis, Mo., Mosby, 1969, pp. 7–17.
5. Chisholm, I. A.: Uncommon retinal vascular anomalies. *Brit. J. Ophthal. 50:*257, 1966.
6. Cogan, D. G.: Development and senescence of the human retinal vasculature. *Trans. Ophthal. Soc. U.K. 83:*465, 1963.
7. Cogan, D. G., and Kuwabara, T.: "Retinal vessels: Anatomy," In *XXth International Congress of Ophthalmology.* Munich, 1966. Part 1, p. 94.
8. Dollery, C. T., Henkind, P., Kohner, E. M., and Paterson, J. W.: Effect of raised intraocular pressure on the retinal and choroidal circulation. *Invest. Ophthal. 7:*191, 1968.
9. Friedenwald, J. S.: A new approach to some problems of retinal vascular disease. *Amer. J. Ophthal. 32:*487, 1949.
10. Hausler, H. R., and Sibay, T. M.: A contribution to the injection technique for studying retinal blood vessels. *Amer. J. Ophthal. 48:*138, 1959.
11. Hayreh, S. S.: The cilio-retinal arteries. *Brit. J. Ophthal. 47:*71, 1963.
12. Helmholtz, H. von: *Beschreilbung eines Augenspiegels z. Untersuch. d. Netzhaut im lebenden Auge,* Berlin, Forstner, 1851.
13. Henkind, P.: The radial peripapillary capillaries of the retina. 1. Anatomy: Human and comparative. *Brit. J. Ophthal. 51:*115, 1967.
14. Henkind, P.: New observations on the radial peripapillary capillaries. *Invest. Ophthal. 6:*103, 1967.
15. Henkind, P.: Microcirculation of the peripapillary retina. *Trans. Amer. Acad. Ophthal. Otolaryng. 73:*890, 1969.
16. Henkind, P., and Dollery, C. T.: Pathophysiology of the retinal vascular bed following acute embolisation. *Invest. Ophthal. 5:*204, 1966.

17. His, W.: Abbildungen uber des Gefass-system der menschlichen Netzhaut und derjenigen des Kaninchens. *Arch. Anat. Entwicklelungsg. 5:*224, 1880.

18. Jaeger, E.: Beitrage zur Pathologie des Auges. Wien, Kaiserlich Koniglichen hof und Staatsdruckerei, 1855.

19. Janes, R. G.: The relationship between eye and kidney pathology in the diabetic rat. *Arch. Path. 67:*386, 1959.

20. Keeney, A. H., and Barlow, F. D.: Histologic methods in the study of retinal vascular patterns. In the albino rat. *Amer. J. Ophthal. 42:*554, 1956.

21. Keys, T. E., and Rucker, C. W.: The atlases of ophthalmoscopy: A bibliography, 1850–1960. *Amer. J. Ophthal. 49:*881, 1960.

22. Knight, G.: Injection-digest method for studying retinal vessels. *Brit. J. Ophthal. 50:*144, 1966.

23. Kornzweig, A. L., Eliasoph, I., and Feldstein, M.: Selective atrophy of the radial peripapillary capillaries in chronic glaucoma. *Arch. Ophthal. 80:*696, 1968.

24. Kuwabara, T., and Cogan, D. G.: Studies of retinal vascular patterns. Part I. Normal architecture. *Arch. Ophthal. 64:*904, 1960.

25. Lerche, W.: "Die Kapillarisierung der menschlichen Retina," In *The Structure of the Eye*, 11. Ed. by J. W. Rohen. Stuttgart, Schattauer-Verlag, 1965, p. 121.

26. Marquardt, R.: Ein Beitrag zur Topographie und Anatomie der Netzhautgefasse des menschlichen Auges. *Klin. Mbl. Augenheilk. 148:*50, 1966.

27. Michaelson, I. C.: *Retinal Circulation in Man and Animals.* Springfield, Ill., Thomas, 1954.

28. Michaelson, I. C., and Campbell, A. C. P.: The anatomy of the finer retinal vessels. *Trans. Ophthal. Soc. U.K. 60:*71, 1940.

29. Michaelson, I. C., and Steedman, H. F.: Injection of the retinal vascular system in enucleated eyes. *Brit. J. Ophthal. 33:*376, 1949.

30. Nettleship, E.: Note on the retinal blood vessels of the yellow-spot region. *R.L.O.H. Rep. 8:*260, 1874.

31. Ruete, C. G. T.: *Bildliche Darstellung der krankheiten des menschlichen Auges.* Leipzig, Tuebner, 1854.

32. Toussaint, D., Kuwabara, T., and Cogan, D. G.: Retinal vascular patterns. 2. Human retinal vessels studied in three dimensions. *Arch. Ophthal. 65:*575, 1961.

33. Van Trigt, A. C.: Dissertatio ophthalmologica inauguralis de speculo oculi. (Thesis, Traj. ad Rhenum, P. W. van de Wecjer, 1853.)

34. Wolff, E., and Penman, G. C.: The position occupied by the peripheral retinal fibers in the nerve fiber layer and at the nerve head. *Acta XVI Concilium Ophthal. 1:*625, 1951.

chapter 3

Structure of Retinal Vessels

This chapter deals with the anatomy of the various components of the retinal vascular system. The function of the different structures will be discussed, and we will consider the role of the endothelium in the blood-retinal barrier, the significance of intramural pericytes in health and disease, and the vasoglial relationship in the retina. The basic premise is that structure and function go hand in hand and an adequate knowledge of structure is essential for understanding disease processes.

ARTERIES

CENTRAL RETINAL ARTERY WITHIN THE OPTIC NERVE

Within the optic nerve, the central retinal artery closely resembles other small muscular arteries (Fig. 3-1). In humans, the diameter of its lumen is approximately 200 μ,[69] varying from a proximal diameter of 245 μ to a distal diameter of 170 μ.[48] In the adult, the thickness of the wall is about 32 μ, increasing in old age to 37 μ. The ratio of wall thickness to lumen diameter is approximately 1:4, but this ratio becomes 1:10 after the artery passes the lamina cribrosa.[8]

A single layer of endothelial cells lines the lumen; the cell nuclei are arranged with their long axes parallel to the length of the vessel. A subendothelial layer, consisting of connective tissue with fine, circularly arranged elastic tissue, is absent at birth, but develops with age. Surrounding this is the internal elastic lamina composed of elastic fibrils. The media consists of multiple layers of smooth muscle interspersed with elastic fibers. There is an ill-defined external elastic lamina surrounding the muscle and merging with the adventitia. The adventitia is the thickest portion of the vessel wall, and is composed mostly of collagen with numerous interspersed circular and longitudinal elastic fibers. This layer is continuous with the pial connective tissue sheath which surrounds the central vessels. In its intraneural course the artery is accompanied by a sympathetic nerve plexus.

Pathologic processes which affect muscular arteries also involve the intraneural portion of the central retinal artery, and include such entities as atheromata and giant cell arteritis.

INTRARETINAL BRANCHES OF THE CENTRAL RETINAL ARTERY

As the central retinal artery enters the retina it divides into its intraretinal branches with the vessel walls losing their elastic tissue.[26] Near the disc, the diameter of the arterial lumen is approximately 100 μ, and the wall is 15-μ thick. As their branches divide, their lumina narrow and their walls thin (Fig. 3-2). Hogan and Feeney provide the most definitive anatomic data on the subject.[26–28]

A layer of endothelium lines the arterial lumen, and the endothelial cells are oriented parallel to the vessel axis. The plasma membranes of these cells may overlap and interdigitate. Except for a sparcity of pinocytotic vesicles, the cells resemble the endothelium of other arteries.

A broad (0.1 to 0.5 μ) basement membrane

Fig. 3-1. *Top right.* Cross section of the human central retinal artery (**A**) and the central retinal vein (**V**) as they lie within the optic nerve. The internal elastic lamina of the artery is darkly stained. The thick common adventitia of both vessels merges with the connective tissue septae of the nerve. Elastic stain, ×120.

Fig. 3-2. *Bottom right.* Retinal artery (**A**) and vein (**V**) at the level of the optic disc. The vessels lie within the tissue of the disc and the retinal layers can be seen at the left of the figure. PAS, ×190.

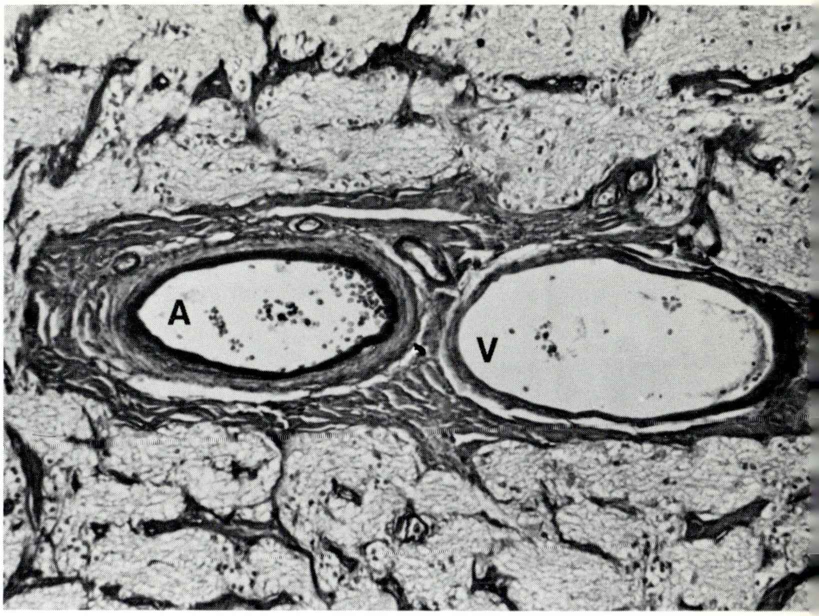

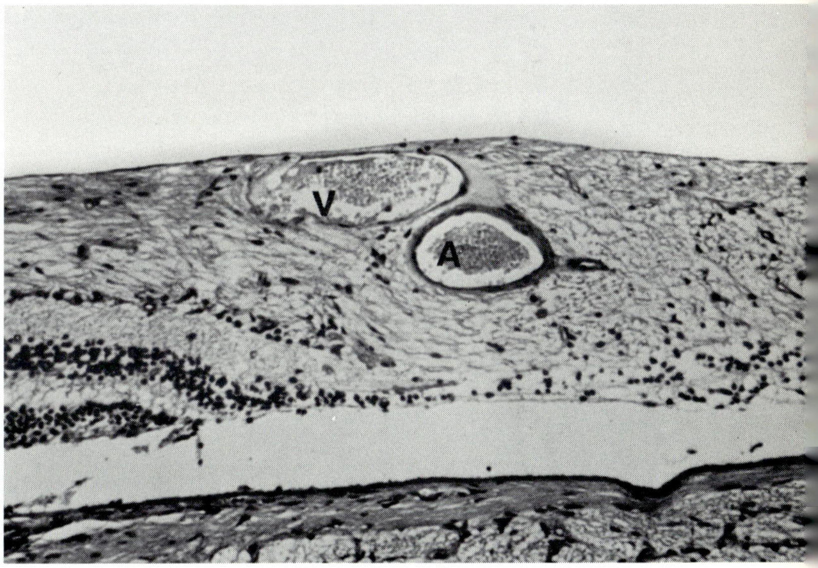

of uniform density lies external to the endothelium. Small clusters of collagen fibers are found within the membrane, but elastin is absent.* The thickness of the membrane varies, and the basement membranes both of the endothelial and smooth muscle cells often appear fused.

The media of the arteries contains five to seven layers of smooth muscle cells near the disc (Fig. 3-3*A* and *B*). This decreases to two or three layers at the equator, and to one or two layers peripherally. Thus, the arterial nature of these main-stem vessels is maintained toward the retinal periphery. The muscle cells are oriented both circularly and longitudinally, and the muscle layers are separated from each other by basement membrane material, which increases in thickness towards the adventitia. Collagen fibrils are present within the basement membrane and become more abundant nearer the adventitia. Cavitation and lami-

* Many previous workers have reported the presence of elastic fibers within intraretinal arteries. It appears that they were misled because of their dependence on the "elastic tissue" stain of Weigert. This resorcin-fuchsin stain has not been shown to be specific for elastin, and indeed it reacts with many substances, including gelatin, altered collagen, and basement membranes. Rodgers, Puchtler, and Gropp[50] have shown by a variety of chemical and optical methods that arteries smaller than 100 μ do not contain elastin in their walls. The so-called "internal elastic lamina" in these smaller arteries is most likely a type of immature collagen, embedded in basement membrane material. These authors feel that such immature collagenous fibers may possess rubber-like elasticity.

It has been suggested that there may be a relationship between the composition of the internal elastic membrane and the type of arteriosclerotic lesions which may affect a vessel. Atherosclerosis seems to be limited to arteries with a "true" internal elastic membrane, i.e., the central retinal artery within the optic nerve. Hyaline deposits are apparently limited (at least in renal arteries[50]) to those segments of the arterial system where the internal "elastic" lamina consists of collagenous fibers embedded in a matrix of basement membrane. Hyalinization of intraretinal arteries is a well-known occurrence.[20] Likewise, giant-cell arteritis affects the central retinal artery within the optic nerve but spares the intraretinal branches.

nation of the basement membranes also become more evident with each succeeding layer. The muscle cells of the retinal arteries are typical of the smooth muscle cells found in other vessels. An unusual feature in these vessels, however, is the frequent displacement of muscle cells into the adventitia. Some muscle cells may in fact be separated from the media by more than a micron of laminated basement membrane and collagen. Dense, feathery, osmiophilic material is found in the media of the larger retinal arteries in man, but is not noted in the arteries of animals.

The adventitia contains loosely arranged collagen fibers which course in different directions, usually aligned somewhat obliquely to the vessel axis. Those fibers closest to the media insert into the laminated basement membranes of the two outer muscle layers.

The caliber of the vessel lumen is not a sufficient guide to determine whether a vessel is an artery or arteriole. Descriptively, at the posterior pole, vessels less than 20 μ in diameter have three or four muscle layers in the media and are considered to be arteries. Hogan and Feeney [26] have noted, however, that in the smaller-caliber vessels of approximately 8 μ found at the retinal periphery, the muscle coat is reduced to one or two layers; here the term arteriole is applicable. In this book we will use the word *arteriole* only to describe the precapillary arterioles, otherwise the terms *artery* and *arterial* will be used.

The retinal arteries lie mainly in the nerve fiber and ganglion cell layer, often just beneath the internal limiting membrane. They may extend downward to the inner and even the outer nuclear layers at points of arteriovenous crossing.[56]

All retinal vessels are separated from the surrounding neural elements by the cytoplasm of Müller and glial cells. This glial tissue, which serves to insulate the mesodermal components of the vessels from the ecto-

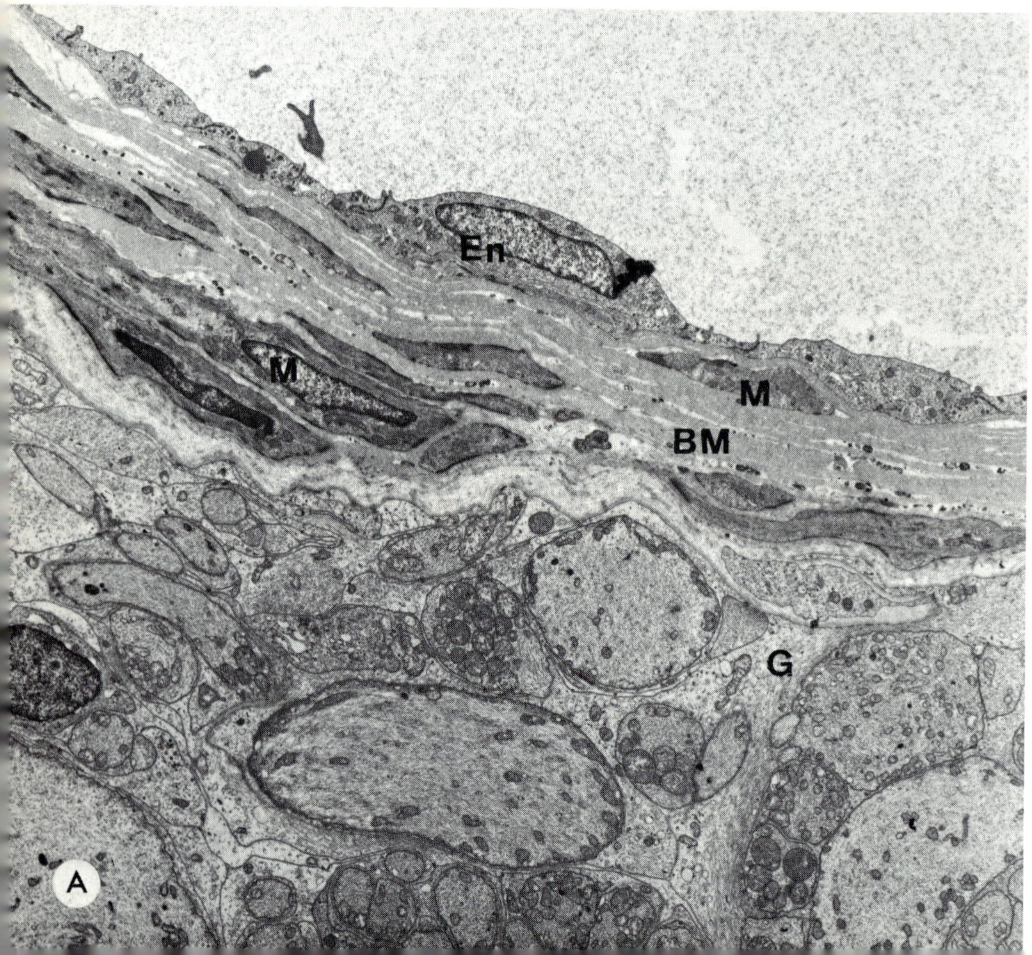

Fig. 3-3. *Left. A,* Electronmicrograph of a human retinal artery near the disc shows endothelium **(En),** basement membrane **(BM),** and several layers of muscle cells **(M).** No internal elastic lamina is present. The adventitia contains loosely packed collagen fibers. Glia **(G)** separates the artery from the surrounding nerve fibers. ×4500.

Opposite page. B, Electronmicrograph of two muscle cells in the wall of a human retinal artery. Their cytoplasm contains abundant glycogen and myofilaments **(arrow).** The basement membrane material **(BM)** separating the muscle cells contains collagen fibers. ×51,000.

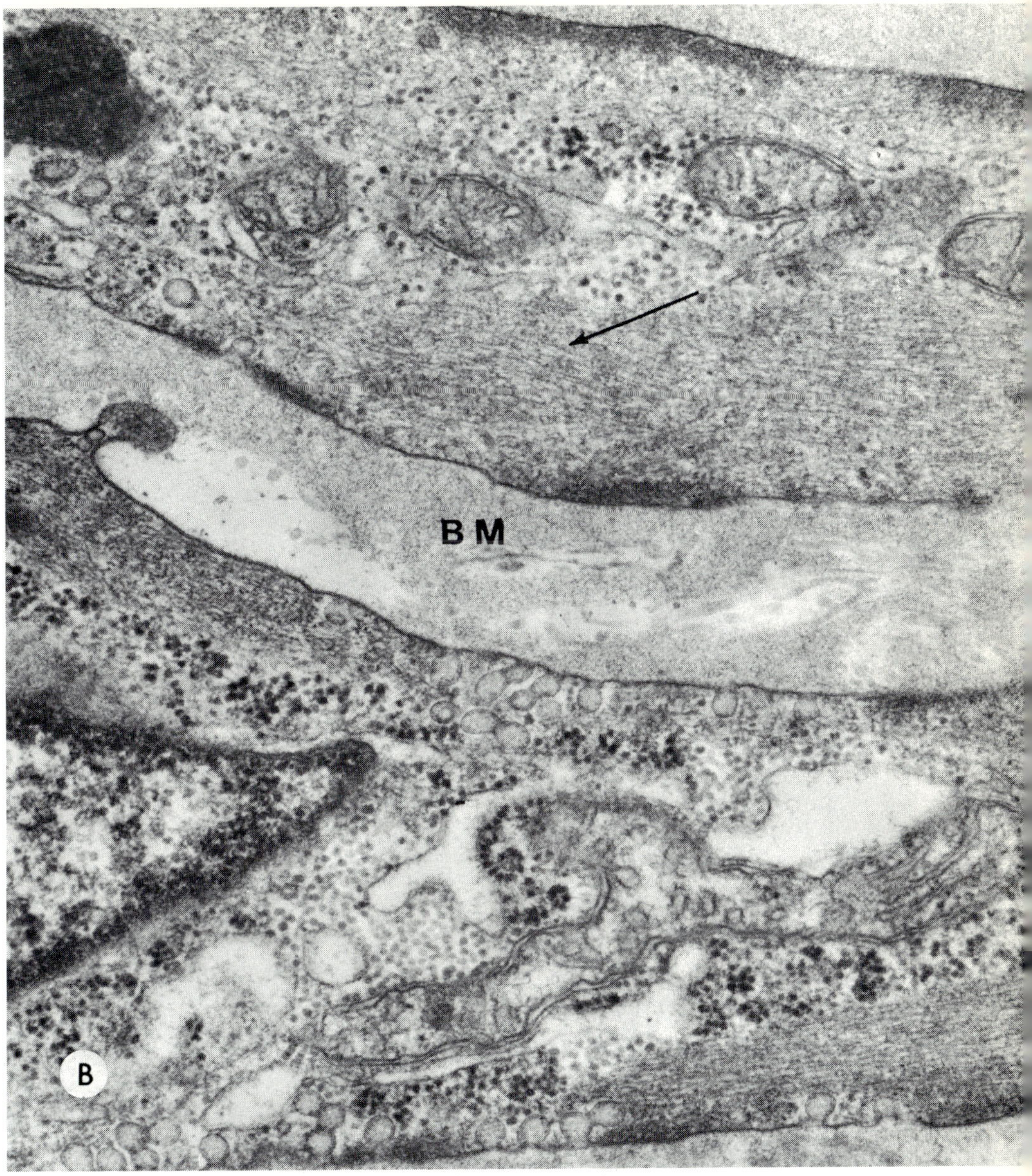

dermal structure of the retina, has been called the "perivascular limiting membrane of Kruckmann."[15] Originally it was thought to surround a perivascular space containing lymphatics. However, electron microscopic study[26] has been unable to demonstrate a perivascular space between the vessel adventitia and the surrounding glia. Nor have the lymph spaces described by other authors[7] been demonstrated by electron microscopy.

It had been assumed, until quite recently, that retinal vessels had a rich sympathetic and parasympathetic nerve supply.[15] Electron microscopy[26] and selective histochemical methods[16,38] have failed to reveal any evidence of sympathetic nerve endings in human or animal retinal vessels. Although the results are conflicting, stimulation or denervation of the cervical sympathetic system causes little or no alteration in the caliber of retinal vessels.[15]

VEINS

CENTRAL RETINAL VEIN WITHIN THE OPTIC NERVE

The central retinal vein usually lies temporally to the central retinal artery within the optic nerve. It has a larger diameter (i.e., a proximal diameter of 245 μ, and a distal diameter of 200 μ), but a thinner wall than the adjacent artery,[48] and it resembles other veins of medium caliber (Fig.3-1). A single layer of endothelial cells line a thin subendothelial coat of connective tissue. The media has few muscle cells, but elastic fibers are abundant. The adventitia is thin, and consists of connective tissue and a few elastic fibers. It merges with the pial connective tissue sheath which surrounds the central vessels.

INTRARETINAL BRANCHES OF THE CENTRAL RETINAL VEIN

The venous system of the retina commences just behind the ora serrata, where it receives blood from enlarged capillary arcades. The veins increase in wall thickness and caliber as they approach the disc; their luminal diameter is approximately 200 μ just before they join to form the central retinal vein.

The lumen is lined by endothelial cells, the basement membrane of which is approximately 0.1 μ in width, thinner than that of the retinal arteries. There is no internal elastic lamina, and instead of muscle cells, which are present only in the larger veins near the disc, the media contains widely spaced cells called "pericytes (Fig. 3-4)."[26] The cytoplasm of these cells differs from that of smooth muscle in that it has fewer cytoplasmic filaments and less dense attachment zones along plasma membranes. The cells resemble smooth muscle cells in size and distribution, and have a similarly flattened nucleus, a rough endoplasmic reticulum, and pinocytotic vesicles along the plasma membrane (Fig. 3-5*A* and *B*). Basement membrane material may be lacking between the pericytes and the endothelial cells. The adventitia comprises the outer two-thirds of the venous wall, and is composed of loosely arranged, longitudinally oriented fibers (Fig. 3-5*A*). The vein is surrounded closely by the basement membranes of glial and Müller cells.

ARTERIOVENOUS CROSSINGS

At their points of crossing, the retinal arteries and veins share a common coat, and only a thin endothelial lining and basement membrane may separate their lumina (Fig. 3-6*A* and *B*). This anatomic configuration is thought to be the cause of various arteriovenous crossing phenomena which may be seen clinically, and in which one diseased vessel can affect the other. For example, branch vein occlusion commonly occurs at an arteriovenous crossing, and is usually initiated by changes in the adjacent artery. Seitz[56] and Kimura[32] feel that most ophthalmoscopically visible changes at arteriovenous crossings are due to alterations in the adventitia and the surrounding glia. While Duke-Elder and Wybar[15] feel that such arteriovenous crossings in the retina are unique because of their intimate relationship, Seitz,[56] who has studied such sites in detail, feels that they are not peculiar to the retina, and can be found in other areas.*

*Tominaga and Ikui[64a,b] found by electron microscopy that at the arteriovenous crossing the basement membranes, which surround the smooth muscle cells both of the retinal arteries and veins, become fused together and a small amount of reticular fibrils are found in the common part of the basement membranes. No neuronal or glial elements are interposed at the arteriovenous crossing.

CAPILLARIES

The capillaries of the retina vary in diameter from 3.5 to 6 μ, and their wall is composed of three distinct elements; endothelial cells, intramural pericytes, and basement membrane (Table 3-1).

ENDOTHELIUM

The capillary is lined by endothelial cells whose nuclei bulge centrally into the lumen, or at least this is the appearance seen on fixed material. It should be remembered that red blood cells are flexible and can fold to pass through vessels of smaller caliber than their largest diameter. The endothelial cell is thickest at the nucleus; elsewhere, it consists of cytoplasmic extensions which encircle the lumen (Fig. 3-7).[31] Tight junctional complexes, with continuous fusion of the outer leaflets of the cell membranes, are found along the opposing surfaces of adjacent endothelial cells.[57] Frequently, the endothelial cell processes overlap, and a lip-like protrusion often marks the junction of two cells.

In cross section the nuclei of endothelial cells have an irregular contour. The chromatin is evenly divided except for a slight concentration along the nuclear membrane; a nucleolus may be prominent. Scattered throughout the cytoplasm are tubular and vesicular components, endoplasmic reticulum, free dense particles, and relatively few small mitochondria. Centrioles and the Golgi apparatus are found near the nucleus, while pinocytotic vesicles are seen along the lumen and basal cell borders.

Function of Endothelium

The function of the blood-retinal barrier depends upon an intact functioning endothelium. Damage to the endothelium alters permeability and allows material, otherwise barred, to enter the retina.

Electron microscopic studies have shown the existence of pinocytotic vesicles within endothelial cells of normal blood vessels. It has been postulated that larger molecules can pass across endothelial cells within these structures. While such vesicles are

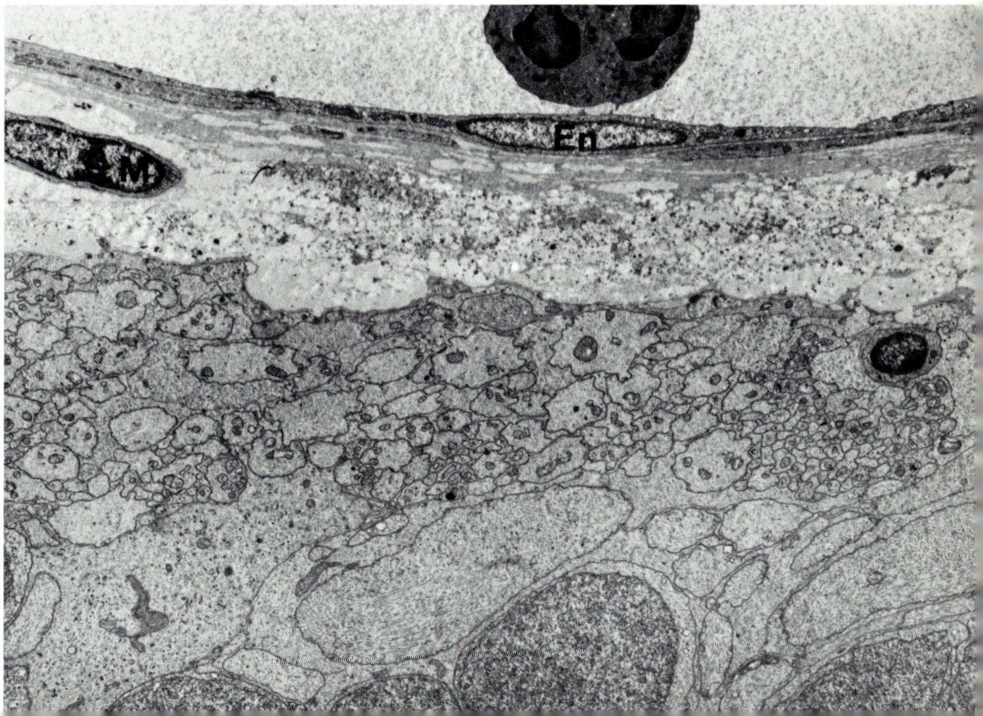

Fig. 3-4. Electronmicrograph of the wall of a human retinal vein shows the endothelium **(En)**, relatively sparse basement membrane material, and a muscle cell **(M)** or pericyte. ×4000.

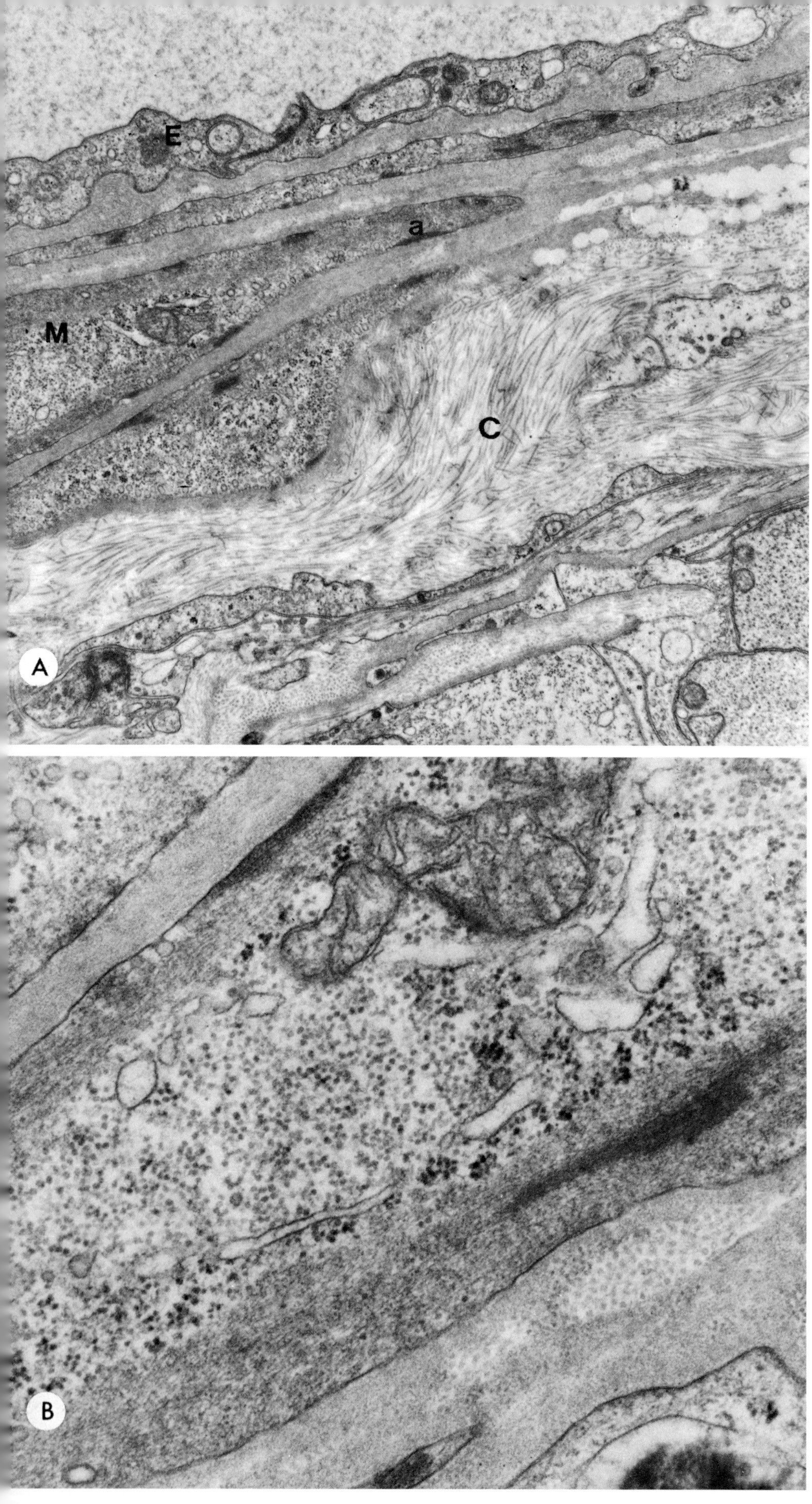

Fig. 3-5. *A*, Electronmicrograph of the wall of a human retinal vein shows the endothelium **(E)** and basement membrane with cavitations and abundant, loosely arranged collagen fibers **(C)**. Note the muscle cells **(M)** with their attachment zones **(a)**. ×14,000.

B, High-power view of a muscle cell or pericyte in the wall of a human retinal vein shows myofilaments. ×45,000.

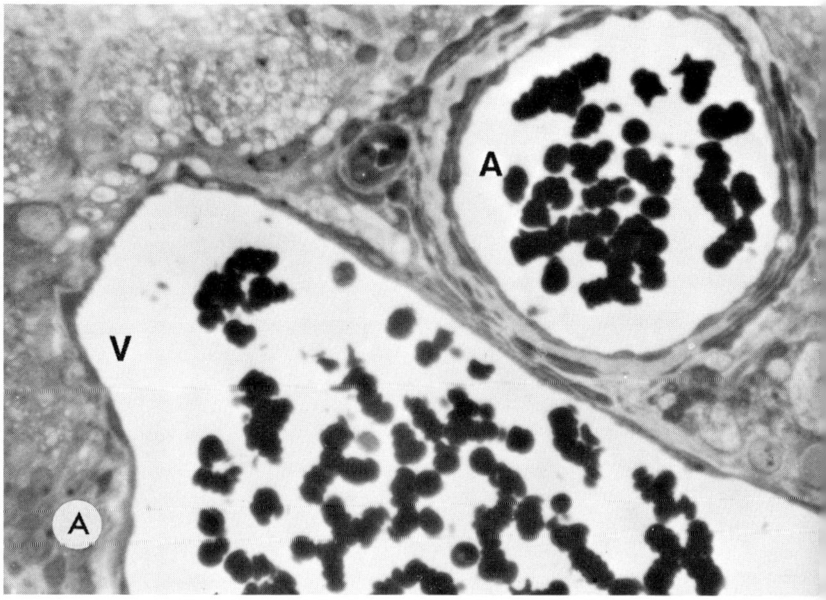

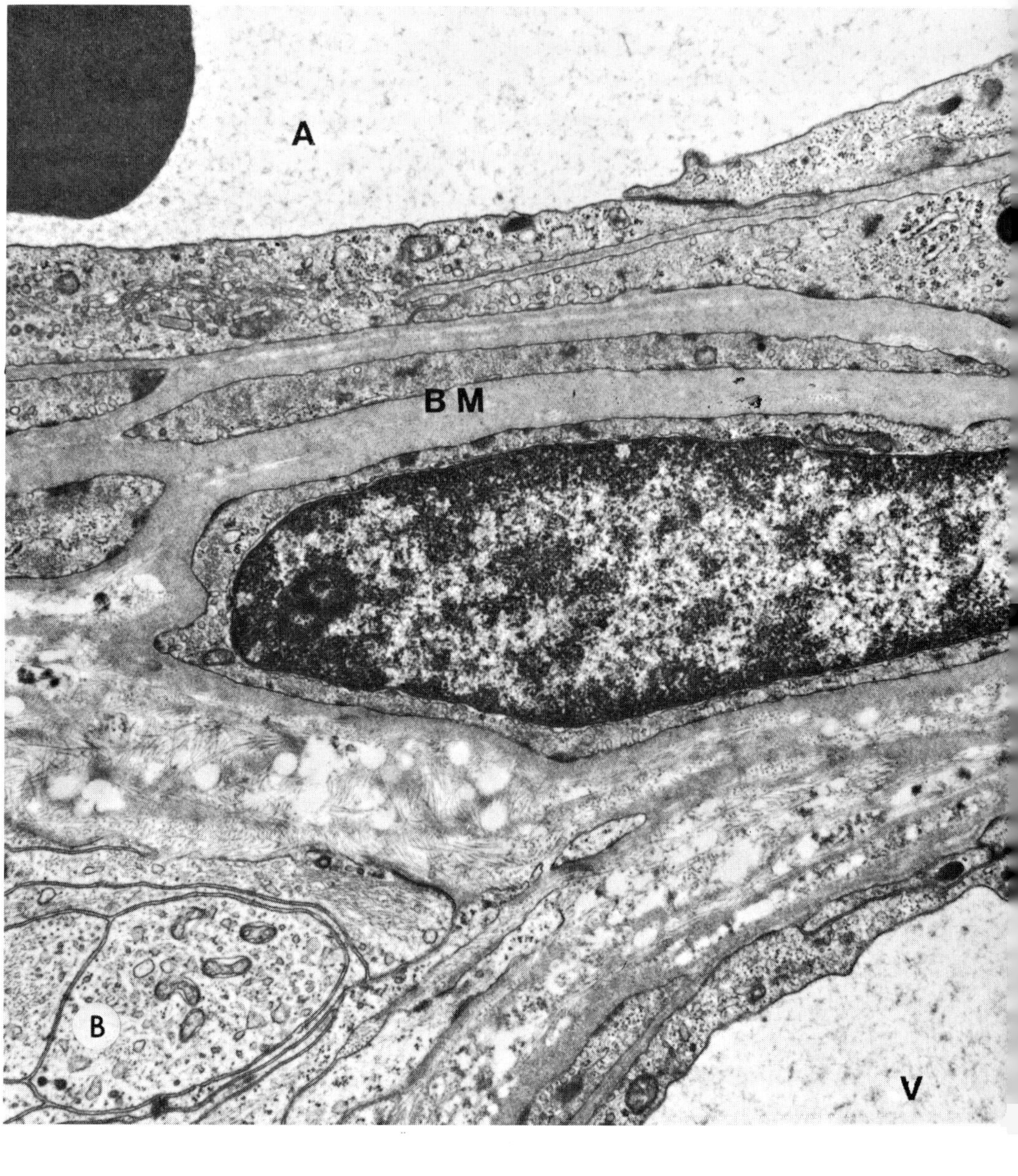

Fig. 3-6. *A*, Section through a retinal arteriovenous crossing in man. Artery **(A)**; vein **(V)**. ×480.

B, Electronmicrograph of an arteriovenous crossing in a human retina. The common wall between the artery **(A)** and the vein **(V)** contains basement membrane material **(BM)** and some muscle cells. ×16,000.

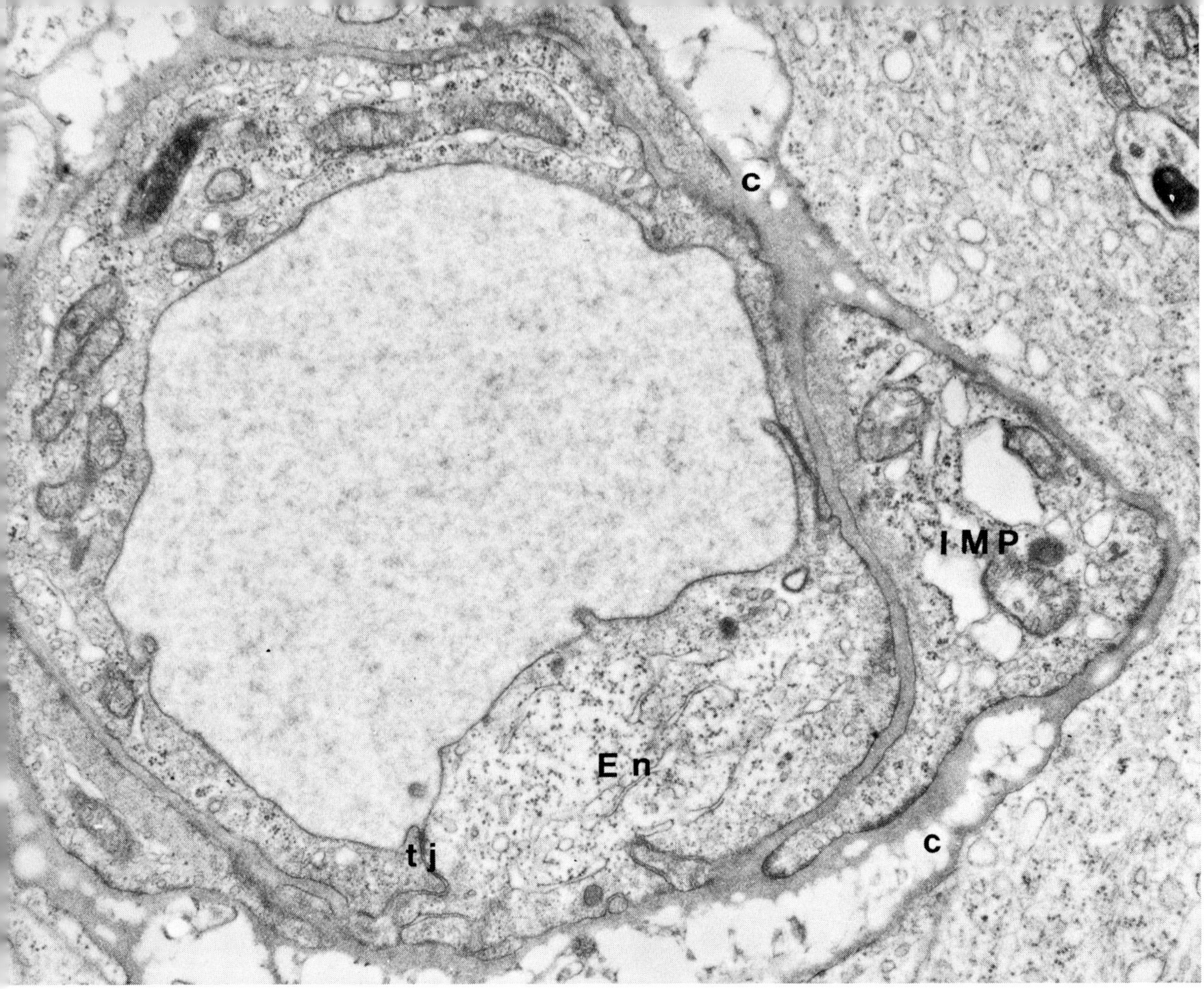

Fig. 3-7. Electronmicrograph of a human retinal capillary shows the endothelium **(En)** with tight junctional complexes between adjacent cells **(tj)**, intramural pericyte **(IMP)**, and basement membrane material with cavities **(c)**. ×22,000.

Fig. 3-8. *A*, Retinal digest preparation shows a rat retinal capillary bed. The small, round, dark intramural pericyte nuclei **(P)** can be distinguished from the larger, paler endothelial cell nuclei **(E)**. Several fine intercapillary strands **(arrows)** can be seen. They represent remnants of the primitive retinal capillary bed. PAS and hematoxylin, ×800.

B, Retinal digest preparation of human retinal capillaries. There are an approximately equal number of small, dark intramural pericyte nuclei **(p)** and larger, paler, oval endothelial cell nuclei **(e)**. PAS and hematoxylin, ×480.

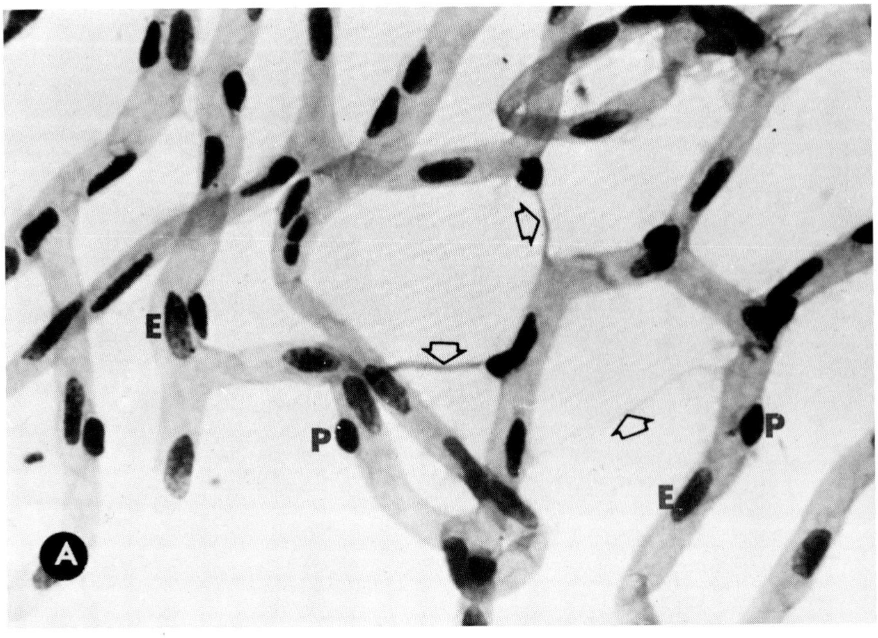

TABLE 3-1
Retinal Endothelial Cells vs Intramural Pericytes

Endothelial cells	Intramural pericytes
Location	
Line the vascular lumen. Covered externally by the basement membrane	Discontinuous, but evenly spaced along the wall. Lie within the basement membrane
Cell Shape	
Polygonal or elongated rhomboidal shape	Irregular, with branching cytoplasmic processes
Nucleus	
Shape: Elongated	Shape: Spherical
Size: Large (compared to intramural cell)	Size: Small
Stain: Light with hematoxylin	Stain: Dark
Relation to capillary wall: Often appears internal to wall	Relation to capillary wall: On outer portion of wall—may appear "stuck on"
Pathology	
Aging: Lost before intramural cells	Aging: Relative sparing
Ischemia: Lost before intramural cells	Ischemia: Relative sparing
Diabetes: Spared	Diabetes: Preferential loss

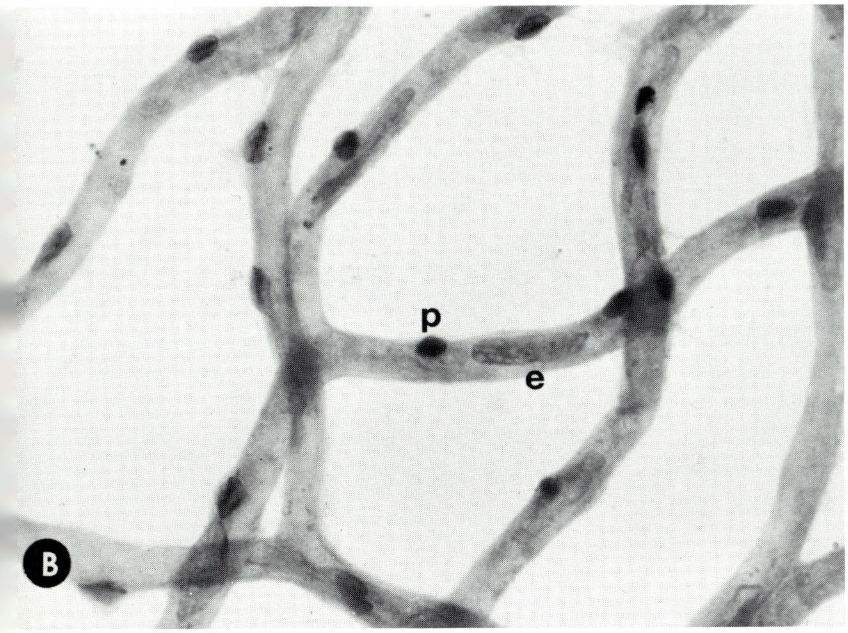

found in normal retinal endothelial cells, tracer particles can rarely be found within them. Fenestrae, gaps in the endothelial lining, have been observed in many vessels, but not those of the retina, nor elsewhere in the central nervous system. Interendothelial junctions, once considered to be the major pathway for material to cross the endothelial surface, may exist in some vessels, but apparently not in the retina. In the latter such junctions are always closed and the membranes of adjacent cells fuse to form zonulae occludentes.[57] The basement membrane of the endothelial cells may act as a barrier to large particles which traverse the endothelium, but it does not appear to hinder smaller particulate matter. Recently, it has been shown that the retinal endothelium contains an active transport system for small cationic and anionic dyes (this is discussed in Chapter 6, Physiologic Principles).

INTRAMURAL PERICYTE (PERICYTE, ROUGET CELL, MURAL CELL)

The pericapillary cellular component, the intramural pericyte, has engendered controversy for almost 100 years. We now know that this cell resides within the basement membrane of the capillary and that it is an integral part of most capillaries.

Rouget[51] has described and illustrated cells within the capillary wall differing from endothelial cells, which he termed "non-pigmented adventitial cells," or cells with ramified protoplasmic processes. Among the tissues which he studied were the hyaloid and capsulopupillary membranes of rabbit and sheep embryos, kittens, puppies, and frogs, as well as the meningeal vessels of embryo calves, and rabbit and human retinal vessels. His material was fresh tissue stained with silver nitrate, gold chloride, or carmine and fuchsin. Examination of Rouget's figures and a reading of his text leaves little doubt that the cells described are the same as the intramural pericytes seen on digest preparations.

Vimtrup[65–67] confirmed Rouget's findings and named the pericapillary cells "Rouget cells." Zimmerman[74] used the term "pericyte" in his work on perivascular components. His preparations, stained with a modification of the Golgi-silver chromate technique, included vessels from many tissues in all classes of vertebrates, and confirmed the universal existence of pericytes. Unfortunately, the stain revealed more than one type of cell: some were identical to those presently accepted as intramural pericytes, and others were definitely external to the vessel wall. Later workers questioned some of Zimmerman's interpretations.[33,60] Schaly[55] described Rouget cells in many vessels of human eyes including those of the retina, choroid, ciliary body, iris, conjunctiva, orbital fat, and even in the newly proliferated vessels within a vitreous abscess. De Oliveira,[13] utilizing electron microscopy and digest preparations, has confirmed the observations of Schaly and Vimtrup.

Electron microscopy has provided new evidence concerning the nonendothelial cell component of capillaries. Farquhar and Hartman[19] have described cellular elements completely enclosed in compartments formed by splitting of the basement membrane in the cerebral capillaries of rats. Maeda[42,43] has studied human retinal vessels and found cells enclosed in the basement membrane which he termed pericytes. In a more recent work Ikui and co-workers[30] have referred to the cells within the basement membrane as pericytes, or Rouget cells. These cells have been noted in electron micrographs of capillaries from numerous organs in a wide variety of species.

Kuwabara and his colleagues[11,34] have coined the term "mural cell" for the pericapillary cells found in the retina by their digest technique. They consider mural cells to be specific for the retina and possibly the brain, and deny their presence on capillaries elsewhere in the eye or body.

There is abundant evidence that mural cells, Rouget cells, pericytes, and intramural pericytes are one and the same, and that they have a wide distribution throughout the body.[59] The term "intramural pericyte" has been suggested as the most appropriate name for the cell under discussion[6] and already it has received acceptance.[4]

Appearance of Intramural Pericytes

Intramural pericytes can be seen in cross sections examined by light and electron microscopy, however, they are most readily observed in digested, retinal flat mounts stained with hematoxylin and periodic acid-Schiff (PAS) reagent. With this last technique the nuclei of endothelial cells and intramural pericytes can be distinguished from one another (Fig. 3-8). The latter have darker, more spherical nuclei which often appear to protrude from the capillary wall. They are spaced regularly along the vessel and are as numerous as endothelial cells.[36] Light and electron microscopy show the intramural pericyte to be completely enclosed by the basement membrane of the capillary (Fig. 3-7). There may be dehiscences in the basement membrane, and in these areas intramural pericytes come in direct contact with endothelial cells.[36]

Staining with hematoxylin and eosin (H & E) fails to reveal the cytoplasm of the intramural pericyte. Retinal incubation with nitro blue tetrazolium, or injection of colloidal carbon, followed by retinal digestion, shows the pattern of the intramural pericyte processes (Fig. 3-9).[36] These are slender, long, longitudinal and circumferential processes which envelop the wall and overlap adjacent cells.[27] Kuwabara and Cogan[36] have suggested that intramural pericytes can be separated from endothelial cells on the basis of certain histochemical stain reactions, but this has been denied by a number of workers who could find no such differences.[2,17,40]

Electron microscopy reveals that the cytoplasm of intramural pericytes contains organelles whose number vary with the developmental stage of the vessel.[58] During the formative stage the cytoplasm is rich in rough-surfaced endoplasmic reticulum, free RNA granules, and mitochondria. Numerous pinocytotic vesicles may also be present. Fewer such organelles are present in the mature intramural pericyte. No desmosomes or attachment plates have been found between adjacent intramural pericytes or between them and endothelial cells. No clear evidence of myofibrils have been found in the cytoplasm of these cells,[36] although they were once reported.[46]

The nuclei of intramural pericytes may vary considerably in size and shape; in man they are usually round or oval. They have a similar electron density to endothelial cell nuclei.

Origin of Intramural Pericytes

Kuwabara and Cogan,[36] and Agrawal,[3] thought that the intramural pericytes arose from the same fetal cell that gave rise to the endothelium. This was confirmed experimentally by Shakib and de Oliveira[58] who have studied the developing retinal capillaries of the kitten. They have found that developing retinal capillaries are formed by one or two layers of undifferentiated cells resembling mesenchyme. These undifferentiated cells contain a large amount of well-developed, rough-surfaced endoplasmic reticulum filled with basement membrane-like material, and actively produce basement membrane. With the appearance of basement membrane in the intracellular spaces the outer cells differentiate into intramural pericytes, while the inner ones, in contact with the blood stream, become endothelial cells.

Function of Intramural Pericytes

A number of functions have been ascribed to pericytes, the two main ones being con-

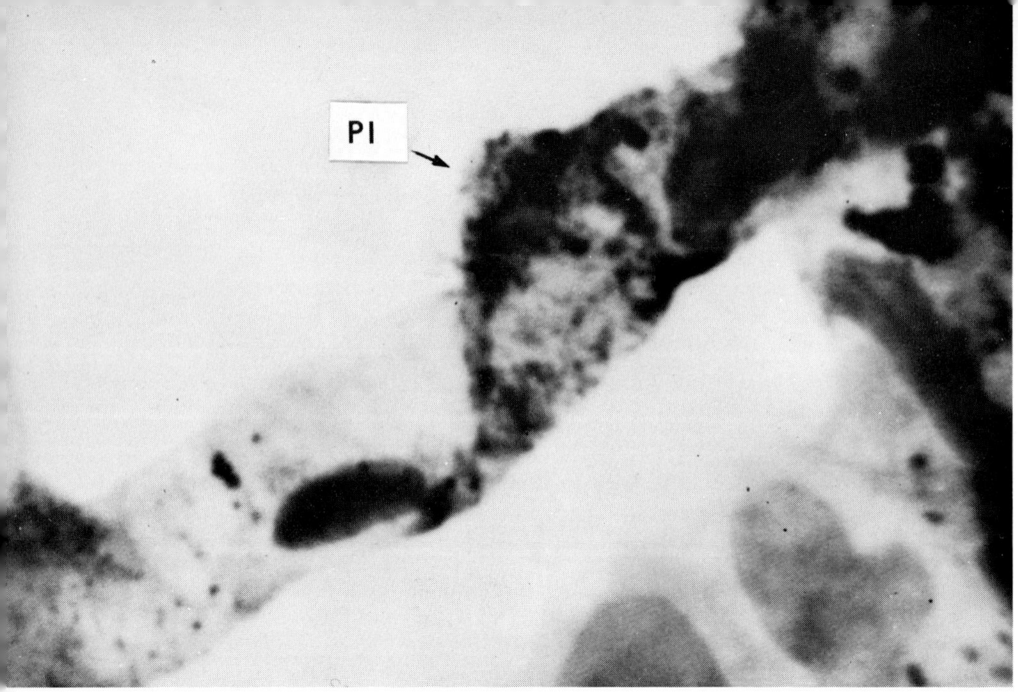

Fig. 3-9. High-power magnification of capillary of a rat retina 4 days after local injection of glycerol and overloading of the reticuloendothelial system with a solution of colloidal carbon. The infiltration around the intramural pericyte nucleus **(PL),** strikingly demonstrates the branched cytoplasm of this cell which looks as if carbon had been actively taken up by the cell. PAS and hematoxylin, ×3000. (From de Oliveira.[13])

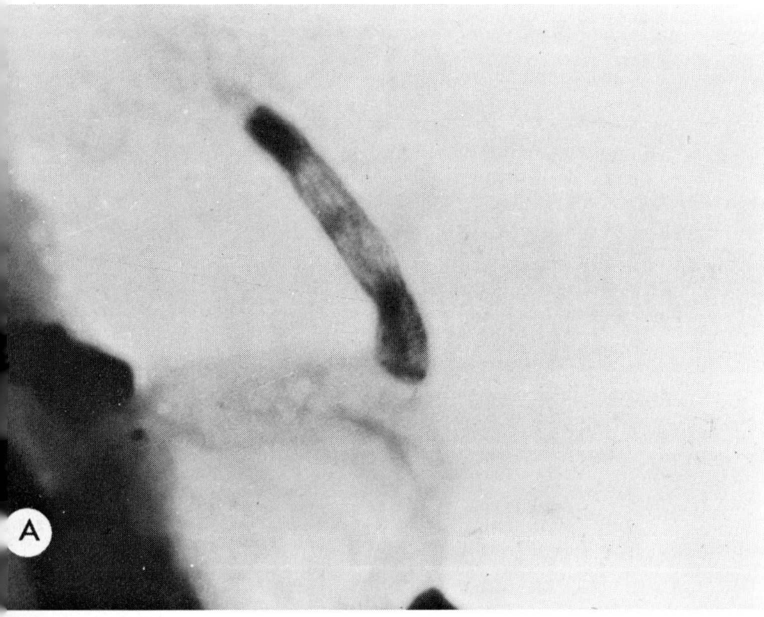

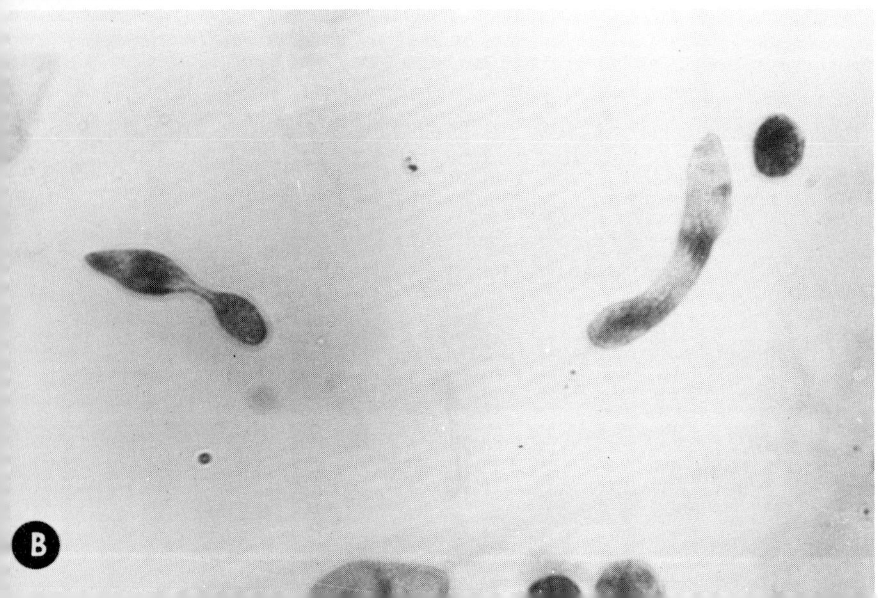

Fig. 3-10. *A*, Endothelial cell of a human retinal capillary which appears to be in mitotic division. ×1200.

B, Endothelial cells of a human retinal capillary which appear to be dividing ×800.

traction and phagocytosis. Contractility was the initial, and still is the most widely discussed attribute of these cells. Rouget[52,53] who was the first to suggest that there was a gradual transition from the muscle cell of the arteriole to the pericyte of the capillary, felt that the latter were contractile elements, analogous to the muscle cells of arteries and veins. Krogh,[33] and Bensley and Vimtrup[9] have supported and extended the observations of Rouget. Unfortunately, all of the direct evidence suggesting that pericytes cause capillary contractility has come from observations in amphibia, and more recent studies of mammalian tissue give no such evidence.[54,68]

There is no direct evidence for the contractile role of intramural pericytes of the retina, indeed, the in vivo observations of Friedman, Smith, and Kuwabara[22] have shown neither retinal capillary contraction, nor changes in the shape of intramural pericytes. Kuwabara and Cogan,[36] however, feel that these cells may play a role in controlling retinal capillary blood flow. In digest preparations they have found that loss of such cells increased significantly the frequency with which red blood cells were found in capillaries. Furthermore, they have postulated that mural cells are lost preferentially in diabetes, and that such loss seems to result in pathologic shunt formation.[10] This preferential loss of intramural pericytes in diabetes has been confirmed by other workers.[61,73] De Oliveira[12] has reported selective degeneration of intramural pericytes in macroglobulinemia, polycythemia, and other disorders, and he has concluded that such degeneration is not specific for diabetes. Agarwal and co-workers[1] have suggested that intramural pericytes act as "cellular valves" and aid in controlling retinal capillary blood flow, but they have provided no evidence for this point of view.

Pericytes apparently can act as phagocytic cells. Phagocytic responses of these cells have been noted in vessels of the frog tongue,[63] rat cremaster muscle,[44] and rat retinal capillaries.[13] It is not known whether human intramural pericytes possess phagocytic properties.

Intramural pericytes may have the capacity to differentiate into muscle cells[24] or endothelium, but these functions have not been established beyond doubt.

Replication of Endothelial Cells and Intramural Pericytes

It is likely that normal endothelial cells and intramural pericytes are capable of reproducing themselves in the retinal vascular bed. In a survey of numerous human retinal digest preparations, a number of endothelial cells and intramural pericytes had nuclei which appeared to be undergoing division (de Oliveira and Henkind, unpublished observations). In some instances the cells appeared to be in mitosis (Fig. 3-10*A*), while at other times unusual nuclear divisions were seen (Fig. 3-10*B*). Whether the latter represented amitotic division, terminal cellular change, or artifact could not be determined.

A combination of retinal vascular digestion and autoradiography utilizing ^{3}H-thymidine was used to study the replication rate of cells composing the retinal capillary bed of the adult rat. In this species the replication rate was found to be approximately 0.09 per cent (Fig. 3-11; Henkind, de Oliveira, and Lyons, unpublished observations). Engerman, Pfaffenbach, and Davis[17a] performed a similar study in mice and found labeling of 0.01 per cent of cells.

BASEMENT MEMBRANE

The presence of a connective sheath around capillaries was first described in the latter part of the nineteenth century: the term "basement membrane" is almost a century old. The initial studies on this tissue component were carried out in the renal glomerulus, but subsequent investigations have shown that virtually all fine vessels are surrounded by a basement membrane. Friedenwald[21] was apparently the first to examine the basement membrane of retinal vessels.

Controversy over the nature, origin, and function of the basement membrane of vessels has been persistent. Some authors have considered it to be a hyaline or homogeneous membrane, others have thought it a fibrillar or granular structure, or even a labile jelly-like material. Recently, electron microscopy has revealed that it is a definite membrane, with characteristic fibrillar structure, and uniform thickness of approximately 500 Å. In osmium-fixed material, the membrane appears as a band of moderate electron density applied to the endothelium. It has been subdivided into three layers: a dense medial zone (lamina densa), bounded by an inner more translucent layer (lamina rara, or lucida), and an outer fuzzy layer (zona diffusa).

Originally it was felt that the membrane was composed primarily of mucopolysaccharide; the fact that it stained red by the PAS reaction was strong evidence for this point of view. Recently, however, several biochemists[14,62] have demonstrated that the bulk of certain basement membrane material consists of collagen. Earlier histochemical and biochemical studies had demonstrated that basement membranes contain a protein-carbohydrate complex.[39] It should be noted that the reason for the success of retinal "digestion," with preservation of vessel architecture, hinges on the fact that both trypsin and pepsin have little effect on the basement membrane. On the other hand, collagenase will hydrolyse it almost completely.

In the human retina, the endothelial basement membrane measures approximately 500 Å, but varies in thickness depending upon the proximity of adjacent intramural pericytes (Fig. 3-7).[27] Where the intramural pericyte is absent it may be two or three times as thick. The basement membrane external to the intramural pericyte is often thick, measuring up to 400 Å in width. It may contain, particularly in later life, irregular-sized spaces which give it a "Swiss cheese" appearance (Fig. 3-7).[27] Occasionally these irregular cavitations are found in the basement membrane between the endothelium and the intramural pericyte. In general, the perivascular membrane thickens with age.

Early workers had believed that the basement membrane was a condensate of the ground substance of connective tissue. Evidence has been provided which suggests that basement membrane is secreted by endothelial cells. Shakib and de Oliveira[58] have shown, in the developing retinal capillaries of the kitten, that the undifferentiated cells destined to become endothelium and intramural pericytes, probably produce basement membrane.

The basement membrane has several functions, the most obvious one is that of support. It acts as a framework for the endothelial cells and intramural pericytes, as well as an anchorage for the vessel to the surrounding tissue. It is a stable structure that will persist after the disappearance of endothelial cells and intramural pericytes,[11,49] and will not dissolve in the process of retinal "digestion." The basement membrane may act as a filter, and there is also some evidence that it possesses enzyme activity. Nucleoside phosphatase (ATPase) activity has been demonstrated in the basement membrane of retinal vessels in the rat, and it has been suggested that such activity is involved in cation transport across cell membranes.[45]

GLIA

In the central nervous system, glial tissue provides the following: a framework for the conducting cells, insulation for the neurons, and, through its intimate contact with blood vessels, nutrition for the neural elements. This is also true for the retina.[5,28]

Glial elements closely invest all retinal vessels. There is no place in the retina where neuronal elements directly abut vessels (Fig. 3-3*A*). Therefore, material from the blood stream must traverse not only the vascular wall, but also the glial cell membranes and cytoplasm in order to reach the surrounding nervous tissue. Electron microscopy has revealed that the basement membranes of the glial cells merge with adjacent smooth muscle cells, intramural pericytes, or endothelial cells.[28]

The cytoplasm of the Müller cells surrounds the major portion of the capillary wall in all layers of the retina. Their processes extend to, and actually form, the inner and outer limiting membranes of the retina, and their nuclei lie mainly within the inner nuclear layer. In the nerve fiber layer broad strips of cytoplasm are seen, but in the inner nuclear layer it may be quite thin. Arterioles and venules are also surrounded by Müller cell cytoplasm, while the larger arteries and veins, lying in the nerve fiber layer, are invested partially by Müller cells and also by astrocytic glial cells.

The Müller cell cytoplasm contains numerous well-developed fibrils 100 Å in diameter without periodicity, smooth-surfaced vesicles averaging 1000 Å in diameter either "empty" or filled with moderately dense material, and dense granules 250 to 300 Å in diameter which are probably glycogen. There are also smaller, denser particles, RNA-rich granules, and smooth-surfaced endoplasmic reticulum. Mitochondria are uncommon, and pinocytotic vesicles have not been found.[28] Abundant dehydrogenase activity has been described in these cells.[37]

Fig. 3-11. Adult rat retinal digest preparation shows presumptive intramural pericyte **(1)** and endothelial cell **(2)** labeled with ^{3}H-thymidine. Hematoxylin, ×2000.

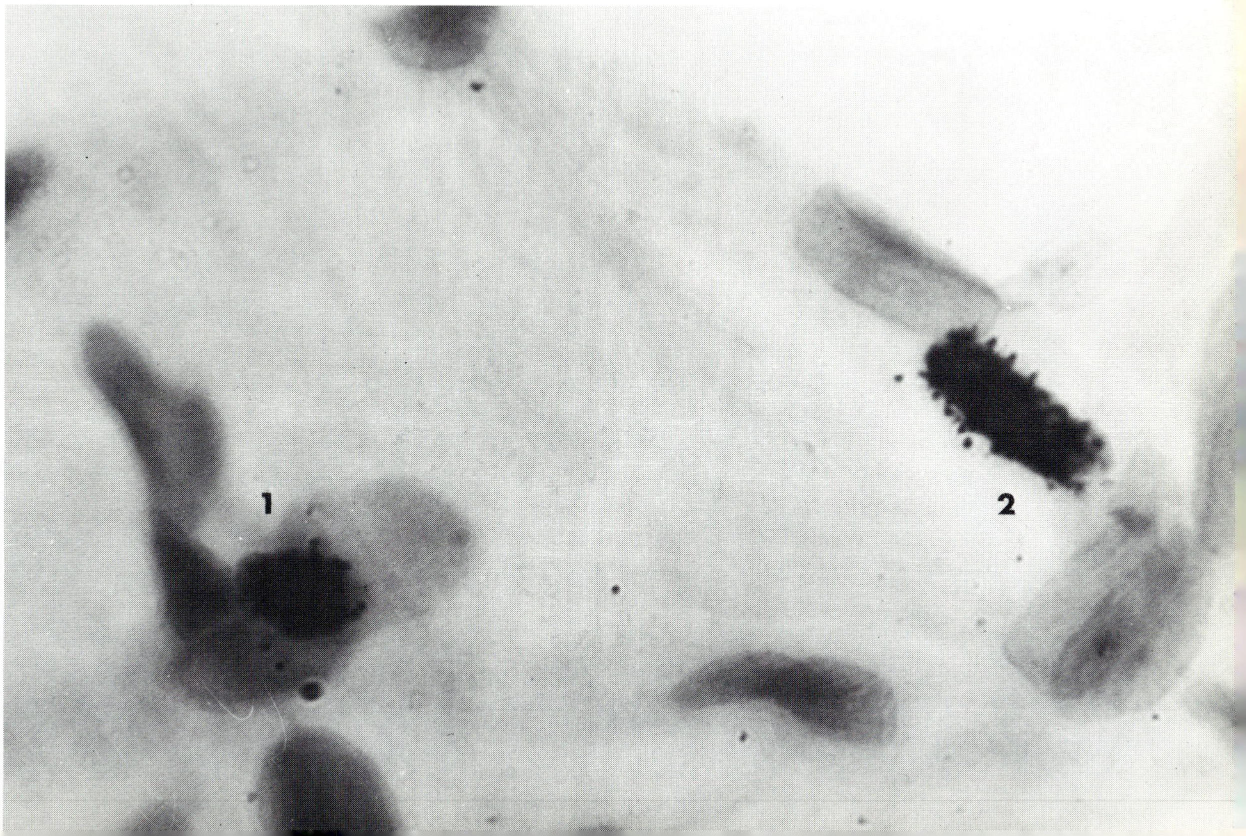

Hogan and Feeney[28] have described two types of astrocytes in the retina. One resembles fibrous astrocytes and contains bundles of fine fibrils in the cytoplasm. This type of cell is found most often around the wall of retinal arteries; near the optic disc similar cells are present around capillary walls in the nerve fiber layer. The second type of astrocyte has paler cytoplasm and more distinct organelles and is likened to a protoplasmic astrocyte. This cell is usually found in contact with retinal veins. Near the disc they are more common and have broad expanses of cytoplasm surrounding capillary walls. They also send processes to capillaries in the inner plexiform layer. Both cells have a basement membrane beneath the portion of cytoplasm that abuts on the vessel.

Wolter, in a series of papers[70–72] has described the perivascular glia of retinal blood vessels as seen by light microscopy of silver-stained sections. It is difficult to be absolutely certain what the cells outlined represent, or how they relate to electron microscopic appearances. Presumably, they are the same as the glia described by Hogan and Feeney.[28] However, Wolter[72] considers "perivascular glia" as a particular type of glia found around capillaries of the human retina, and assigns to them and the retinal astroglia the role of covering the capillary wall, a function now ascribed primarily to Müller cells.

ARTERIOLAR ANNULI

For some time there has been a question of how the retinal circulation is regulated, and whether there are specific anatomic structures that can alter flow in the retinal vessels. Evans[18] has described precapillary arteriolar sphincters in human retinas, but his work has not been confirmed. Similarly, the precapillary "cushion cells" of Loewenstein[41] have not been demonstrated by electron microscopy or in digest preparations of human and animal retinae.

Thuránszky[64] has published pictures of constrictions at arteriolar branch points in the retina of the cat. His studies were performed on open eyes lacking an anterior segment. Initially, it was thought that these constrictions might have their anatomic counterpart in the arteriolar annuli described by Kuwabara and Cogan.[35] However, Friedman, Smith, and Kuwabara,[22] by utilizing a sclerouveal window and high magnification in the living cat, were able to visualize arteriolar annuli, but did not see them acting as sphincters.

Arteriolar annuli occur at the side-arm branches of retinal arteries in a number of animals, but cannot be demonstrated in man (Fig. 3-12*A* and *B*).[25] The annuli are PAS-positive, and also stain with Masson's, elastic-van Gieson's, and Gridley's quadruple stains. In most instances the annuli are hypercellular, and some of the cells have small dark nuclei which appear to be different from those of surrounding cells (Fig. 3-13). There is no evidence at present that annuli contain muscular or elastic tissue components; most likely they are composed of basement membrane or immature collagen.[25] Their role in retinal circulation is unknown.

CHEMICAL COMPOSITION AND METABOLIC ACTIVITY OF RETINAL VESSELS

Only a limited amount of information is available about the composition and metabolism of retinal vessels.

Futterman and Kupfer[23] using gas chromatography, have analyzed human retinal

Fig. 3-12. *Right. A*, Appearance of retinal arteriolar annuli **(arrows)** in the cat (PAS and Hematoxylin, ×480); dog (Masson's, ×480); pig (PAS and hematoxylin, ×480); and *Aotes trivirgatus* or owl monkey (PAS and hematoxylin, ×615). In *Aotes* the annulus is at a secondary side-arm branch. (From Henkind and de Oliveira.[25])

Below. B, Absence of arteriolar annuli at the side-arm branchings of a human retina. PAS and hematoxylin, ×250.

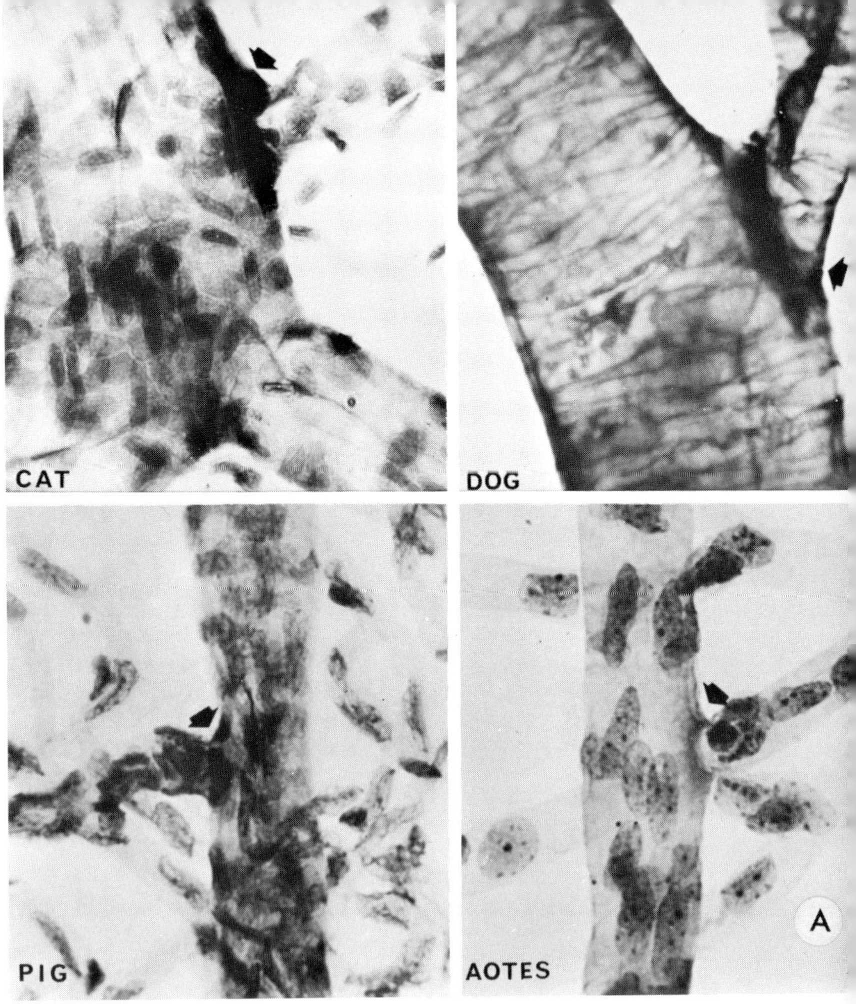

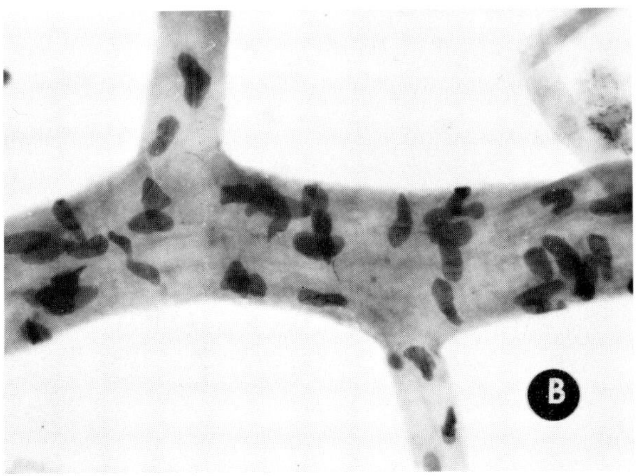

Fig. 3-13. *Right.* Schematic drawing of a primary side-arm branch annulus showing the morphology and cellular components. (From Henkind and de Oliveira.[25])

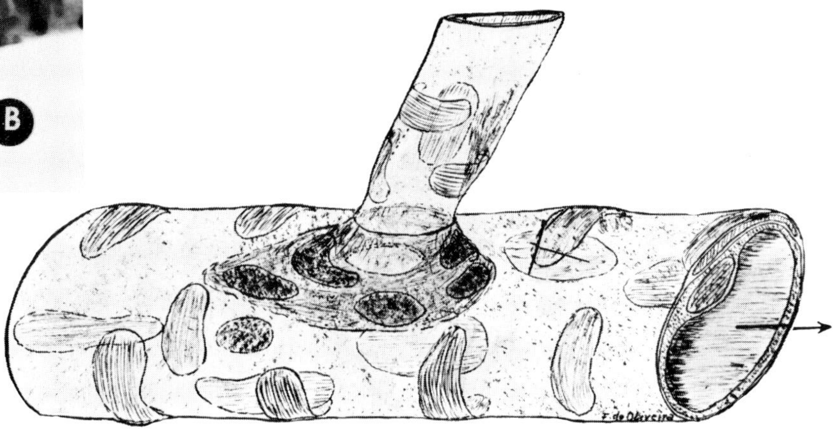

digests for their lipid content. The major fatty acids found were: oleate, palmitate, stearate, and arachnidate. No major alterations in fatty acid composition were found with aging, or in diabetes.

Using Cartesian diver microrespirometers, Howard and Sears[29] have measured the respiration and determined the respiratory quotients of isolated vessels from adult humans and rhesus monkeys. They found that human retinal arteries consume oxygen at a rate of 0.5 to 28 μ liters per milligram of dry tissue per hour. Veins have a similar rate of consumption. The larger arteries and veins are less active than smaller vessels. The extremely wide range of oxygen uptake found by these authors makes interpretation difficult.

Pandolfi[47] using a histochemical fibrin slide method, has studied the fibrinolytic activity of the central retinal vessels and their branches in man and monkeys. He found high fibrinolytic activity in the endothelium of the central retinal artery and vein and their intraocular branches. These findings in the retinal arteries differ from the pattern seen in other systemic arteries which usually lack fibrinolytic activity. This observation suggests that retinal vessels are able rapidly to dissolve fibrin deposited within their lumina.

REFERENCES

1. Agarwal, L. P., Singh, K., and Dayal, Y.: Retinal vascular patterns. 3. Physio-pathological evaluation. *Orient. Arch. Ophthal. 4:*63, 1966.
2. Agarwal, L. P., and Tandon, H. D.: Histochemical studies of the retinal blood vessels. 1. (Normal adult rats). *Orient. Arch. Ophthal. 3:*299, 1965.
3. Agrawal, P. K.: The cellular structure and development of the retinal vessels of the rat. *Orient. Arch. Ophthal. 3:*23, 1965.
4. Anderson, B., Jr., and McIntosh, H. D.: Retinal circulation. *Ann. Rev. Med. 18:*15, 1967.
5. Ashton, N.: The blood-retinal barrier and vaso-glial relationships in retinal disease. *Trans. Ophthal. Soc. U.K. 85:*199, 1965.
6. Ashton, N., and de Oliveira, L. F.: Nomenclature of pericytes. *Brit. J. Ophthal. 50:*119, 1966.
7. Ballantyne, A. J., and Michaelson, I. C.: *Textbook of the Fundus of the Eye.* Baltimore, Md., Williams & Wilkins, 1962.
8. Becker, B., and Ley, A. P.: "Retinal Arteriosclerosis." In *Arteriosclerosis*, ed. by Cowdry, E. V. Springfield, Ill., Thomas, 1966, p. 401.
9. Bensley, R. R., and Vimtrup, B. J.: On the nature of the Rouget cells of capillaries. *Anat. Rec. 39:*37, 1928.
10. Cogan, D. G., and Kuwabara, T.: Capillary shunts in the pathogenesis of diabetic retinopathy. *Diabetes 12:*293, 1963.
11. Cogan, D. G., and Kuwabara, T.: The mural cell in perspective. *Arch. Ophthal. 78:*133, 1967.
12. de Oliveira, L. F.: Pericytes in diabetic retinopathy. *Brit. J. Ophthal. 50:*134, 1960.
13. de Oliveira, L. F.: "Form, Function and Pathology of Pericytes (Intramural Cells)." (Ph.D. thesis, University of London, 1965.)
14. Dische, Z.: "Glycans of the Lens Capsule – A Model of Basement Membranes," in *Small Vessel Involvement in Diabetes Mellitus*, ed. by Siperstein, M. D., Colwell, A. R., and Meyer, K. Washington, D.C., American Institute of Biological Science, 1964, pp. 201–213.
15. Duke-Elder, S., and Wybar, K. C.: *The Anatomy of the Visual System. System of Ophthalmology.* St. Louis, Mo., Mosby, 1961, vol. 2.
16. Ehinger, B.: Adrenergic nerves to the eye and to related structures in man and in the cynomolgus monkey (*Macaca Irus*). *Invest. Ophthal. 5:*42, 1966.
17. Engerman, R. L., Molitor, D. L., and Bloodworth, J. M. B.: Vascular system of the dog retina: Light and electron microscopic studies. *Exp. Eye Res. 5:*296, 1966.

17a. Engerman, R. L., Pfaffenbach, D., and Davis, M. D.: Cell turnover of capillaries. *Lab. Invest. 17:*738, 1967.

18. Evans, J. N.: The capillary sphincter in the human retina. *Arch. Ophthal. 37:*182, 1947.
19. Farquhar, M. C., and Hartman, J. F.: Elec-

tron microscopy of cerebral capillaries. *Anat. Rec. 124:*288, 1956.

20. Friedenwald, J. S.: "Retinal Arteriosclerosis" in *Arteriosclerosis,* ed. by Cowdry, E. V. New York, MacMillan, 1933, p. 363.
21. Friedenwald, J. S.: A new approach to some problems of retinal vascular disease. *Amer. J. Ophthal. 32:*487, 1949.
22. Friedman, E., Smith, T. R., and Kuwabara, T.: Retinal microcirculation in vivo. *Invest. Ophthal. 3:*217, 1964.
23. Futterman, S., and Kupfer, C.: The fatty acid composition of the retinal vasculature of normal and diabetic human eyes. *Invest. Ophthal. 7:*105, 1968.
24. Henkind, P.: Ballotini occlusion of retinal arteries. Collateral vessels. *Brit. J. Ophthal. 50:*482, 1966.
25. Henkind, P., and de Oliveira, L. N. F.: Retinal arteriolar annuli. *Invest. Ophthal. 7:*584, 1968.
26. Hogan, M. J., and Feeney, L.: The ultrastructure of the retinal blood vessels. 1. The larger vessels. *J. Ulstruct. Res. 9:*10, 1963.
27. Hogan, M. J., and Feeney, L.: The ultrastructure of the retinal vessels. 2. The small vessels. *J. Ulstruct. Res. 9:*29, 1963.
28. Hogan, M. J., and Feeney, L.: The ultrastructure of the retinal vessels. 3. Vascular-glial relationships. *J. Ulstruct. Res. 9:*47, 1963.
29. Howard, R. O., and Sears, M. L.: Metabolism of retinal blood vessels of humans and rhesus monkeys studied with the cartesian diver. *Invest. Ophthal. 3:*432, 1964.
30. Ikui, H., Mimatsu, T., Maeda, J., and Tomita, I.: Fine structure of the blood vessels in the iris. Light and electron microscopic studies (preliminary report). *Kyushu J. Med. Sci. 11:*113, 1960.
31. Ishikawa, T.: Fine structure of retinal vessels in man and the macaque monkey. *Invest. Ophthal. 2:*1, 1963.
32. Kimura, T.: Studies on fine structure of retinal blood vessels in arteriolar sclerosis of the human retina. *Jap. J. Ophthal. 11:*91, 1967.
33. Krogh, A.: *The Anatomy and Physiology of Capillaries.* New Haven, Conn., Yale University Press, 1929.
34. Kuwabara, T., Carrol, J. M., and Cogan, D. G.: Retinal vascular patterns. III. Age, hypertension, absolute glaucoma, injury. *Arch. Ophthal. 65:*708, 1961.
35. Kuwabara, T., and Cogan, D. G.: Studies of retinal vascular patterns. I. Normal architecture. *Arch. Ophthal. 64:*904, 1960.
36. Kuwabara, T., and Cogan, D. G.: Retinal vascular patterns. VI. Mural cells of the retinal capillaries. *Arch. Ophthal. 69:*492, 1963.
37. Kuwabara, T., Cogan, D. G., Futterman, S., and Kinoshita, J. H.: Dehydrogenases in the retina and Müller's fibres. *J. Histochem. Cytochem. 7:*67, 1959.
38. Laties, A. M.: Central retinal artery innervation. Absence of adrenergic innervation to the intraocular branches. *Arch. Ophthal. 77:*405, 1967.
39. LeBlond, C. P., Glegg, R. E., and Eidinger, D.: Presence of carbohydrates with free 1,2 glycol groups in sites stained by the periodic acid-Schiff technique. *J. Histochem. Cytochem. 5:*455, 1957.
40. Levene, R. Z., Horton, G., and Einaugler, R.: Retinal vessel dehydrogenase enzymes. *Arch. Ophthal. 72:*99, 1964.
41. Loewenstein, A.: Cushion cells in retinal precapillaries and capillaries. *Nature 160:*229, 1947.
42. Maeda, J.: Electron microscopy of the retinal vessels. *Acta Soc. Ophthal. Jap. 62:*1002, 1958.
43. Maeda, J.: Electron microscopy of the retinal vessels. Report 1. Human retina. *Jap. J. Ophthal. 3:*37, 1959.
44. Majno, G., and Palade, G. E.: Studies on inflammation. 1. The effect of histamine and serotonin on vascular permeability: An electron microscopic study. *J. Biophys. Biochem. Cytol. 11:*571, 1961.
45. Marchesi, V. T., Sears, M. L., and Barrnett, R. J.: Electron microscopic studies of nucleoside phosphatase activity in blood vessels and glia of the retina. *Invest. Ophthal. 3:*1, 1964.
46. Missotten, L.: Etude des capillaires de la rétine et de la choriocapillaire au microscope electronique. *Ophthalmologica 144:*1, 1962.
47. Pandolfi, M.: Fibrinolytic activity of retinal vessels in man and monkey. *Amer. J. Ophthal. 63:*428, 1967.
48. Parsons, J. H.: *The Pathology of the Eye.* London, Hodder & Stoughton, 1905, vol. 2, p. 659.
49. Reinecke, R. D., Kuwabara, T., Cogan, D. G., and Weis, D. R.: Retinal vascular patterns. 5. Experimental ischemia of the cat eye. *Arch. Ophthal. 67:*470, 1962.

50. Rodgers, J. C., Puchtler, H., and Gropp, S.: Transition from elastin to collagen in internal elastic membranes. *Arch. Path. 83:*557, 1967.

51. Rouget, C.: Mémoire sur le développement, la structure, et les propriétés physiologiques des capillaires sanguins et lymphatiques. *Arch. Physiol. Norm. Path. 5:*603, 1873.

52. Rouget, C.: Mémoire sur le développement de la tunique contractile des vaisseaux. *C. R. Acad. Sci. 79:*559, 1873.

53. Rouget, C.: Sur la contractilite des capillaires sanguins. *C. R. Acad. Sci. 88:*916, 1879.

54. Sandison, J. C.: Contraction of blood vessels and observations on the circulation in the transparent chamber of the rabbit's ear. *Anat. Rec. 54:*105, 1932.

55. Schaly, G. A.: "Over het Vorkamen van de Cellen van Rouget op den Wand van de Capillaren in het Oog van den Mensch." (Dissertation, Groningen, 1926.)

56. Seitz, R.: *The Retinal Vessels* (Trans. by Blodi). St. Louis, Mo., Mosby, 1964.

57. Shakib, M., and Cunha-Vaz, J. G.: Studies on the permeability of the blood-retinal barrier. IV. Junctional complexes of the retinal vessels and their role in the permeability of the blood-retinal barrier. *Exp. Eye Res. 5:* 229, 1966.

58. Shakib, M., and de Oliveira, L.: Studies on developing retinal vessels. X. Formation of the basement membrane and differentiation of intramural pericytes. *Brit. J. Ophthal. 50:*124, 1966.

59. Simon, G.: "Ultrastructure des Capillaires," in *Morphology and Histochemistry of the Vascular Wall.* Basel, Karger, 1966, p. 370.

60. Spalteholz, W.: "Blutgefasse der Haut, in *Handbuch der Haut und Geschlechtskranlecheiten.* Berlin, Jadassohn, 1927.

61. Speiser, P., Gittelsohn, A. M., and Patz, A.: Studies on diabetic retinopathy. 3. Influence of diabetes on intramural pericytes. *Arch. Ophthal. 80:*332, 1968.

62. Spiedel, E., and Lazarow, A.: "Chemical Composition of Glomerular Basement Membrane Material in Diabetes," in *Small Vessel Involvement in Diabetes Mellitus,* ed. by Siperstein, M. D., Colwell, A. R., and Meyer, K. Washington, D.C., American Institute of Biological Sciences, 1964, pp. 127–150.

63. Stilwell, F.: On the phagocytic capacity of the blood vessel endothelium of the frog's tongue and its presumed transformation into wandering cells. *Folia Haemat. 33:*81, 1926.

64. Thuránszky, K.: *Der Blutkreislauf der Netzhaut.* Budapest, Ungarischen Akademie der Wissenschaften, 1957.

64a. Tominaga, Y., and Ikui, H.: The fine structure of the blood vessels of the human retina. *Acta Soc. Ophthal. Jap. 67:*1481, 1963.

64b. Tominaga, Y., and Ikui, H.: The fine structure of the arterio-venous crossing parts in the human retina (The preliminary report). *Acta Soc. Ophthal. Jap. 68:*148, 1963.

65. Vimtrup, B.: Beitrage zur Anatomie der Capillaren. I. Ueber Kontractile Elemente in der Gefasswand der Blutcapillaren. *Z. Ges. Anat. 65:*150, 1922.

66. Vimtrup, B.: Sur les éléments contractiles dans la paroi des capillaires sanguins. *C.R. Soc. Biol.* (Paris), *87:*761, 1922.

67. Vimtrup, B.: Beitrage zur Anatomie der Capillaren. II. Weitere Untersudmugen uber Kontraktile Elemente in der Gefasswand der Blutcapillaren. *Z. Anat. Entwicklungsgesch. 68:*469, 1923.

68. Wiedeman, M. P.: "Patterns of Arteriovenous Pathways," in *Handbook of Physiology,* Sec. 2: *Circulation.* Washington, D.C., American Physiological Society, 1963, vol. 2, p. 924.

69. Wolff, E.: *The Anatomy of the Eye and Orbit,* 4th ed. London, Lewis, 1958.

70. Wolter, J. R.: The cells of Remak and the astroglia of the normal human retina. *Arch. Ophthal. 53:*832, 1955.

71. Wolter, J. R.: Perivascular glia of the blood vessels of the human retina. *Amer. J. Ophthal. 44:*766, 1957.

72. Wolter, J. R.: Glia of the human retina. *Amer. J. Ophthal. 48:*370, 1959.

73. Yanoff, M.: Diabetic retinopathy. *New Eng. J. Med. 274:*1344, 1966.

74. Zimmerman, K. W.: Der feinere Bau der Blutcapillaren. *Z. Anat. Entwicklungsgesch. 68:*29, 1923.

chapter 4

Choroidal Vessels, Bruch's Membrane and Papillary Angioarchitecture

CHOROID

The choroid is a thin, highly vascularized membrane lying between the retina and sclera (Fig. 4-1). Its primary function is to supply the outer avascular layers of the retina with oxygen and nutriment. Lower vertebrates possess a choroid which is made up largely of a single layer of vessels. In mammals, however, the vascular components tend to be stratified.[16] Larger veins are found external to a middle layer of arteries and smaller veins. Innermost is a two-dimensional network of large-caliber, sinusoidal capillaries which make up the choriocapillaris. In addition to vessels, the choroid contains elastic and collagenous tissue, ground substance, nerves, melanocytes, fibroblasts, and a variety of cellular elements including mast cells, plasma cells, lymphocytes, and phagocytes. The thickness of the choroid is not constant and may vary with the level of intraocular pressure. According to Hogan[7] the blood-filled living choroid of man probably has a thickness of approximately 0.25 mm (250 μ) in most areas, increasing to 0.30 mm in the peripapillary and macular regions, and thinning to 0.12 mm at the periphery.

ARTERIES

Two arterial systems supply the choroid. Posteriorly there are six to eight short posterior ciliary arteries which divide into many branches as they pierce the sclera around the optic nerve. Anteriorly one finds a combination of recurrent arteries from the major circle of the iris, long posterior ciliary arteries and anterior ciliary arteries. The systems approach one another at the equator of the eye, and anastomose either through an intervening capillary network or by direct intercommunication.[17] The short posterior ciliary arteries are arranged segmentally with each branch supplying a localized area of choroid with an arteriolar-capillary network; there is, however, no anatomic evidence that these are end-arteries. Wybar[18] has found no evidence to suggest that the selective localization of choroidal disease was due to anatomic peculiarities or zonal differences. It should be noted that occlusion of a short posterior ciliary artery in man can produce patchy destruction of the choroid,[10] and embolization of choroidal arteries in the cat creates a similar situation[5] (Fig. 4-2). Furthermore, fluorescein angiographic studies in the pig reveal that the choriocapillaris fills in a patchy manner[3] (Fig. 4-3 *A* through *D*). Neither Ashton,[1] Wybar,[17] nor Hogan and Feeney[9] have found any arteriovenous anastomoses or shunts such as have been described by other workers. Glomus cells, large polyhedral cells at the periphery of large and medium-sized choroidal arteries, supposedly acting to shunt choroidal blood flow, have been reported by Loewenstein.[13] Ashton,[1] in an exhaustive histologic study, was unable to confirm their presence.

Hogan and Feeney,[9] in their study of the ultrastructure of choroidal vessels, have found the small arteries and arterioles to be identical in structure to those of other tissues. They also have provided measurements of the luminal diameter of the arteries. The larger vessels average $35 \times 60\ \mu$ while the smaller stromal arteries average

25 × 40 μ. Arterioles, distinguished by the thinning and disappearance of the internal elastic lamina and discontinuity of the muscularis, average 29 μ in diameter.

VEINS

Four main vortex veins, formed by the confluence of converging venous tributaries, drain the choroid in the region of the equator. Subsidiary vortex veins are occasionally found. From their origin in the choriocapillaris the venous tributaries either pass directly into the closest vortex vein or pass backwards toward the peripapillary region and then sweep around to join the main vessels. According to Wybar [17] this leads to a marked concentration of venules in the posterior part of the choroid. Kiss and Orban [11] had described swellings or bulbiculi in the walls of choroidal venules, and they thought that these represented sites of arteriovenous anastomoses. Ashton,[1] however, has shown that the swellings are simply sites of venous compression by the overlying arteriole.

The wall of the choroidal veins is thin and consists of an endothelial layer and a surrounding basement membrane. Pericytes are scattered along the wall and large areas are devoid of such cells. Only a small amount of collagen is present outside of the basement membrane, and muscle cells are absent.[9] The luminal diameter of the veins of the outer posterior choroid average 20 × 100 μ, while those in the stroma measure 20 × 30 μ.

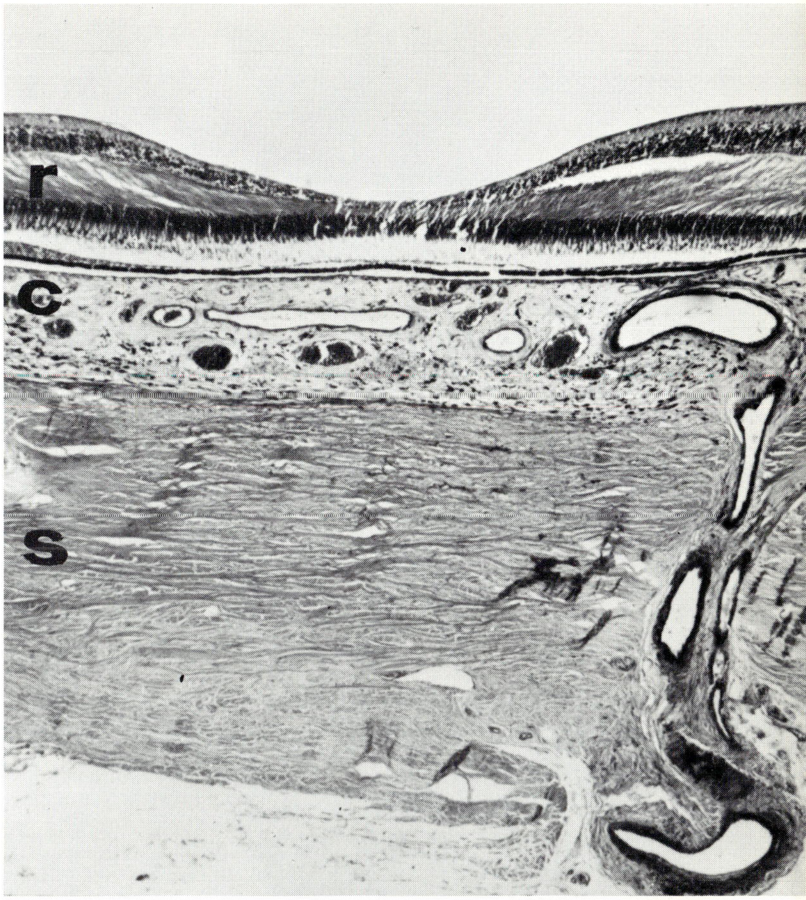

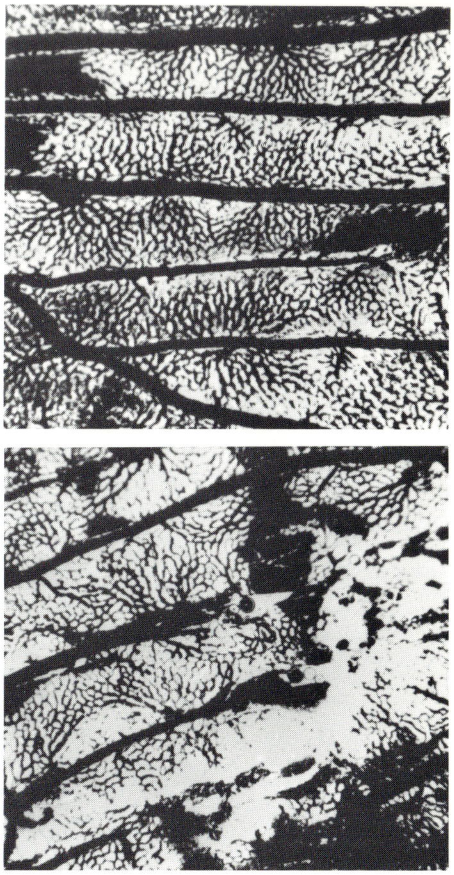

A

B

Fig. 4-1. *Top.* Section of human eye through the posterior pole at the macula. In this instance the ganglion cells are missing from the retina **(r)** for the patient had ischemic optic neuritis with retrograde neuronal degeneration. The retinal pigment epithelium is artifactually detached from the underlying choroid **(c)**. Ciliary arteries can be seen running through the sclera **(s)** at the right of the figure. Verhoeff's elastic stain, ×50.

Fig. 4-2. *Bottom. A*, India-inked specimen of the choriocapillary network in an adult cat. The arteries run as thick parallel lines above the capillaries. The venules have mainly been removed.

B, Same eye as *A*. Several areas of choriocapillary bed obliteration are seen following embolization of choroidal arteries. Note the irregular filling defects in the capillary bed.

(From Henkind.[5])

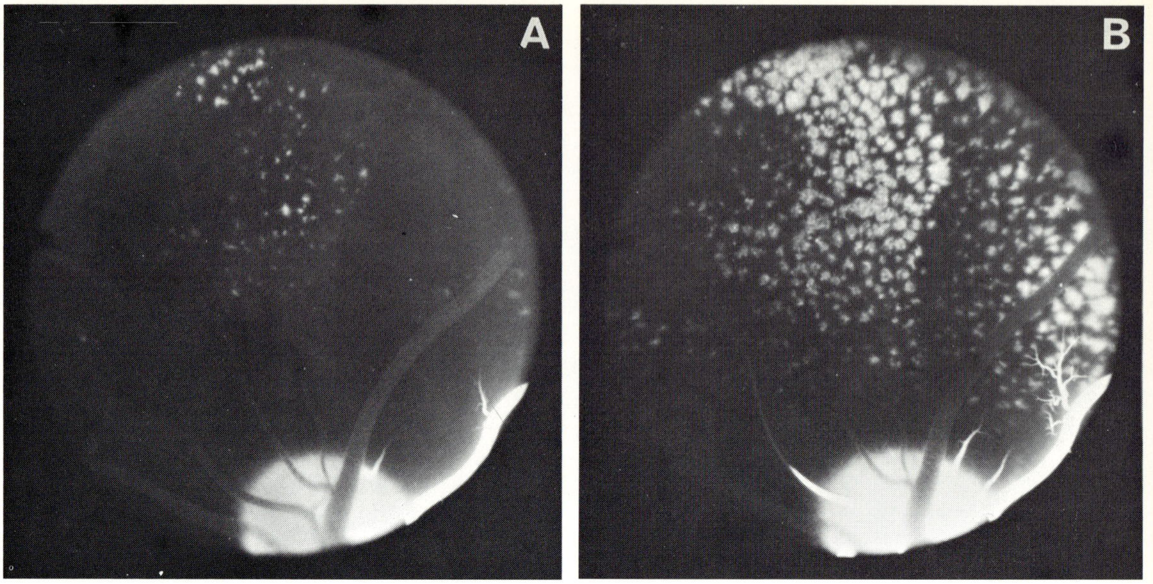

Fig. 4-3. *A–D*, Choroidal filling in a pig with an intraocular pressure of 36 mmHg and systemic arterial mean pressure of 67 mmHg. A series of pictures taken at 3.0, 3.7, 4.2, and 5.5 seconds after injection of fluorescein into the carotid artery shows choroidal fluorescence appearing as a series of islands which later coalesce. (From Dollery, C. T., Henkind, P., Kohner, E. M., and Paterson, J. W.[3])

Fig. 4-4. Section through a human choroid. The choriocapillaris **(C)** lies as a continuous vascular meshwork of large caliber, thin-walled vessels beneath Bruch's membrane **(B).** The larger choroidal vessels lie below the choriocapillaris. The retinal pigment epithelium **(P)** lines the inner surface of Bruch's membrane. Epon-embedded, toluidine blue, ×320.

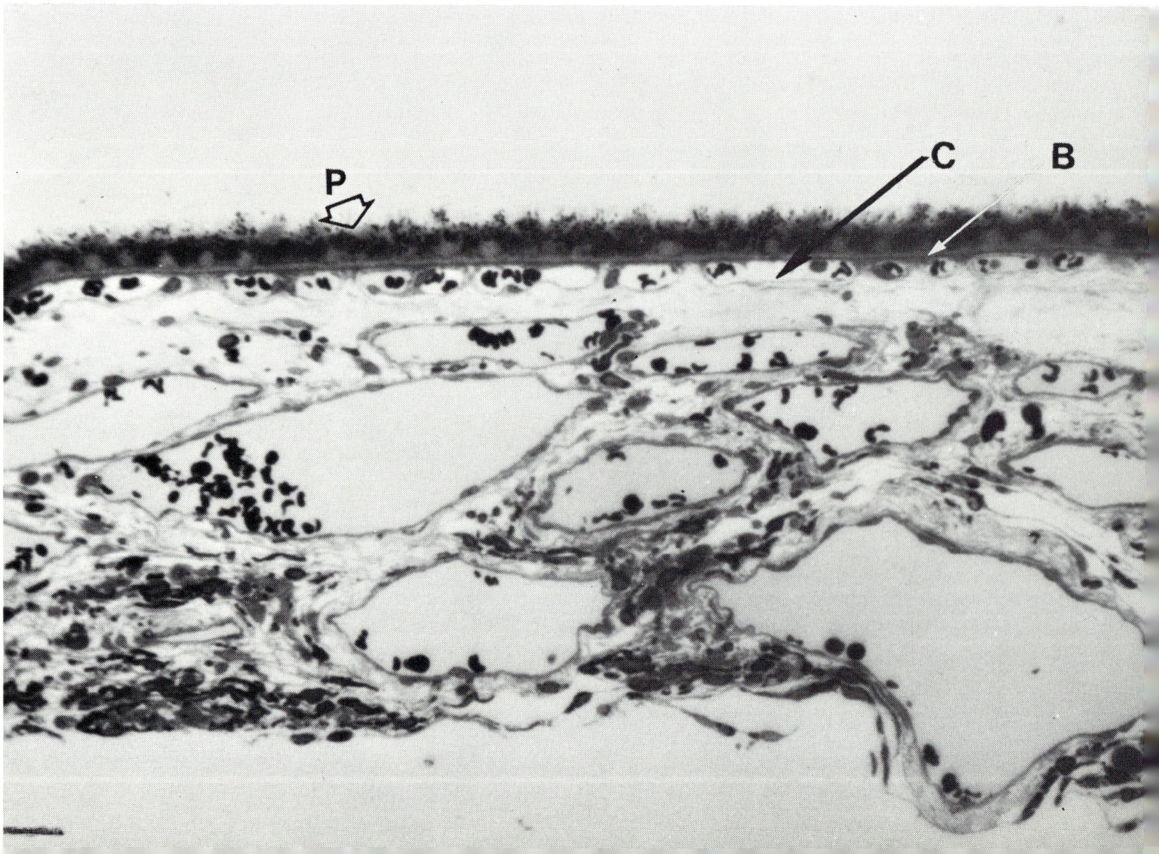

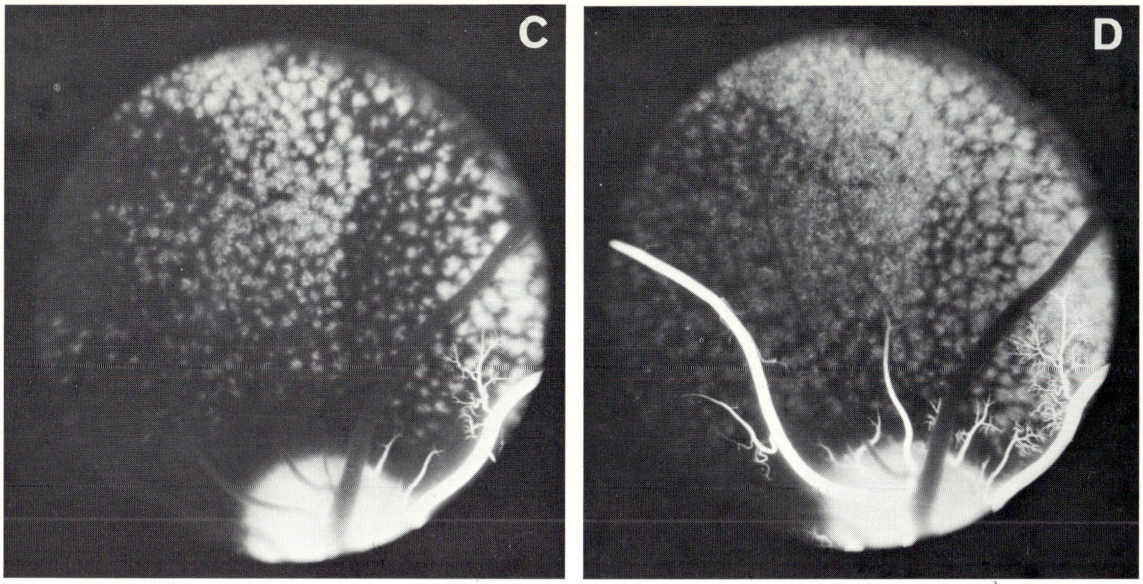

CHORIOCAPILLARIS

The choroidal capillaries lie in a single plane at the innermost surface of the choroid, and together form the vascular meshwork termed the choriocapillaris (Fig. 4-4). They are fed by relatively large-caliber arterioles (Fig. 4-5). While they possess the thin wall one associates with capillaries, their luminal diameter is larger than that of other capillaries. Leber [12] has noted that their diameter ranges from 10 to 36 μ, while Sattler [15] has provided figures of 18 to 38 μ in the neighborhood of the ora serrata. These vessels form a very tight meshwork which measures 3 to 18 μ at the posterior pole, and 6 to 36 μ anterior to the equator.[12] Beneath the macula the capillary lumina are broader than the spaces between the vessels, however, the vessel density in this region does not differ appreciably from that of any other portion of the choriocapillaris situated at an equal distance from the optic nerve.[4]

The ultrastructure of the choriocapillaris is different from that of the retinal capillaries. While the latter have a continuous or unfenestrated cytoplasm, the choroidal capillaries have a fenestrated or discontinuous cytoplasm.[2] Their inner surface, adjacent to Bruch's membrane is attenuated and fenestrated, while the endothelial cell nuclei and surrounding, richly vesiculated cytoplasm are found primarily on the choroidal side (Fig. 4-6). According to Bernstein and Hollenberg [2] the attenuated capillary wall forms part of a surface across which massive fluid transport occurs, and presumably this configuration facilitates the movement of fluid and dissolved solutes. These authors have demonstrated that ferritin particles migrate more readily through the choriocapillaris than through retinal capillaries.

BRUCH'S MEMBRANE

Bruch's membrane lies in between and separates the retinal pigment epithelium from the choroid. Long considered to be a "glass membrane," similar to the capsule of the lens and Descemet's membrane of the cornea, it has recently been shown by electron microscopy to be composed of five layers: (*1*) The basement membrane of the

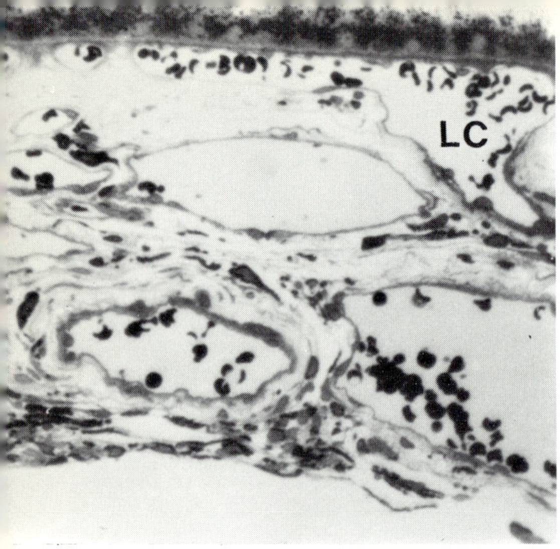

Fig. 4-5. A large-caliber **(LC)** channel entering into the choriocapillaris. Presumably this is an arteriole, but the possibility that it represents a venous drainage channel cannot be ruled out. ×320.

Fig. 4-6. *Below.* Electronmicrograph of the inner wall of the choriocapillaris **(C)** shows Bruch's membrane **(Br),** and the retinal pigment epithelium **(Pi)** in man. Note the fenestrated attenuated endothelium **(fe)** of the choriocapillaris. The fenestrae appear to be covered by an electron-dense material continuous with the cell membrane. ×13,000.

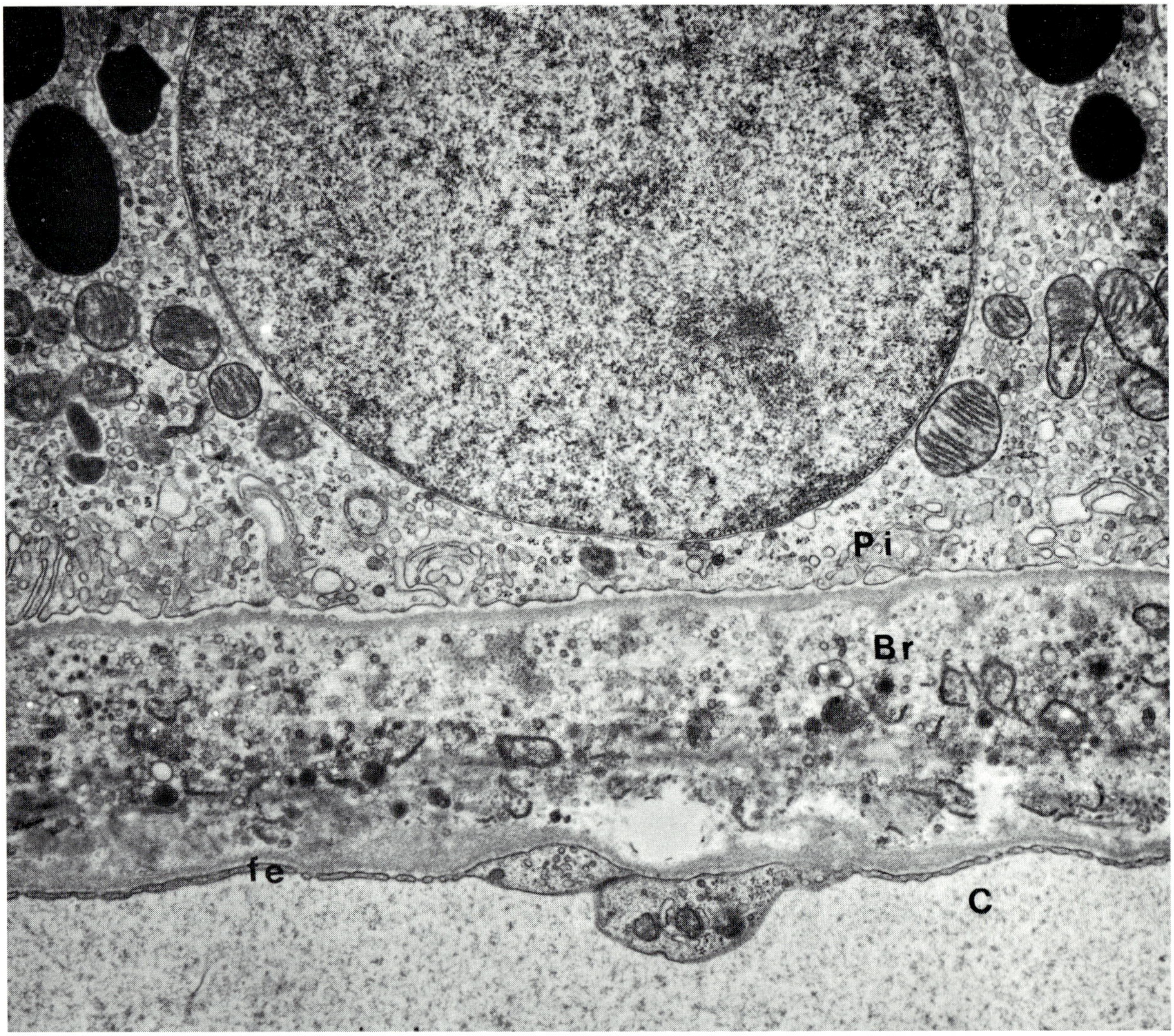

Fig. 4-7. Electronmicrograph of Bruch's membrane **(Br)** lying between the retinal pigment epithelium **(Pi)** and the choriocapillaris **(C)** with its fenestrated endothelium **(fe).** Five layers can be discerned; **1,** basement membrane of the retinal pigment epithelium; **2,** inner collagenous zone, **3,** elastic tissue zone; **4,** outer collagenous zone; **5,** basement membrane of the choriocapillaris. Vesicles and tubules within Bruch's membrane indicate that this specimen comes from an older individual. ×39,000.

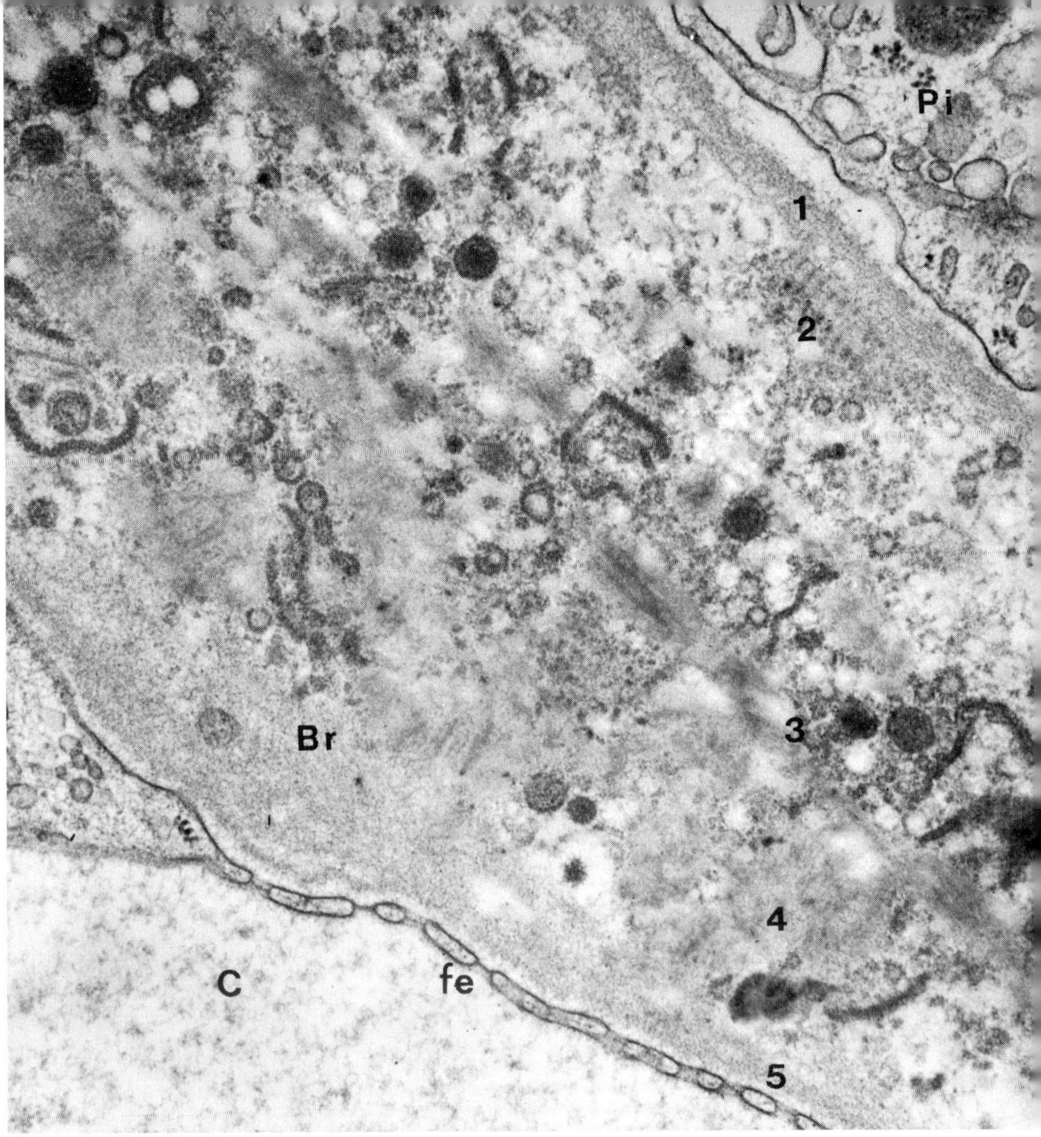

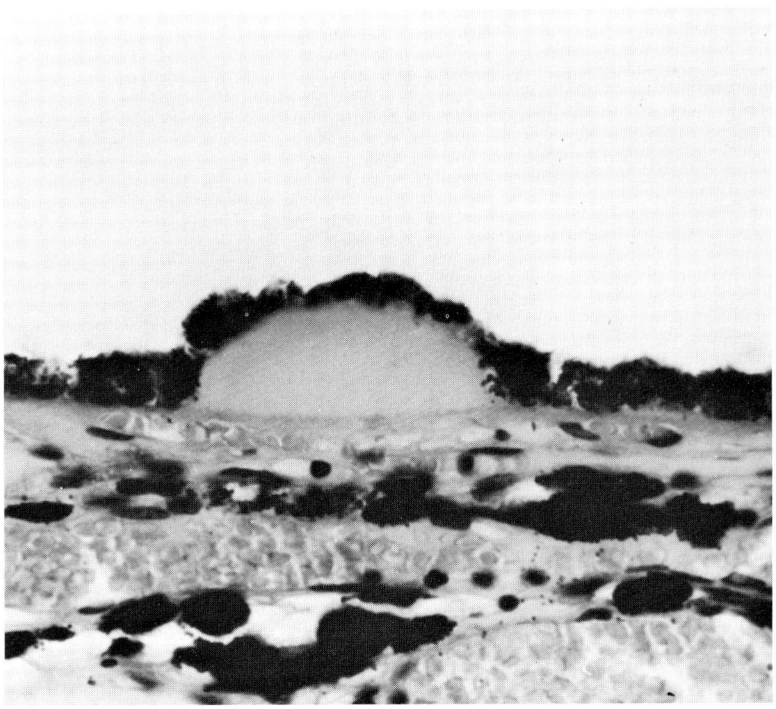

Fig. 4-8. A drusen lying upon Bruch's membrane. H&E, ×560.

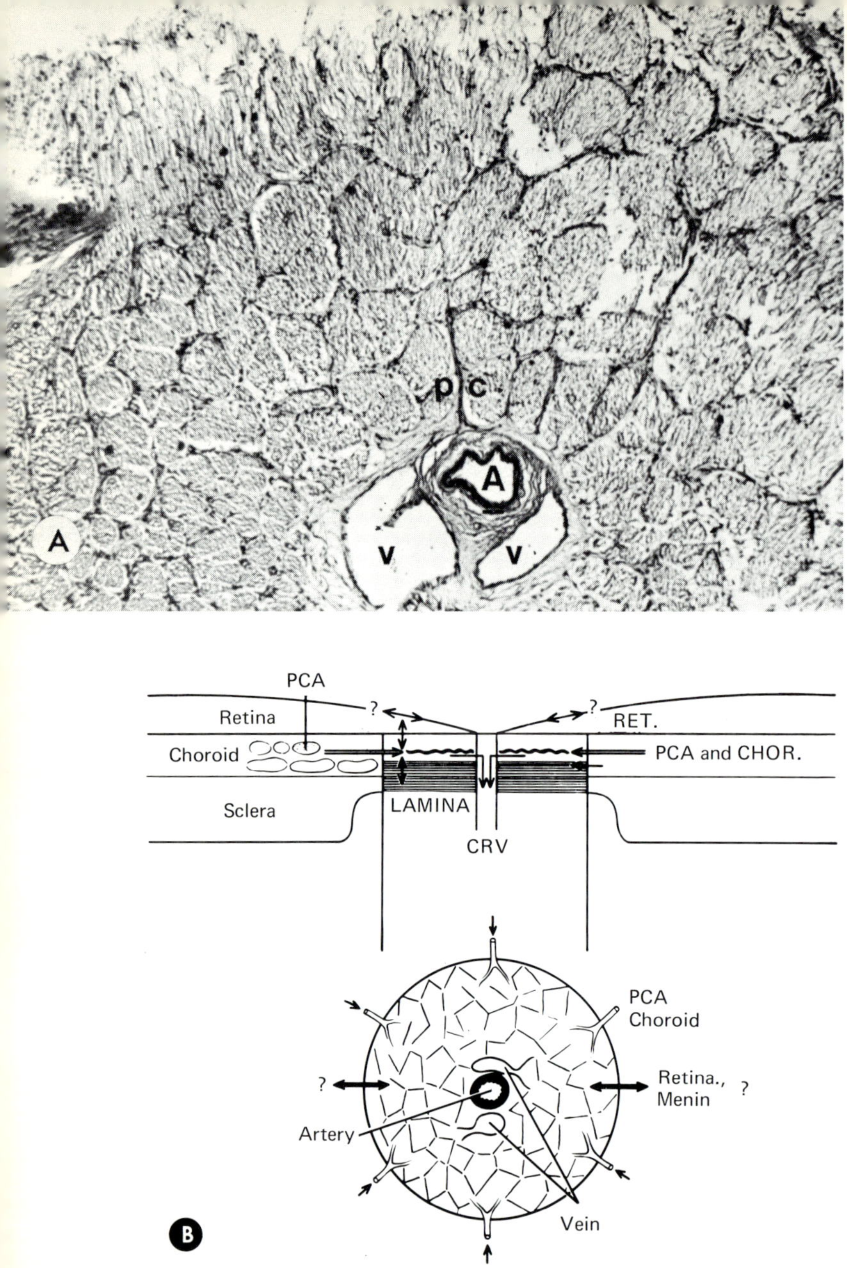

Fig. 4-9. *A*, Flat section of a little more than half of the papilla of an adult human. The capillaries and their surrounding glia are visible as a meshwork of polygonal spaces. At the bottom of the figure are the central retinal artery **(A)** and the central retinal vein **(v)**. A postcapillary venule **(pc)** can be traced from the papillary capillary bed into a branch of the central retinal vein. PAS, ×87.

B, Schematic diagram of the microcirculation of the papilla. The afferent vessels are mainly choroidal via short posterior ciliary arteries **(PCA)** and the major efferent channel is the central retinal vein **(CRV)**. Note other potential vascular connections, such as possible communications with the retinal and meningeal circulation. *Top,* longitudinal section; *Bottom,* transverse section.

(From Henkind and Levitzky.[6])

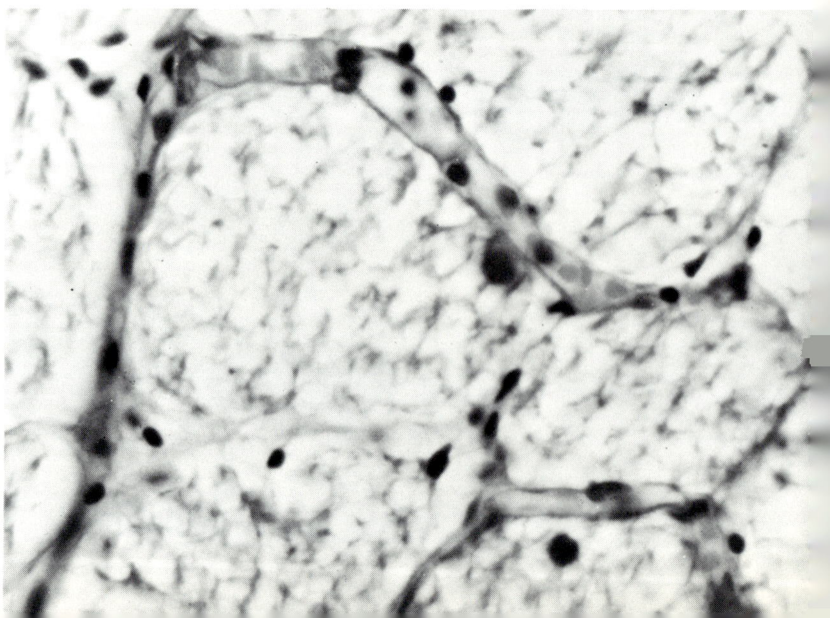

Fig. 4-10. Higher-power view of Figure 4-9*A* shows the thin-walled vessels of the papillary meshwork. The upper vessel may be a postcapillary venule—note the several red cells lying side by side, while the lower vessel is a capillary. PAS, ×560.

retinal pigment epithelium; (*2*) an inner collagenous zone; (*3*) a central elastic layer; (*4*) an outer collagenous zone; and (*5*) the basement membrane of the capillary endothelium (Fig. 4-7).[8] The elastic fibers do not form a continuous layer, rather they are arranged in an interlacing network with spaces through which collagen bundles can intermingle. Ring and Fujino[14] recently have reported finding round holes, 15 to 30 μ, in flat preparations of Bruch's membrane. They occur mainly at the posterior pole, particularly in the region of the macula, and are more frequent in older individuals. If such defects really exist they may play a role in various maculopathies such as central serous retinopathy, detachment of the retinal pigment epithelium, and disciform macular degeneration.

In infancy Bruch's membrane is thin and contains only small amounts of collagen and elastic tissue. It reaches its maximum thickness in late childhood, and this is due to the addition both of collagen and elastic fibers. With aging there is an accumulation of vesicles in the inner collagenous zone. After age 40 the collagen becomes more electron dense, and the elastic fibers thicken, show fibrillary changes and develop calcific foci. In the elderly, collagen extends down between the choriocapillaries. The above ultrastructural observations[8] correspond with the light microscopic findings of aging of Bruch's membrane which include thickening and hyalinization, intercapillary thickening, and basophilia. Drusen, a frequent finding in many fundi after age 20, have been shown to arise from the pigment epithelium and may either remain in the pigment cells or be deposited upon the inner surface of Bruch's membrane (Fig. 4-8). Hogan[8] has concluded that it is disease of Bruch's membrane, mainly aging changes of the collagenous and elastic tissue components, which is responsible for most cases of senile macular degeneration. Most such patients have little or no retinal vascular disease, but do show alterations in Bruch's membrane and the underlying choriocapillaris.

Fig. 4-11. Flat section of the border of a human optic papilla. A vessel, presumably a choroidal artery **(CA),** crosses the border tissue of Elschnig **(E)** and bifurcates to supply the papillary capillaries. PAS, ×320. (From Henkind and Levitzky. *Amer. J. Ophthal. 68:* 979, 1969.)

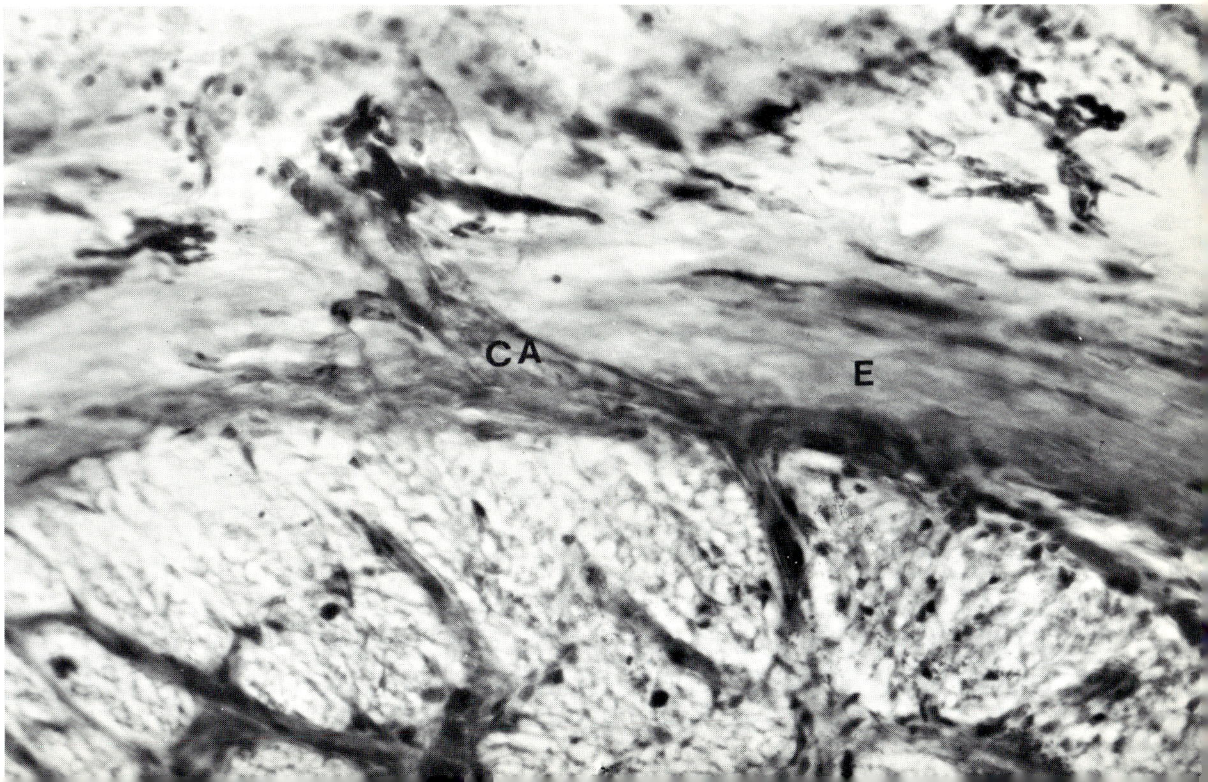

PAPILLARY ANGIOARCHITECTURE

From the standpoint of descriptive anatomy we find that the capillary bed lying within the human optic disc head is essentially in the form of a meshwork with vessels enclosing polygonal spaces of varying size ranging from 30×50 and 50 to 85 μ (Fig. 4-9). The meshwork is best seen in flat or slightly oblique sections.[6]

The capillaries making up the papillary or disc network range in size from 7 to 10 μ. So far as can be determined these vessels have a typical capillary structure with a basement membrane lined by endothelium (Fig. 4-10). Astroglial cells surround these capillaries, but the perivascular cellularity is less than that found in the deeper lying capillary plexus of the lamina cribrosa. There may be capillary connections between the retinal circulation and the disc capillaries, but these are not prominent. Capillary intercommunications exist between the disc capillaries and those of the underlying lamina cribrosa.

The major afferent or inflow channels for the capillary bed of the disc arise at the level of the choroid from choroidal arteries. Such channels can be traced at many points crossing the border tissue of Elschnig (Fig. 4-11). There is little or no contribution from the central retinal artery or its major branches on the disc. It has not yet been determined whether any of the feeding arterioles are meningeal in origin. The channels considered to be afferent arterioles range in size from 7 to 17.5 μ.

The major efferent or outflow channel for the papillary capillary mesh is the central retinal vein or its major branches on the disc. It is possible that some venous drainage also takes place via choroidal veins or veins of the optic nerve sheaths. In most instances capillaries were found to join a thin-walled channel leading to one of the major branches of the central retinal vein.

REFERENCES

1. Ashton, N. Observations on the choroidal circulation. *Brit. J. Ophthal. 36:*465, 1952.
2. Bernstein, M. H., and Hollenberg, M. J.: Fine structure of the choriocapillaris and retinal capillaries. *Invest. Ophthal. 4:*1016, 1965.
3. Dollery, C. T., Henkind, P., Kohner, E. M., and Paterson, J. W.: Effect of raised intraocular pressure on the retinal and choroidal circulation. *Invest. Ophthal. 7:*191, 1968.
4. Duke-Elder, W. S., and Wybar, K: *System of Ophthalmology: The Anatomy of the Visual System,* London, Kimpton, 1961, vol. 2.
5. Henkind, P.: Discussion of Goldor and Gay. Chorioretinal vascular occlusion with latex microspheres (A long-term study) Part 2. *Invest. Ophthal. 6:*56, 1967.
6. Henkind, P., and Levitzky, M.: Angioarchitecture of the optic nerve. 1. Papilla. *Amer. J. Ophthal. 68:*979, 1969.
7. Hogan, M. J.: Ultrastructure of the choroid. Its role in the pathogenesis of chorioretinal diseases. *Trans. Pacif. Coast Otoophthal. Soc. 42:*61, 1961.
8. Hogan, M. J.: Bruch's membrane and disease of the macula. Role of elastic tissue and collagen. *Trans. Ophthal. Soc. U.K. 87:*113, 1967.
9. Hogan, M. J., and Feeney, L.: Electron microscopy of the human choroid. 3. The blood vessels. *Amer. J. Ophthal. 51:*1084, 1961.
10. Irvine, A. R., Jr.: Discussion of Hogan, M. J. See Reference 7.
11. Kiss, F., and Orban, T.: New contributions to the circulation of the eye. *Acta Morph. Acad. Sci. Hung. 1:*23, 1951.
12. Leber, T.: "Die Circulations und Ernahrungsverhaltnisse des Auges," in *Handbuch der gesamten Augenheilkunde,* 2. ed., ed. by Graefe, A. von, and Saemisch, T. Leipzig, Englemann, 1903, vol. 2.
13. Loewenstein, A.: Glomus cells in the human

choroid as the basis of arteriovenous anastomoses. *Amer. J. Ophthal. 32:*1651, 1949.

14. Ring, H. G., and Fujino, T.: Observations on the anatomy and pathology of the choroidal vasculature. *Arch. Ophthal. 78:*431, 1967.

15. Sattler, H.: Ueber den feineren Bau der Chorioidea des Menschen nebst Beitragen zur pathologischen und vergleichenden Anatomie der Aderhaut. *Graefe. Arch. Ophthal. 22* (*2*)*:*1, 1876.

16. Vilstrup, G.: *Studies on the Choroid Circulation.* Copenhagen, Munksgaard, 1952.

17. Wybar, K. C.: A study of the choroidal circulation of the eye of man. *J. Anat. 88:*94, 1954.

18. Wybar, K.: Vascular anatomy of the choroid in relation to selective localization of ocular disease. *Brit. J. Ophthal. 38:*513, 1954.

chapter 5

Phylogeny and Retinal Vessels in Selected Animals

PHYLOGENY

The pattern of vessels supplying the retina varies among vertebrates. Depending upon the species, one may find intraretinal, preretinal, choroidal vessels, or various combinations of these. The retinal vasculature of the different species are compared below.

FISH

Many of the Teleostii possess a vascular network which lies on the posterior surface of the vitreous. This membrane (membrana vasculosa retinae) has a widespread distribution among vertebrates; a similar structure is seen in certain amphibians and snakes. The arteries arise from a branch of the internal ophthalmic artery and enter the eye through the optic disc. The veins drain anteriorly into an annular vein which leaves the eye in the region of the ciliary body. Virchow [58] and Schultze [55] noted that in the superficial vitreous network a capillary-free zone was present around each artery only; this observation has been confirmed by Michaelson.[47] Other teleosteans have a falciform process which is a prominent ridge of highly vascularized choroidal tissue extending through the inferior part of the retina in the region of the fetal fissure.

The eel appears to be unique among Teleostii in possessing superficial vitreous vessels which extend into the retina. Michaelson [47] has shown in india-ink injection studies that the larger vitreous vessels are arterial in nature, while the larger retinal vessels are venous. Denissenko [1] and Virchow [58] demonstrated that the eel has two vascular layers within the retina; the superficial, situated in the inner nuclear layer; and the deep, lying in the outer nuclear layer in front of the external limiting membrane. The eel, which possesses the most highly developed retinal circulation of any animal, lacks a choroid.

The Selachii (sharks) do not have vitreous vessels.

AMPHIBIANS

Anurans or untailed amphibians (which include frogs and toads) have a network of vitreous vessels (membrana vasculosa retinae) lying upon the retina. There is a capillary-free zone only around the arteries.[47] The capillaries of this membrane form a close meshwork at the posterior pole, but become sparse at the periphery.

Urodeles or tailed amphibians (such as salamanders) have an avascular retina, and lack a membrana vasculosa retinae. Members of this group, however, usually have a pecten-like structure extending into the vitreous cavity.

REPTILES

Among reptiles, only snakes possess a preretinal vascular network. In the colubrid snake, Tarbophis, these vessels penetrate into the retina itself. Other reptiles, including lizards, derive their retinal nutrition from a conus papillaris, an outgrowth of vascularized glial tissue from the optic disc which is derived from the hyaloid vascular system.[2]

BIRDS

Birds have no retinal blood vessels, but do have a pecten, a structure similar to the falciform process of teleostean fish, or the conus of lizards.[60] This structure appears in the lower half of the fundus, arises from the optic disc, and is generally heavily pigmented (Fig. 5-1). Essentially, it is a dense capillary network lying within a stroma of supporting tissue. While many functions have been ascribed to the pecten, most investigators feel that its main function is to assist in retinal nutrition.

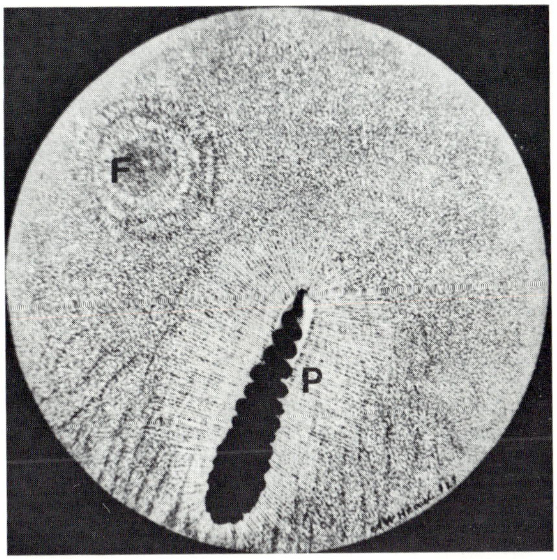

Fig. 5-1. Fundus painting of the glossy ibis (*Plegadis falcinellus*). The dark, club-shaped pecten **(P)** partially covers the elongated, obliquely slanted disc. **F** indicates fovea. (From Wood.[60])

MAMMALS

With the exception of the eel and a colubrid snake, only mammals have intraretinal capillaries.[2] However, there is great variation among mammals. Some placental animals, for example, have no vessels within the retina, while others have marked intraretinal vascularization. Johnson[38] divided the circulation of the retina of placental animals into four groups and Leber[44] proposed a similar classification (his terminology is in parentheses).

1. Euangiotic (Holangiotic). The entire retina is supplied by either a central retinal artery or branches of cilioretinal arteries emerging from the optic disc. This type of vascularization is present in some insectivores, rodents, and carnivores, in several ungulates, and in all the primates (Fig. 5-2).

2. Angiotic (Merangiotic). Only part of the retina is supplied by vessels. This pattern is found in the Lagomorpha (rabbit and hare), in which the vessels are present upon

Fig. 5-2. Fundus painting of a Tasmanian devil (*Sarcophilus ursinus*) an animal with a holangiotic type of retinal vascularization. (After G. L. Johnson.[38])

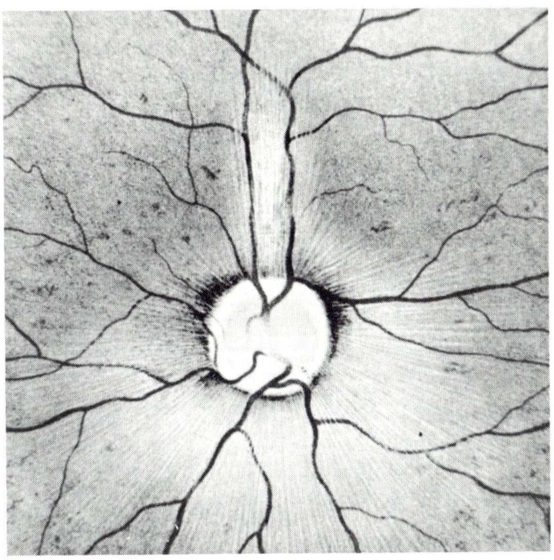

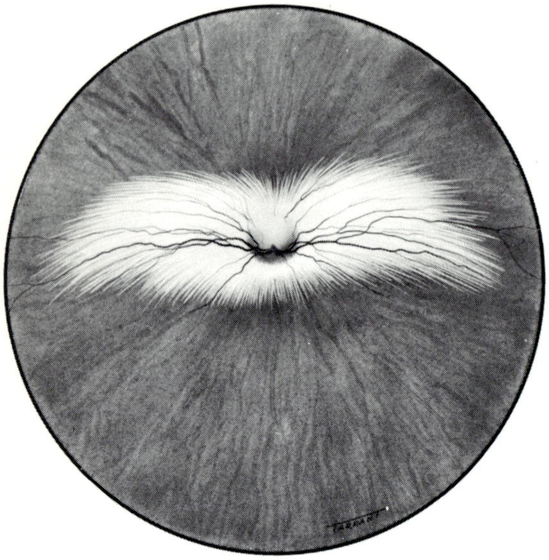

Fig. 5-3. *Top left.* Fundus painting of a rabbit, an animal with a merangiotic type of retinal vascularization. The vessels are confined to the horizontal leashes of opaque nerve fibers and are usually not intraretinal.

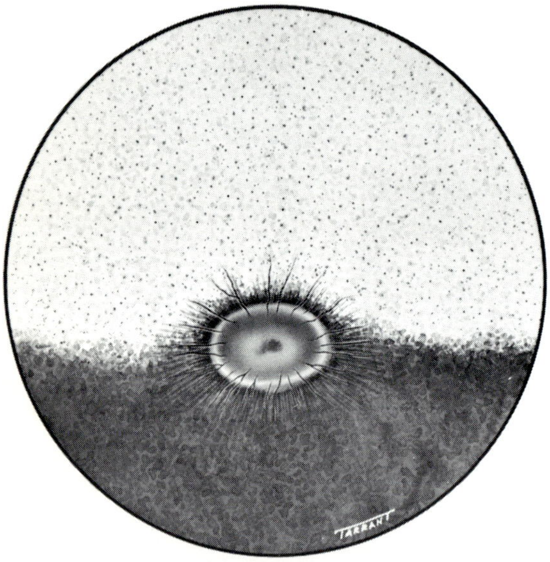

Fig. 5-4. *Middle left.* Fundus painting of Burchell's zebra, an animal with a paurangiotic type of retinal vascularization. Vessels are present only for a short distance around the optic disc. The light-colored upper portion of the fundus is the tapetum.

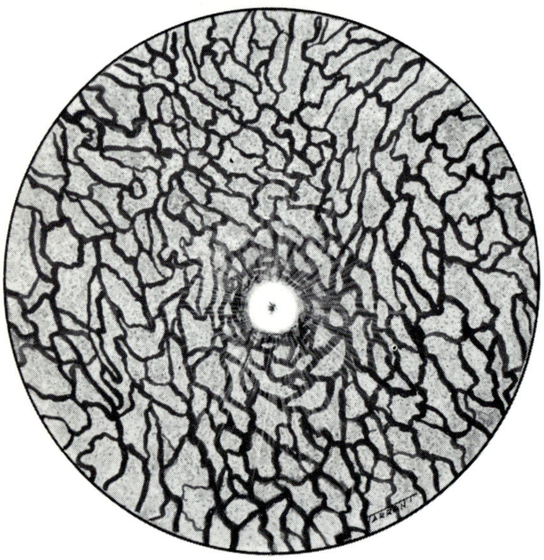

Fig. 5-5. *Bottom left.* Fundus painting of a chinchilla, an animal with an anangiotic type of fundus. The retina is avascular.

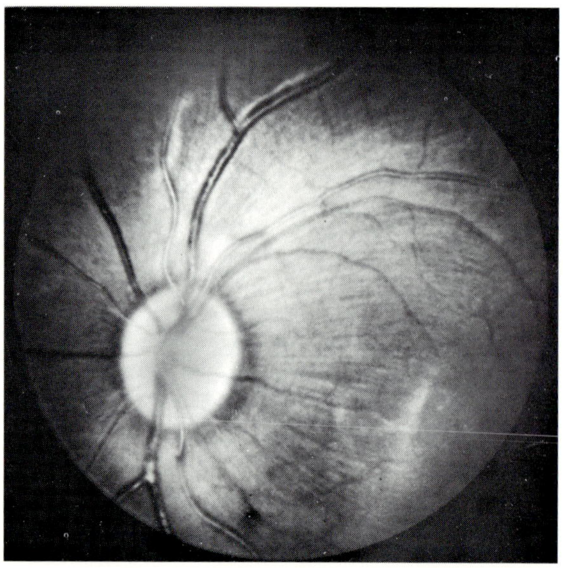

Fig. 5-6. *Below.* Fundus photograph of the posterior pole of a rhesus monkey (*Macaca mulatta*). Note the similarity to a human fundus. The arteries are narrower and have a brighter light reflex than do the veins.

the horizontal leashes of the opaque nerve fibers (Fig. 5-3).

3. Pseudoangiotic (Paurangiotic). The vessels are minute and are present only around the disc. The horse, elephant, manatee, and guinea pig are examples of mammals having vasculature of this type (Fig. 5-4).

4. Anangiotic (Anangiotic). The retina is avascular. The group of mammals lacking retinal vessels comprise the more primitive mammals and certain rodents. Included are *Echidna hystrix,* and other monotremes, hippopotamus, rhinocerus, and marsupials (Fig. 5-5).

FEATURES OF RETINAL VASCULATURE

The major retinal vessels, i.e., the arteries and veins, tend to lie in the innermost retinal layers, and can usually be found just beneath the internal limiting membrane. Except in the eel and Myoxidea, capillaries are not normally found more deeply in the retina than the inner nuclear–outer plexiform layer boundary.

Two retinal areas lack capillaries: the far periphery just posterior to the ora, and, where present, the foveal region. Some capillaries do traverse the pseudofoveal areas of the cat [29] and *Aotes,*[18] however, they are sparser in that location than in the immediately adjacent retina. A capillary-free zone of varying size around retinal arteries is evident in most species.

RETINAL VESSELS IN SELECTED ANIMALS

Detailed studies of retinal vessel pattern and structure have been carried out in relatively few animals. In this section we describe briefly the anatomic findings in those species which have been used in experimental situations, and the areas of research in which work has been done. A number of other animals may prove suitable for experimental purposes, but anatomic data should be gathered before they are utilized.

All of the animals noted below, with the exception of the rabbit, possess a complete intraretinal vascular supply.

MONKEYS

Monkeys, primates with the exception of man, possess a holangiotic retinal vascular tree, and for the most part, the pattern, distribution, and structure of the vessels is similar to that of the human. The fundus of the monkey has been studied in a wide variety of experimental disorders.

Of the commonly used experimental animals the rhesus monkey (*Macaca mulatta*) is one with a fundus most closely resembling that of man (Fig. 5-6). It possesses radial peripapillary capillaries,[30] has an avascular fovea,[18] and its arteriolar side-arm branchings lack annuli.[33] Papilledema,[27,28] hypertensive retinopathy [11] and arterial [31] and venous [47] retinal occlusions have been experimentally produced in this animal.

The owl monkey (*Aotes trivirgatus*) has some features which distinguish its retinal vascular bed both from that of man and the rhesus monkey. While there appears to be a macular region temporal to the disc there is no capillary-free foveal region [18] (Fig. 5-7). Radial peripapillary capillaries are absent, but faint arteriolar annuli are present at points of side-arm branching.[33] The capillary meshwork is relatively sparse and the capillary-free zone around arterioles is broad. Studies of experimental glaucoma and retinal arterial embolization have been conducted in this species.

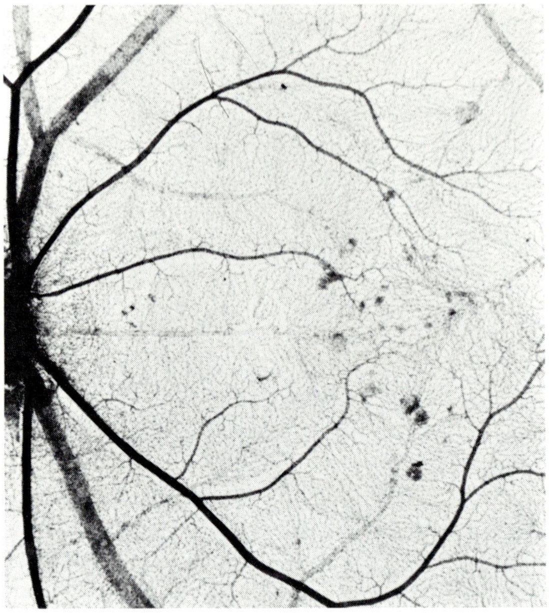

Fig. 5-7. Retinal digest preparation of an owl monkey (*Aotes trivirgatus*). The macular region has no avascular zone centrally, but the retinal capillary bed is thinner in the central macular zone. The retinal arteries are darker and narrower than the retinal veins. The optic disc is at the far left. PAS and hematoxylin.

Fig. 5-8. Fundus painting of the domestic cat (*Felis domestica*). This is a view of a left eye with the "macular" or central zone up and to the right of the optic disc. The tapetum appears bright, and the vessels coursing over it stand out, while those passing over the pigmented portion of the fundus are barely visible. (From Henkind.[29])

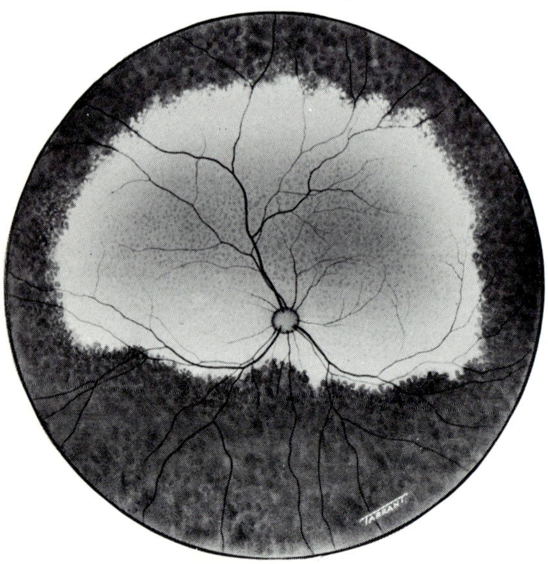

CAT

The retina of the cat is often utilized in research due to the ease with which it can be visualized, and because its holangiotic circulation is considered to closely resemble that of man.[29]

The arterial supply is derived from a series of cilioretinal arteries, and unlike man, its central retinal artery is either absent or vestigal. The internal carotid artery is also atrophic, the eye receiving the majority of its blood from the internal maxillary artery. The ciliary artery is a branch of the internal maxillary and gives rise to the cilioretinal arteries. A small ophthalmic artery may arise from the circle of Willis and join the ciliary artery before it reaches the globe; however, it is often absent, and appears to play only a minor role in normal ocular circulation in the cat.

The fundus of the cat may be divided into two halves: the upper half, with the exception of the far periphery, is occupied by the glistening, yellowish green tapetum lucidum; the lower half and the periphery consists of a heavily pigmented layer (Fig. 5-8). The optic nerve head, which appears pale and cupped (this is a spurious impression due to the marginal position of the vessels), lies near the center of the posterior pole just within the lowermost portion of the tapetal zone. The retinal vessels arise from the margin of the disc; those coursing over the tapetal zone are clearly visible against the lighter background, while those traversing the inferior retina blend into the dark surround. The major vessels may be traced, with the direct ophthalmoscope, to their third or fourth bifurcations, but the smaller vessels are invisible. The veins are darker, broader, and less tortuous than adjacent arteries, and generally lie superficially to arteries at points of crossing.

The greater portion of the retina is served

by three pairs of vessels designated superior, temporal, and nasal. In addition, the macular region is supplied by small vessels from the temporal portion of the optic disc. Arteries of intermediate size often arise from the inferior and superior temporal borders of the optic nerve head and extend to the periphery of the retina.

The larger arteries and veins lie superficially in the nerve fiber layer, and where they cross they share a common adventitia. Small arterioles, venules, and capillaries are found not only in this layer, but also in the ganglion cell, inner plexiform, and inner nuclear layers; the outer retinal layers are devoid of vessels. Near the disc, where the retinal tissue is thickest, three layers of small vessels are present: (*1*) within the nerve fiber layer; (*2*) within the inner plexiform and ganglion cell layers; and (*3*) within the inner nuclear layer. At the equator, only two strata of vessels are discernible, while the periphery is thin and contains but a single layer of vessels.

Arteries divide by bifurcating or by right-angle branching. From the latter are derived the precapillary arterioles and capillaries. Most precapillary arterioles lie in the superficial retina, but some may feed the deeper capillary nets directly. The venous pattern is similar, and postcapillary venules drain both superficial and deep capillary nets, being more obvious in the latter. Michaelson[47] has suggested that the deep network is more venous in character than the superficial one. The capillaries can be divided into two groups: a superficial net lying in the layer of nerve fibers and ganglion cells, and a deeper one lying predominantly in the inner and outer aspects of the inner nuclear layer.[47] The deep net is denser (area of mesh 2000 μ^2) than the superficial one (7000 μ^2).[47] The superficial capillaries are absent on either side of the arterioles with the capillary-free zone measuring 100 to 200 μ.[44] Such a capillary-free zone is not present around venules, and indeed some capillaries may enter large veins directly. Although it has been reported that the foveal zone lacks capillaries,[47] this has not been confirmed.[29] There is, however, a prominent avascular zone approximately 500 μ in width at the retinal periphery.

A plexus of radially arranged, superficially placed, elongated capillaries is prominent above and below the disc. These capillaries, which are derived from intraretinal arterioles, are similar to the radial peripapillary capillaries of man (Fig. 5-9).[30]

At the retinal periphery a series of broad capillary arches link the terminal arteriolar branches with venules (Fig. 5-10). These peripheral channels appear larger than ordinary capillaries, and Thuránszky[57] considers them to be "shunt capillaries" which act as preferential channels. Other authors have described preferential channels linking small arterioles and venules at the posterior pole or equator of the cat retina.[39,45] They have been noted in instances where the anterior segment of the eye was removed for in vivo studies, but they are not evident on inspection of injected material. The concept

Fig. 5-9. Photomicrograph of the peripapillary region of an adult cat. Fine radial capillaries can be seen running obliquely in the inner retina. India ink, ×65. (From Henkind.[29])

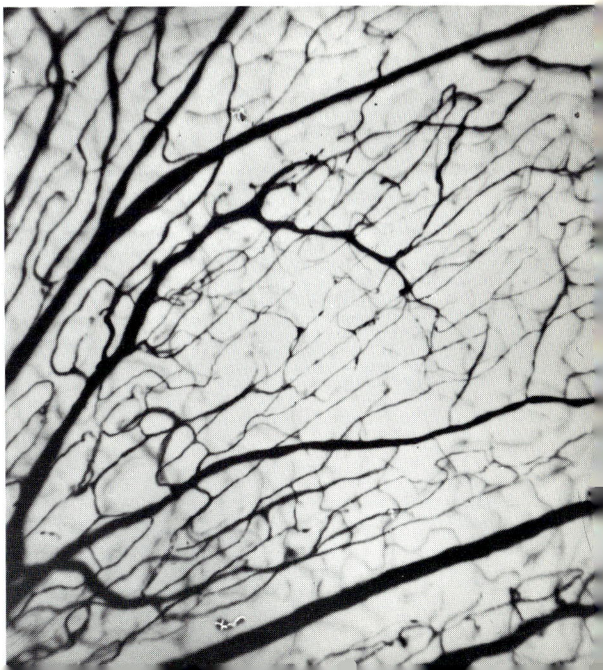

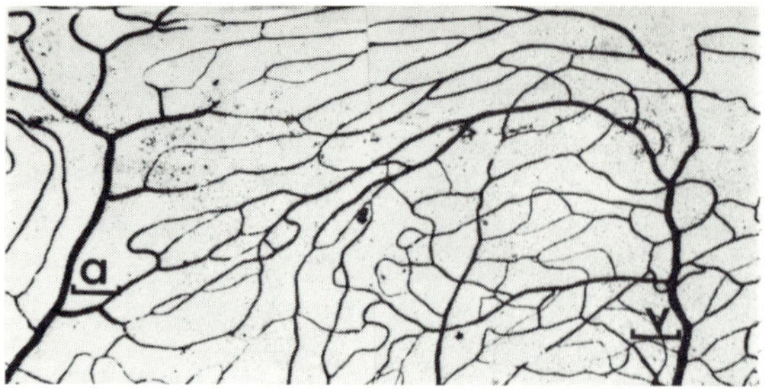

Fig. 5-10. Photomicrograph of retinal periphery of an adult cat. Note that all the capillaries appear to lie at one level, that they form a wide meshwork, and that broad capillary arches link the terminal branches of the artery **(a)** and vein **(v)**. India ink, ×25. (From Henkind.[29])

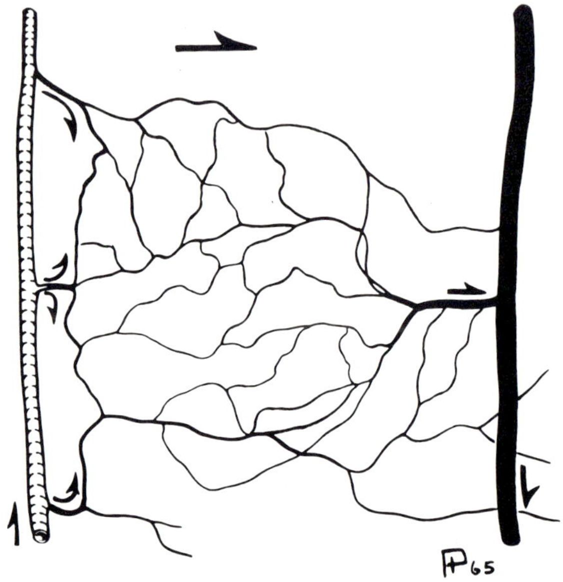

Fig. 5-11. Drawing based on the equatorial region of an india-inked cat retina. Note the arcuate channels between adjacent precapillary arterioles. The concept of multiple arteriolar feedpoints for the retinal capillary bed is easily discerned in this diagram. The **arrows** suggest the paths of blood flow. The major feeding artery is striped and the vein is solid black. (From Henkind.[29])

Fig. 5-12. Photomicrograph of an india-ink injected retina (*left*) and the immediately underlying choriocapillaris (*right*) of a young cat. The figures demonstrate that the choriocapillary network is much denser and more evenly distributed than the retinal capillary bed. ×75. (From Henkind.[29])

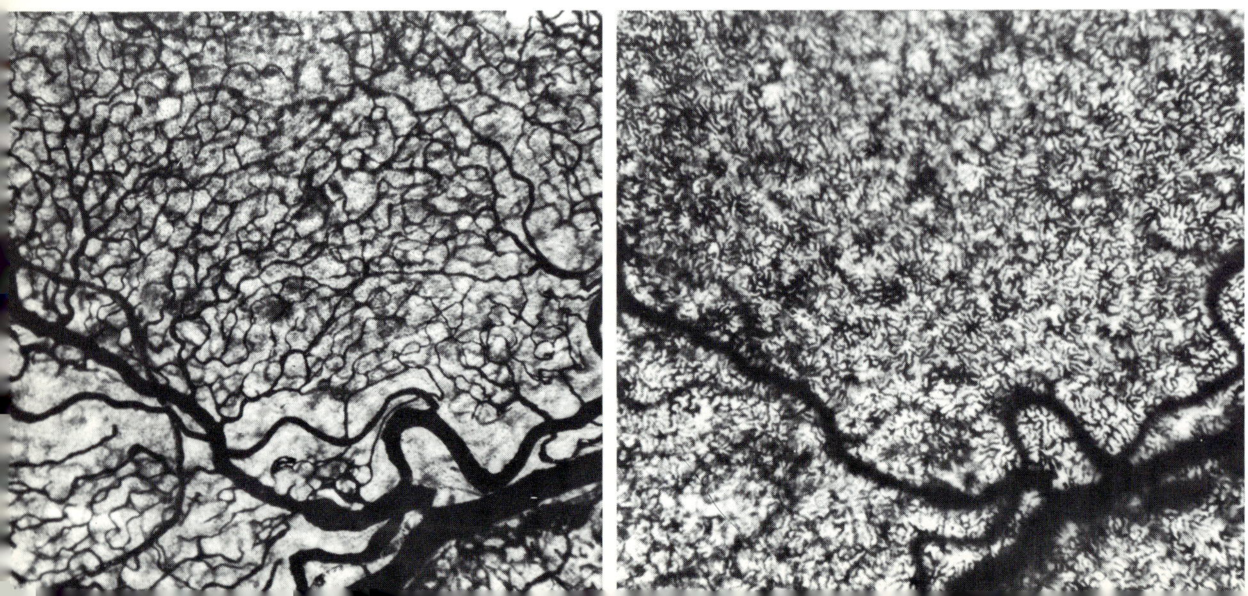

Fig. 5-13. *Right.* Digest preparation of arterial annuli at primary **(black arrow)** and secondary **(open arrows)** side-arm branches of a retinal artery in a cat. PAS and hematoxylin, ×320. (From Henkind and de Oliveira.[33])

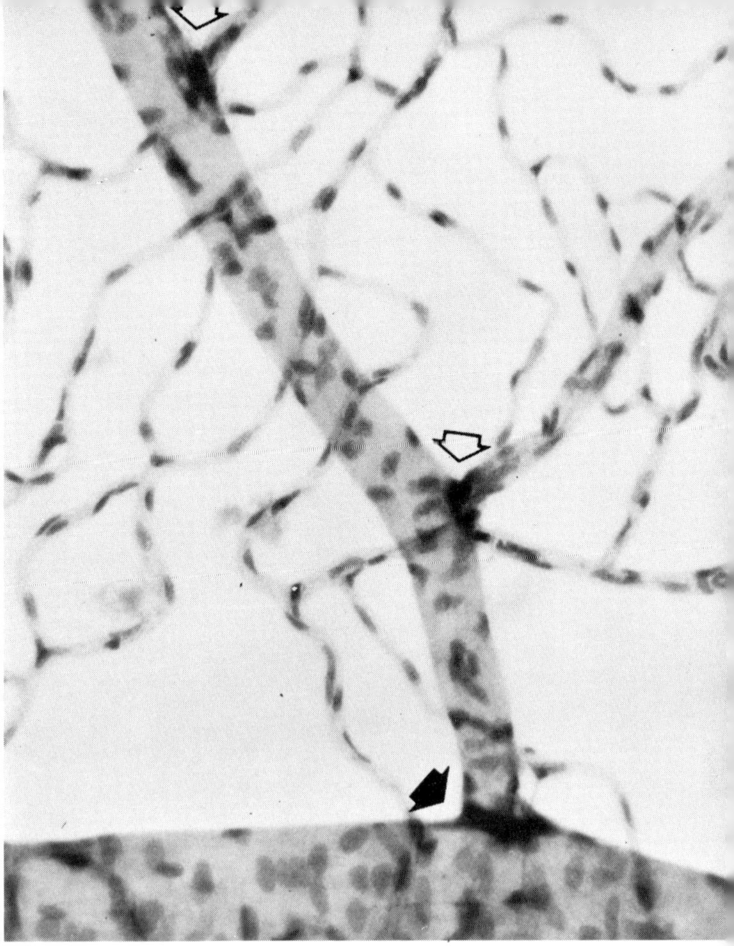

Fig. 5-14. *Below.* Electronmicrograph of a retinal capillary in an adult cat. Both the endothelial cell **(E)** and intramural pericyte **(P)** nuclei are seen. Basement membrane completely surrounds the intramural pericyte. Müller cell processes **(M)** completely surround the capillary wall. **(L)** represents the vascular lumen. ×17,000. (From Henkind.[29])

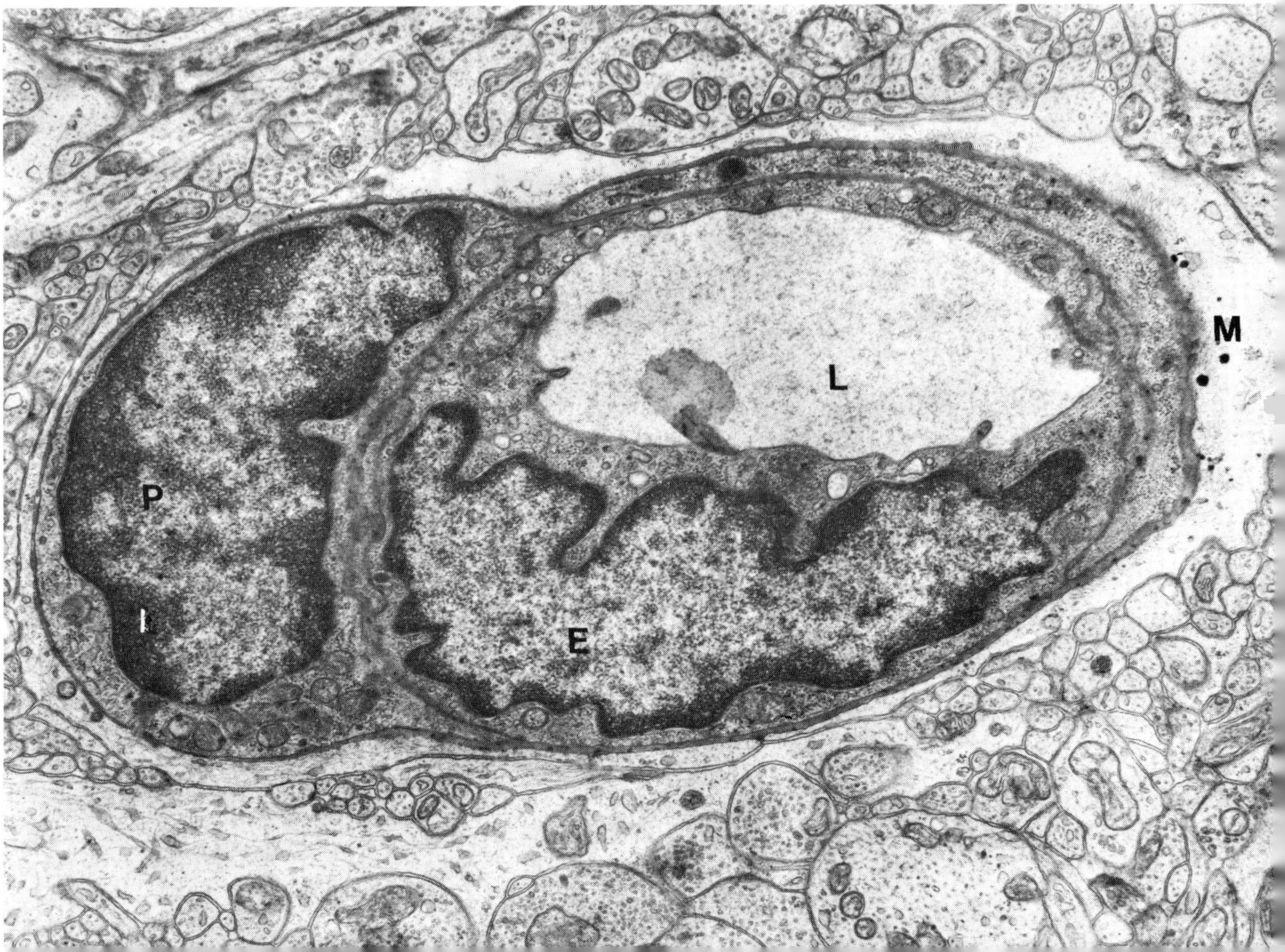

of the retinal capillary bed being fed by many arteriolar feedpoints[29] is well demonstrated in the cat retinal vascular system (Fig. 5-11).

In this species it has been possible to compare the density of the retinal capillary with the underlying choriocapillary bed. The latter is by far more compact, and its close-knit nature lends support to the idea that a large portion of retinal nutrition is derived from the choriocapillaris (Fig. 5-12).

Retinal digest preparations stained with periodic acid-Schiff (PAS) reagent and hematoxylin reveal that the arteries are narrower, more cellular, and deeper staining than adjacent venules. Endothelial cells and pericytes are found with equal frequency. PAS-positive arteriolar annuli can be seen at sites of side-arm branching, but not at dichotomous branchings nor anywhere along the venous portion of the vascular tree (Fig. 5-13.[33]

The ultrastructure of the vessels is much like that of man (Fig. 5-14).

The retinal vascular system of the cat has been used in a wide variety of studies including: studies of experimental retrolental fibroplasia,[7] venous[15] and arteriolar occlusion,[10] alterations in vascular permeability and the development of the concept of the blood-retinal barrier,[6,16] and the effect of raised intraocular pressure on retinal vessels.[5]

DOG

The fundus of the dog bears some resemblance to that of the cat; it has a tapetum, a holangiotic retinal vascular supply, and multiple cilioretinal rather than a single central retinal artery (Fig. 5-15).

Instead of a central retinal artery[59] three or four large (up to 70 μ in diameter), and numerous smaller cilioretinal arteries enter the retina at the margin of the optic nerve head. The arteries, especially the larger ones, pursue tortuous paths. They divide by dichotomous and right-angle branching to form a dense capillary network. The retinal veins are fewer in number and broader in caliber, the largest being approximately 100 μ in diameter. They usually unite to form a central retinal vein; this vein has a very short course in the optic nerve, leaving it at the level of the lamina cribrosa.[59] At points of crossing, either the artery or vein may take the inner position. Occasionally an arteriole will cross another arteriole, a situation rare in other species.[24] No vascular configuration suggesting a macular zone or fovea has been noted.

The capillaries occupy the inner retina down to the border of the outer plexiform and inner nuclear layers. Although the capillaries form layers in the various inner retinal strata, they have numerous intercommunications. At the posterior pole both an inner and outer capillary network can be seen. Anteriorly, the networks are less prominent, and near the ora serrata only a single layer of widely spaced capillaries is present. In the nerve fiber layer at the posterior pole superficial radial capillaries have been noted.[24]

In retinal digest preparations there are, at points of arteriolar side-arm branching, PAS-positive annuli.[33] Focal narrowing of the lumen has also been described at this site,[24,49] but we have been unable to confirm its presence.[33] A capillary-free zone is visible around arteries, but is not evident around veins. The cellular components of the capillaries are endothelial cells and intramural pericytes with the former outnumbering the latter by as much as five to one.[24] This is distinctly unlike the situation in man and most other species where both cell types are found with about equal frequency.

The ultrastructure of the vessels is similar to that of other species.[24] A vacuolated basement membrane resembling that reported in man was found in two mature dogs.[24]

Spontaneous diabetes occurs in the dog

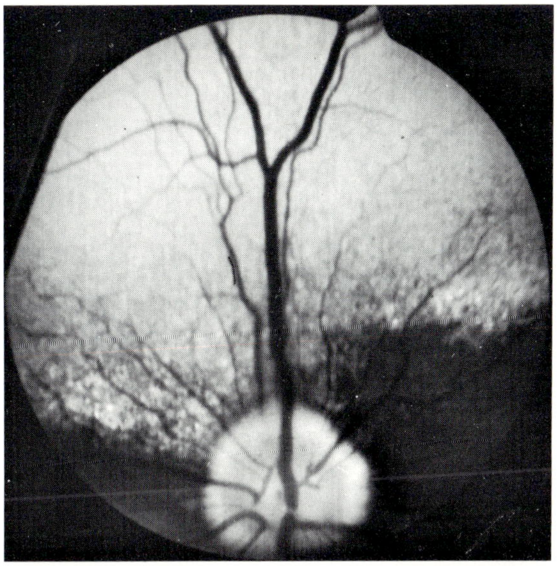

Fig. 5-15. Fundus photograph of a dog. Medullated nerve fibers surround the optic disc giving its margin a fuzzy appearance. The retinal arteries are thinner, more tortuous, and more numerous than the retinal veins. (Courtesy of Dr. Roy Bellhorn.)

Fig. 5-16. Fundus photograph of a rat taken by means of applanation ophthalmoscopy. (For a further description see Chapter 8.) The arteries and veins radiate in spoke-like fashion from the center of the disc. (Courtesy of Dr. Roy Bellhorn.)

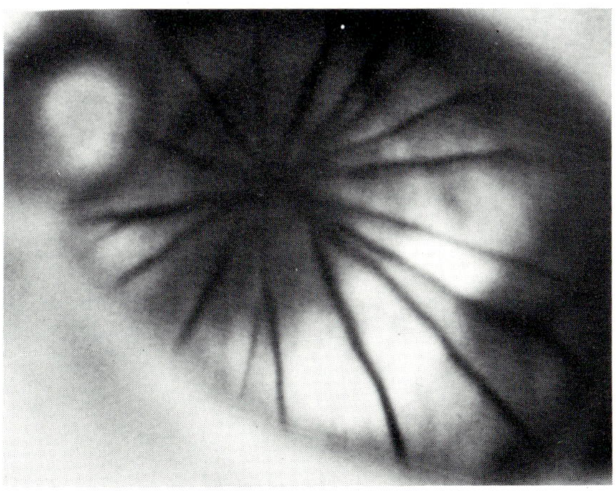

and aneurysms of the retinal capillaries have been noted on several occasions.[21,26,52] Hypertensive retinopathy has been produced in the dog.[41]

RAT AND MOUSE

The rat has a holangiotic retinal vascular supply, central retinal vessels, and no tapetum. Although the eye of the rat is small, its fundus can be examined clinically without difficulty. The retinal vessels of the mouse are comparable to those of the rat.[7]

A varying number of major retinal vessels, usually five to seven arteries and a like number of veins, derived from the central retinal vessels, radiate from the disc towards the retinal periphery (Fig. 5-16). Arteries alternate with veins, the former having a lighter color and narrower blood column. The main arteries, approximately 50 μ in diameter, divide by dichotomous and right-angle branching, and precapillary arterioles come off from the smallest arteries and pass into the superficial (innermost) network of capillaries.

The superficial capillaries lie in the nerve fiber layer. According to Michaelson,[47] precapillary arterioles (arteriae afferentes) do not pass directly into the deep capillary plexus, rather there are capillary channels which pass perpendicularly or obliquely from the superficial into the deep plexus. The latter lies within and on either side of the inner nuclear layer. In the mature rat, the superficial network of capillaries is essentially arterial, while the deeper vessels are mainly venous.[47] The average diameter of the mesh of the superficial capillaries is approximately 130 μ, compared to 80 μ for the denser, more regular, deep plexus.[47]

Postcapillary venules form in the deep capillary plexus and slope upward to join the veins which lie in the nerve fiber layer. Capillaries from the superficial net may join directly with veins, or more commonly, then

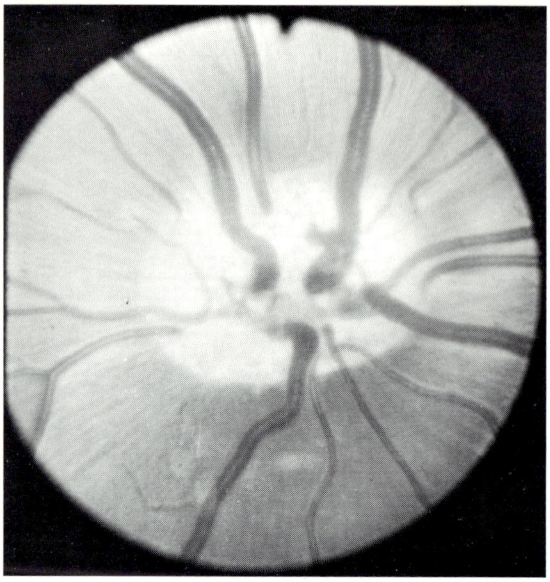

Fig. 5-17. Fundus photograph of the posterior pole of a domestic farm pig.

Fig. 5-18. Cross section through the peripheral retina of a pig. A large venous arcade (**V**) encircles the retinal periphery. H & E.

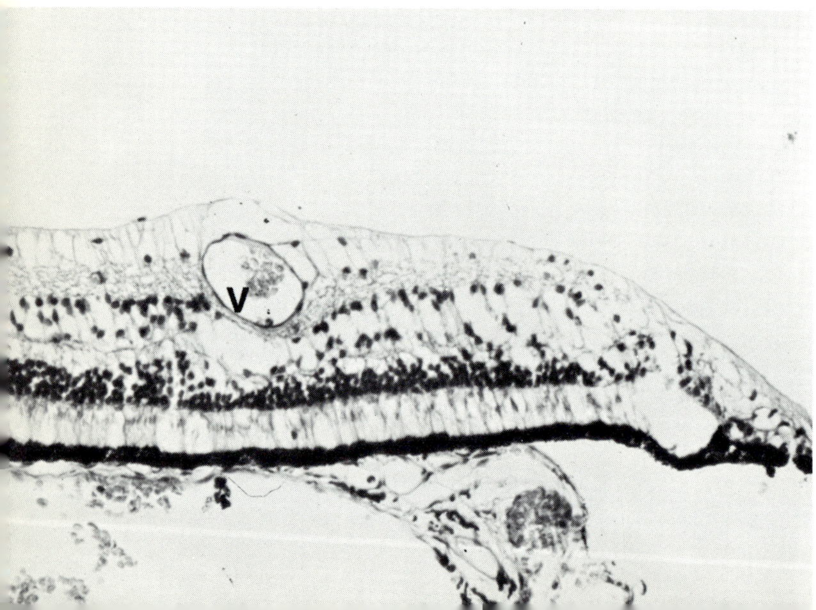

pass into postcapillary venules before these vessels enter the larger, superficial veins. As the retinal veins join to form the central retinal vein at the nerve head, they are posterior to the arteries. Janes and Bounds [37] have noted that the central retinal vein lies temporal to the artery in the nerve.

The structure of retinal capillaries resembles that of other species; flat endothelial cells line the lumen and lie upon a homogeneous basement membrane which surrounds intramural pericytes. Although the retinal arteries of the rat possess abundant basement membrane material their walls lack mature collagen and elastin, and there is no adventitia.[35] The principal branches near the disc may have several layers of muscle cells in the wall. Cellular annuli have been found at sites of arterial side-arm branching.[33]

Studies on the development of retinal vessels have been conducted in the rat.[2,8,22,32,40,47,56] A number of workers have examined the effect of various concentrations of oxygen on the developing retinal vessels of this animal in order to duplicate the human condition of retrolental fibroplasia.[3,8,51] Agrawal and coworkers [4] have stated that they were able to produce experimental diabetic retinopathy in albino rats, and a number of workers have studied the effects of induced hypertension on the retinal blood vessels of this animal.[1,14,23] Retinal vessel cell turnover has been studied in the mouse.[25]

PIG

The eye of the pig has a holangiotic retinal vascular supply, lacks a tapetum, and is similar in size and shape to the human eye.

Instead of a central retinal artery the pig has three or four major retinal arteries derived from the ciliary artery of the orbit. They enter the retina from the nerve head, and have been termed supero- and inferotemporal, and supero- and inferonasal arteries (Fig. 5-17). One or more of the major vessels may divide before the retina is reached, in which case multiple smaller cilioretinal arteries are seen. As the arteries travel outward from the disc they divide dichotomously and by right-angle branching. From the latter are derived the precapillary arterioles and the capillary bed. The major veins follow a similar pattern, however, they are fewer in number, of larger caliber, and darker than adjacent arteries. In general, the arteries lie internally to the veins at sites of crossing. Although the arteries often appear to bulge into the vitreous, they are invariably covered by some nerve fibers and the internal limiting membrane. A broad venous arcade encircles the retinal periphery (Fig. 5-18).

The capillary bed of the pig has the closest-set mesh that we have encountered in any retina, and this is consistent with the measurements made by Bruns.[13] Lateral to the nerve head three layers of capillaries can be defined.[12] The first is at the outer edge of the nerve fiber layer, the second at the outer edge of the inner plexiform layer, and the third within the inner nuclear layer. Peripherally, only two layers are found; one stratifying at the junction of the ganglion cell layer and the inner plexiform layer, and the other at the junction of the inner nuclear and outer plexiform layer. There are numerous intercommunications between the layers. Recently, a very superficial layer of radial peripapillary capillaries has been described in the pig[30] (Fig. 5-19).

A capillary-free zone has been described around retinal arteries in the pig, however, this has not been obvious in our inked or digested preparations of young farm pigs (unpublished observations). In the temporal retina, several millimeters from the disc, we have observed an area where small arterioles and venules converge in a configuration reminiscent of that seen in the macular region of other species (Fig. 5-20). This is probably the same area that Prince et al.[53] has noted to be "sufficiently free of blood ves-

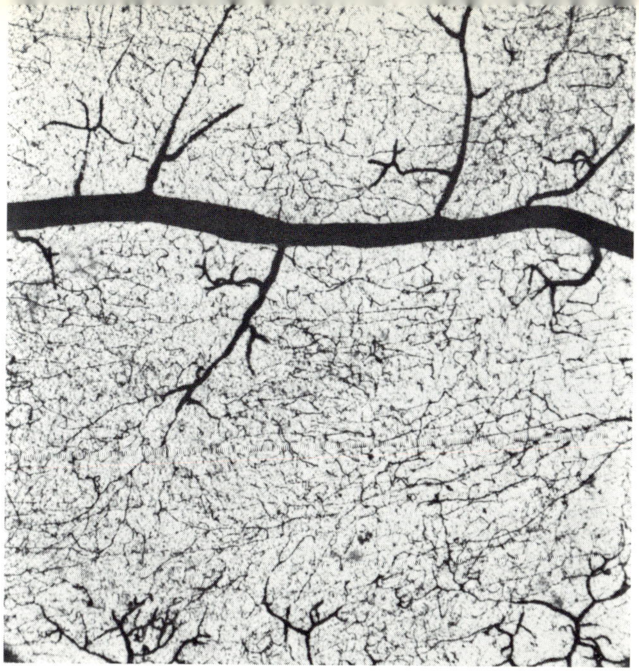

Fig. 5-19. India-ink injected retina of a domestic farm pig in the region adjacent to the disc. Radial capillaries lie parallel to the artery traversing the field. ×35.

Fig. 5-20. Digested retina of a domestic farm pig in the region temporal to the disc. Note that the arteries and veins seem to converge on a central region, but there is no capillary-free zone. ×35.

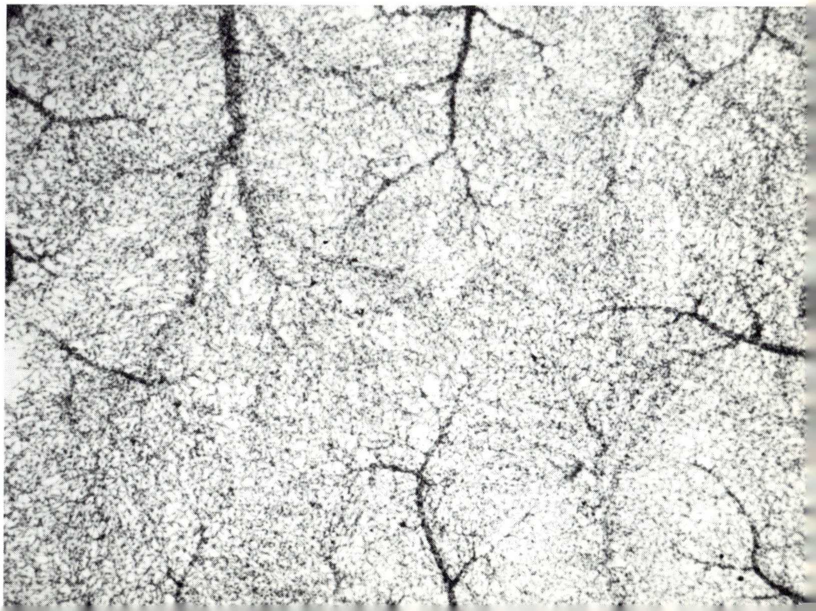

sels to suggest macular qualities." Bloodworth and co-workers [12] have found no such area in their specimens.

Cellular, PAS-positive annuli at the sites of right-angle branching of retinal arterioles recently have been described.[33] The ultrastructural morphology of the retinal vessels closely resembles that of man. One exception, is the absence of a vacuolated, or "Swiss cheese" appearance at the periphery of the basement membrane in the pig.[12]

The pig has been used in experimental studies of retinal circulation including: arteriolar occlusion,[9] venous occlusion,[42] retinal burns,[43] platelet emboli,[50] and effect of altered intraocular pressure on retinal circulation.[19]

RABBIT

The rabbit does not possess a true retinal vascular system. The visible vessels are confined to wing-shaped areas of medullated nerve fibers extending horizontally on either side of the disc (see Fig. 5-3). According to Ashton [7] and Rohen [54] the vessels can best be considered as a modified vascular system of the optic nerve rather than as retinal vessels.

Developmentally, the vessels grow outwardly from the disc and extend along the inner surfaces of the retina, but not within its substance. Only a limited number of capillaries project down to the retina, and even these may only lie within pockets bounded by the internal limiting membrane rather than entering the neural tissue.[7]

The main vessels run from the disc to the periphery of the medullated area; the artery and vein may be parallel to, or cross each other. The major artery has a diameter ranging from 29 to 57 μ (with an average of 38 μ), while the main vein is 38 to 95 μ in diameter (with an average of 61 μ).[36] According to Hyvärinen [36] the structure of the main arterial stem and its first branches is of arteriolar character; the endothelium is surrounded by a well-defined internal elastic lamina; the muscle layer is two cells thick and there is a thin adventitia. The large veins have a thin adventitia and scattered muscle cells in their media. Dichotomous, or more commonly small side-arm branches,[36] of both the arteries and veins occur in all portions of the vessel complex. There are marked variations both in the number and caliber of the vascular branches. Short capillary segments link the artery and vein.

Four different types of capillary nets have been described in the rabbit; (*1*) the central superficial net capillaries; (*2*) the central deep capillaries in the nerve fiber layer; (*3*) the peripheral capillary loops; and (*4*) the peripapillary network.[36] Those of the central superficial net form short capillary loops which have an aneurysm-like appearance in digest preparation—this could lead to confusion if one attempts to study diabetic retinopathy in this species. The various capillaries range from 6 to 18 μ in diameter. Hyvärinen [36] found that there was an unequal distribution of red blood cells in different parts of the capillary net; more red cells were found in the deep than the superficial capillaries. Both endothelial cells and mural cells (intramural pericytes) have been described in the wall of the capillaries. The latter are not as easily distinguished here as in man or in other species,[36,48] and they have oval or elongated rather than spherical nuclei. Furthermore, they are irregularly distributed along the capillary wall, and are easily lost in the process of retinal digestion.

Studies both of retinal arterial [34] and venous [46] occlusion have been conducted in this animal. The rabbit fundus is a poor choice for the study of retinal vascular disease and other experimental animals should be used whenever possible.

REFERENCES

1. Abt, K. and Bruckner, R.: Netzhautgefass-spasmen bei artifizell hypertonischen Ratten. *Ophthalmologica 119:*17, 1950.
2. Agrawal, P. K.: The cellular structure and development of the retinal vessels of the rat. *Orient. Arch. Ophthal. 3:*23, 1965.
3. Agrawal, P., Agarwal, L. P. and Tandon, H. D.: Experimental diabetic retinopathy in albino rats. *Orient. Arch. Ophthal. 4:*68, 1966.
4. Agrawal, P. K., Agarwal, L. P., and Tandon, H. D.: Oxygen and retinal blood vessels. Reaction of immature retina. *Orient. Arch. Ophthal. 4:*77, 1966.
5. Alterman, M., and Henkind, P.: Radial peripapillary capillaries of the retina. 2. Possible role in Bjerrum scotoma. *Brit. J. Ophthal. 52:*26, 1968.
6. Ashton, N.: The blood-retinal barrier and vaso-glial relationships in retinal disease. *Trans. Ophthal. Soc. U.K. 85:*199, 1965.
7. Ashton, N.: Some aspects of the comparative pathology of oxygen toxicity in the retina. Donders Lecture. *Brit. J. Ophthal. 52:*505, 1968.
8. Ashton, N., and Blach, R.: Studies on developing retinal vessels. 8. Effect of oxygen on the retinal vessels of the ratling. *Brit. J. Ophthal. 45:*321, 1961.
9. Ashton, N., Dollery, C. T., Henkind, P., Hill, D. W., Paterson, J. W., Ramalho, P. S., and Shakib, M.: Focal retinal ischemia. Ophthalmoscopic, circulatory and ultrastructural changes. *Brit. J. Ophthal. 50:*281, 1966.
10. Ashton, N., and Henkind, P.: Experimental occlusion of retinal arterioles. *Brit. J. Ophthal. 49:*225, 1965.
11. Ashton, N., Peltier, S., and Garner, A.: Experimental hypertensive retinopathy in the monkey. *Trans. Ophthal. Soc. U.K. 88:*167, 1968.
12. Bloodworth, J. M. B., Gutgesell, H. P., and Engerman, R. L.: Retinal vasculature of the pig. Light and electron microscope studies. *Exp. Eye Res. 4:*174, 1965.
13. Bruns, L.: Vergleichend-anatomische Studies uber des Blutegefass-system der Netzhaut. *Z. Vergl. Augenheilk 2:*77, 1882.
14. Byrom, F. B.: The nature of malignancy in hypertensive disease. Evidence from the retina of the rat. *Lancet 2:*516, 1963.
15. Campbell, F.: Retinal vein occlusion. An experimental study. *Arch. Ophthal. 65:*2, 1961.
16. Cunha-Vaz, J. G. F.: "Permeability of the Retinal Vessels in Health and Disease." (Ph.D. thesis, University of London, 1966.)
17. Denissenko, G.: Einiges uber den Bau der Netzhaut des Aales. *Arch. Mikr. Anat. 21:*1, 1882.
18. de Oliveira, L. F. N. and Ripps, H.: The "area centralis" of the owl monkey (*Aotes trivirgatus*). *Vis. Res. 8:*223, 1968.
19. Dollery, C. T., Henkind, P., Kohner, E., and Paterson, J. W.: Effect of raised intraocular pressure on the retinal and choroidal circulation. *Invest. Ophthal. 7:*191, 1968.
20. Duke-Elder, W. S.: *System of Ophthalmology, Vol. I: The Eye in Evolution.* London, Kimpton, 1958.
21. Engerman, R. L., and Bloodworth, J. M. B.: Experimental diabetic retinopathy in dogs. *Arch. Ophthal. 73:*205, 1965.
22. Engerman, R. L., and Meyer, R. K.: Development of retinal vasculature in rats. *Amer. J. Ophthal. 60:*628, 1965.
23. Engerman, R. L., Meyer, R. K., and Buesseler, J. A.: Effects of alloxan diabetes and steroid hypertension on retinal vasculature. *Amer. J. Ophthal. 58:*965, 1964.
24. Engerman, R. L., Molitor, D. L., and Bloodworth, J. M. B.: Vascular system of the dog retina: Light and electron microscopic studies. *Exp. Eye Res. 5:*296, 1966.
25. Engerman, R. L., Pfaffenbach, D., and Davis, M. D.: Cell turnover of capillaries. *Lab. Invest. 17:*738, 1967.
26. Hausler, H. R., Sibay, T. M., and Campbell, J.: Retinopathy in a dog following diabetes induced by growth hormone. *Diabetes 13:*122, 1964.
27. Hayreh, S. S.: Pathogenesis of edema of the optic disc (papilledema) *Brit. J. Ophthal. 48:* 522, 1964.
28. Hayreh, S. S.: Pathogenesis of edema of the optic disc. *Docum. Ophthal. 24:*289, 1968.
29. Henkind, P.: The retinal vascular system of the domestic cat. *Exp. Eye Res. 5:*10, 1966.
30. Henkind, P.: The radial peripapillary capillaries of the retina. 1: Anatomy, human and comparative. *Brit. J. Ophthal. 56:*115, 1967.
31. Henkind, P., and Dollery, C. T.: Pathophysiology of the retinal vascular bed following

acute embolisation. *Invest. Ophthal. 5:*204, 1966.

32. Henkind, P., and de Oliveira, L. N. F.: Development of retinal vessels in the rat. *Invest. Ophthal. 6:*520, 1967.
33. Henkind, P., and de Oliveira, L. N. F.: Retinal arteriolar annuli. *Invest. Ophthal. 7:*584, 1968.
34. Hirose, K., and Baba, K.: A study of Takayasu-Ohnishi's (pulseless) disease. *Amer. J. Ophthal. 55:*554, 1963.
35. Hogan, M., and Feeney, L.: The ultrastructure of the retinal blood vessels. I. The larger vessels. *J. Ultrastruct. Res. 9:*10, 1963.
36. Hyvärinen, L.: Vascular structures of the rabbit retina. *Acta Ophthal. 45:*852, 1967.
37. Janes, R. G., and Bounds, G. W.: The blood vessels of the rat's eye. *Amer. J. Anat. 96:* 357, 1955.
38. Johnson, G. L.: Contributions to the comparative anatomy of the mammalian eye, chiefly based on ophthalmoscopic examination. *Phil. Trans. Roy. Soc. B:*194, 1901.
39. Keith, G. C., Cunha-Vaz, J. G. and Shakib, M.: Studies of the effects of osmotically active substances on the circulation and structure of the retina. I. Observations in vivo. *Invest. Ophthal. 6:*192, 1967.
40. Kessler, L. *Zur Entwickelung des Auges der Wirbeltwiere.* Leipzig, Vogel, 1877.
41. Keyes, J. E. L., and Goldblatt, H.: Experimental hypertension. 4. Clinical and pathologic studies of eyes: preliminary report. *Arch. Ophthal. 17:*1040, 1937.
42. Kohner, E. M., Dollery, C. T., Shakib, M., Henkind, P., et al.: Experimental retinal branch vein occlusion. *Am. J. Ophthal. 69:*778, 1970.
43. Kohner, E., Dollery, C. T., Henkind, P., Paterson, J. W., and Ramalho, P. S.: Retinal vascular changes following exposure to high-intensity light. *Amer. J. Ophthal. 63:*1748, 1967.
44. Leber, T.: "Die Circulations und Ernahrungsverhaltnisse des Auges," in *Handbuch der gesamten Augenheilkunde,* 2. ed., ed. by Graefes, A. von and Saemisch, T., Leipzig, Englemann, 1903, vol. 2.
45. Lemmingson, W.: Zur tierexperimentellen Lebendbeobechtung der Netzhautgefasse im Auglichtverfahren. *Ber Deutsch Ophth. Ges. 63:*441, 1960.
46. Linner, E.: Occlusion of the retinal veins in rabbits induced by light coagulation. *Acta Ophthal. 39:*739, 1961.
47. Michaelson, I. C.: *Retinal Circulation in Man and Animals.* Springfield, Ill., Thomas, 1954.
48. Mutlu, F., and Leopold, I. H.: Structure of retinal vascular system of cat and rabbit. *Amer. J. Ophthal. 57:*804, 1964.
49. Mutlu, F., and Leopold, I. H.: Structure of retinal vascular systems of the dog, monkey, rat, mouse and cow. *Amer. J. Ophthal. 58:* 261, 1964.
50. Paterson, J. W., Dollery, C. T., Ramalho, P. S., and Kohner, E. M.: The effects of platelet aggregates on the retinal microcirculation. *Bibl. Anat. 9:*85, 1967.
51. Patz, A.: Oxygen studies in retrolental fibroplasia. 4. Clinical and experimental observations. *Amer. J. Ophthal. 38:*291, 1954.
52. Patz, A., and Maumenee, A. E.: Studies on diabetic retinopathy. 1. Retinopathy in a dog with spontaneous diabetes mellitus. *Amer. J. Ophthal. 54:*532, 1962.
53. Prince, J. W., Diesem, C. D., Eglitis, T., and Ruskell, G. L.: *Anatomy and Histology of the Eye and Orbit in Domestic Animals.* Springfield, Ill., Thomas, 1961.
54. Rohen, J.: Uber des Gefass-system der Retina beim Kaninchen. *Ophthalmologica 128:*307, 1954.
55. Schultze, O.: *Zur entwickelungesgeschichte des Gefass-systems im Saugetierauge.* Kollicker's Festschrift gewidmet vom. Anat. Instit. zu Wurzberg, Leipzig, 1892.
56. Shakib, M., de Oliveira, L. N. F., and Henkind, P.: Development of retinal vessels. 2. Earliest stages of vessel formation. *Invest. Ophthal. 7:*689, 1968.
57. Thuránszky, K.: *Der Blutreislauf der Netzhaut.* Budapest, Ungarischen Akademie der Wissenschaften, 1957.
58. Virchow, H.: Ueber die Glaskorper-und Netzhautgefasse des Aales. *Morphol. Jahrb. 7:*573, 1882.
59. Wolff, E., and Davies, F.: A contribution to the pathology of papilledema. *Brit. J. Ophthal. 15:*609, 1931.
60. Wood, C. A.: *The Fundus Oculi of Birds Especially as Viewed by the Ophthalmoscope.* Chicago, Ill., Lakeside Press, 1917.

chapter 6

Physiologic Principles

Scientific advances usually depend upon the ability to make measurements and so proceed upon a secure basis of numerical information. In vascular beds this means the ability to measure pressure and flow, vessel tone, blood viscosity, and numerous other factors.

In a simple system of rigid tubes with fluid driven under a steady pressure it is easy to make predictions about how the system will respond to change. Unfortunately, the vascular system is not so simple for the vessels can alter their size and tone, the blood is a complex fluid, and the applied pressure is not steady but pulsatile.

In the eye the problems are a little simpler than in other systems with larger channels because the vessels are more nearly uniform in structure and the flow has a smaller pulsatile component. It is worth knowing the principles that underlie a mathematical analysis of vessel behavior for the improved understanding it gives of vascular physiology in both health and disease.

This chapter is intended only as an introduction to vascular dynamics. The circulatory physiologist can safely pass it by and the research worker will need to refer to more complete analyses such as McDonald's book *Blood Flow in Arteries*,[44] Burton's writing[11] on vascular tone and Zierler's papers[62] on indicator-dilution curves from which this account is largely derived.

MICROCIRCULATION

The term "microcirculation" is used to describe blood flow through capillaries and the immediately adjacent arterioles and venules. This portion of the circulation is concerned with metabolic exchange of respiratory gases, nutrients, and waste products between blood and tissues. These vessels, particularly the precapillary arterioles, form a major part of the systemic vascular resistance.

Much of the research on the microcirculation has been carried out on preparations such as the hamster cheek pouch, bat wing, and rat mesoappendix, all of which can be spread out on a microscope stage and examined at high magnification.[14,38,46,63] Deep organ circulations are difficult to examine in this way because the vessels are arranged in three dimensions and it is a problem to illuminate and focus upon them properly. The retinal circulation is unique because it is so easily accessible and its thin structures lie in a single optical plane. Unfortunately, the retinal vessels cannot easily be examined at very high magnification in the intact eye. Individual capillaries can be resolved on fluorescein angiograms but no details of individual cells in the vessel wall or blood column can be seen.

CAPILLARY FLOW

Blood flow is defined as the total volume passing a point in a vessel in unit time. In capillaries the flow of cells and plasma may not be the same. Cells flow faster in the axial stream while the plasma near the wall moves more slowly. The relative volume of cells and plasma (hematocrit) is lower in capillaries than in larger vessels because the cells are in lower concentration near the wall.

In many vascular beds the flow through capillaries appears to be intermittent. Some capillaries with a contracted feeding arteriole may have only plasma flow while others are plugged occasionally by leukocytes. Spontaneous rhythmical contraction of terminal arterioles has been described in many vascular beds and is believed to exert an important role in the regulation of the microcirculation.[46] The flow of blood through capillaries appears to be controlled chiefly by the activity of their terminal arteriole. The numerous terminal arterioles supplying one capillary bed often contract and relax asynchronously permitting the flow through the capillaries to be continuous despite the variations in individual arterioles. Some capillaries including those of the retina are narrower in diameter than one erythrocyte and the cell must fold or assume a thimble shape to pass through.

Several investigators have described preferential or thoroughfare channels in the capillary bed. Chambers and Zweifach[14] have suggested that the capillary bed consists of a main through channel or preferential channel with surrounding branches which they have termed "nutritional capillaries." Later work has shown that preferential channels are found in some vascular beds, such as the rat mesoappendix, the outer edge of the rat skeletal muscle and the serosa of the small intestine but not in others such as the skin, and bladder, etc.

It is possible that preferential channels are a feature of capillary beds which are relatively avascular or have wide alterations in flow with variations in activity. Preferential channels have been described in the cat retina by Thuránzsky[59] who used a water objective in an eye with the anterior segment removed. However, this preparation disturbs the normal pressure relations of the retina and other workers such as Friedman, Smith, and Kuwabara[27] who have observed retinal capillaries under more physiologic circumstances, have found no evidence of intermittent flow through them. Fluorescein angiographic studies also show that retinal capillaries are continuously perfused, even when the systemic arterial pressure is reduced in hemorrhagic shock.[18] However, the fluorescein method would not distinguish between flow of plasma and flow of plasma and red cells together.

VASOMOTION AND VASOMOTOR NERVES

Vasomotion is the term used to describe active changes in the diameter of blood vessels. It is seen in one form or another wherever there is vascular smooth muscle, e.g., in arteries, arterioles, precapillary sphincters, venules, and veins.[47] Capillaries are generally regarded as being incapable of vasomotion but this is by no means certain. Such contraction can be initiated or modified by the central nervous system, by local smooth muscle autoregulatory activity, and by other local factors. In many beds it is difficult to be sure which mechanisms control vasomotion although in most microcirculations local factors are probably more important than changes in vasomotor tone effected by nervous or humoral influences.

For many years there has been disagreement about the innervation of the retinal vessels. The matter seems now to have been settled by the use of the technique devised by Falck[24] which renders catecholamines fluorescent. Most arteries, arterioles, and veins have a rich adrenergic innervation which can be demonstrated due to the fluorescence of the neurotransmitter norepinephrine. The ophthalmic artery has an adrenergic innervation up to the point where it enters the eye. Thereafter, no sympathetic adrenergic vasomotor nerves to the retinal vessels can be demonstrated.[39,43] This finding has now been confirmed in the rabbit, monkey, and man.

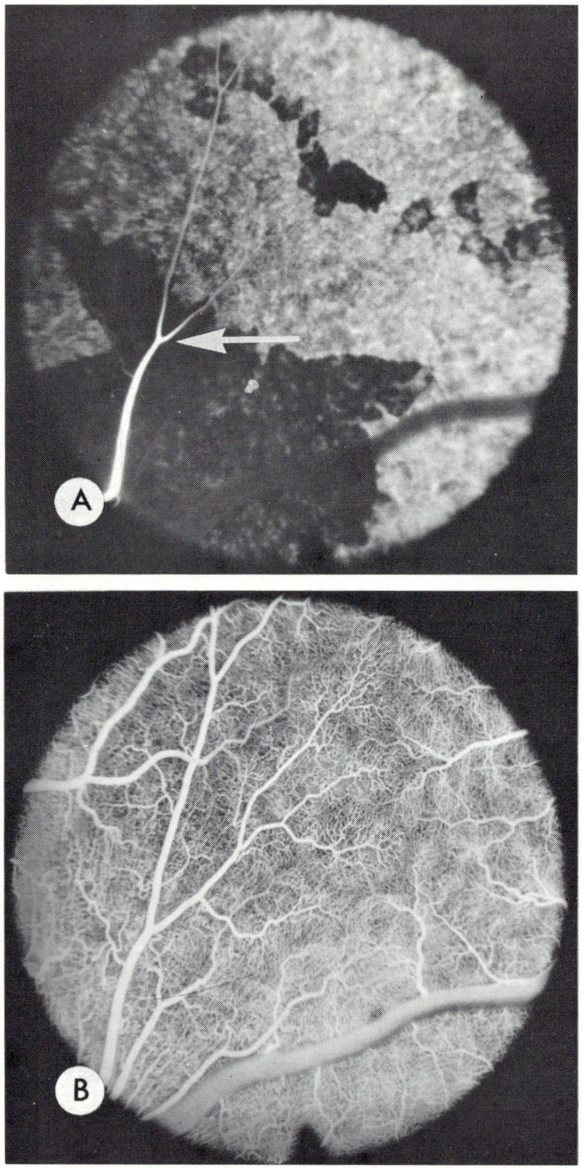

Fig. 6-1. *A*, Fluorescein angiogram shows early filling of a retinal artery in a pig. A thin tongue of dye moves down the center of the vessel and divides onto the inner aspects of a dichotomous junction **(arrow).** *B*, A later stage of dye transit when the lumen is completely filled and the fluorescent stream is wider.

The lack of vasomotor nerves in the eye has important consequences for understanding the control of the retinal circulation. Changes observed in the retinal vessel caliber must be the result of locally controlled vasomotion and systemic vasomotor activity can have no effect, except as it acts via alterations in the blood pressure. It is conceivable that changes of vasomotor tone in the ophthalmic artery are of sufficient magnitude to alter the pressure applied to the retinal circulation, but the measurements made by Duke-Elder[22] suggest that the pressure gradient along this vessel is normally small. Thus the eye provides an opportunity to observe vessels that are responding only to local regulatory factors and possibly to humoral ones.

The retinal circulation is one of the most precarious vascular beds as it has a high arteriovenous oxygen difference and the perfusion pressure is opposed by the intraocular pressure. It is interesting to speculate on the reason for the lack of vasomotor nerves in the retinal circulation. The sympathetic vasomotor system may have evolved to protect animals against blood and fluid loss and so preserve the blood supply to the brain. Embryologically the retina is an outgrowth of the brain and this may explain why there is no nervous mechanism for restricting its blood supply.

HYDRODYNAMIC PRINCIPLES

The circulation consists of a series of branching cylindrical pipes. The simplest hydrodynamic system is a long straight pipe with a steady flow through it. In such a pipe the head of pressure (Δp) is directly proportional to the length (L), the flow (F), the viscosity of the fluid (μ), and inversely to the fourth power of the radius (R). This is the law of Poiseuille which may be stated in mathematical symbols:

$$\Delta p = \frac{8L\mu F}{\pi R^4} \qquad (6\text{-}1)$$

Dye injected into such a pipe moves faster near the axis and more slowly towards the wall, a phenomenon easily seen on fluorescein angiograms of retinal arterioles (Fig. 6-1). The flow in this pipe can be regarded as a series of concentric laminae moving fastest at the axis and with a fall in velocity away from it. The shell of fluid in contact with the wall is stationary. Each lamina is slipping over an adjacent one and this type of flow is termed "laminar." When two such pipes join, dye at one wall will not mix with the fluid in the other and the two streams run side by side. This phenomenon is demonstrated at the junction of the Blue and White Niles and by the fluorescein pattern in retinal veins (Fig. 6-2); it is termed "streamlining." As the rate of flow through pipes increases there comes a point when mixing begins to occur and the regular lines of laminar flow are lost. This type of flow is called "turbulent" and Poiseuille's law no longer applies.

TURBULENCE AND REYNOLDS NUMBER

The breakdown of laminar flow depends upon the diameter of the tube (D), the mean velocity of flow ($\bar{V}$), the density (ρ) and the viscosity (μ) of the fluid. The point of transition from laminar to turbulent flow depends upon the value of the Reynolds number (R_e). Thus:

$$R_e = \frac{\bar{V}D\rho}{\mu} \qquad (6\text{-}2)$$

The fraction μ/ρ is known as the kine-

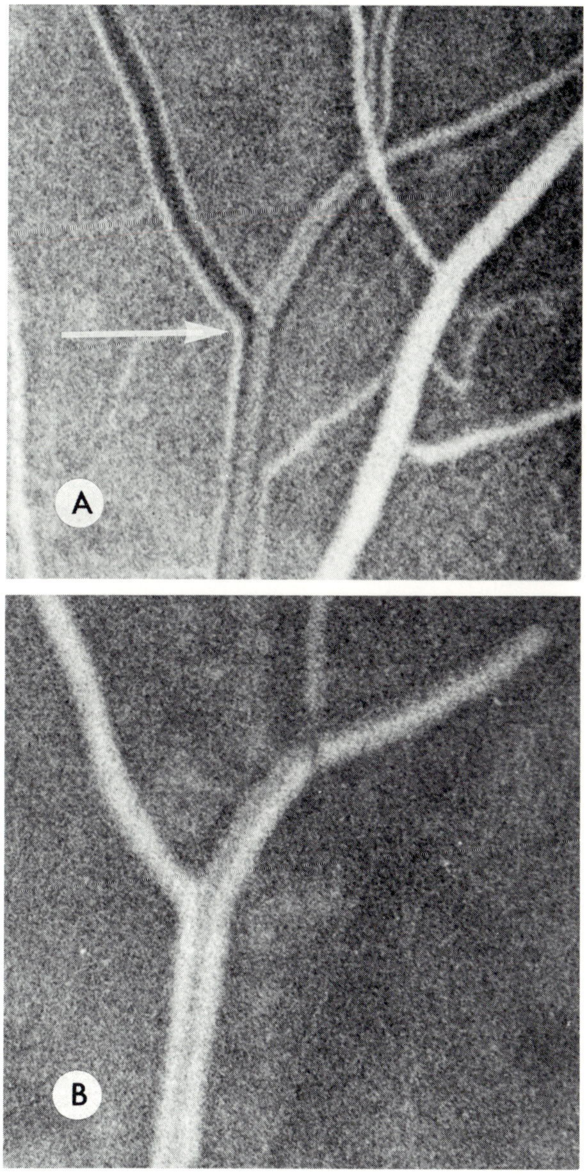

Fig. 6-2. *A*, Early venous phase of a fluorescein angiogram in man showing early appearance of dye at the edge of the vessel. At the junction dye from the two adjacent margins forms the axial stream **(arrow).** *B*, Later in the venous phase the pattern is reversed. The marginal streams carry undyed blood and these unite to form a dark layer in the center of the vessel.

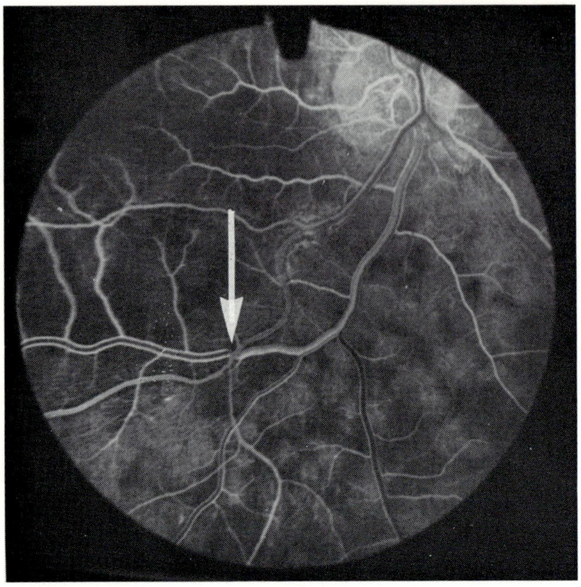

Fig. 6-3. Venous-phase fluorescein angiogram of a hypertensive patient showing a nipped vein with mixing of the laminar streams **(arrow).**

Fig. 6-4. Schematic diagram of a shell of fluid with radius, **r,** and length, **L,** moving through a tube driven by a pressure gradient $P_1 - P_2$.

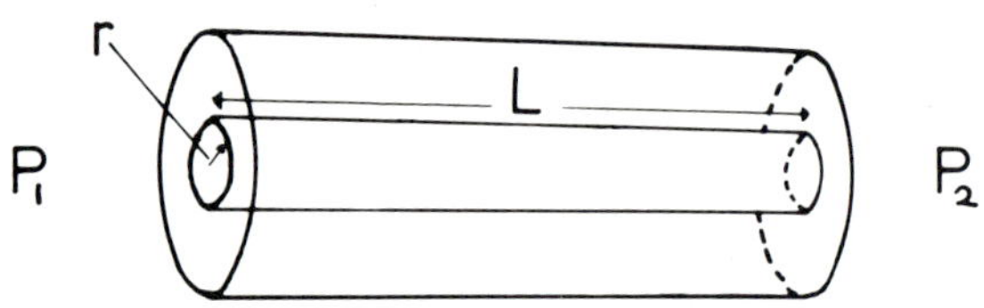

matic viscosity and is written as ν. The formula can therefore be rewritten as:

$$R_e = \frac{\bar{V}D}{\nu} \qquad (6\text{-}3)$$

The kinematic viscosity of blood at body temperature is about 3.8×10^{-2} stokes. The stoke is a unit whose dimensions are cm^2 per second. For a main retinal arteriole of 0.1-mm diameter with mean blood velocity 2 cm per second, the Reynolds number is approximately 0.52.

As the critical value of Reynolds number for breakdown of laminar into turbulent flow is about 2000 for any fluid, including blood, pure laminar flow would be expected in the retinal vessels under almost all conditions. The only condition in which turbulent flow has been observed in the retinal circulation is at crossings where the vein is severely nipped (Fig. 6-3). If it is assumed that the cross-sectional area in such a nip might be reduced to 2 per cent of normal and that flow is unchanged the Reynolds number can be calculated. The result is about 4, still much too small to expect turbulence. The explanation may lie in eddy formation beyond the narrowing.

The viscosity of a fluid is a property akin to the frictional resistance to motion of solids. In a pipe with laminar flow the adjacent shells of fluid are slipping over one another as they move at different velocities (Fig. 6-4). This velocity gradient is called the "rate of shear." If we consider a cylindrical shell of fluid, with length (L) and radius (r), the viscous force opposing its movement will be the product of its surface area ($2\pi rL$), viscosity (μ) and the velocity gradient $\frac{dV}{dr}$,

$$Force = 2\pi rL\mu\frac{dV}{dr} \qquad (6\text{-}4)$$

The driving force is the pressure drop along the vessel ($p_1 - p_2$) multiplied by the cross-sectional area across which the force is applied.

Under conditions of steady flow these forces balance one another.

$$\pi r^2(p_1 - p_2) = 2\pi r L\mu \frac{dV}{dr} \qquad (6\text{-}5)$$

or

$$\frac{dV}{dr} = \frac{r(p_1 - p_2)}{2L\mu}$$

If this equation is integrated the result is:

$$V = \frac{-r^2(p_1 - p_2)}{4L\mu} + Constant \qquad (6\text{-}6)$$

We have assumed that the boundary layer of fluid against the wall is stationary and in this case we can calculate the constant by substitution. The velocity, **V**, is zero when the term, **r**, which is the distance from the axis of the tube, is equal to the radius, **R.** Thus:

$$V = \frac{(p_1 - p_2)}{4L\mu}(R^2 - r^2) \qquad (6\text{-}7)$$

This is the equation of a parabola. As $\frac{(p_1 - p_2)}{4L\mu}$ is constant for conditions of steady flow, the velocity at any point in the tube depends upon the square of the distance from the axis subtracted from the square of the radius. Thus at the axis where r^2 is zero, the velocity is a maximum and at the edge where r equals R, and $R^2 - r^2$ is zero, the velocity is zero.

The volume flow rate can be calculated by integrating this equation and substituting for V. The average velocity, $\bar{V}$, across the vessel is half the axial velocity. This is a useful property because it makes possible the calculation of volume flow rate if the vessel diameter and the axial velocity can be measured. Both of the latter may be obtained from frame analysis of cine-fluorescein retinal angiograms (Fig. 6-5). Although this equation does not hold in a pulsatile flow system, the pulsatile element in normal retinal vessels is so small that the error should not be serious.

In larger vessels, greater than 300 μ in diameter, blood behaves as a Newtonian fluid, i.e., it has a viscosity which is independent of the rate of shear. The apparent viscosity of blood is less in smaller tubes than in larger ones. For example, the viscosity in a vessel 20 μ in diameter is only about two-thirds of that measured in a vessel of larger size, while in a vessel with a 10-μ diameter viscosity is only about half. For the same reason viscometer readings do not give an accurate measure of viscosity in small vessels.

This variation in viscosity has its origin in factors which are common to flow of suspensions whose particles are large enough to be comparable with the radius of the tube through which they pass. The particles of a suspension cannot penetrate into the wall of the vessel in which they are flowing. Thus, with blood there is bound to be a relative deficiency of cells within one red cell diameter from the wall. Measurements of the optical properties of blood flowing in small vessels suggest a marginal zone of greater optical transmittance which contains plasma but not red cells. Experimental evidence suggests that the width of this zone is somewhat less in blood than predicted theoretically and the width of this zone may be somewhere between 1 and 3 μ. This wall effect accounts for the reduced viscosity of blood in small vessels. It also explains the greater width of retinal vessels on fluorescein photographs than in color studies. Color photographs show the width of the red cell column while fluorescein, which is in the plasma, reveals the outer limit of the plasma zone surrounding it (Fig. 6-6). The width of this plasma zone in retinal vessels can be measured by difference from such photographs.[10a]

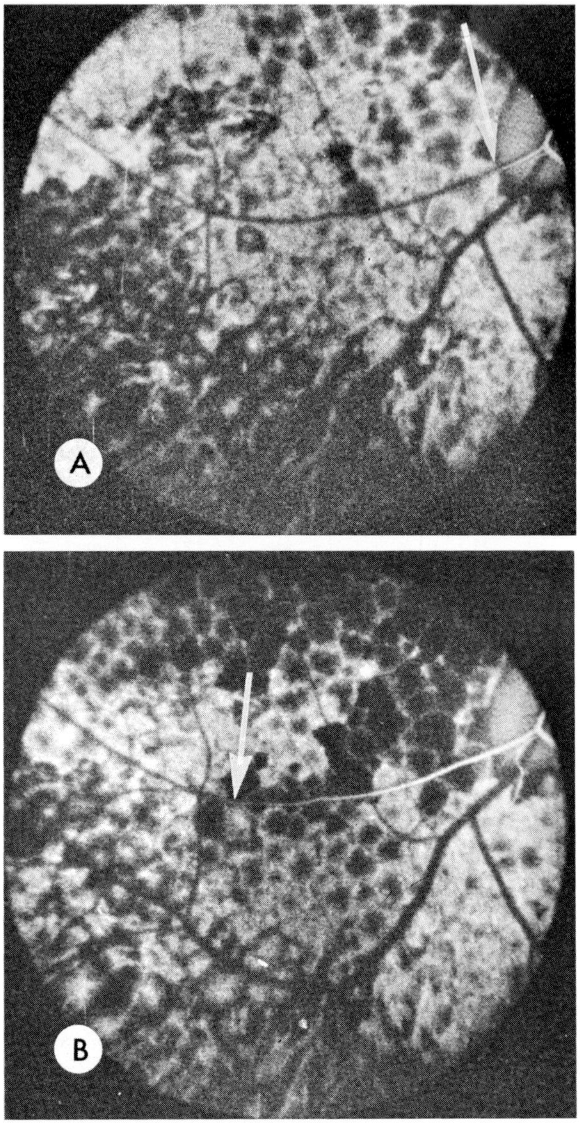

Fig. 6-5. *A*, A 16-mm cine sequence shows the dye front entering an artery **(arrow)**. *B*, Three frames later (at 32 frames per second) the dye front movement **(arrow)** can be measured and the flow velocity calculated.

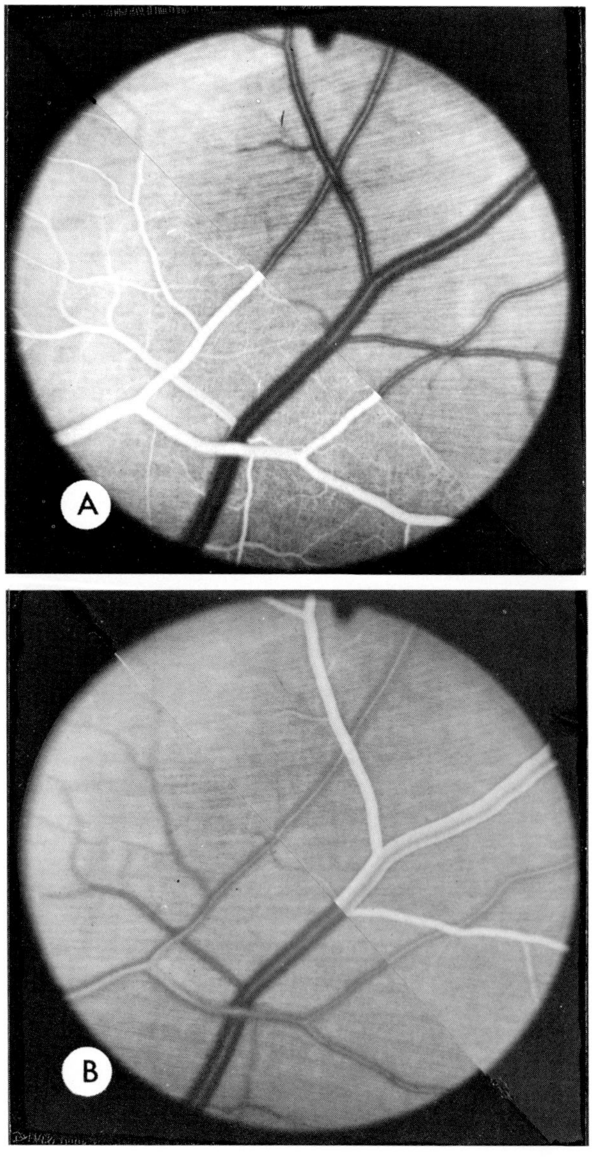

Fig. 6-6. *Right,* Composite figure from a color transparency and fluorescein angiogram. The width of the artery is greater on the fluorescein picture. *B*, Composite color and fluorescein figure in the venous phase showing the greater apparent width of the vein when it contains fluorescein.

COHERENCE RESISTANCE AND SLUDGING

Coherence resistance is a property which depends upon the aggregation of red cells into clumps which offer a greater resistance to flow than single cells.

As blood flow through a retinal vessel is slowed the first visible change is a shimmering reflection from the blood column as the red cells lose their alignment in the stream and take up a random orientation. Further reduction in flow allows the red cells to adhere together in clumps and the blood column breaks into a series of granular segments of red cells separated by plasma. In the eye, this situation only occurs at very low flow rates such as may be seen in terminal hemorrhagic shock or vascular obstruction. As the blood flow increases again the red cells are dragged apart as soon as the shearing stress exceeds the coherence forces.[8,20]

Coherence resistance may partly explain some alinearities in the relationship between blood pressure and blood flow. The graph relating pressure and flow in most vascular beds is linear at higher flows and pressures. As the pressure is reduced to low values, the relationship becomes alinear and the flow slows more than would be predicted from the reduction in pressure. Red cell clumps may offer a greater resistance to flow than single cells but as the aggregates only form in the eye at very low flows they are unlikely to be important in most circumstances.

Knisely et al.[37] have suggested that the greater tendency of the red cells to adhere together in many systemic diseases may cause obstruction to small blood vessels. Red cell clumps or "blood sludge" have been observed in the retinal vessels of pigs with terminal hemorrhagic shock but capillary flow remained uniform even when hypotension was extreme. Blood transfusion and restoration of the systemic pressure returned the retinal circulation to normal.[37]

The importance of blood sludging, which can be observed in the vessels of the bulbar conjunctiva, is controversial. Present evidence suggest it is of no significance in the retinal circulation, or human skin.[8,21]

Platelet aggregates may be of greater importance. In pathologic states in man white bodies probably composed of clumped platelets may cause transitory obstruction of the retinal vessels.[5] This situation can be reproduced experimentally by infusing clumped platelets or adenosine diphosphate (ADP) into the carotid circulation of animals.[51]

MECHANICAL PROPERTIES OF VESSEL WALLS

The walls of retinal vessels are not rigid tubes and in appropriate circumstances they can dilate, constrict, or collapse. The properties of the vessel wall depend, in part, upon the mechanical characteristics of the fibers and other elements of which they are formed. Besides these factors there is the added effect of smooth muscle tone which varies the resistance of the vessel and may even cause it to close. These purely mechanical properties can be examined by plotting a length-tension diagram (Fig. 6-7).

Fig. 6-7. Length-tension diagram of the aortic wall at different ages. (Adapted from Burton.[11])

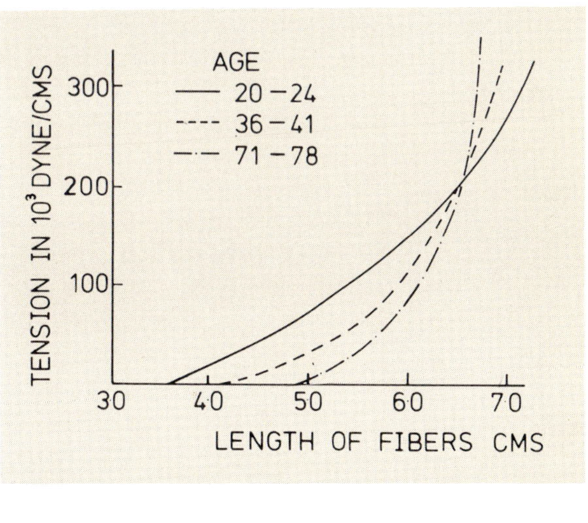

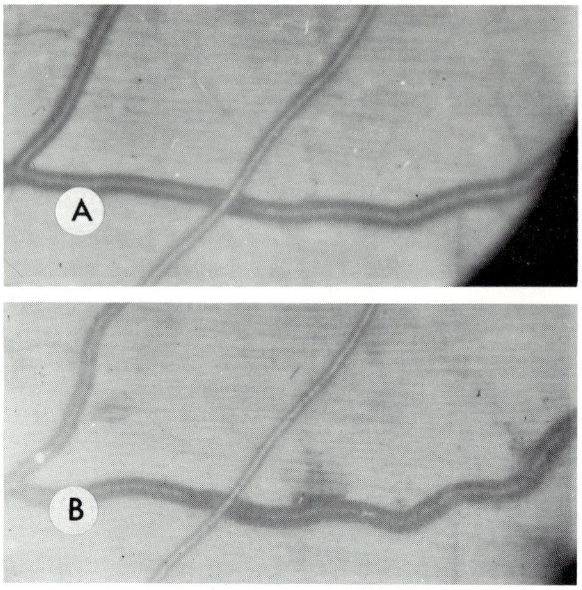

Fig. 6-8. *A*, Retinal vein of a pig before obstruction. *B*, After obstruction the vein stretches both circumferentially and lengthwise so it becomes dilated and tortuous.

The vessel walls resist stretching more strongly as the degree of stretch increases. This is due to the mixture of collagen and elastin in most vessel walls and to the variation in the degree of stretch of different fibers. The initial part of the length-tension diagram represents elastic tissue stretching and a small number of collagen fibers that are fully straightened at this length. The steeply rising part of the curve is caused by successive collagen fibers reaching their maximum unstretched length.

Aging is accompanied by an increase in the number of collagen fibers and a tightening up of individual fibers so that they exert a more powerful force with a smaller degree of stretch to the wall. In the human retina the vessels possess little or no elastic tissue, but collagen is present in the walls both of arterioles and veins. The length-tension diagram of retinal vessels has not been determined, but it is probably similar to that of larger vessels.

Increases in vascular transmural pressure increase the tone in a vessel wall and in the case of a thin-walled structure, such as a retinal vein, they will cause it to dilate. Besides the increase in circumference there will also be an increase in length caused by the increased longitudinal tone.

Thus, when a retinal vein is occluded the diameter of the vessel may increase by 20 per cent and the length by 10 per cent. As the vessel cannot elongate because it is tethered at various points it adopts a tortuous, looped configuration (Fig. 6-8).

PRESSURE-FLOW RELATIONSHIPS AND ROLE OF VASCULAR TONE

In almost all vascular beds flow ceases before the perfusion pressure reaches zero (Fig. 6-9). This positive intercept on the pressure axis at no-flow may be as little as 5 mmHg but can be much larger. The highest values observed in man has been 94 mmHg in the forearm of a patient with hypertension. Burton [11] has defined the pressure at which flow ceases as the "critical closing pressure (CCP)." A small value of CCP ($>$ 5 mmHg) is found even in vascular beds where all vasomotor activity has been

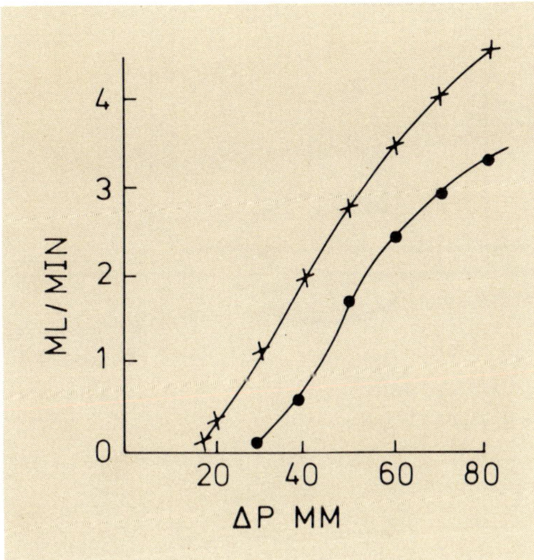

Fig. 6-9. Plot of pressure versus flow in the vascular bed of a rabbit leg. Flow ceases before the pressure reaches zero, without vasomotor tone **(x—x).** After sympathetic stimulation the closing pressure is higher (•—•). (From Burton.[11])

abolished by cyanide. Thus, this small residual CCP seems to depend upon "the interfacial tension," between blood and the vessel wall. It can be reduced experimentally by using Tween 80, an agent which lowers surface tension.

In small vessels a CCP of about 5 mmHg could be theoretically accounted for by the coherence resistance of the blood cells at low velocity. However, for blood it has not been possible to find a positive value of pressure at which flow through rigid tubes ceases.

ACTIVE TONE AND CLOSING PRESSURE

In a blood vessel there is tension (T) in the wall as a result of elastic stretch (T_E) and vasomotion (T_A). If the vessel of radius (R) is in equilibrium, the transmural pressure (P_{TM}) must be balanced by the tension in the wall (Fig. 6-10). This is the law of Laplace:

$$P_{TM} = \frac{T}{R} \tag{6-8}$$

The law of Laplace means that active tension exerted by smooth muscle may produce instability. Suppose that the tension is slightly increased in a vessel in equilibrium.

Fig. 6-10. The tension in the vessel wall **(T)** which balances the transmural pressure **(P_{TM})** is related to the radius, **R.**

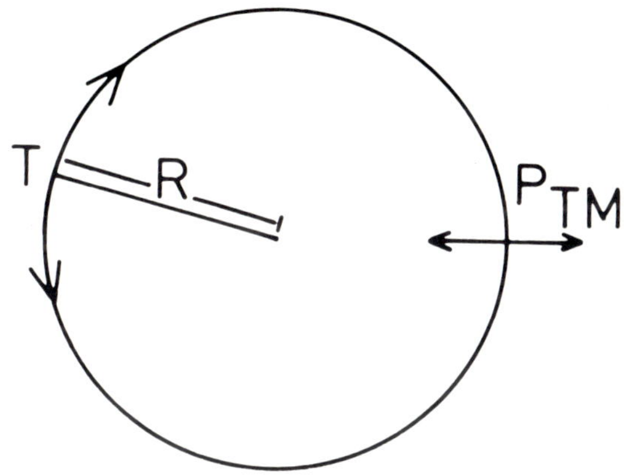

The radius of the vessel will be slightly decreased by the increase of tension so that the pressure it is capable of opposing will be higher. If the intravascular pressure is unchanged a small increase in tension might close the vessel because as the radius decreases a smaller and smaller tension is needed to balance the transmural pressure in the vessel. The same phenomenon is illustrated by two soap bubbles connected by a tube. Whichever bubble is the smaller will pump up the larger one and collapse itself. The tension in the two soap films will be the same so that whichever has the smaller radius will be able to exert a higher pressure and so blow up the other. As the smaller bubble gets still smaller its radius decreases and it exerts a bigger pressure, while the larger bubble whose radius is increasing requires less and less pressure to inflate it. Burton [11] has expressed this tendency of vessels to close in the equation:

$$CCP = \frac{T_A}{r_o} \qquad (6\text{-}9)$$

If this analysis should be correct one would expect a vessel whose wall is mainly composed of smooth muscle to be fully open or fully closed. This prediction is not fulfilled by microscopic observations of terminal vascular beds. In some beds alternate opening and closing of precapillary sphincters is observed; while in others graded variations of size occur. The elastic stretch (T_E) provides a stabilizing influence by its reduction in tension as the lumen diameter is reduced.

It is difficult to measure CCP in practice because it requires that flow should be reduced to zero which will often change vascular tone. Furthermore, this concept neglects the influence of wall thickness. Constriction of a vessel with finite wall thickness, increases thickness and internal stresses develop. As a result very large tensions will be required to close the vessel completely.[25]

In the eye there is little evidence for a significant closing pressure. In experimental hemorrhagic shock the no-flow point was reached at a mean systemic blood pressure of 15 mmHg, about the level of the intraocular pressure. This puts an upper level on the CCP although it may have been affected by reactive hyperemia under these circumstances.

The nearest approach to arteriolar closure caused by active tone in the retinal vessels occurred in the eyes of rats with experimental malignant hypertension. In these animals severe, but reversible, focal narrowing was a frequent finding.[12] The smooth muscle tone must have been high enough to approach closure despite the high transmural pressure. Closure of human retinal vessels by "spasm" has not been demonstrated although reversible focal narrowing has been observed in toxemia of pregnancy.

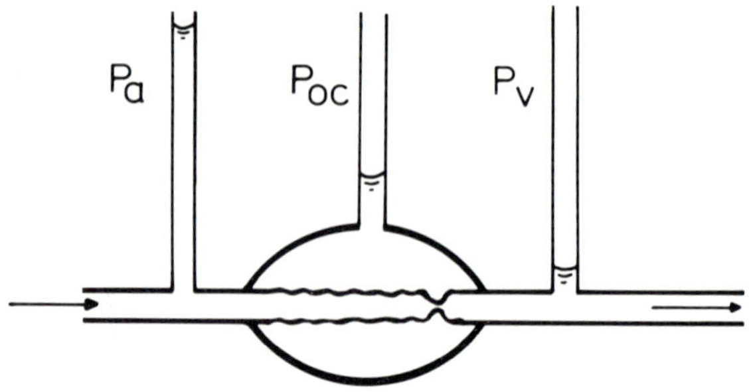

Fig. 6-11. The retinal vessels are collapsible tubes within a relatively rigid sphere. The arterial pressure (**P**$_a$) exceeds the intraocular pressure (**P**$_{oc}$), which in turn exceeds the downstream venous pressure, **P**$_v$.

THE VASCULAR WATERFALL OR SLUICE

The resistor used in the Starling heart-lung preparation is a collapsible tube within a rigid sphere. Resistance is increased by raising the pressure in the rigid sphere (Fig. 6-11). The hydrodynamic characteristics [53] of such a tube are applicable to some hemodynamic problems in the eye. The pressure-flow relationship is linear, but flow ceases not when arterial pressure, P_a, reaches zero but when it reaches the intraocular pressure, P_{oc}. This occurs because the pressure surrounding the tube tends to collapse it and the transmural pressure (P_{TM}) reaches zero when $P_a = P_{oc}$. The situation is more complex if the vascular bed has active vasomotor tone and exhibits a CCP phenomenon. In this case both P_{oc} and CCP have an additive effect in opposing P_a: Thus when the vessel closes and the radius, r_o, reaches zero [53]

$$P_{TM} = P_a - \left(\frac{T_A}{r_o} + P_{oc}\right) \qquad (6\text{-}10)$$

The Starling resistor also has interesting properties in terms of downstream pressure effects upon resistance and flow. It is usual to calculate vascular resistance as the arterial, P_a, minus the venous, P_v, pressure divided by the flow. However, in the Starling resistor variations in downstream venous pressure have no effect upon flow unless the downstream pressure exceeds P_{oc}. The driving pressure for calculating resistance is $P_a - P_{oc}$ not $P_a - P_v$. Thus, the pressure in the retinal veins at the outflow from the eye will depend upon the value of P_{oc}. The flow over a waterfall or sluice is independent of downstream pressure so long as it is lower than the upstream pressure. The vascular waterfall is so named because of this. In the eye, in most circumstances, downstream venous pressure will be less than P_{oc} but in conditions of increased intracranial tension the downstream pressure might exceed it and thus lead to a rise in retinal venous pressure and dilatation of the veins.

The second possible site for a vascular waterfall lies in the vessels with active tone. Here P_{TM} is higher but in small vessels with active tension there is a possibility that the CCP added to P_{oc} may be sufficient to close the vessel under some circumstances. This has the interesting consequence that obstruction of individual capillaries in a bed may not alter the driving pressure applied to the capillary bed so long as some channels of the network are patent, and the capillary pressure does not rise above the closing pressure.

PULSATILE PRESSURE AND BLOOD FLOW

Poiseuille's law applies only to steady flow but in most parts of the arterial tree both pressure and flow are oscillatory. Different concepts are needed to handle this situation and those who understand the difference between the electrical theory of direct (dc) and alternating (ac) current will find the analogy helpful. In a dc circuit the current varies directly with the applied voltage and inversely with the resistance of the circuit. This is true in an ac circuit if it is purely resistive, but if the circuit contains inductive or capacitative elements there will be a phase difference between voltage and current.

If pulsatile pressure and flow are measured in a large artery the maximum flow precedes the maximum pressure. This is because large arteries have a capacitative input impedance at low frequencies.

A phase difference between pressure gradient and flow occurs because of the inertia of the blood. As the pressure gradient increases the flow lags behind it and when the pressure gradient declines or reverses the momentum of the blood tends to keep it moving in the original direction for a short time.

An oscillatory pressure creates an oscillatory pressure gradient and as the wave may be reflected from the periphery, further difficulties in analysis are created.

The mathematical solution of the problem of pulsatile flow was proposed as long ago as 1914 and one of the clearest analyses is that of Womersley.[61]

The arterial pressure pulse has a complex waveform, very different from a pure sine wave. Mathematical analysis is much easier for sine waves so it is usual to analyze a complex waveform into a fundamental frequency and different proportions of harmonics. By this means, known as "Fourier analysis," any periodic wave form can be reproduced.

Full details of Womersley's equations, which are used for analysis of oscillatory flow, need not concern us, but it is of great importance that in small vessels the formula simplifies to:

$$Flow = \frac{\pi R^4}{8\mu L} \times (P_1 - P_2)$$

This is a restatement of Poiseuille's law so that in smaller vessels the deviation from it caused by pulsatile pressure is small. The phase difference between pressure and flow can be calculated from the nondimensional constant, α.[44] For a vessel of radius, R, blood density, ρ, viscosity, μ, order of harmonics, n, and fundamental frequency, f, α equals:

$$\alpha = R\sqrt{\frac{2\pi n f \rho}{\mu}} \qquad (6\text{-}11)$$

In a retinal arteriole of man with a radius of 0.006 cm, fundamental frequency of 60 beats per minute, blood density 1.054 gm per milliliter, and viscosity of 0.02 P at 37°C the value of α will be about 0.11.

At such a low value of α the phase lag of flow with respect to pressure will be very small, probably less than two degrees[44] while the relationship between the maximum and steady flow will approach unity. Thus, there should be little deviation from Poiseuille's formula in the retinal vessels.

METHODS OF STUDYING CIRCULATION

Direct methods of measuring pressure and flow in retinal vessels are impractical. Although Duke-Elder[22] succeeded in making direct retinal vascular punctures, most research in animals and man must rely upon standard methods of measuring systemic blood pressure and in the eye, upon ophthalmodynamometry and tonometry. Direct-flow measurements with devices such as the drop counter or electromagnetic flow meter are not applicable to such tiny vessels as are found in the retina. Lack of direct-flow measurements make it particularly important to understand the advantages and limitations of dye-dilution curves for studying retinal hemodynamics.

INDICATOR-DILUTION CURVES

Colored dyes and other substances have been used to study the velocity of flow and circulation time, for many years. Dyes are now used to measure both blood flow and blood volume by sampling downstream to a point of sudden or constant injection. The time-concentration curve of the indicator is recorded by withdrawing blood at a constant rate through a cuvette sampling device with a photoelectric system which gives a linear response to changes in concentration. The use of these techniques in physiology and cardiology is well understood and much work has been done on the theoretical basis of the interpretation of the curves. A particularly thorough account is that of Zierler.[62]

The eye can be used as a cuvette by recording a time-concentration curve of dye either from the whole retina or from individual vessels. If the response of the recording system can be calibrated in terms of dye concentration, the curves can be used to calculate cardiac output, and blood volume between the point of injection and points on the arterial tree equivalent to the sampling point in the eye. However, there is no advantage in using the eye and indeed many disadvantages as compared with an arterial cuvette. The shape of the curve recorded by a cuvette is altered by the rate of blood flow through it, but the flow through the cuvette cannot be calculated from the curve. Thus, retinal blood flow cannot be calculated from a single indicator curve recorded from a retinal vessel. However, curves recorded separately from an artery and a vein in the eye can be used to calculate differences in transit time and changes in retinal blood volume and/or flow thus inferred (Fig. 6-12).

To understand something more of these problems it is necessary to consider the theoretical basis of their interpretation.

BLOOD FLOW

Stewart[58] was the first to employ indicator methods for measuring blood flow. He injected sodium chloride solution into the blood stream at a constant rate for several seconds and measured the concentration in a downstream artery. If the amount, q, injected over time, t, is known it is only necessary to measure the concentration of the indicator, c, after it is fully mixed downstream to calculate the flow, F. Unfortunately, this simple method is difficult to apply in man because early recirculation of the indicator through vascular beds with a high flow, such as the kidney and heart, causes an alteration to the baseline. The method can be used in segments of the circulation where the measurement can be completed before there is recirculation. Flow is calculated from the relationship:

$$q/t = F \times c \qquad (6\text{-}12)$$

The alternative, and more widely used method of measuring the flow, introduced by Hamilton et al.[29] is by instantaneous injection of the indicator. When an indicator is injected suddenly into a flowing system the concentration at the outflow will be some function of time, $c(t)$. The rate at which indicator leaves the system at any moment, t, is a product of its concentration at that moment and the unknown flow. Over a period of time all the indicator will leave the system. Thus, if the product of concentration $c(t)$ and flow (F) are summed this must be equal to the total amount of indicator (q).

$$q = F \int_0^\infty c(t)\, dt \qquad (6\text{-}13)$$

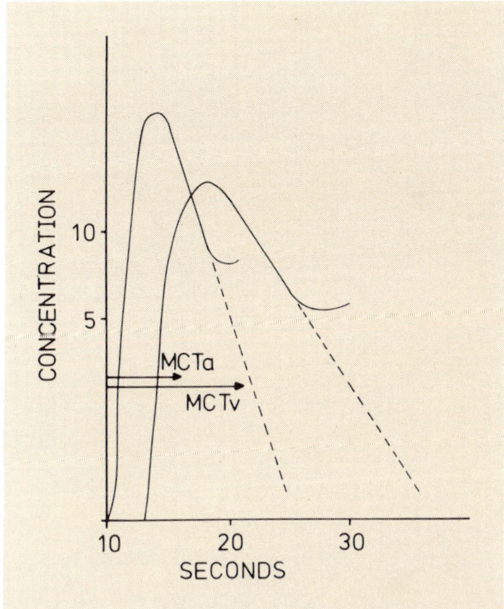

Fig. 6-12. Mean circulation time can be calculated from separate dye curves recorded from a branch retinal artery (**MCT**$_a$) and vein (**MCT**$_v$) to the same quadrant. The difference between these times is the mean transit time through that part of the retinal circulation.

Fig. 6-13. Dye-dilution curve on a semilogarithmic plot. The time between injection and the arrival of dye is the appearance time **(AT).** The curve area can be calculated by extrapolating the downslope to infinity.

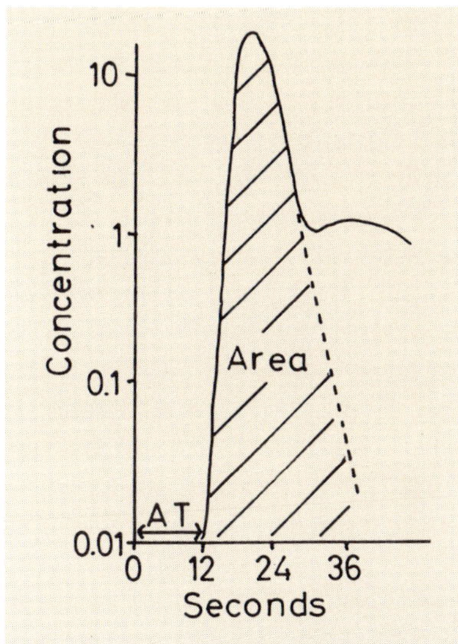

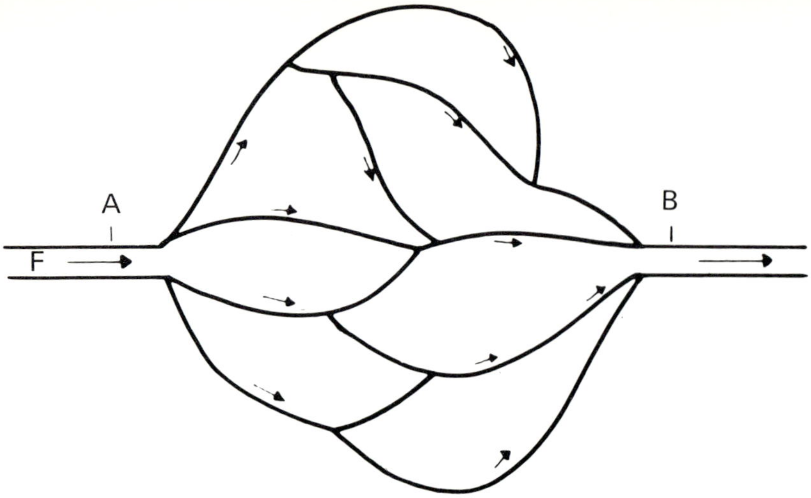

Fig. 6-14. Diagram of a branching system of blood vessels with different path lengths which are followed by fluid flowing from **A** to **B.**

The integral between zero and infinity of $c(t)\ dt$ is equivalent to the area (A) under the curve and Equation 6-2 can be rewritten:

$$q = F \times A \text{ or } F = q/A \qquad (6\text{-}14)$$

The area under a dye-dilution curve can be calculated by summing. The problem of recirculation is overcome by extrapolating the exponential downslope to infinity (Fig. 6-13).

BLOOD VOLUME AND MEAN TRANSIT TIME

The method of deriving volume from indicator-dilution curves is not so straightforward as flow. Consider a system of tubes with a single inflow point (**A**), outflow (**B**), a blood volume (**V**) and flow (**F**) (Fig. 6-14). Dye molecules entering **A** may take a variable time to reach **B** depending upon the length of the path they follow and their velocity. Thus, the dye does not have a single transit time but a range of transit times. If flow, volume, and the distribution of transit times (stationarity) are constant the volume can be calculated from the time-concentration curve.

If a quantity of dye, q, is injected at point **A** and the concentration at **B** at time t is $c(t)$ the amount of indicator leaving the system in a small interval of time dt is given by Equation 6-13 above. This can be restated as:

$$F = \frac{q}{\int_0^\infty c(t)\ dt}$$

It is now necessary to calculate the function which describes the distribution of transit times, $h(t)$; $h(t)$ is the fraction of indicator leaving the system per unit time at time, t.

$$h(t) = \frac{Fc(t)}{q} \qquad (6\text{-}15)$$

The fraction of indicator leaving the eye in unit time represents the frequency with which that transit time occurs. The sum of all these fractions when all the indicator has left the system must equal unity. Let us assume that a small element of the volume initially present, dV, leaves the system in the time interval t to $t + dt$ and the fraction of the dye having this transit time is $h(t)\ dt$. Then, as the rate at which fluid enters and leaves is the total flow, F, the rate at which dV leaves the system will be $Fh(t)\ dt$. The volume of such particles is the time required for them to leave is the rate multiplied by the time, t.

$$dV = tFh(t)\ dt$$

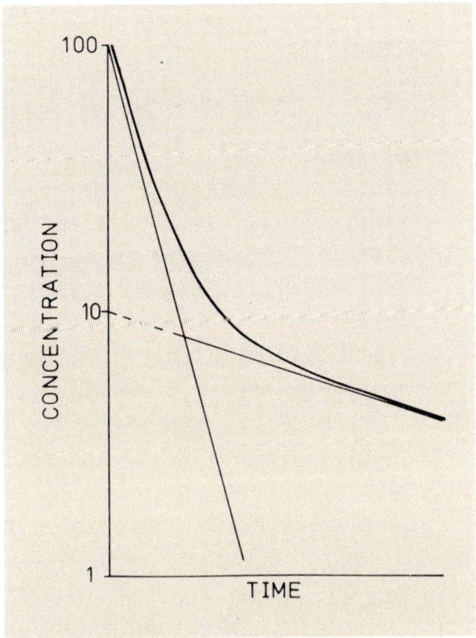

Fig. 6-15. The individual components of double-exponential washout can be evaluated by stripping the longest lived from the mixed curve and replotting the remainder which is the short-lived component.

the volume of the system will be therefore the sum of all the elements dV.

$$V = F \int_0^\infty th(t)\, dt \qquad (6\text{-}16)$$

As $h(t)$ is the frequency function of the transit time, this integral is the mean of the transit times, $\bar{t}$.

Thus, volume = flow × mean transit time:

$$V = F\bar{t} \qquad (6\text{-}17)$$

In a system where flow is constant and an indicator curve can be recorded at two points without loss of indicator between them, the differences in mean transit time can be used to calculate the volume. Alternatively, if the volume can be measured or assumed to be unchanged, the alterations in mean transit time between two sampling points on the same closed vascular system can be used to calculate changes in flow.

When indicator-dilution curves are applied to the eye there are a number of practical difficulties. Fluorescence is only related to concentration of dye in blood over a limited range of concentrations. It is necessary to ensure that the peak concentration achieved remains within this linear range and that the film exposure and processing give a linear change in optical density in relation to changes in fluorescein concentration.[10,31] It is then necessary to scan across the width of the vessel to determine the mean concentration on each frame.[10] A further difficulty is that fluorescent light is strongly absorbed by the red pigment hemoglobin. This means that a greater proportion of the light falling on the film will come from fluorescein in the more superficial layers of the blood column than from the deeper layers. Such a sample may not be representative of events across the whole thickness of the vessel and may lead to errors.

INERT GAS WASHOUT

There are similarities between the inert gas washout methods and other indicator-dilution techniques. It is assumed that the dissolved gas, both xenon 133 (^{133}Xe) or krypton 85 (^{85}Kr) are widely used, diffuses readily into the tissues and the relative concentration in blood and tissue depends only upon the solubility of the gas in them. The radioactive gas may be introduced into the tissue either by rebreathing air which contains trace amounts of the isotope or by intraarterial injection of the gas dissolved in saline. Once the administration of the isotope ceases the amount in the tissue is washed out by the blood flow. In each unit of time a fixed proportion of the isotope will be removed depending upon the volume of blood flowing through the tissue in that time, the volume of the tissue, and the relative solubility of the gas in blood and tissue. Thus, the rate of change of concentration with time, *dc/dt,* will be proportional to a constant, *K,* relating blood flow to tissue volume. The rate of fall of concentration will be exponential since a fixed proportion is lost per unit time. The initial concentration, C_o, is related to the concentration at time, t, C_t, by the formula:

$$C_t = C_o\, e^{-Kt} \qquad (6\text{-}18)$$

The advantage of this method is that it is unnecessary to measure the absolute amount of radioactivity in the tissue, only the rate of change is needed. The rate constant, *K,* can be measured from the exponential slope of decline in tissue radioactivity and the blood flow per unit of tissue volume can be calculated if the relative solubilities are known. The solubility of the isotope in the blood and the tissue being studied can be measured on a separate occasion.

In many tissues there is nonuniform distribution of blood flow and in this case the downslope will contain more than one exponent. If the rate constants are well separated the change in slope can be detected on the graph and they can be read off separately by extrapolating the line (Fig. 6-15). Friedman, Kopald, and Smith have used this method to measure the retinal and choroidal blood flow in cats.[26]

PRESSURE AND FLOW MEASUREMENTS IN RETINAL VESSELS

Measurements of retinal vascular resistance requires knowledge of the retinal blood flow and of the arterial and venous pressure in the central retinal vessels. The measurements available for all these quantities are inexact.

PRESSURE

The pressure in the central retinal artery can be measured by the technique of ophthalmodynamometry. In this method the intraocular pressure is raised either by pressing on the globe with a spring-loaded plunger or, in animals, by placing a needle in the anterior chamber and raising the pressure by introducing fluid. As the pressure is raised visible pulsation in the artery increases and the point of first complete collapsing pulsation is taken as the diastolic pressure, and the point at which pulsation disappears is taken as the systolic pressure.[6] Many formulas have been suggested for relating the brachial artery pressure measured with the sphygmomanometer to the retinal arterial pressure measured by ophthalmodynamometry.[60] There is no physiologic reason why the relationship should be constant and such efforts are misdirected.

Duke-Elder[22] undertook direct measurements in cats using a micropuncture technique. In five cats the average intraocular pressure was 24 mmHg, the retinal arterial systolic pressure 88.5 mmHg, and diastolic pressure 64 mmHg. Duke-Elder has pointed out that as ophthalmodynamometry requires that flow should be arrested to secure a reading it therefore cannot be taken as a measure of pressure in the retinal vessels but should approximate to the value in the ophthalmic artery as it enters the eye. Duke-Elder's measurements show that the pressure gradient between the carotid artery and the retinal artery under normal circumstances is small. The gradient may be increased in hypertension.[41] The pressure in both the carotid and retinal arteries is decreased by carotid artery ligation in the neck, but ophthalmodynamometry has not proved a completely reliable method for diagnosing carotid artery occlusions, presumably because of the formation of effective collaterals.[57] It may be concluded that the retinal arterial pressure at the disc is only a little less than the carotid pressure but there is no method of measuring it in man of sufficient precision to quantitate small changes.

Duke-Elder went on to measure the intraocular venous pressure and found that it was about 2 mmHg above the intraocular pressure. He has pointed out that there must be a rapid change in pressure in the retinal veins as they emerged from the eye. As we have already seen (on p. 94) there must be a vascular waterfall or sluice at the outflow from the eye, and Duke-Elder's measurements fulfill the prediction that the retinal venous pressure will always be very slightly above the intraocular pressure. This finding has important consequences for interpreting changes in the caliber of retinal veins, for the transmural pressure in the veins will depend chiefly upon the flow and the rheology of the blood in the retinal veins. Increase in blood flow or viscosity would be expected to increase the transmural pressure in the veins while decreases would reduce it. If the wall of the vein behaves as a purely passive structure, changes in vein diameter should be a reliable indication of flow changes. The amount of vasomotion that the vein wall can achieve is unknown. There is relatively little smooth muscle in the wall of large retinal veins but it remains to be seen whether they are entirely inactive. Many caliber changes can be explained by an increase in pressure gradient in veins following a change in blood flow or viscosity. Thus, moderate degrees of hemorrhagic hypotension cause arteriolar dilatation, presumably as an attempt at autoregulation. Here the diameter of the veins decreases, probably because the flow falls.[21] Conditions which increase blood viscosity, such as the dysproteinemias, are associated with dilated retinal veins and this dilatation can be reversed by plasmapheresis which reduces viscosity.[13] The decrease in caliber of veins during oxygen breathing may be a response to changes in oxygen pressure in the retinal tissue or venous blood, but it may also be a reflection of the drop in blood flow which takes place.

FLOW

There is virtually no data, reliable or otherwise, on retinal blood flow. Several authors have measured transit times from retinal artery to veins using fluorescein angiograms. Thus, Oberhoff, Evans, and Delaney[48] have recorded that the artery to vein time was 1.8 to 1.9 seconds in the temporal vessels, 2.3 to 2.4 seconds in the nasal vessels, and 1.2 seconds at the macula. Hart and co-workers[30] have suggested that the artery to vein time was about 5 seconds for large vessels where they crossed the disc edge. Such measurements are of limited value and should not be confused with mathematically acceptable measurements of mean transit time.

Hickam and Frayser[31] have measured the mean time between the injection of fluorescein dye and its transit through the main veins and arterioles at the disc. The difference between these two times is the mean transit time of the retinal circulation. In 29 normal men the figure was 4.7 ± 1.1 seconds. This time was measured from all the vessels around the optic disc and is not the same as the mean transit time for one quadrant. Bulpitt and Dollery[10] have recorded dilution curves of fluorescein from an artery and vein to one quadrant of the retina using film processing and dye concentrations within a linear range, and scanning the negative with a recording microdensitometer. In the superior temporal quadrant the mean transit time was about 2.5 seconds in normals and about half this in patients with severe anemia. It is not possible to translate mean transit time measurements into bulk flow rates unless the volume of the system is known and this cannot be measured at present.

Direct measurements of flow using high-speed, cine-fluorescence photography seem promising.[18] The velocity of flow is greatly reduced in animals with hypotension due to blood loss.[21] Thus, the axial velocity of flow in an artery of about 160 μ diameter was 44 mm per second at a mean arterial pressure of 110 mmHg, 28 mm per second at 45 mmHg and 3.6 mm per second at 20 mmHg. It is also reduced by increasing the intraocular pressure using a limbal suction cup.[20] Thus, in one experiment when the mean systemic blood pressure averaged 88 mmHg the axial velocity dropped from 38.5 mm per second at an intraocular pressure of 5 mmHg to 3.0 mm per second when the pressure in the eye was raised to 50 mmHg.

Conversion of these axial velocity measurements to bulk flow involves assumptions about the velocity profile and measurement of the internal diameter of the vessel. In animals the axial velocity in an artery of about 120 μ diameter is about 30 mm per second. If the velocity profile were parabolic this would indicate a blood flow rate of about 10 μL per minute. However, recent unpublished work by Bulpitt suggests that the velocity profile is relatively flat and this velocity with plug flow corresponds to about 5 μL per minute. The measurements made in man by this method have larger errors but velocities in vessels of the same size are comparable to those found in animals.

Under normal circumstances flow in retinal arteries is pulsatile but the relationship between mean and peak flow has not been measured. Calculations for the normal eye suggest that difference would be small. If the intraocular pressure is raised the difference is exaggerated and backflow in diastole is prominent.[20]

OXYGEN UPTAKE

The color of blood changes as the proportions of oxyhemoglobin and reduced hemoglobin are varied. Most laboratory methods for measuring oxygen saturation depend upon the color change. Hickam and Frayser have made use of a photographic method to measure the oxygen saturation of the hemoglobin in retinal veins.[31] They passed the image of the large vessels at the disc through a beam splitter fitted with red and green interference filters.

The retina proved to have a fairly high arteriovenous oxygen difference as the saturation in the retinal veins averaged 55 per cent. If the flow through the superior temporal artery in man is 10 μl a minute the oxygen uptake of the quadrant of retina which it supplies will be about 0.8 μl a minute. We have used a similar beam splitting device to record images of the same retinal vessels side-by-side through red and green interference filters (Fig. 6-16).

OXYGEN DIFFUSION

The retina is supplied by oxygen from both the retinal and choroidal capillaries. Given the oxygen tension in the blood vessels, the diffusion constant of oxygen in the tissues and the oxygen uptake per unit mass of tissue, it is possible to calculate the oxygen tension at any point in the retina.[19] Such calculations have interesting consequences because of the special characteristics of the choroidal circulation. They may explain the exaggerated response of the retinal vessels to oxygen and the paradox that the oxygen uptake of the normal retina appears to fall to only 44 per cent of the resting value during oxygen breathing at 1 atmosphere.[31]

To calculate the proportion of the retina supplied by the retinal and choroidal circulations under different circumstances it is necessary to make a number of assumptions. These include values for the retinal and choroidal blood flow. Friedman, Kopald, and Smith[26] have used an inert-gas washout technique in anesthetized cats and found the choroidal blood flow to be 1200 ml/100 gm of

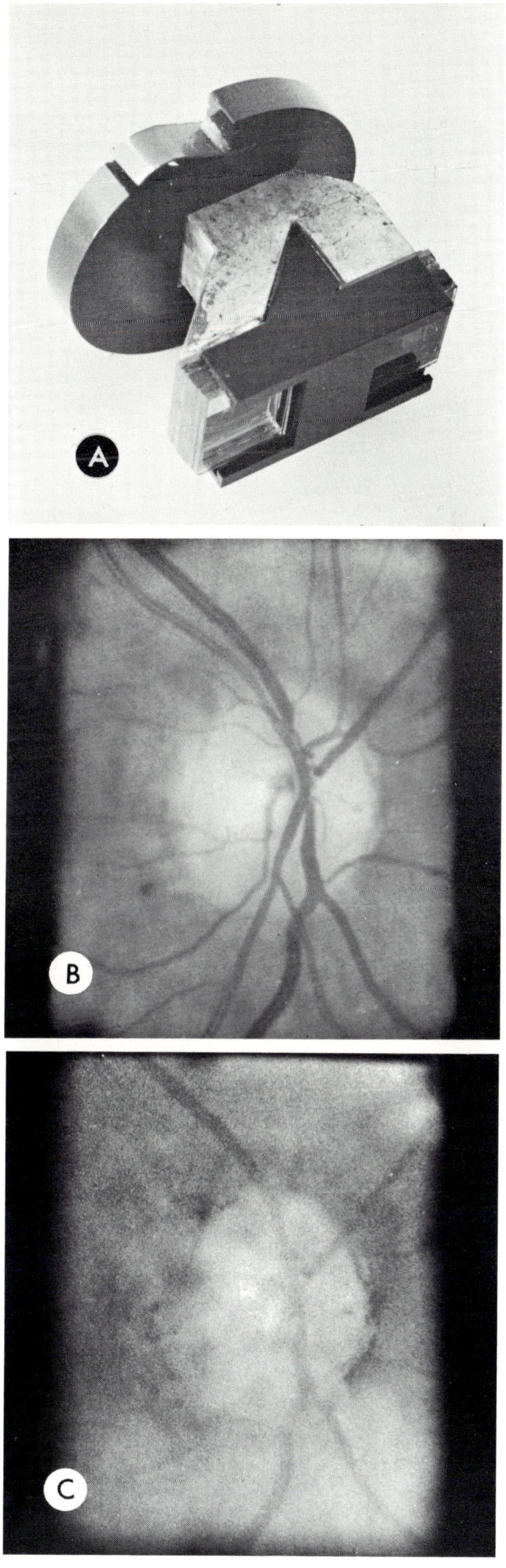

Fig. 6-16. *A*, Beam splitter used to form side-by-side image of retinal vessels through red and green interference filters. *B*, Image recorded through the beam splitter and green filter shows both arteries and veins clearly. *C*, Through the red filter only the veins have appreciable optical density because of their bluer color.

tissue per minute and the retinal blood flow to be 166 ml/100 gm of tissue per minute. Bill has calculated the blood flow in the rabbit choroid and retina to be 1000 ml/100 gm of tissue per minute.[7] The second assumption is the hemoglobin saturation of the retinal venous and choroidal venous blood. This has been measured in the human retinal circulation by Hickam and Frayser.[31] These authors have found that the retinal venous saturation was 55 per cent during air breathing and 82 per cent during oxygen breathing at 1 atmosphere. At pH 7.4 these saturations are equivalent to retinal venous pO_2 values of 28.5 and 48 mm. The arteriovenous difference across the uveal tract of the dog eye has been measured by Elgin.[23] He has found an arterial oxygen tension of 85 mm and a uveal venous tension of 69 mm during air breathing. During oxygen breathing the average arterial oxygen tension was 419 mm and the average uveal venous tension 252 mm. As the arterial oxygen tension in anesthetized animals does not rise as high as it does in a normal man breathing oxygen these figures must be adjusted. We have assumed a figure of 600 mmHg for the arterial oxygen tension in man during oxygen breathing at 1 atmosphere. We have assumed that the arteriovenous oxygen difference in the human choroid would be the same as in the dog uveal circulation, namely 167 mm. This gives a figure for choroidal oxygen tension during oxygen breathing at 1 atmosphere of 433 mmHg. It is also necessary to make assumptions about the thickness of the retina. The retina varies from approximately 300-μ thick near the optic disc to less than half that thickness at the periphery. Furthermore, the retinal capillaries do not run on the surface of the retina but penetrate into it forming a deep layer from which the retinal veins drain (Fig. 6-17). That part of the human retina which lies between the deep layer of retinal capillaries and the choriocapillaris is about 100 μ thick. The diffusion constant for oxygen has not been measured in the retina and we have used the value measured by Krogh in muscle, 1.7×10^{-5} ml of oxygen per minute per square centimeter of retina at 37°C in a concentration gradient of 1 atmosphere per cm.[33]

It is necessary to calculate the oxygen consumption per a 100-gm retina per minute. Assuming a choroidal blood flow of 1200 ml per 100 gm of tissue per minute and an arteriovenous difference of 0.5 ml of oxygen per 100 ml of blood the oxygen uptake is 6 ml per 100 gm of tissue per minute. The corresponding calculation for the retinal circulation gives a figure of 13 ml per 100 gm per minute. It is difficult to know how much overlap there is between the retinal and choroidal tissue pools whose blood flow is measured by the inert gas washout method. We have assumed they are separate and have therefore taken an average value of 9.5 ml of oxygen per 100 gm per minute to represent the oxygen uptake.

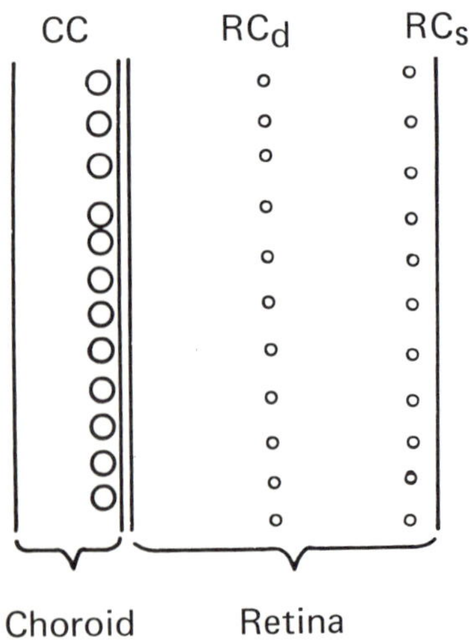

Fig. 6-17. Diagram showing the relationship between the superficial (**RC**$_s$) and the deep (**RC**$_d$) retinal capillaries and the choriocapillaris, **CC**.

CALCULATION OF RETINAL OXYGEN DIFFUSION

The rate of diffusion across a square centimeter of retina parallel to the surface is $\frac{Ddp}{dx}$ where D is the diffusion constant and $\frac{dp}{dx}$ is the rate of change of oxygen pressure with depth. The rate of accumulation of oxygen at a point x cm from the surface will be $D\frac{d^2p}{dx^2}$ and under steady-state conditions this must equal the amount of oxygen consumed by the tissue, M ml O_2 per 100 gm of tissue per minute.

$$M = D\frac{d^2p}{dx^2} \qquad (6\text{-}19)$$

The solution of this equation is:

$$p = \frac{Mx^2}{2D} + Bx + p_o \qquad (6\text{-}20)$$

where p_o is the oxygen pressure constantly maintained at the surface and B is a constant of integration. When $x = 0$, $p = p_o$.

In a tissue consuming oxygen the value of p will fall as the distance from the blood supply increases and a point will be reached either were $p = 0$, or in the case of the retina which is supplied from both sides, where the pressures from the choroidal and the retinal circulations balance. At this point diffusion of oxygen must stop and the concentration gradient $\frac{dp}{dx}$ becomes zero. If x_b cm is the distance from the choroidal surface where the pressures balance then:

$$\frac{dp}{dx} = 0 = \frac{Mx_b}{D} + B \qquad (6\text{-}21)$$

$$B = -\frac{Mx_b}{D}$$

and by substitution in Equation 6-20

$$p = \frac{Mx^2}{2D} - \frac{Mxx_b}{D} + p_o$$

At the point where the pressures balance $x = x_b$ and the equation simplifies to:

$$p = \frac{Mx_b^2}{2D} - \frac{Mx_b^2}{D} + p_o$$

or

$$p = p_o - \frac{Mx_b^2}{2D} \qquad (6\text{-}22)$$

If the oxygen pressure constant maintained at the choroidal surface is p_c and at the retinal surface it is p_r the point of balance, x_b cm from the choroidal surface, can be calculated. If the thickness of retina between the choroid and the deep retinal capillaries is 0.01 cm, the distance between the point of balance and the deep retinal capillaries will be $0.01 - x_b$. Thus:

$$p_c - \frac{Mx_b^2}{2D} = p_r - \frac{M(0.01 - x_b)^2}{2D}$$

This equation simplifies to:

$$x_b = \frac{2D}{0.02M}(p_c - p_r) - 0.005 \qquad (6\text{-}23)$$

As all the other values have been measured this equation can be solved at different values of p_c and p_r. During air breathing 40 per cent of the retina between the two circulations is supplied by the retinal vessels (Fig. 6-18), while if the arterial oxygen tension, p_aO_2, is increased to 400 mmHg, 97 per cent of the thickness of the retina between the two circulations can be supplied from the choroid (Fig. 6-19). At higher pressures there is a net delivery of oxygen from the choroid to the deep retinal capillaries.

OXYGEN SUPPLY FROM THE CHOROID ALONE

If the retinal vessels are interrupted the tissue oxygen tension will fall as distance from the choroid increases and a point will

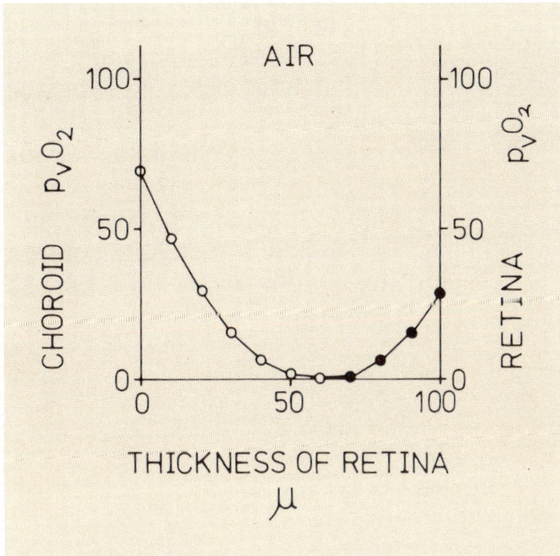

Fig. 6-18. Diagram of the calculated oxygen tension at different points in the retina between the deep retinal capillaries and the choriocapillaris during air breathing.

Fig. 6-19. Diagram of the calculated oxygen tension at different points in the retina between the deep retinal capillaries and the choriocapillaris during 70% oxygen breathing.

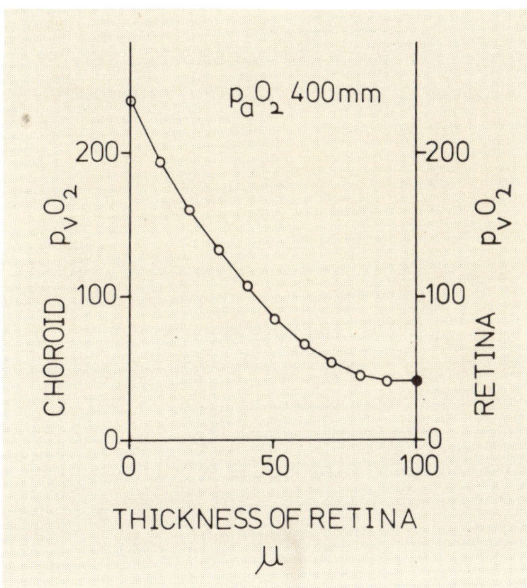

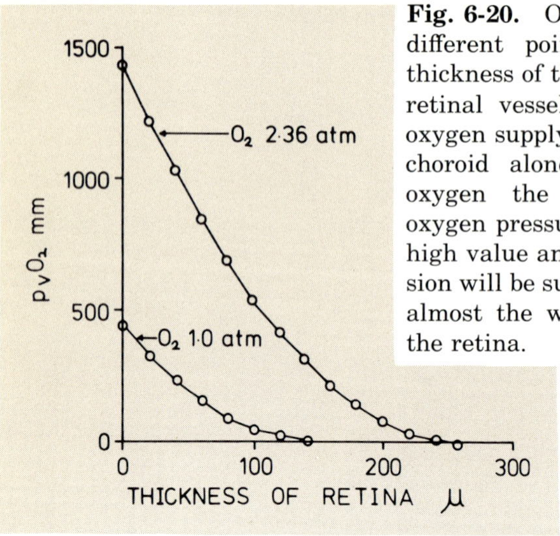

Fig. 6-20. Oxygen tensions at different points through the thickness of the retina with the retinal vessels obstructed and oxygen supply coming from the choroid alone. In hyperbaric oxygen the choroidal-venous oxygen pressure rises to a very high value and the oxygen tension will be sufficient to nourish almost the whole thickness of the retina.

be reached where $p = 0$. At this point diffusion of oxygen must stop and the concentration gradient $\frac{dp}{dx}$ becomes zero. If x_a is the distance from the choroid where $p = 0$ then from Equation 6-21:

$$\frac{dp}{dx} = \frac{Mx_a}{D} + B$$

so when $\frac{dp}{dx} = 0$

$$B = -\frac{Mx_a}{D}$$

substituting this value of B in Equation 6-2 when $x = x_a$ gives the value of x_a which is the greatest depth to which oxygen can penetrate in a tissue supplied from one surface.

$$x_a = \sqrt{\frac{2Dp_o}{M}} \tag{6-24}$$

During oxygen breathing at 1 atmosphere this distance is 143 μ from the choroidal surface and at 2.36 atmospheres with an assumed choroidal venous oxygen pressure of 1430 mmHg the distance is 260 μ. Thus, at this high oxygen pressure, the choroid can supply oxygen to almost the whole thickness of the retina. Hickam and Frayser[31] observed that the oxygen saturation in the retinal veins rose to about 94 per cent during oxygen breathing at 2.36 atmospheres which suggests that almost all the oxygen consumption of the retina was met from the choroid.

The oxygen tension at different points in the thickness of retina can be calculated by substituting for B in Equation 6-21 since

$$B = -\frac{Mx_a}{D} \quad \text{and} \quad x_a = \sqrt{\frac{2Dp_o}{M}}$$

$$B = -\sqrt{\frac{2Mp_o}{D}}$$

from Equation 6-20:

$$p = \frac{Mx^2}{2D} - x\sqrt{\frac{2Mp_0}{D}} + p_0 \tag{6-25}$$

Calculated pressures at different depths in the retina during oxygen breathing at normal temperature and pressure (NTP) and at 2.36 atmospheres are shown in Figure 6-20.

CLINICAL IMPLICATIONS

These calculations, which have clinical implications, explain the exaggerated response of the retinal vessels to increased oxygen concentrations in the inspired gas. If the oxygen concentration in the inspired gas is increased to about 70 per cent the proportion of the retina between the two capillary beds supplied with oxygen from the choroid rises to 97 per cent. It is not surprising that the oxygen uptake from the retinal circulation is reduced.

To calculate the proportional change in oxygen uptake from the retinal vessels during the change from air to oxygen breathing it is necessary to make an assumption about the amount of oxygen supplied to the retina which lies between the superficial and deep retinal capillaries. This tissue is almost as thick as the tissue lying between the deep retinal capillaries and the choroidal vessels. If it is assumed that this retinal tissue receives an amount of oxygen equivalent to that supplied to the deep retinal tissues from the retinal capillaries during air breathing it is possible to calculate the proportional change in oxygen uptake. The oxygen uptake from the retinal vessels while breathing 70% oxygen with an arterial pO_2 of about 400 mm would fall to about 50 per cent of that observed during air breathing and on 100% oxygen to less than 50 per cent. This figure agrees well with the value measured by Hickam and Frayser but too much should not be made of this agreement because the assumptions have been chosen with their measurements in mind.

Most of the assumptions on which these calculations are based seem reasonable. Experimental verification may be difficult because of the inaccessibility of the choroidal vessels. The assumption least likely to be correct is the one concerning the uniformity of oxygen uptake through the retinal tissue. However, nonuniformity would alter the point at which the oxygen supplied by the two circulations balances but not the principle underlying the calculations.

The effect depends upon the high flow and low arteriovenous oxygen difference in the choroidal circulation. The ability of unsaturated hemoglobin to buffer changes in oxygen pressure is lost as soon as the venous hemoglobin saturation becomes complete. Increasing the proportion of oxygen in the inspired air to about 40 per cent allows the whole of the oxygen extraction from the choroidal blood to be met from dissolved oxygen and beyond this point the choroidal venous pO_2 will mount rapidly.

The calculations suggest that the major part of the oxygen supply of the retina could be met from the choroid under conditions of increased oxygen pressure. In practice oxygen therapy has not proved of much value in retinal arterial obstruction but it may be diffusion of other molecules which is the limiting factor.

The severe and apparently disproportionate vasoconstriction observed in the retinal circulation may after all be an autoregulatory response to a raised tissue pO_2. It is not clear why the choroidal vessels do not autoregulate[49] but their large caliber and high flow suggest that they may have another function besides oxygenation of the retina. This function may be cooling the retinal pigment epithelium which is the main site of energy absorption in the eye.

The potential ability of the choroid to oxygenate almost the whole thickness of the retina has interesting implications for understanding the physiologic problem of retrolental fibroplasia. If premature human infants or newborn kittens are exposed to high oxygen concentrations in the inspired gas, severe vasoconstriction occurs in retinal vessels.[2,4] The retina of a 7-month human fetus is about 175 μ thick, a little thinner than that of the adult, and the vasoconstriction is most severe at the periphery where the retina is thinnest. In 80% oxygen at NTP the choroid could supply retinal tissue about 135 μ thick, which would suffice for all except the area close to the posterior pole.

In adults the retinal vessels narrow when exposed to oxygen but return to their original caliber on return to air. Immature retinal vessels are obliterated by exposure to high oxygen tensions for only a few hours.[4] It is interesting to note that others have suggested that the choroidal circulation might be responsible for the vasoconstriction in the retinal vessels during oxygen breathing[52] but they were unable to propose a physiologic mechanism to account for it. Confirmation of the importance of choroidal circulation comes from the work of Ashton and Cook[2] who showed that vasospasm and retrolental fibroplasia did not develop in detached areas of the kitten retina and furthermore that vasospasm that had already occurred could be reversed by detaching the retina.

AUTOREGULATION IN THE RETINAL VASCULAR BED

The term "autoregulation" is used to define processes which operate locally in a vascular bed to maintain a factor such as blood flow constant in the face of external stresses such as changes in blood pressure. The cerebral circulation is able to maintain flow nearly constant over a range of mean arterial pressure from 35 to 90 mmHg when autoperfused although this regulation is lost if a pump is used to supply the blood.[42] In dog skeletal muscle there appears to be autoregulation between about 40 and 90 mmHg but this is lost if the pressure rises above normal.[28]

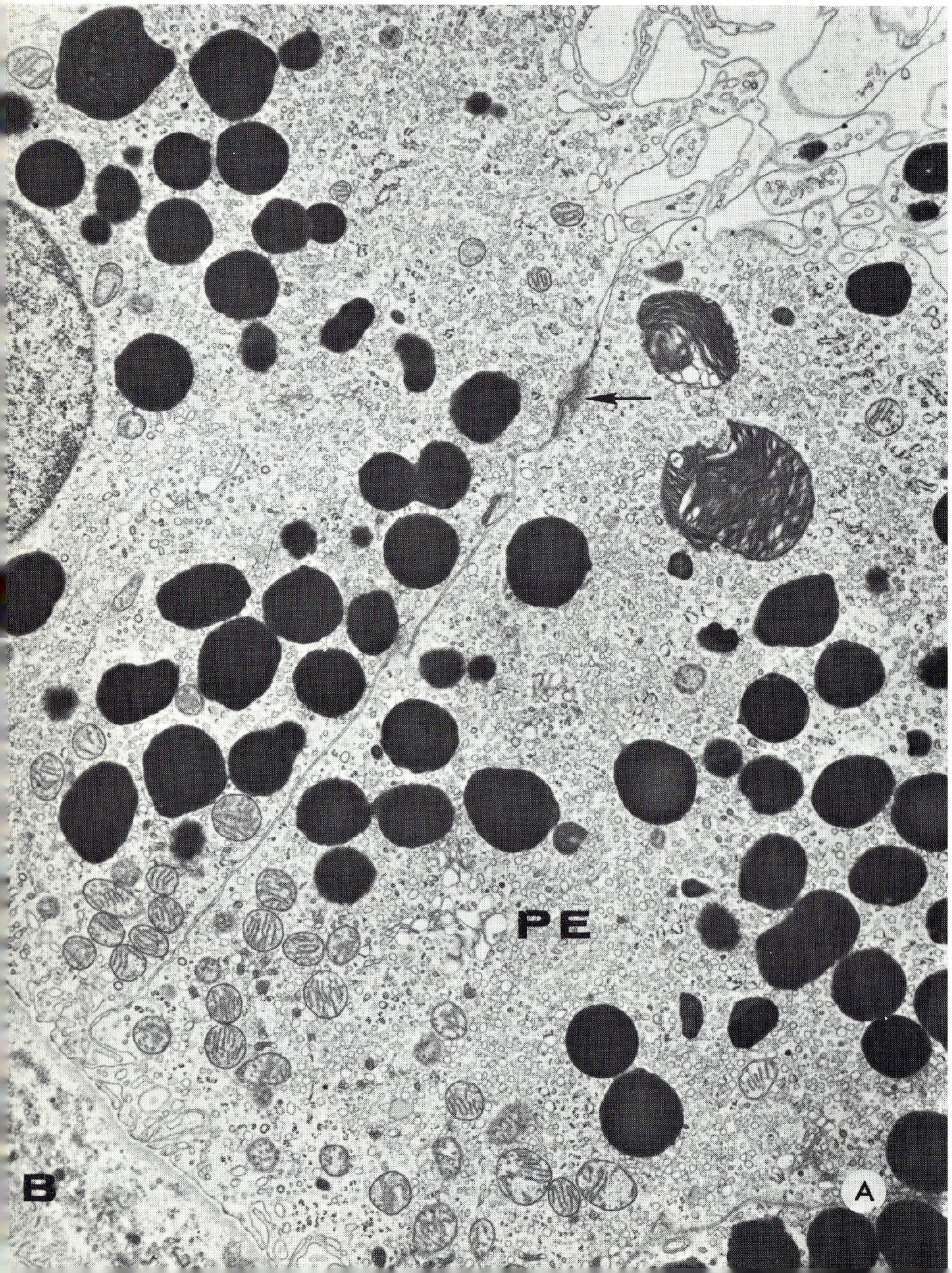

Fig. 6-21. *Opposite page. A*, Electronmicrograph from human adult shows Bruch's membrane **(B)**, pigment epithelium **(PE)**, and tight junction **(arrow)**. ×12,600.

Below. B, Higher magnification of *A* at region of tight junction of the pigment epithelium. There is a marked desmosomal component **(1)** and a small zonula occludens **(2)**. ×49,500.

Following page. C, Electronmicrograph from adult rat shows Bruch's membrane **(B)**, pigment epithelium **(PE)**, intercellular space **(arrow)**, and tight intercellular junction **(TJ)** of the pigment epithelium. ×21,600.

D, Higher magnification of *C*. Note the two components of the tight junction; desmosomal component **(1)**, zonula occludens **(2)**. The intercellular space **(arrow)** is empty. ×60,800.

(Courtesy of Drs. M. Shakib and E. D. MacDonald.)

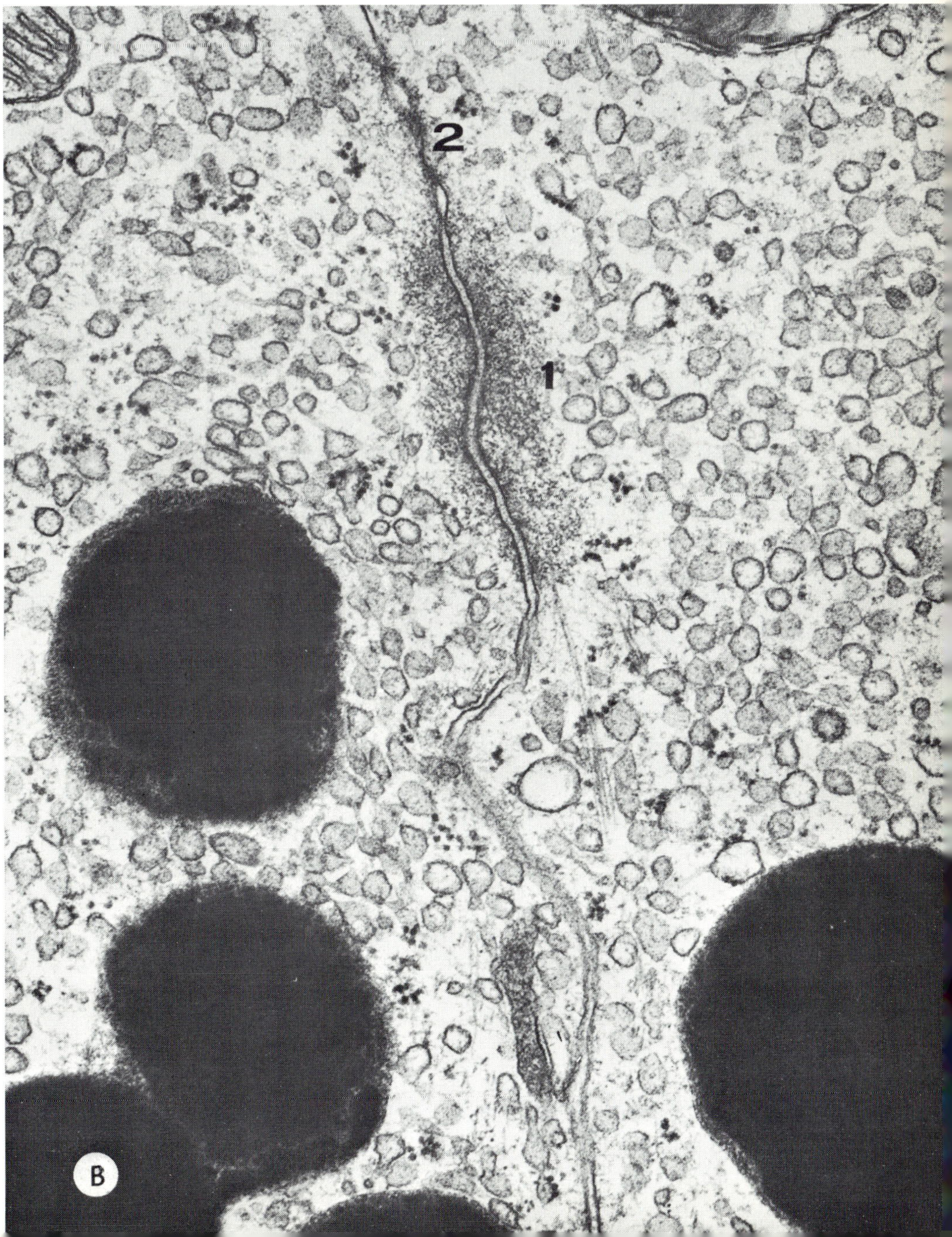

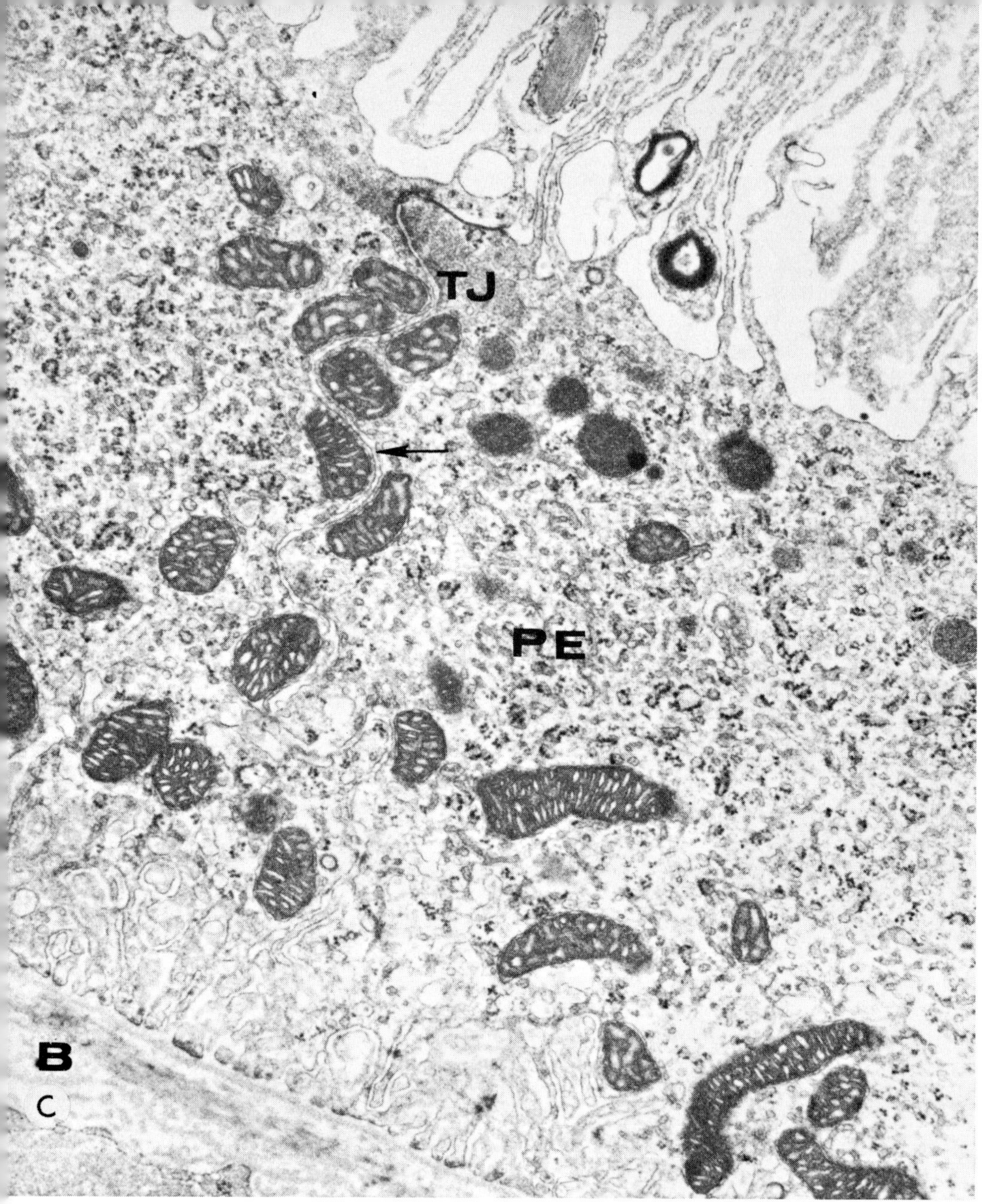

Fig. 6-21*C*

The general concept of autoregulation is that of the engineer's feedback loop. The detector senses the magnitude of the variable, it is compared with the desired value and the resulting signal is fed to an effector, in this case vascular smooth muscle.

In many circumstances the caliber changes observed in the retinal arteries are in the direction anticipated from an autoregulatory response. Thus, elevation of blood pressure causes vessel narrowing, and reduction of pressure, dilatation. Breathing oxygen causes constriction and hypoxic mixtures cause dilatation. However, caliber changes in larger vessels are not necessarily a reliable guide to changes in vascular resistance and it is resistance changes which are important in the concept of autoregulation.

Fig. 6-21*D*

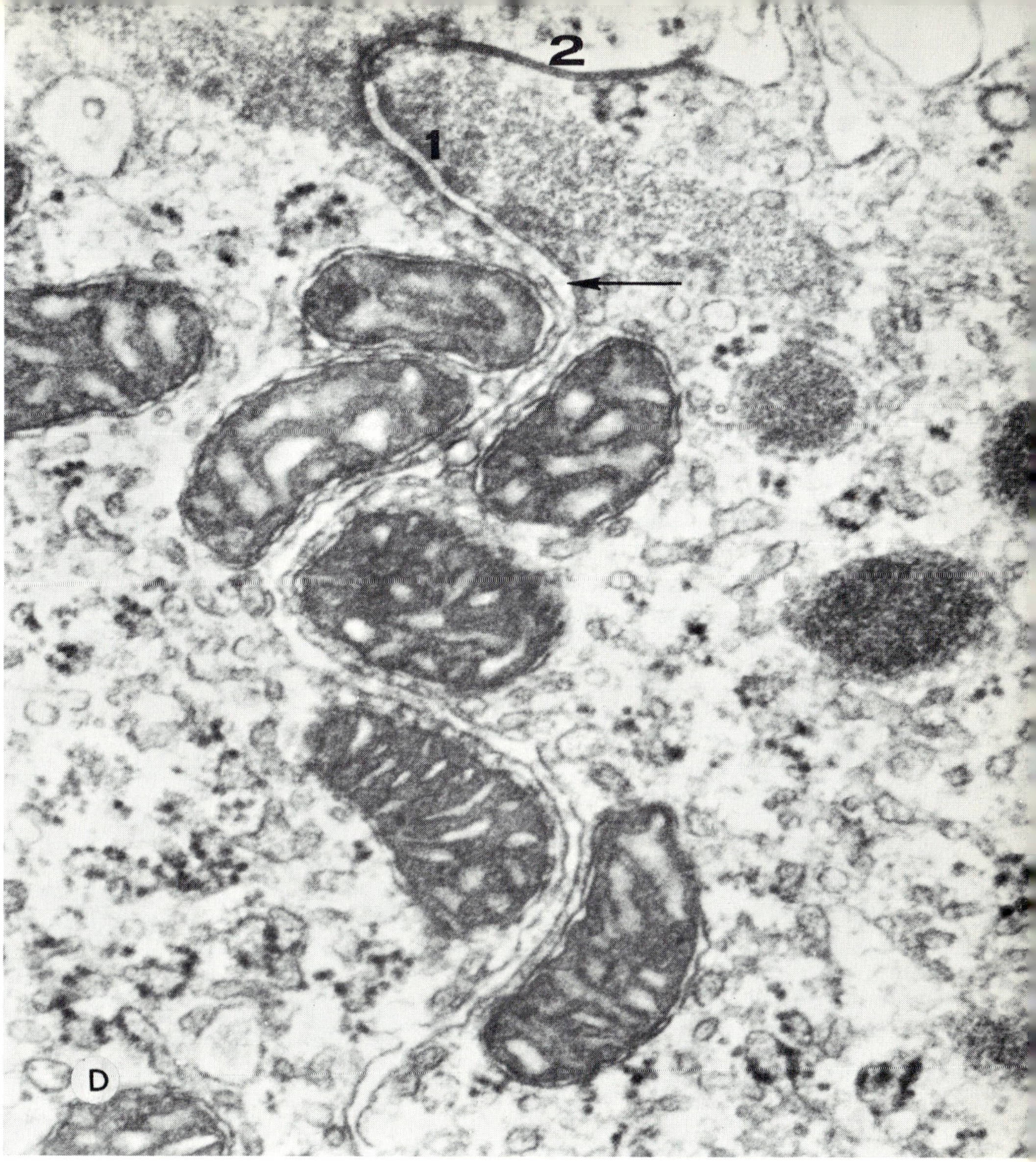

Present evidence suggests that the retinal circulation does autoregulate, but the effectiveness of this mechanism is not known.

DIFFUSION AND TRANSPORT THROUGH RETINAL VESSELS

In 1947 Palm[50] demonstrated a barrier between the blood and retinal tissue similar to that between blood and brain. In his study trypan blue was injected in high dosage (up to 25 ml per kilogram) for several days into animals. All the tissues were stained a deep blue except the central nervous system and the retina. The endothelium of the retinal vessels was not stained. The choroid was deeply stained but not the retina immediately in contact with it. Rodriquez-Peralta[55] has reported similar findings with diamino-acridine fluorescent dye. The dye did not penetrate the blood vessel walls of the visual retina. Dye penetrated into but

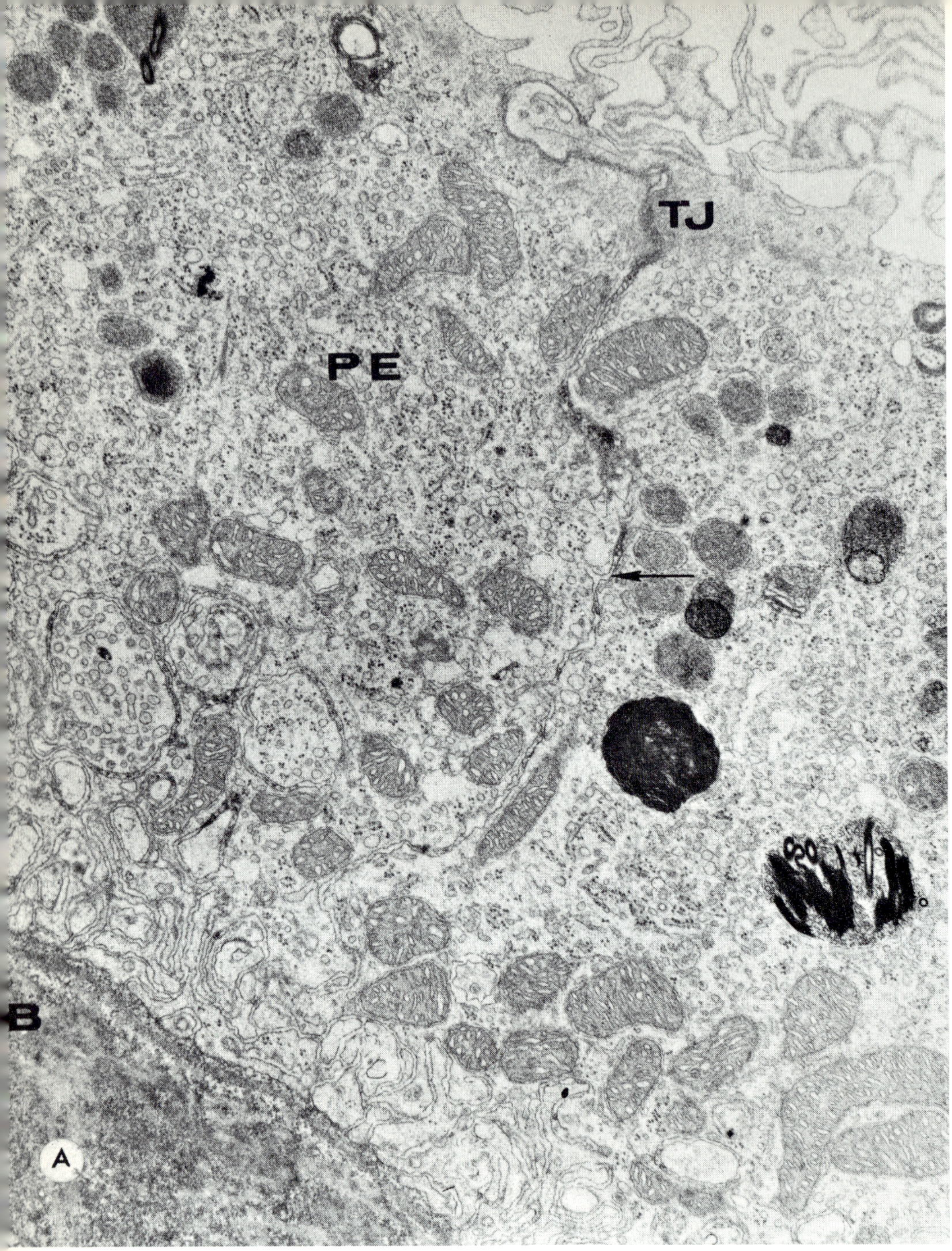

Fig. 6-22. *Above. A*, Electronmicrograph from rat given horseradish peroxidase by intravenous injection. Note fine peroxidase particles in Bruch's membrane **(B)** and in the intercellular space **(arrow). (TJ)** tight junction and **(PE)** pigment epithelium. ×19,200.

Opposite page. B, Higher magnification of *A* shows peroxidase particles within intercellular space **(arrow).** Note that the tight junction acts as a barrier to passage of particles beyond the pigment epithelial cells. ×60,800.

(Courtesy of Drs. M. Shakib and E. D. MacDonald.)

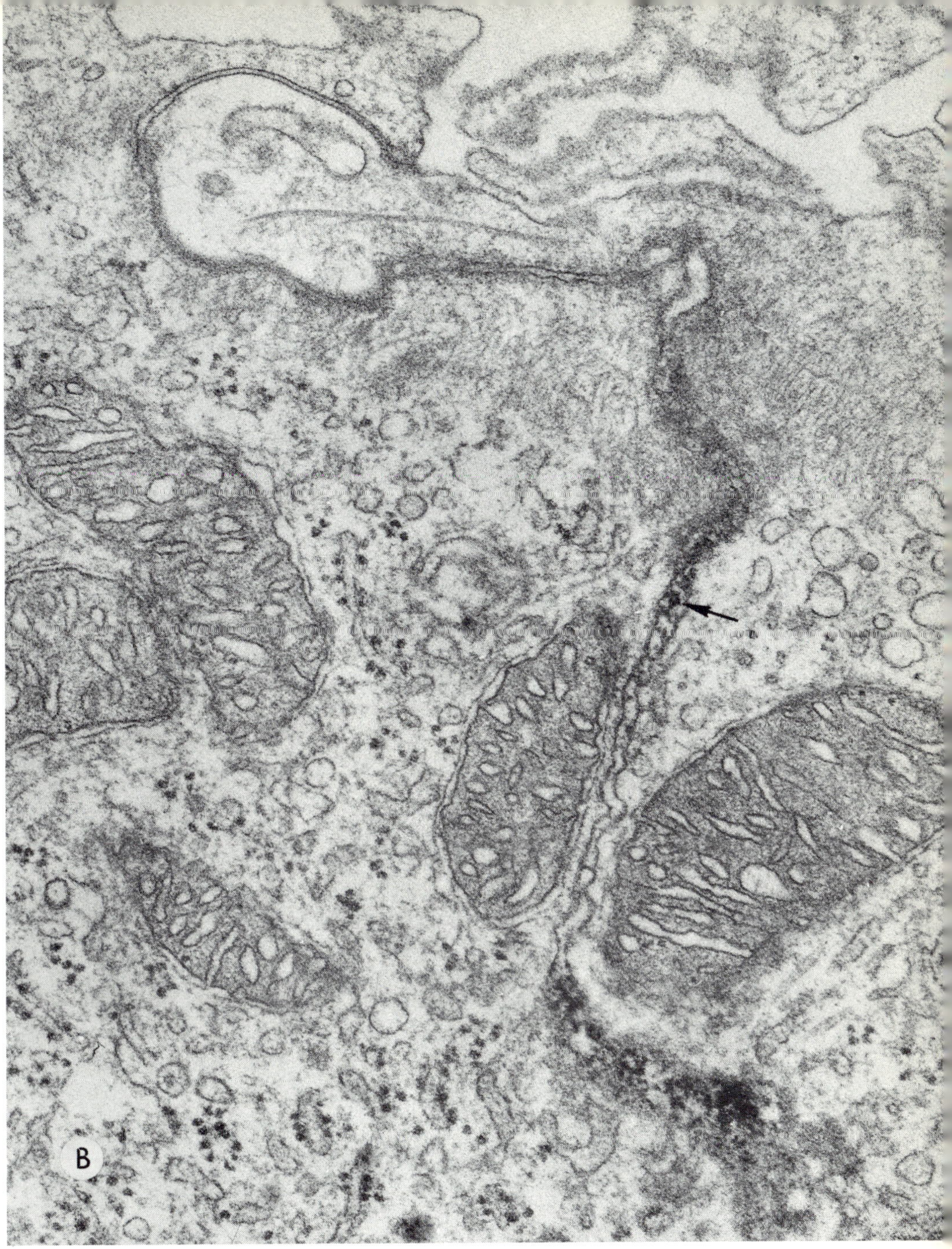

not beyond the retinal pigment epithelial cells and this author concluded that the site of the barrier must be on the retinal aspect of these cells. Recent work of Weinstein, Henkind, and Grant (to be published) does not confirm these findings. Indeed, acridine orange has been shown to stain retinal cells in rabbits, cats, and monkeys within 1 hour after intravenous administration.

There are important structural differences between the retinal and choroidal capillaries. Missoten[45] has shown that the endothelial cells of the retinal capillaries form a continuous lining with tight overlapping junctions like the pieces of a jigsaw puzzle. Shakib and Cunha-Vaz [17,56] have described junctional complexes between endothelial cells with complete occlusion of the intercellular space. They found that these tight junctions were not disrupted by treatment with distilled water, hypertonic saline, or histamine.[3]

In contrast, the choriocapillaris has many pores of about 0.2 μ in diameter between the endothelial cells. Missoten [45] has estimated these might form 5 per cent of the surface area of a choroidal capillary. He theorized that the choroidal capillaries would readily allow the passage of hydrophilic materials through the pores. In the retinal capillaries, the respiratory gases which are lipid soluble could diffuse easily across the cells and he thought that hydrophilic substances would not easily pass the lipid membrane of the endothelial cells. However, Missoten did note many membrane-bound vesicles of about 700 Å diameter within the endothelial cell cytoplasm and considered that these were probably pinocytotic vesicles transporting material across the cell.

Cunha-Vaz and Maurice [15] have published an interesting study of fluorescein transport across the "retinal" vessels of the rabbit. By injecting dye intraperitoneally and into the vitreous they were able to show that fluorescein was transported out of the vitreous against a concentration gradient. Competitive inhibitors blocked this transport system. Thus, systemic administration of probenecid or intravitreal injection of benzylpenicillin both allowed the entry of fluorescein into the retina and vitreous from the blood. Transport out of the eye was also blocked by metabolic inhibitors such as dinitrophenol ($1 \times 10^{-5} M$) and sodium fluoride ($3 \times 10^{-5} M$). Occlusion of the retinal vessels in the rabbit largely prevented transport and suggested that the major part of this activity was carried out by the cells lining these vessels. In the rabbit the walls of most retinal vessels are in contact with the vitreous without the intervention of glial cells and it seems that in this species these cells are the only ones that could be responsible for the active transport of fluorescein. However, transport also takes place over parts of the retinal surface which are not vascularized and in this case the retina itself must transport the dye. The structure responsible is probably the pigment epithelium.

Cunha-Vaz and Maurice [15] have suggested that the function of the transport system is to prevent the entry of potentially toxic organic anions and to provide a mechanism for removal of metabolic products.

It is of interest to note that the enzyme alkaline phosphatase is present in high concentration in the endothelial cells of the retinal blood vessels.[40,54] The only other vessels containing appreciable amounts of this enzyme are those of the brain and the choroid.

The integrity of the blood-retinal barrier is disrupted by many pathologic processes and experimental procedures which damage the vessels. (See section on Pigment Epithelial-Retinal Barrier.) Thus, new vessels and microaneurysms in diabetes, and many minute arteries in malignant hypertension leak fluorescein into the retina. Cunha-Vaz and Shakib [16] have shown in rats that a period of ischemia increased the permeability first of the retinal arterioles and later of the veins. Experimental retinal vein obstruction causes leakage from small venular branches.[36] Exposure to high intensity light causes deep leakage of dye, probably by damaging the pigment epithelium.[35] Presumably these different circumstances all either cause separation of the endothelial or pigment epithelial cells or render them permeable to the dye.

PIGMENT EPITHELIAL-RETINAL BARRIER

A barrier similar to the blood-retinal one exists at the level of the retinal pigment epithelium and its presence is essential for the maintenance of a constant retinal milieu. Tight junctional complexes between the plasma membranes of the pigment epithelial cells were first described by Cohen.[14a] These junctions, like those between endothelial cells of the retinal vessels, have a zonula occludens (Fig. 6-21). In addition, there is a marked desmosomal component. The connections between adjacent cells of the retinal pigment epithelium make it possible to dissect intact large portions of the epithelium from the underlying Bruch's membrane in the laboratory, and also account for the rather large areas of pigment epithelial detachment seen in a number of disease entities such as the group of disciform macular degenerations and subpigment epithelial hematomas.

The permeability of the tight junctional complexes at the level of the retinal pigment epithelium has been studied in experimental animals[56a] (Shakib, M., and MacDonald, E. D., unpublished studies). Peroxidase particles were injected intravenously in rats and within several minutes the particles could be found in the pores of the choriocapillaris, within Bruch's membrane, and in the intercellular space between adjacent pigment epithelial cells; at the tight junctions the particles were arrested (Fig. 6-22).

REFERENCES

1. Ashton, C. H. Personal Communication.
2. Ashton, N., and Cook, C.: Studies on the developing retinal vessels. 1. The influence of retinal detachment. *Brit. J. Ophthal. 39:*449, 1955.
3. Ashton, N., and Cunha-Vaz, J. G.: Effect of histamine on the permeability of the ocular vessels. *Arch. Ophthal. 73:*211, 1965.
4. Ashton, N., Ward, B., and Serpell, G.: The role of oxygen in the genesis of retrolental fibroplasia. *Brit. J. Ophthal. 37:*513, 1953.
5. Ashby, M., Oakley, N., Lorentz, I., and Scott, D.: Recurrent transient monocular blindness. *Brit. Med. J. 2:*894, 1963.
6. Baillart, P.: Circulation arterielle retinienne, Essais de determination de la tension arterielle dans les branches de l'arterie centrale de la retine. *Ann. Oculist 154:*257, 1917.
7. Bill, A.: "Uveal Circulation, a Review of Methods and Results," in *Glaucoma Symposium*, Tutzing Castle, 1966. Basel, Karger, 1967, p. 52.
8. Branemark, P–I.: "Rheological Shock," in *Microcirculation as Related to Shock,* ed. by Shepro, D., and Fulton, G. P., New York, Academic Press, 1968.
9. Van Breemen, V. L., and Clemente, C. D.: Silver deposition in the central nervous system and the haematoencephallic barrier studied with the electron microscope. *J. Biophys. Biochem. Cytol. 1:*161, 1955.
10. Bulpitt, C. J., and Dollery, C. T.: The estimation of retinal blood flow by measurement of the mean circulation time. *Cardiovasc. Res. 5:*406, 1971.

10a. Bulpitt, C. J., Dollery, C. T., and Kohner, E. M.: The marginal plasma zone in the retinal microcirculation. *Cardiovasc. Res. 4:* 207, 1970.

11. Burton, A. C.: "Physical Principles of Circulatory Phenomena: The Physical Equilibrium of the Heart and Blood Vessels," in *Handbook of Physiology, Section 2: Circulation.* Washington, D.C., American Physiological Society, 1962, vol. I, p. 85.
12. Byrom, F. B.: The nature of malignancy in hypertensive disease, evidence from the retina of the rat. *Lancet 1:*516, 1963.
13. Carr, R. E., and Henkind, P.: Retinal findings associated with serum hyperviscosity. *Amer. J. Ophthal. 56:*23, 1963.

14. Chambers, R., and Zweifach, B. W.: The topography and function of the mesenteric capillary circulation. *Amer. J. Anat. 75:*173, 1944.

14a. Cohen, A. I.: A possible cytological basis for the "R" membrane in the vertebrate eye. *Nature 205:*1223, 1965.

15. Cunha-Vaz, J. G., and Maurice, D. M.: The active transport of fluorescein by the retinal vessels and the retina. *J. Physiol. 191:*467, 1967.

16. Cunha-Vaz, J. G., and Shakib, M.: Ultrastructural mechanisms of breakdown of the blood-retinal barrier. *J. Path. Bact. 93:*645, 1967.

17. Cunha-Vaz, J. G., Shakib, M., and Ashton, N.: Studies on the permeability of the blood-retinal barrier. I. On the existence, development and site of a blood-retinal barrier. *Brit. J. Ophthal. 50:*441, 1966.

18. Dollery, C. T.: Dynamic aspects of the retinal microcirculation. *Arch. Ophthal. 79:*336, 1968.

19. Dollery, C. T.: An explanation for the exaggerated response of retinal blood vessels to oxygen, *J. Physiol. 201:*86P, 1969.

20. Dollery, C. T., Henkind, P., Kohner, E. M., and Paterson, J. W.: Effect of raised intraocular pressure on the retinal and choroidal circulation. *Invest. Ophthal. 7:*191, 1968.

21. Dollery, C. T., Kohner, E. M., Paterson, J. W., and Ramalho, P. S.: "The Retinal Microcirculation in Shock," in *Microcirculation as Related to Shock,* ed. by Shepro, D., and Fulton, G. P., New York, Academic Press, 1968.

22. Duke-Elder, S.: The ocular circulation: its normal pressure relationships and their physiological significance. *Brit. J. Ophthal. 10:*513, 1926.

23. Elgin, S. S.: Arterio-venous oxygen difference across the uveal tract of the dog eye. *Invest. Ophthal. 3:*417, 1964.

24. Falck, B.: Observations on the possibilities of the cellular localisation of monoamines by a fluorescence method. *Acta Physiol. Scand.* Suppl. *197,* 1962.

25. Folkow, B., and Lofving, B.: The distensibility of the systemic resistance blood vessels. *Acta Physiol. Scand. 38:*37, 1957.

26. Friedman, E., Kopald, H. H., and Smith, T. R.: Retinal and choroidal blood flow determined with krypton-85 in anesthetised animals. *Invest. Ophthal. 3:*539, 1964.

27. Friedman, E., Smith, T. R., and Kuwabara, T.: Retinal microcirculation in vivo. *Invest. Ophthal. 3:*217, 1964.

28. Green, H. D., Rapela, C. E., and Conrad, M. C.: "Resistance (Conductance) and Capacitance Phenomena in Terminal Vascular Beds," in *Handbook of Physiology, Section 2: Circulation.* Washington, D.C., American Physiological Society 1963, vol. 2, p. 935.

29. Hamilton, W. F., Moore, J. W., Kinsman, J. M., and Spurling, R. G.: Studies on the circulation. IV. Further analysis of the injection method, and of changes in hemodynamics under physiologic and pathologic conditions. *Amer. J. Physiol. 99:*534, 1932.

30. Hart, L. M., Heyman, A., Linhart, J. W., McIntosh, H., and Davies, N. J.: Fluorescein motion picture photography of retinal circulation. *J. Lab. Clin. Med. 62:*703, 1963.

31. Hickam, J. B., and Frayser, R.: Studies of the retinal circulation in man: Observations on vessel diameter, arterio-venous oxygen difference and mean circulation time. *Circulation 33:*302, 1966.

32. Hickam, J. B., Schieve, J. F., and Wilson, W. P.: The relation between retinal and cerebral vascular reactivity in normal and arteriosclerotic subjects. *Circulation 7:*84, 1953.

33. Hill, A. V.: The diffusion of oxygen and lactic acid through tissues. *Proc. roy. Soc. B. 135:*446, 1947–48.

34. Kety, S. S., and Schmidt, C. F.: The effect of altered arterial tensions of carbon dioxide and oxygen of cerebral blood flow and cerebral oxygen consumption of normal young men. *J. Clin. Invest. 27:*484, 1948.

35. Kohner, E. M., Dollery, C. T., Henkind, P., Paterson, J. W., and Ramalho, P. S.: Retinal vascular changes following exposure to high intensity light. *Amer. J. Ophthal. 63:*1748, 1967.

36. Kohner, E. M., Dollery, C. T., Shakib, M., Henkind, P., Paterson, J. W., de Oliveira, L. N. F., and Bulpitt, C. J.: Experimental retinal branch vein occlusion. *Amer. J. Ophthal. 69:*778, 1970.

37. Kniseley, M. H., Bloch, E. H., Eliot, T. S., and Warner, L.: Sludged blood. *Science 106:* 431, 1947.

38. Krogh, A.: *The Anatomy and Physiology of Capillaries.* New Haven, Conn., Yale Univer. Press, 1929.

39. Laties, A. M.: Central retinal artery innervation: Absence of adrenergic innervation to the intraocular branches. *Arch. Ophthal. 77:*405, 1967.

40. Lessel, S., and Kuwabara, T.: Phosphatase histochemistry of the eye. *Arch. Ophthal. 71:*851, 1964.

41. Lobstein, A., and Nordmann, J.: Modern Ophthalmodynamometry. Docum. *Ophthal. 13:*397, 1959.

42. Machowicz, P. P., Sabo, G., Lin, G., Rapela, C. E., and Green, H. D.: Effect of varying cerebral arterial pressure on cerebral venous flow. *Physiologist 4:*68, 1961.

43. Malmfors, T.: The adrenergic innervation of the eye as demonstrated by fluorescence microscopy. *Acta Physiol. Scand. 65:*259, 1965.

44. McDonald, D. A.: *Blood Flow in Arteries.* London, Arnold, 1960.

45. Missoten, L.: Etude des capillaire de la retine et de la chorio-capillaire au microscope electronique. *Bull. Soc. Belg. Ophtal. 129:*382, 1962.

46. Nicoll, P. A., and Webb, R. L.: Blood circulation in the subcutaneous tissue of the living bat's wing. *Ann. N.Y. Acad. Sci. 46:*697, 1946.

47. Nicoll, P. A., and Webb, R. L.: Vascular patterns and active vasomotion as determines of flow through minute vessels. *Angiology 6:*291, 1955.

48. Oberhoff, P., Evans, P. Y., and Delaney, J. F.: Cinematographic documentation of retinal circulation times. *Arch. Ophthal. 74:*77, 1965.

49. O'Rourke, J., and Berghoffer, B.: Uveal extraction and clearance of oxygen in normal, inflamed and hyperthermic eyes. *Ophthalmologica 155:*205, 1968.

50. Palm, E.: On the occurrence in the retina of conditions corresponding to the blood-brain barrier. *Acta Ophthal. 25:*295, 1947.

51. Paterson, J. W., Dollery, C. T., Ramalho, P. S., and Kohner, E. M.: The effect of platelet aggregates on retinal circulation. 4th European Congress on Microcirculation. *Bibl. Anat. 9:*85, 1967.

52. Patz, A.: Oxygen studies in retrolental fibroplasia. IV. Clinical and experimental observations. *Amer. J. Ophthal. 38:*291, 1954.

53. Permutt, S., and Riley, R. L.: Hemodynamics of collapsible vessels with tone: Vascular waterfall. *J. Appl. Physiol. 18:*924, 1963.

54. Reis, J. L.: Histochemical localisation of alkaline phosphatase in the retina. *Brit. J. Ophthal. 38:*35, 1954.

55. Rodriquez-Peralta, L. A.: Experiments on the site of the blood-ocular barrier. *Anat. Rec. 142:*273, 1962.

56. Shakib, M., and Cunha Vaz, J. G.: Studies on the permeability of the blood-retinal barrier. 4. Junctional complexes of the retinal vessels and their role in the permeability of the blood-retinal barrier. *Exp. Eye Res. 5:*229, 1966.

56a. Shiose, Y.: Electron microscopic studies on blood-retinal and blood aqueous barriers. *Jap. J. Ophthal. 14:*73, 1970.

57. Smith, V. H.: Carotid insufficiency. *Trans. Ophthal. Soc. U.K. 80:*253, 1960.

58. Stewart, G. N.: Researches on the circulation time and on the influences which affect it. IV: The output of the heart. *J. Physiol. 22:*159, 1897.

59. Thuránzsky, K.: *Der Blutkreislaut der Netzhaut.* Budapest, Ungarischen Akademie der Wissenschaften, 1957.

60. Weigelin, E.: Hat die Netzhautdruchmessung bei der hypertonie einer Sinn. *Docum. Ophthal. 10:*303, 1956.

61. Womersley, J. R.: Method of calculation of velocity, rate of flow and viscous drag in arteries when the pressure gradient is known. *J. Physiol. 127:*553, 1955.

62. Zierler, K. L.: "Circulation times and the Theory of Indicator-Dilution Methods for Determining Blood Flow and Volume," in *Handbook of Physiology, Section 2: Circulation,* Washington, D.C., American Physiological Society, 1962, vol. 1, p. 585.

63. Zweifach, B. E.: The character and distribution of the blood capillaries. *Anat. Rec. 73:*475, 1939.

chapter 7

Pharmacology of Retinal Circulation

There is relatively little information about the response of the retinal blood vessels to drugs.[16,17,32]

To calculate changes in vascular resistance it is necessary to know the retinal arterial pressure, the intraocular pressure or intraocular venous pressure, and blood flow. In many cases none of this information is available and inferences about vascular effects of drugs have been drawn from measurements of vessel caliber alone. Vessel caliber can be measured accurately from high-quality photographs and if the changes are uniform throughout all orders of vessel size it would be reasonable to infer resistance changes from them. However, the easiest vessels to observe clinically and to measure are the large arteries and veins on or near the optic disc but the main resistance lies in the smallest vessels, especially the precapillary arterioles which are invisible with the ophthalmoscope.

Retinal mean circulation time, measured from the arterial and venous phases of fluorescein angiograms has also been used for evaluating the effects of vasoactive drugs. Unfortunately, the circulation time is altered by both flow and volume changes and it is difficult to make an accurate estimate of changes in the retinal blood volume.

The position is much more difficult in studies where caliber changes have been assessed by eye, by using a scale in an ophthalmoscope, or by measuring the width of the angioscotoma.[42] It is impossible to give much weight to such observations which were usually not controlled and have no estimate of the errors involved.

Caution is essential in interpreting the data presently available. Most studies of drug action on the retinal vessels will need to be repeated once better methods of measuring their action have been devised.

RESPIRATORY GASES

There is more published quantitative information about the effects of respiratory gases on the retinal vessels than there is about drugs. Much of this information has come from the careful quantitative work of Hickam and Frayser.[20,22,26,27,39]

OXYGEN

Oxygen breathing causes narrowing of the retinal vessels. The earliest report was that of Cusick, Benson, and Boothby[9] who measured caliber changes in the largest retinal arteries and veins. They reported that arterial narrowing averaged 24 per cent and venous narrowing averaged 28.2 per cent when normal people breathed oxygen at 1 atmosphere. Frayser and Hickam[21] and Hickam, Frayser, and Ross[27] have extended these observations using more reliable methods and found a narrowing of larger vessels averaging 11.6 per cent for arteries and 14.9 per cent for veins in 50 normal subjects when they changed from breathing air to 100% oxygen. Oxygen breathing also increases the retinal venous oxygen saturation. Hickam and his colleagues found an increase of venous saturation from 55 per cent in air, to 79 per cent with oxygen in 37 subjects whom they studied. These authors have also calculated the retinal mean circulation time from a series of fluorescence photographs.[26] They used an average time derived from the large vessels around the optic disc. In five subjects studied during oxygen breathing the mean circulation time increased from 4.8 seconds in air to 6.1 seconds with oxygen.

As changes in the circulation time are proportional to both flow and volume Hickam and Frayser went on to estimate volume changes from the diameter of the large veins. From this figure they calculated a relative change in retinal blood flow and oxygen uptake during oxygen breathing. In five subjects they estimated that flow decreased to 57 per cent of control and oxygen uptake to 44 per cent of control during oxygen breathing at 1 atmosphere.

The degree of retinal arterial and venous constriction during oxygen breathing is proportional to the inspired oxygen pressure. A significant narrowing occurs when the normal inspired oxygen pressure is doubled. The degree of constriction of vessels varies in relation to their size, being greatest in the smallest measurable vessels of about 30 to 40 μ in diameter.[12]

HYPERBARIC OXYGEN

Breathing oxygen at higher than atmospheric pressure causes even more severe retinal vasoconstriction than is observed at normal pressure. Dollery et al.[12] have reported that small retinal arterioles narrowed by a mean of 42.3 per cent while breathing oxygen at 2 atmospheres (Fig. 7-1). Frayser et al.[22] have measured vessel caliber, mean circulation time, and retinal venous oxygen saturation at 2.36 and 3.7 atmospheres inspired oxygen pressure. The mean circulation time increased from 4.2 seconds in air to 6.3 seconds with 3.7 atmospheres oxygen while the arterial caliber was reduced to less than half the diameter while breathing air. The retinal venous saturation rose from 58 per cent in air to 94 per cent with oxygen at 2.36 atmospheres. Calculated blood flow was reduced to about 30 per cent of the value on air. After taking into account the dissolved oxygen in blood at these high pressures the reduction in calculated blood flow derived from the alterations in transit time is disproportionate to the amount required to keep oxygen delivery constant.

Recently it has been suggested that the apparent sensitivity of the retinal vessels to oxygen can be explained by some special features of the choroidal circulation.[11] The choroid has a high blood flow with a very small difference in oxygen saturation between the arterial and venous blood. When the arterial oxygen tension is increased the dissolved oxygen becomes capable of supplying the amount normally extracted and the hemoglobin in the choroidal venous blood is fully saturated with oxygen. The ability of unsaturated hemoglobin to buffer changes in oxygen tension is then lost and the oxygen tension in both the tissues and the venous blood will rise rapidly. This theory is supported by the measurements of Elgin[15] who found that during air breathing the choroidal arterial and venous oxygen tensions were 85.5 and 66 mmHg respectively. During oxygen breathing the arterial tension rose to 419 mmHg and the venous to 253 mmHg. The very high tissue-oxygen tension in the choroid would establish a diffusion gradient of oxygen from the choroid into the retina that would enable it to supply a larger proportion of the retinal tissue and decrease the amount extracted from the retinal blood.

One consequence of this situation is that the retinal elements, particularly the visual receptors, which are closest to the choroid, are exposed to very high oxygen pressures. Noell[34,35] has noted degeneration of the visual receptors in rabbits exposed to oxygen concentrations as low as 60 per cent for several days. Bresnick[6] has confirmed these findings and shown that the earliest structural change is vesicular swelling of the endoplasmic reticulum and Golgi complex of the inner segment.

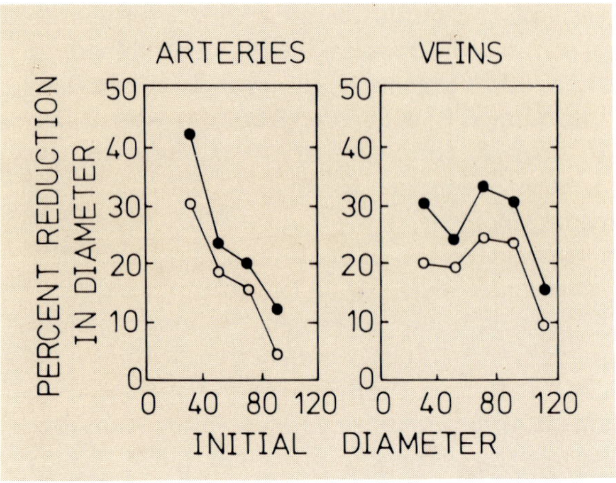

Fig. 7-1. Narrowing of normal retinal arteries and veins of different sizes during oxygen breathing at 1 (○—○) and 2 (•—•) atmospheres. (From Dollery et al.[12])

Fig. 7-2. Percentage change in caliber of retinal arteries and veins during oxygen breathing at 1 atmosphere in 13 normals ranging in age from 19 to 62 years. (From Ramalho and Dollery. Hypertensive retinopathy: Calibre changes in retinal blood vessels following blood-pressure reduction and inhalation of oxygen. *Circulation 37*:580, 1968. By permission of the American Heart Association, Inc.)

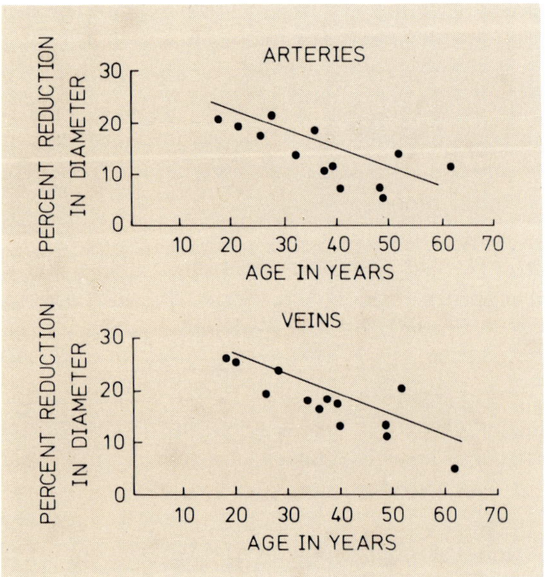

REDUCED OXYGEN PRESSURE

If inspired oxygen pressure is reduced the retinal arteries and veins dilate. Cusick, Benson, and Boothby[9] have noted that the vascular dilatation at oxygen pressures simulating 18 to 20,000 feet of altitude was 10 to 20 per cent, being more marked in the veins. Sieker and Hickam[39] have used 10% oxygen and found a dilatation averaging 10.1 per cent in large arteries and 10.0 per cent in large veins.

EFFECT OF AGE AND VASCULAR DISEASE ON OXYGEN REACTIVITY

The narrowing of retinal vessels caused by oxygen is reduced by aging and by diseases such as hypertension and diabetes. Presumably, structural changes take place in the walls of the vessels under these conditions which involve replacement of smooth muscle by fibrous tissue and lessens the ability of the vessel to constrict. There is a linear relationship between age and the degree of narrowing that takes place during oxygen breathing at 1 atmosphere (Fig. 7-2). Quantitative studies of retinal vascular reactivity to oxygen in babies show that their vessels react with a greater degree of constriction than adult vessels to moderate increases in arterial oxygen.[5]

In the 1940s an epidemic of infant blindness occurred caused by retrolental fibroplasia following retinal vasoconstriction induced by oxygen treatment.[8,19] Experimental studies in kittens showed that severe vasospasm could be induced in the immature retinal vessels and if exposure was prolonged this became irreversible. Proliferative changes in the region of vasospasm caused the clinical condition of retrolental fibroplasia.[3] In the following decade the use of oxygen was restricted and retrolental fibroplasia became rare, but unfortunately there has been an increase in mortality among premature infants caused by hypoxia.[4] Recently it has been recognized that some infants require high concentrations of oxygen to achieve adequate arterial oxygenation. It is important to monitor the arterial oxygen tension, because when these infants improve and the right-to-left shunting ceases the arterial oxygen tension may rise quickly to levels which cause retinal vasospasm.[36]

CARBON DIOXIDE

Several authors have reported that carbon dioxide causes retinal vasodilatation, which might be expected by analogy with cerebral vessels, but recent quantitative measurements have not confirmed this. Frayser and Hickam[20] have reported that the caliber of the larger retinal arteries increased by 2 per cent and the veins by 1 per cent when 10 normal subjects switched from air breathing to a mixture containing 10% CO_2 and 21% O_2. These changes are not significant. The retinal mean circulation time is decreased by breathing a mixture of 7% CO_2 and 21% O_2. Hickam and Frayser reported a reduction from 5.0 to 4.2 seconds but this change was also not significant. They calculated that flow increased by 22 per cent during 7% CO_2 breathing and oxygen uptake fell by 6 per cent. It seems clear that CO_2 has relatively little effect on the retinal circulation but it is of interest to note that there may be an increase in flow while the caliber of the larger vessels does not change. This surprising finding may be explained by recent work in our laboratory[7] which shows that carbon dioxide increases the width of the plasma zone surrounding the red cell column in retinal vessels although it does not increase the width of the red cell column itself. Measurement of vessel caliber from color pictures give the width of the red cell column and not the total internal diameter of the vessel.

Recent work in pigs shows that breathing CO_2 mixtures that raise arterial pCO_2 to approximately 80 mmHg cause blood flow through the retinal vessels to double (Archer et al., unpublished).

Hyperventilation caused no significant alteration in the caliber of the retinal vessels, but prolonged the mean retinal circulation time from 5.5 to 8.6 seconds in five normal subjects. The retinal arteriovenous difference of oxygen saturation increased from 37 to 47 per cent during hyperventilation presumably as a result of a decreased retinal blood flow.

Sevel and Freedman[38] have reported a patient who died in coma after carbon dioxide poisoning. The retina showed absence of ganglion cells, atrophy of the nuclear layers, and loss of the endothelial cells of the retinal capillaries.

MIXTURES OF CARBON DIOXIDE AND OXYGEN

Although carbon dioxide has little effect on vessel caliber or blood flow at normal oxygen pressures it has a profound effect in preventing the vasoconstriction caused by oxygen at high pressures. Frayser and Hickam[20] found that the normal arterial constriction of 11.6 per cent caused by oxygen was reduced to 3 per cent by breathing 10% CO_2 in 90% oxygen. Similar figures for veins were −14.9 with 100% oxygen reduced to −7 per cent on 10% CO_2 in 90% oxygen. Carbon dioxide also prolongs the time taken for ischemic visual blackout.[1] The ability of CO_2 to reverse the vasoconstriction of extra oxygen is of great theoretical interest and may have applications to therapy.

However, it is extremely unpleasant to breathe high concentrations of carbon dioxide for more than a few minutes. Some instances where patients appear to have tolerated breathing 7% to 10% CO_2 for prolonged periods may have been because plastic face masks were used which allowed considerable dilution of the inhaled gas with air. As a useful therapeutic effect would have to be maintained for hours or days it is unlikely that mixtures of carbon dioxide and oxygen will prove of value.

NITROGEN

Nitrogen has a narcotic effect on the brain at high pressures. No vascular effects of changes in nitrogen pressure, if PCO_2 and PO_2 are constant, have been described for the retina or other organs. One study in which caliber changes induced by oxygen breathing at 1 atmosphere were compared with the effects of air at 5 atmospheres did not suggest any effect of nitrogen for the vasoconstriction was the same under both circumstances. It seems likely that nitrogen has no effect on the retinal vessels.[12]

VASODILATOR DRUGS

Reliable data concerning drug effects on the retinal circulation are scanty.

GLYCERYL TRINITRATE

Glyceryl trinitrate (nitroglycerin) is a powerful vasodilator drug which is widely used in the treatment of angina pectoris. The effect of this drug on retinal vessel caliber and the mean transit time of dye has been studied in normal subjects.[21] The retinal veins dilated by a mean of 5 per cent while the mean circulation time increased from 4.8 to 6.9 seconds. The calculated retinal blood flow fell to 77 per cent of control and the oxygen uptake to 93 per cent of control. In these studies there was little change in blood pressure yet vessels dilated and flow decreased. It is possible that changes in larger vessels upstream are responsible for this paradoxical response but the results emphasize the difficulty in interpreting caliber changes in retinal vessels without data on blood flow.

HYDRALAZINE

Hydralazine is a vasodilator, used as a hypotensive agent, which acts directly on smooth muscle. Ramalho and Dollery[37] have studied the blood pressure and retinal vascular response to intravenous administration in patients with severe hypertension. Following an average dose of 37 mg in six patients, which reduced the mean blood pressure from 168 to 121 mmHg, all retinal vessels dilated but the response was much greater in the smaller arteries than the larger ones (Fig. 7-3). These results suggest that hydralazine dilates the retinal vessels as the response, particularly in the larger vessels, was greater than occurred with other methods of lowering blood pressure. No measurements of flow were made in this study.

PAPAVERINE

Papaverine acts directly upon vascular smooth muscle and is a spasmolytic agent.

Frayser and Hickam[21] have studied the response of retinal vessels in five normal subjects given 64 mg of papaverine intravenously. The arteries dilated by a mean of 4 per cent while the veins did not change. The retinal venous oxygen saturation fell from 52 per cent to 41 per cent. These results suggest that retinal blood flow may have fallen, if it is assumed that the oxygen uptake remained constant. Ellis and Lende[18] have applied papaverine to the retinal vessels of the opened eye after the vessels had been put into spasm by mechanical or electrical stimulation. Papaverine caused the vessels to dilate. Papaverine was used in a 1.6% solution (16 mg per milliliter) and such a concentration could never be approached in therapy. Recent studies in pigs (Ffytche et al., unpublished) have shown that infusion of papaverine 0.3 mg per kilogram per minute into the carotid artery or 0.6 mg per kilogram per minute into a systemic vein cause a substantial increase in retinal blood flow.

AMINOPHYLLINE

Aminophylline is a smooth-muscle relaxing agent widely used for the treatment of bronchospasm.

Frayser and Hickam[21] gave 500-mg intravenous doses to five normal subjects. The caliber of arterioles and veins both fell by 4 per cent while the retinal venous hemoglobin saturation was unchanged. It does not appear from these results that aminophylline has any effect on the retinal vessels.

TOLAZOLINE

Tolazoline is a vasodilator used in the treatment of peripheral vascular disease.

Ellis and Lende[18] used a 2.5% solution of tolazoline applied directly to the exposed retinal vessels and caused vasodilatation. Such a high concentration can have little relevance to use in intact animals or man.

ADRENERGIC BLOCKADE

Ramalho and Dollery[37] have studied blood pressure and retinal vascular responses in groups of hypertensive patients given adrenergic neurone-blocking drugs such as bethanidine, guanethidine, and methyldopa to lower their blood pressure. The smaller retinal arteries dilated and the larger ones became narrower as the blood pressure fell. As the same type of change occurred in patients whose blood pressure was lowered by renal surgery, Ramalho and Dollery concluded that the response was probably autoregulatory and resulted from the change in blood pressure, rather than as a direct effect of the drugs on the vessels.

OTHER DRUGS

There are reports that the caliber of retinal vessels has been observed to increase after administration of a number of other drugs such as nicotinic acid, amitriptylline and acetylcholine. These reports are not substantiated by measurements and it is impossible to evaluate them.

THERAPEUTIC USE OF VASODILATOR DRUGS AND RESPIRATORY GASES IN RETINAL VASCULAR DISEASE

The evidence is so inadequate that it is difficult to give any opinion about the usefulness of vasodilators in therapy of acute retinal artery occlusion. As the retinal vessels have no adrenergic supply it would be surprising if agents that act by blockade of the sympathetic nerves or neurotransmitter had any effect. There is no evidence that they do. It would be more reasonable to anticipate that some vasodilators which act directly on vessels may exert an effect. Of these drugs, hydralazine appears to be the most active but more data is needed for a definite evaluation.

In the present state of knowledge it is not possible to recommend any of these drugs in the therapy of occlusive retinal vascular disease.

Hyperbaric oxygen has been used for the treatment of retinal arterial insufficiency. Calculations show that the oxygen supply to almost the whole thickness of the retina could be met from the choroid alone if the inspired oxygen pressure was about 2.5 atmospheres. However, in practice hyperbaric oxygen has not proved of much value.[2,24] There may be several reasons. Oxygen is toxic and there is a risk of convulsions with prolonged exposure. Because of the risk of oxygen poisoning, treatment with hyperbaric oxygen for the period required would probably be impractical. Unless an efficient demand-valve system is used with a gas-tight mouthpiece the concentration of oxygen administered may be much less than it appears. Conceivably, the diffusion of other factors besides oxygen into the ischemic tissue may be important and the concentration of these in blood cannot be increased in the same way as oxygen. Animal experiments suggest that prolonged exposure to high concentrations of oxygen may be toxic for the retina[33,34] but there is no data on this point in man.

VASOCONSTRICTOR DRUGS

NOREPINEPHRINE

Dollery, Hodge, and Hill[13] have infused norepinephrine intravenously in six normal humans and elevated their blood pressures from an average of 114/73 mmHg to 173/104 mmHg. The retinal arteries narrowed by about 7 μ on average.

Subsequent work in animals anesthetized with chloralose has shown that retinal blood flow increases slightly as the blood pressure is raised with systemic norepinephrine although the vessels narrow. Norepinephrine infused locally into the carotid circulation had little effect on either vessel caliber or blood flow.[7] These results suggest that the drug does not have a direct vasoconstrictor effect on retinal vessels in these dosages and that the changes observed during systemic administration may be in response to the rise in blood pressure.

ANGIOTENSIN

The position with angiotensin is similar to that with norepinephrine.[13] In seven normals, angiotensin infusions increased their blood pressures from 115/72 mmHg to 166/114 mmHg and brought about a narrowing of the retinal arteries by a mean of 9.5 μ (Fig. 7-4).

Studies in animals suggest that retinal flow increases when the blood pressure is raised with angiotensin given systemically but there is no response when it is infused in subpressor doses into the carotid circulation.

NICOTINE

In a study of five men who were particularly sensitive to nicotine and who responded by a rise in blood pressure to smoking a cigarette[10] it has been reported that the retinal arteries narrowed by a mean of 21.9 per cent. As the blood pressure rose the change in vessel caliber may have occurred because of autoregulation.

VASOCONSTRICTOR DRUGS IN THERAPY

There do not appear to be any therapeutic uses for retinal vasoconstrictor drugs. The

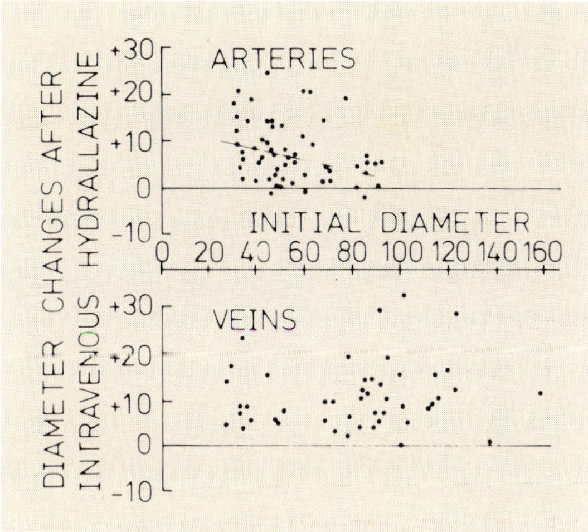

Fig. 7-3. Caliber changes in retinal arteries and veins in hypertensive patients treated with a mean of 37.5 mg of intravenous hydralazine. Mean blood pressure fell from 168 to 121 mmHg. Each **point** represents the change in caliber of a single vessel compared with its initial diameter before blood pressure was reduced. (From Ramalho and Dollery. Hypertensive retinopathy: Calibre changes in retinal blood vessels following blood pressure reduction and inhalation of oxygen. *Circulation 37:*580, 1968. By permission of the American Heart Association, Inc.)

Fig. 7-4. Changes in caliber of normal human retinal arteries during intravenous infusion of angiotensin and norepinephrine. Both drugs caused general narrowing of the vessels. (From Dollery, Hodge, and Hill.[13])

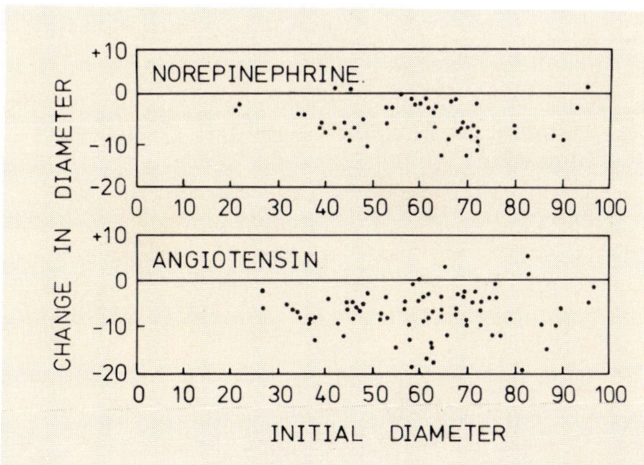

possibility of long-term effects of nicotine on retinal vessels in heavy cigarette smokers needs to be further evaluated.

ANTICOAGULANTS IN RETINAL VASCULAR DISEASE

If the central retinal artery or one of its branches is obstructed the retina suffers irreversible damage in a few minutes to hours. Anticoagulant drugs are unlikely to be of use in this situation.

The use of anticoagulants in retinal vein occlusion appears more promising because the circulation is less severely impaired and improvement may continue for several weeks. Following Holmin and Plomans' report in 1938[28] many patients have been treated, and most publications claim favorable results[14,29–31] although some have been less enthusiastic.[23,40] Vannas and Raitta[41] have treated 179 patients with central vein occlusion and 144 with branch vein occlusion. They claim that patients with central vein occlusion who were given anticoagulants had a better result than those who did not receive them. The visual acuity of the patients treated with anticoagulants lay between 1.0 to 0.1 in 55 to 57 per cent of cases while only 40 per cent of those treated with other agents reached this acuity. The incidence of hemorrhagic glaucoma was 35 per cent among the patients treated with anticoagulants and 48 per cent among those who did not receive them. It is interesting to note the reasons quoted why some patients were not treated with anticoagulants. These included therapeutic nihilism between 1951–52, the patients' unwillingness to cooperate, and the presence of other diseases such as malignant hypertension, polycythemia, etc. It is not surprising that the group who did not receive anticoagulants did worse than the others. Until a controlled therapeutic trial is carried out the value of anticoagulants in central retinal vein occlusion must be regarded as unproved.

Similarly, there is no evidence that various forms of fibrinolytic therapy are of value.[25]

REFERENCES

1. Anderson, B., Saltzman, H. A., and Barbee, J. Y.: Effect of carbon dioxide on delay in ischemic visual blackout. *Invest. Ophthal. 4:*955, 1965.
2. Anderson, B., Saltzman, H. A., and Heyman, A.: The effects of hyperbaric oxygenation on retinal arterial occlusion. *Arch. Ophthal. 73:* 315, 1965.
3. Ashton, N., Ward, B., and Serpell, G.: Role of oxygen in the genesis of retrolental fibroplasia. *Brit. J. Ophthal. 37:*513, 1953.
4. Avery, M. E., and Oppenheimer, E. H.: Recent increase in mortality from hyaline membrane disease. *J. Pediat. 57:*553, 1960.
5. Baum, J. D., and Bulpitt, C. J.: Retinal vasoconstriction in premature infants with increased arterial oxygen tensions. *Arch. Dis. Child. 45:*350, 1970.
6. Bresnick, G. as quoted by Ashton, N.: Donders Lecture. Some aspects of the comparative pathology of oxygen toxicity in the retina. *Brit. J. Ophthal. 52:*505, 1968.
7. Bulpitt, C. J., Dollery, C. T. and Kohner, E. M.: The marginal plasma zone in the retinal microcirculation. *Cardiovasc. Res. 4:*207, 1970.
8. Campbell, K.: Intensive oxygen therapy as a possible cause of retrolental fibroplasia. A clinical approach. *Med. J. Aust. 2:*48, 1951.
9. Cusick, P. L., Benson, O. O., and Boothby, W. M.: Effect of anoxia and of high concentrations of oxygen on retinal vessels. *Proc. Mayo Clin. 15:*500, 1940.
10. Cusick, P. L., and Herrell, W. E.: Retinal arteriolar changes as part of an induced general vasospastic reaction. Effect of tobacco and cold. *Arch. Ophthal. 21:*111, 1939.
11. Dollery, C. T.: An explanation for the exaggerated response of the retinal vessels to oxygen. *J. Physiol. 201:*86P, 1969.
12. Dollery, C. T., Hill, D. W., Mailer, C. M., and Ramalho, P. S.: High oxygen pressure and the retinal blood vessels. *Lancet 1:*291, 1964.
13. Dollery, C. T., Hodge, J. V., and Hill, D. W.: The response of normal retinal blood vessels to angiotensin and noradrenaline. *J. Physiol. 165:*500, 1963.
14. Duff, I. F., Falls, H. F., and Linman, J. W.: Anticoagulant therapy in occlusive vascular disease of the retina. *Arch. Ophthal. 46:*601, 1951.
15. Elgin, S. S.: Arterio-venous oxygen difference across the uveal tract of the dog eye. *Invest. Ophthal. 3:*417, 1964.
16. Ellis, P. P.: Annual Review: Ocular pharmacology and toxicology. *Arch. Ophthal. 76:* 117, 1966.
17. Ellis, P. P.: Annual Review: Ocular pharmacology and toxicology. *Arch. Ophthal. 78:* 524, 1967.
18. Ellis, P. P., and Lende, R. A.: Induced spasm in the retinal arteries of cats. II. Influence of physical factors and drugs. *Arch. Ophthal. 71:*706, 1964.
19. Evans, P. J.: Retrolental fibroplasia. *Trans. Ophthal. Soc. U.K. 71:*613, 1951.
20. Frayser, R., and Hickam, J. B.: Retinal vascular response to breathing increased carbon dioxide and oxygen concentrations. *Invest. Ophthal. 3:*427, 1964.
21. Frayser, R., and Hickam, J. B.: Effect of vasodilator drugs on retinal blood flow in man. *Arch. Ophthal. 73:*640, 1965.
22. Frayser, R., Saltzman, H. A., Anderson, B., Hickam, J. B., and Sieker, H. O.: The effect of hyperbaric oxygenation on retinal circulation. *Arch. Ophthal. 77:*265, 1967.
23. Glees, M.: Ueber Erfahrungen mit Thrombozid bei der Zentralvenen thrombose. *Klin. Mbl. Augenheilk. 134:*807, 1959.
24. Haddad, H. M., and Leopold, I. H.: Effect of hyperbaric oxygenation on microcirculation. Use in therapy of retinal vascular disorders. *Invest. Ophthal. 4:*1141, 1965.
25. Hawkey, C., and Howell, M.: Intravenous streptokinase in the treatment of retinal vascular occlusion. *J. Clin. Path. 17:*363, 1964.
26. Hickam, J. B., and Frayser, R.: A photographic method for measuring the mean reti-

nal circulation time using fluorescein. *Invest. Ophthal. 4:*876, 1965.

27. Hickam, J. B., Frayser, R., and Ross, J. C.: A study of retinal venous blood oxygen saturation in human subjects by photographic means. *Circulation 27:*375, 1963.
28. Holmin, H., and Ploman, K. G.: Thrombosis of central vein of retina treated with heparin. *Lancet 1:*664, 1938.
29. Klien, B. A.: Anticoagulant therapy of occlusion of central vein of retina. *Arch. Ophthal. 26:*699, 1943.
30. Klien, B. A., and Olwin, J. H.: A survey of the pathogenesis of retinal vein occlusion. *Arch. Ophthal. 56:*207, 1956.
31. Larsson, S., and Nord, B.: Some remarks on retinal vein thrombosis and its treatment with anticoagulants. *Acta Ophthal. 28:*187, 1950.
32. Macri, F. J.: Pharmacology and toxicology of ophthalmic drugs. *Arch. Ophthal. 80:*506, 1968.
33. Margolis, G.: Hyperbaric oxygenation: The eye as a limiting factor. *Science 151:*466, 1966.
34. Noell, W. K.: Metabolic injuries of the visual cell. *Amer. J. Ophthal. 40:*60, 1955.
35. Noell, W. K.: Differentiation, metabolic oxygenation and viability of the visual cell. *Arch. Ophthal. 60:*702, 1958.
36. Patz, A.: New role of the ophthalmologist in the prevention of retrolental fibroplasia. *Arch. Ophthal. 78:*565, 1967.
37. Ramalho, P. S., and Dollery, C. T.: Hypertensive retinopathy: Caliber changes in retinal blood vessels following blood-pressure reduction and inhalation of oxygen. *Circulation 37:*580, 1968.
38. Sevel, D., and Freedman, A.: Cerebro-retinal degeneration due to carbon dioxide poisoning. *Brit. J. Ophthal. 51:*475, 1967.
39. Sieker, H. O., and Hickam, J. B.: Normal and impaired retinal vascular reactivity. *Circulation 7:*79, 1953.
40. Tilburtius, H.: Ueber Venenverschlusse der Netzhaut. *Klin. Mbl. Augenheilk. 136:*604, 1960.
41. Vannas, S., and Raitta, C.: Anticoagulant therapy of retinal venous occlusion. *Amer. J. Ophthal. 62:*874, 1966.
42. Zahnd, K.: The effect of vasoactive drugs on the retinal circulation. *Trans. Ophthal. Soc. U.K. 86:*529, 1966.

chapter 8

Diagnostic Methods and Clinical Applications

This chapter outlines a number of the methods used for observing the fundus and detecting vascular abnormalities. Aside from direct visualization we have included ophthalmodynamometry, a manipulative procedure for eliciting retinal vascular pulsation, and electroretinography, an objective test of retinal function. The most important of the methods to be described in evaluating the retinal vasculature is direct ophthalmoscopy. Indirect ophthalmoscopy and biomicroscopy are also very important tools in the diagnosis of retinal disease. Of course, no written description of the various techniques can approach the usefulness of personal experience gained by looking at the fundus.

OPHTHALMOSCOPY

DIRECT OPHTHALMOSCOPY

Use of a direct ophthalmoscope permits one to view the fundus and obtain a virtual image which is erect and magnified. The magnification depends upon the dioptric power of the eye examined. In an individual without refractive error, an emmetrope, the apparent magnification is approximately 15 times. In the myopic individual, whose eye has a greater dioptric power, the image size is larger and the field of view smaller. The hyperope, possessing an eye of lesser dioptric strength, presents a smaller image and a larger field of view. In the aphakic individual, one without a lens, the field of view is large but magnification is small. Vessels, which would normally be invisible to the naked eye, can easily be seen by direct ophthalmoscopy. It is possible to examine small arteries and veins 15 to 20 μ in diameter because their apparent size will be 225 to 300 μ. Similarly, Wolff[31] noted that it is possible to see individual retinal pigment epithelial cells by this technique.

The fundus is usually viewed with white light, and the more intense it is the better can detail be appreciated. Electric ophthalmoscopes provide more light than battery-operated ones and are particularly useful in cases where the ocular media are hazy. Restricted spectral light may be useful in some instances. For example, red-free light, and more particularly yellow green light, shows up the blood vessels as black against a light background. Red light, such as obtained with a Wratten # 29 filter, helps to delineate alterations in the pigment epithelium, but makes the small retinal vessels and hemorrhages virtually invisible. Potts[25] has provided a discussion of monochromatic ophthalmoscopy which should be consulted by those interested in the subject.

Pupillary dilatation with mydriatics is essential for adequate evaluation of the fundus by any form of ophthalmoscopy. Neo-Synephrine in a 10% solution may suffice to dilate the pupils of patients with blue or light brown eyes, but stronger mydriatics such as cyclopentolate (Cyclogyl) or tropicamide (Mydriacil) are used in patients with darker irides. Through a well-dilated pupil it is possible to examine the fundus of the eye to the equator or just beyond by the direct method.

Both direct illumination and indirect illumination are utilized in the examination of the fundus. In the former, light is played over the surface to be examined. Depth can be appreciated by the use of parallax, here the ophthalmoscope is steadied and the observer moves his eye across the pupillary aperture of the ophthalmoscope. In indirect illumination the tissue to the side of the illuminated area is examined. By this means it is possible to detect small alterations in the pigment epithelium, and to determine whether a fundic mass is solid or serous. For example, a choroidal melanoma will appear dark when the ophthalmoscope light is directed towards its edge, while serous elevations will transilluminate.

The examination of the fundus should commence at the optic nerve head or disc, and then each quadrant should be examined in turn by having the patient rotate his eye into the field viewed (i.e., examination of the superotemporal retina requires the eye to be rotated up and out). The shape, color, configuration, and the vessel pattern of the disc should all be noted. The disc measures about 1.5 mm in diameter and provides a good standard for comparison of the relative size of the retinal vessels and of fundus lesions. The size of the disc also serves as a marker for distances within the fundus. For example, it is common usage to note that a lesion is so many disc diameters (dd) from the disc margin, or that a fundus lesion is so many dd in size. The fovea is approximately 2 dd from the temporal edge of the disc just below the horizontal meridian. If present, retinal vascular pulsation will be seen at or adjacent to the disc, and its presence or absence may be significant.

RETINAL VASCULAR PULSATION

Retinal arteries and veins exhibit pulsation which is related to the general phenomenon of systemic vascular pulsation, but with certain modifications due to the location of the retinal vessels within a closed pressure chamber—the eye. The retinal vascular pulsation is synchronous with the contraction of heart. Thus, the pulse rate and its regularity can often be detected on routine ophthalmoscopy.

Arterial Pulsation

Two types of rhythmic pulsation of retinal arteries have been described; expansile and serpentine.[8] The former, a rhythmic alteration in caliber-reflecting transmission of the pressure-pulse from the heart through the systemic arteries, is best seen upon or near the disc. It is infrequent to detect such pulsation in the normal human by monocular direct ophthalmoscopy. However, with increased magnification, such as provided by the Gullstrand type of binocular ophthalmoscope, expansile arterial pulsation can be detected in the majority of people. Enhanced arterial pulsation is seen in the following:

1. Conditions which are associated with an exaggerated systemic pulse pressure such as aortic insufficiency, aortic aneurysm or thyrotoxicosis
2. Elevated intraocular pressure; i.e. glaucoma, ophthalmodynamometry
3. Decreased systemic or carotid artery blood pressure; i.e. anemia, shock, etc.
4. Increased distensibility of the globe, i.e. high myopia

Serpentine pulsation, also called arterial locomotion, can, with appropriate magnification, be detected in all normal eyes. It consists of rhythmic lateral movements or variations in curvature of a segment of a retinal artery. It is most easily seen in dilated and tortuous arteries, but never in a perfectly straight one. An elevated systolic blood pressure and a large pulse pressure enhance its appearance. The phenomena is similar to that seen in any flexible tube which is subject to intermittent flow.

TABLE 8-1
Retinal Vein Pulsation

Incidence:
Commonly seen or easily elicited in normal individuals.

Prominent Appearance:

A. Increased intraocular pressure
   1. Glaucoma
   2. Ophthalmodynamometry

B. Increased systemic arterial pressure or widened pulse pressure
   1. Hypertension
   2. Aortic insufficiency

Diminished or Absent:

A. Occasionally absent in normal eyes, but easily elicitable

B. Decreased intraocular pressure

C. Increased venous pressure
   1. Impending CRV occlusion
   2. Frank CRV occlusion
   3. Mechanical elevation of venous pressure: pressure on jugulars, Valsalva maneuver, lateral rotation of eyes.
   4. Secondary to increased cerebral spinal fluid pressure. Pulse generally absent in papilledema and difficult to elicit.

D. Decreased arterial pressure.

Venous Pulsation

Spontaneous expansile pulsation of the central retinal vein (CRV) at the optic disc can be observed in almost all normal humans if observations are made with the binocular direct ophthalmoscope. With the ordinary direct ophthalmoscope it can be appreciated in a high proportion of individuals. Spontaneous pulsation was seen in 68 per cent of 200 consecutive nondiseased eyes (Henkind, unpublished data). The incidence increased directly with age (Fig. 8-1), and was more common in eyes with higher intraocular pressure (Fig. 8-2). Gentle digital pressure invariably produced a venous pulse in those eyes without a spontaneous one. The rate of pulsation corresponds directly to the rate of ventricular contraction and is independent of the auricular rate; in auricular-ventricular dissociation, the ventricular rate determines the retinal venous pulse rate.

More data will have to be accumulated before any definite statements regarding the significance of absent or present venous pulsation can be made. However, some general statements may be of value (Table 8-1).

An abnormal pulsatile rhythm may indicate a cardiac arrhythmia. Increased visibility of venous pulsation may indicate either increased intraocular pressure or an abnormal state of the general circulation (e.g., hypertension, aortic insufficiency). Absent pulsation occurs in ocular hypotension, sclerosis of the central retinal artery, and particularly if not elicitable by gentle digital pressure, in increased intracranial pressure. Unilaterally decreased or absent venous pulsation may be an early sign of partial or impending venous obstruction. In the pseudochoked disc normal venous pulsation is either present or easily elicitable. On the other hand, in true papilledema, even in the early state, the pulse is generally absent and difficult to elicit. However, this sign is not invariable and in rare instances of frank papilledema there may be a spontaneous CRV pulse. In certain diseases such as diabetes and conditions with serum hyperviscosity the retinal veins may be dilated and the venous pulse diminished or absent.

INDIRECT OPHTHALMOSCOPY

In indirect ophthalmoscopy a strong convex lens is held in front of the patient's eye. The lens focuses emergent rays from the eye and the observer obtains a real inverted image which is formed at the principal focus of the lens. This focus lies between the plus

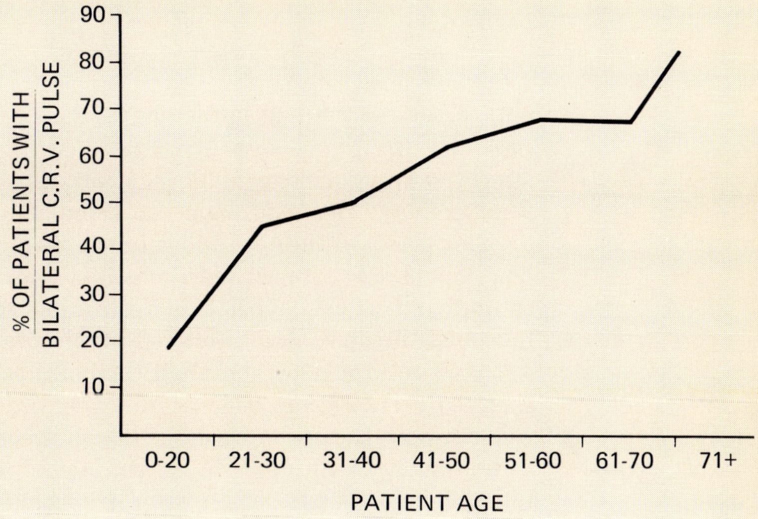

Fig. 8-1. Chart showing the percentage of patients exhibiting bilateral spontaneous CRV pulsation at various age groups.

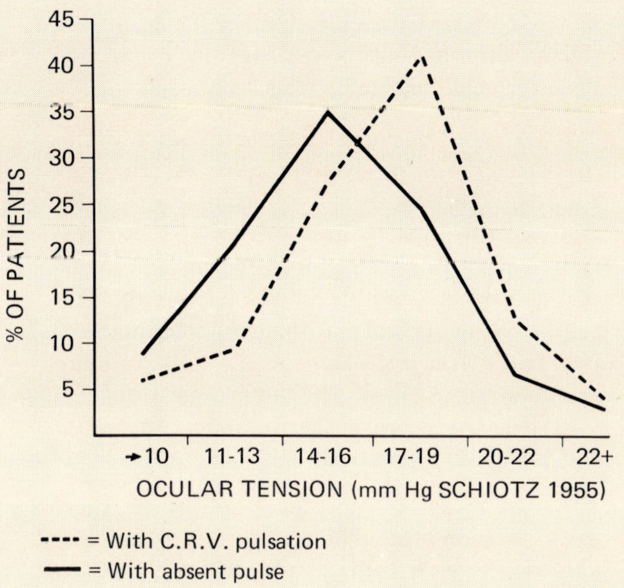

Fig. 8-2. Comparison of ocular tensions in patients with and without spontaneous CRV pulsation. Patients with spontaneous pulsation tended to have slightly higher ocular tensions that those without spontaneous pulsation.

(convex) lens and the observer. In this form of ophthalmoscopy the magnification of the retinal image depends primarily on the lens used; i.e., with the +13 diopter lens the magnification is approximately five times. Stronger lenses produce a smaller magnification, but provide a larger and brighter field of view. With a widely dilated pupil it is possible, by proper positioning of the patient's eye, to see well beyond the equator. The addition of the technique of scleral indentation permits observation of the entire fundus beyond the ora serrata.

The advantages of binocular indirect ophthalmoscopy are stereopsis, large field of view, and excellent illumination. This is of particular value in retinal detachment surgery, in evaluation of large and elevated fundus lesions, and in patients with cloudy media. On the other hand, the lesser magnification of this method compared to direct ophthalmoscopy is a marked disadvantage when studying retinopathies characterized by small retinal lesions and when evaluating retinal vascular alterations. Furthermore, the method is not easily learned and is little used outside of ophthalmology.

APPLANATION OPHTHALMOSCOPY

Eliminating the dioptric power of the cornea, either by flattening it or by applying a contact lens with a flat anterior surface permits one to view the interior of the eye by ordinary illumination, such as a penlight. A number of workers, dating back to the latter half of the nineteenth century, found that the application of a glass cover slip to the cornea was sufficient for fundoscopy. By this method a large field can be surveyed rapidly. The magnification of the fundus image depends upon the remaining dioptric power of the eye, and is in the neighborhood of five times. We have had some limited experience with this technique in humans. A specially designed applaning glass on a handle was applied to the anesthetized cornea and observations were carried out with the use of a bright illuminating source such as an electric ophthalmoscope light. In most instances a drop of methylcellulose was placed on the undersurface of the glass before it was applied to the eye. The method was useful for examining the fundi of high myopes and fundi with extensive lesions. With a widely dilated pupil one gets the feeling of looking into a "fish bowl." Applanation ophthalmoscopy has been particularly valuable in examining the fundi of animals with small eyes. Here the method is combined with use of the lighting and magnification of an operating microscope.

SLIT-LAMP BIOMICROSCOPY

Slit-lamp biomicroscopy is invaluable for studying the vitreous and retina. With this method one obtains a magnified, bright, stereoscopic image which in combination with the slit beam permits accurate localization of anatomic structures and pathologic features.

In order for the posterior vitreous and retina to be viewed some type of lens must be used to bring the image of the posterior segment within the focusing range of the microscope. Three different methods have been used to resolve this problem:

1. Use of a contact lens, such as the Goldmann lens. This lens with its flat anterior surface eliminates the corneal refraction and permits a virtual image of the fundus. The magnification depends on that of the biomicroscope; 25 times is about the highest useful magnification. Aside from its other virtues the contact lens can be used to steady the eye in a patient with nystagmus, thus permitting a fundus evaluation unobtainable by other means.

2. Use of a concave lens to negate the dioptric power of the eye converts the corneal microscope into a telescope with a focus on the retina and provides a virtual image. In the Hruby lens system a −55 diopter lens is used in front of the eye. The field of view and magnification obtained are less than that with the contact lens, but the advantage is that the eye need not be touched. Only the posterior pole can be observed by this method.

3. In a technique, described by El Bayardi,[7] which corresponds to indirect ophthalmoscopy, a high plus lens is placed in front of the cornea. In this case a real, inverted image of the fundus is obtained.

Goldmann has modified the contact lens by the addition of three internal mirrors each placed at a different angle. This permits observation of the entire fundus out to the periphery.

According to Goldmann [9] the examination is carried out as follows:

1. In direct illumination with the focused light either white or red-free the desired site is examined. With red-free light nerve fibers, changes in the retina, and the yellow color of the macula are well seen. To estimate depth, the angle between the illuminating beam and the microscope should be as wide as possible.

2. By indirect illumination the tissue surrounding the illuminated site is examined. This procedure permits evaluation of the details and abnormalities of the pigment epithelium and underlying choroid.

OPHTHALMODYNAMOMETRY

Normally the amplitude of the retinal artery pulse is too slight to be observed by ordinary direct or indirect ophthalmoscopy. In ophthalmodynamometry the intraocular pressure is increased by a calibrated external force. The first visible pulsation of the retinal arteries caused by the applied force is considered diastolic while the first pulse following complete collapse of the arteries signifies it is systolic. Thus, the eye is converted into a visible sphygmomanometer. As Duke-Elder[6] has emphasized, the compression of the central retinal artery to the point of collapse actually *measures the lateral pressure in the ophthalmic artery.* He states, "The technique thus elucidates the state of the cerebral rather than the ocular circulation. Its interest is therefore almost entirely non-ophthalmological."

The ophthalmodynamometer is a device for exerting pressure upon the globe. Bailliart's instrument, or variations of it, is the most commonly used. It consists of a spring-loaded plunger with a slightly convex footplate. The force exerted by the footplate upon the lateral aspect of the globe is indicated on a scale calibrated in grams. Another instrument, the suction cup, uses negative pressure to deform the globe and thus increase intraocular pressure.

For ophthalmodynamometry the patient's pupil should be dilated. The footplate of the instrument is placed over the lateral rectus muscle of the anesthetized eye and pressure is applied toward the center of the globe while the nerve head is being observed with the ophthalmoscope. Readings may be taken both at diastole and systole, but many clinicians feel that the diastolic readings alone are sufficient for most purposes. The values obtained need not be converted into mmHg, for the test is used primarily to compare the differences between the eyes. Normally there is less than a 15 per cent difference in the readings of the two eyes.

The major use of ophthalmodynamometry has been in the diagnosis of carotid artery stenosis or occlusion. A difference of more than 15 or 20 per cent suggests carotid disease on the side of the lower recording. It is also useful for assessing the probable effect of carotid ligation in cases of aneurysms of the carotid system. If preoperative compression of the carotid artery results in a drop of the pressure reading to less than 30 per cent of the initial value, ligation may be dangerous.

ELECTRORETINOGRAPHY

All of the previous material has dealt with tests or procedures that directly examine the retinal vessels, and can thus be considered subjective methods. Objective electrophysiologic tests may also be used to gain some useful information regarding the state of the retinal circulation, with the most common of the tests being the electroretinogram (ERG).

After a brief consideration of the ERG we will consider some aspects of its response to various agents and its use in retinal vascular disease.

Electroretinography is a technique for eliciting a transient electrical response from the outer retinal layers by means of a light flash. A corneal electrode is used to pick up the electrical response which is then amplified and displayed on an oscilloscope, multichannel recorder, or computer. In the testing procedure the light stimulus may be controlled with regard to wavelength, in-

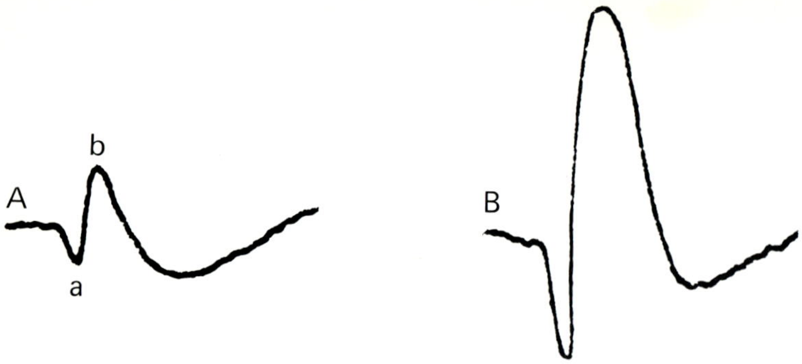

Fig. 8-3. Electroretinographic responses obtained from an ink-writing galvanometer. *A*, Light-adapted, white light: **a,** a-wave; **b,** b-wave, *B*, Dark-adapted, red light. (Courtesy of Dr. Ronald Carr.)

tensity, and frequency, and for maximum information, testing is conducted under both light-adapted (photopic) and dark-adapted (scotopic) conditions.

The normal response in man consists of a series of electrical oscillations which form a distinctive type of two-dimensional trace on an oscilloscope or on the paper of an appropriate recorder (Fig. 8-3). The components of the ERG in the order which they appear have been designated as follows: a-wave (or late receptor potential), which appears as a sharp downward deflection; b-wave (or on-effect) which follows the a-wave as a more pronounced upward or positive deflection; and c-wave (secondary rise) which is a sluggish positive wave usually appearing before the b-wave has returned to the baseline. Of these waves, the a and the b are the most important in relation to retinal vascularization. The a-wave is thought to arise from the inner segments of the photoreceptors (rods and cones), an area nourished primarily by the choriocapillaris, while the b-wave originates in the bipolar layer (inner nuclear layer), an area supplied directly by the deep strata of retinal capillaries.

PHYSIOLOGIC RESPONSES

Alpern and co-workers [1] and Jayle, Boyer, and Saracco [16] have demonstrated that hyperventilation caused an increase in the amplitude of the b-wave with the increase being noted after 1 minute of increased respiration. The a-wave has been found to vary and may decrease or increase in amplitude.

A number of workers [2,26] have noted a diminution of the b-wave in hypoxia, and this loss in the positive potential was particularly marked on stimulation with red light.[2]

According to Jayle, Boyer, and Saracco [16] only Sverak [30] has studied the effect of hypercapnia on the ERG. Using 8% CO_2 and 92% O_2 he found a significant elevation in the amplitude of the b-wave.

Henkes, in 1951,[11] was the first to demonstrate that vasodilating drugs caused an elevation in the amplitude of the b-wave. Shortly thereafter, Jacobson and his colleagues [14,15] showed that 1.2 mg of nitroglycerin given sublingually; 120 mg of papaverine given intravenously; 50 mg of Priscoline given intravenously; 12 mg of nylidrin given orally, all caused a marked increase in the amplitude of the scotopic b-wave in normal individuals. The maximum effect was observed 15 minutes after administration of the drug. A 100-mg dose of nicotinic acid given intravenously, or stellate ganglion block with lidocaine, had no appreciable effect on the ERG. The authors have suggested that the increased amplitude of the b-wave reflected an increase in blood flow in either the retinal or choroidal circulation.[15] However, there is no proof that the changes in the b-wave were the result of changes in blood flow.

Zewi and Vainio-Mattila [33] have published findings similar to those of Jacobson and Lincoln [15] except that they have noted an increment in the b-wave after oral administration of 100 mg of nicotinic acid. In a 37-

TABLE 8-2
ERG in Retinal Circulatory Abnormality

	ERG findings
Extraocular	
Carotid artery occlusion	Diminished b-wave, especially to flicker [23]
Temporal arteritis	Most commonly diminished b-wave, but may have enhanced a-wave [4,32]
Ophthalmic artery occlusion	Absent ERG [5]
Intraocular	
Hypertension	Normal in grade 1 or 2, normal or subnormal ERG in grades 3 or 4 K–W [18]
Arteriosclerosis	No typical picture, most commonly a diminished b-wave [13,28]
Retinal artery occlusion	
Central	Generally reduced or negative ERG [12,18,22] May find initial elevation of b-wave [3,10]
Branch	Generally normal
Retinal Vein Occlusion	
Central	Varies from sub- to supernormal. Prognosis better in cases with normal or supernormal ERG [18,19]
Branch	Normal
Diabetic Retinopathy	Usually normal, occasionally supernormal possibly due to venous stasis.[21] Abnormal oscillatory potentials even before visible retinopathy [27]

K–W = Keith-Wagener classification of hypertensive retinopathy

year-old female with retinal arterial spasm they noted a beneficial effect of vasodilating agents on the visual acuity and an increase in b-wave amplitude in a case of retinal angiospasm due to quinine poisoning, but only during the initial phase of the disease.

Papst and Heck [24] found that small doses of vasodilators (0.08-mg dose of nitroglycerin given sublingually; 5 mg of Dilatol given subcutaneously; 25 mg of Nepresol given intramuscularly or orally), 96% O_2 or glucose loading caused no alteration in the ERG in normal individuals. Patients with "moderate" retinal circulatory disturbances showed an increased b-wave amplitude when given Nepresol, nitroglycerin, or glucose.

Nicotine, a vasoconstrictor, has been noted [29] to cause, paradoxically, an increased amplitude of the b-wave, but this may be due to factors other than vascular.

As a result of the above findings, Jayle, Boyer, and Saracco [17] concluded that the amplitude of the ERG seems closely linked to the retinal circulation. Particularly impressive are the b-wave responses. The association of the bipolar cells which probably generate the b-wave and their surrounding capillaries certainly bears further investigation. At present there is no direct evidence that the capillary blood flow is enhanced, or the capillaries are directly dilated by vasodilating agents.

ERG IN RETINAL CIRCULATORY ALTERATIONS

The ERG has been studied in a wide variety of disorders which affect the retinal circulation either directly or secondarily[20] in retinal vascular disease. (Table 8-2.)

REFERENCES

1. Alpern, M., Faris, J., Eskildsen, P., and Garnett, P.: Effect of hyperventilation on the human electroretinogram. *Science 121:*101, 1955.
2. Brown, J., Hill, J., and Burke, R.: The effect of hypoxia on the human electroretinogram. *Amer. J. Ophthal. 44:*57, 1957.
3. Burian, H.: Clinical electroretinography. *Int. Ophthal. Clin. 2:*21, 1962.
4. Burian, H.: Electroretinography in temporal arteritis. *Amer. J. Ophthal. 56:*796, 1963.
5. Carr, R. E., and Siegel, I.: Electrophysiologic findings in several retinal disorders. *Amer. J. Ophthal. 58:*95, 1964.
6. Duke-Elder, W. S.: *System of Ophthalmology. The Foundations of Ophthalmology.* London, Kimpton, 1962, vol. 7, p. 356.
7. El Bayardi, G.: New method of slit-lamp microophthalmoscopy. *Brit. J. Ophthal. 37:*625, 1953.
8. Friedenwald, J. S.: Retinal vascular dynamics. *Amer. J. Ophthal. 17:*387, 1934.
9. Goldmann, H.: Biomicroscopy of the eye. *Amer. J. Ophthal. 66:*789, 1968.
10. Heck, J.: Das Elektroretinogramm bei Verschluss der Arteria centralis retinal. *Graefe. Arch. Ophthal. 158:*17, 1956.
11. Henkes, H.: Use of electroretinography in measuring the effects of vasodilatation. *Angiology 2:*125, 1951.
12. Henkes, H.: ERG in circulatory disturbances of the retina. 1. ERG in cases of occlusion of the central retinal artery or one of its branches. *Arch. Ophthal. 51:*42, 1954.
13. Henkes, H.: ERG in circulatory disturbances of the retina. 4. ERG in cases of retinal and choroidal hypertension and arteriosclerosis. *Arch. Ophthal. 52:*30, 1954.
14. Jacobson, J. H., and Basir, D.: The effects of a new drug, nylidrin, upon the electroretinogram. *Arch. Ophthal. 56:*865, 1956.
15. Jacobson, J. H., and Lincoln, M. W.: Effect of vasodilator drugs and stellate ganglion block upon the electroretinogram. *Arch. Ophthal. 52:*917, 1954.
16. Jayle, G. E., Boyer, R. L., and Saracco, J. B.: *L'Electroretinographie. Bases physiologiques et donnees cliniques.* Paris, Masson et Cie, 1965, p. 427.
17. Jayle, G. E., Boyer, R. L., and Saracco, J. B.: *L'Electroretinographie. Bases physiologiques et donnees cliniques.* Paris, Masson et Cie, 1965, p. 437.
18. Jayle, G. E., Boyer, R. L., and Saracco, J. B.: *L'Electroretinographie. Bases physiologiques et donnees cliniques.* Vol. 2, pp. 811–852.
19. Karpe, G.: The basis of clinical electroretinography. *Acta Ophthal. Suppl. 24,* 1945.
20. Karpe, G.: Indications for clinical electroretinography. *Arch. Ophthal. 60:*889, 1958.
21. Karpe, G., Kornerup, T., and Wulfing, B.: The clinical electroretinogram. 8. The electroretinogram in diabetic retinopathy. *Acta Ophthal. 36:*281, 1958.
22. Karpe, G., and Uchermann, A.: The ERG in circulatory disturbances of the retina. *Acta Ophthal. 33:*493, 1955.
23. Krill, A. E., Diamond, M., and Iser, G.: The electroretinogram in carotid artery disease. *Arch. Ophthal. 68:*42, 1962.
24. Papst, W., and Heck, J.: Das Elektroretinogramm bei Zirkulationsstörungen der Netzhaut und seine Beeinflussung durch gefässerweiternde Mittel, Sauerstoffbeatmung und Hyperglykämie. *Klin. Mbl. Augenheilk. 131:*598, 1957.

25. Potts, A.: Monochromatic ophthalmoscopy. *Trans. Amer. Ophthal. Soc. 63:*276, 1965.
26. Schubert, G., and Bornschein, H.: Elektroretinogramm und Helligkeitswahrnehmung bei Hypoxie. *Wien Z. Nervenheilk. 4:*393, 1951.
27. Simonsen, S. E.: "ERG in Juvenile Diabetics: A Prognostic Study," in *Treatment of Diabetic Retinopathy.* Ed. by Goldberg, M. F., and Fine, S. L. U.S. Washington, D. C., Public Health Service Publication No. 1890, 1969, p. 681.
28. Straub, W.: Elektroretinographie Befunde bei sklerotischen Fundusveränderungen. *Ber. Deutsch Opth. Ges. 61:*203, 1957.
29. Straub, W. and Winkelman, J.: Versuche über die Beeinflussung der b-Wellenamplitude des Menschlichen Elektroretinogramms durch Zigaretten rauchen, Kaffeegenus und Lachgasinhalation. Symp. Luhacovice. 1959: Acta Facult. Med. Univ. Brunensis. *4:*179, 1960.
30. Sverak, J.: Prispevek ke klïnicke fysiologii lidskeho ERG. Suppl. Sborniku vedeckych praci Lekarske fakuly KUV Hradci Kral *2:*3, 1959. Quoted by Jayle et al.[16]
31. Wolff, E.: Can the network formed by the retinal pigment epithelium be seen by the ophthalmoscope? *Proc. R. Soc. Med. 31:*1104, 1938.
32. Younessian, S.: L'ERG dans l'arterite temporale. *Ophthalmologica 143:*288, 1962.
33. Zewi, M., and Vainio-Mattila, B.: The effect of vasodilation on the electroretinogram. *Acta Ophthal. 33:*53, 1955

resolution of about 80 line pairs per millimeter on the film which is equivalent to about 5 μ on the retinal surface.

CAMERA

Several cameras are available for fluorescein work, but the most widely employed is the Carl Zeiss apparatus fitted with a rapid-fire electronic flash pack and a motorized Robot camera for film transport. Our own cameras have been modified to use motorized Nikon F 36 camera bodies (Fig. 9-2). It is important that film transport should be automatic and the electronic flash should recycle at least every second. A timing device which prints the time elapsed since the dye injection onto each frame is essential. For animal work and some clinical purposes such as photography of retinal lesions in neonates it is convenient to have a vertically mounted camera (Fig. 9-3). The retinal camera can also be fitted with a device for automatically taking stereoscopic fluorescein pictures if this facility is needed.[1,2]

TECHNIQUE

Before dye injection, the camera is set up and focused using white light and the blue filter switched in. Injections are usually made into a forearm vein in doses of 0.5 to 1 gm using 5 or 10% solution. We generally use 10% solution for venous injections. Errors can easily occur in a darkened room and it is important to have a foolproof checking system to ensure that the correct fluid is given. If several injections are to be given it is our practice to insert a plastic catheter in an antecubital vein through a needle. The Intracath available commercially is suitable.

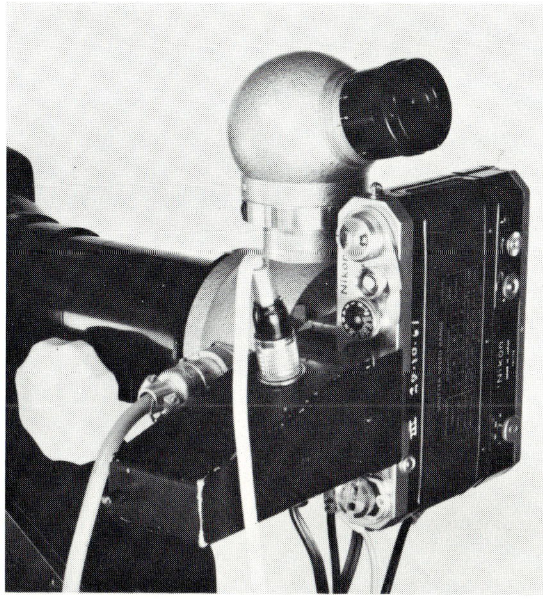

Fig. 9-2. Zeiss retinal camera modified to accept a Nikon F36 electrically driven camera. The light path in the eyepiece has been lengthened to compensate for the greater thickness of the Nikon camera. The pentaprism and reflex mirror of the Nikon have been removed and a timing unit inserted which prints the time on each frame to the nearest 1/100th second.

Fig. 9-3. Zeiss retinal camera mounted vertically for fluorescein work in recumbent patients or anesthetized animals. The table movement controls have been extended to facilitate operation of the apparatus.

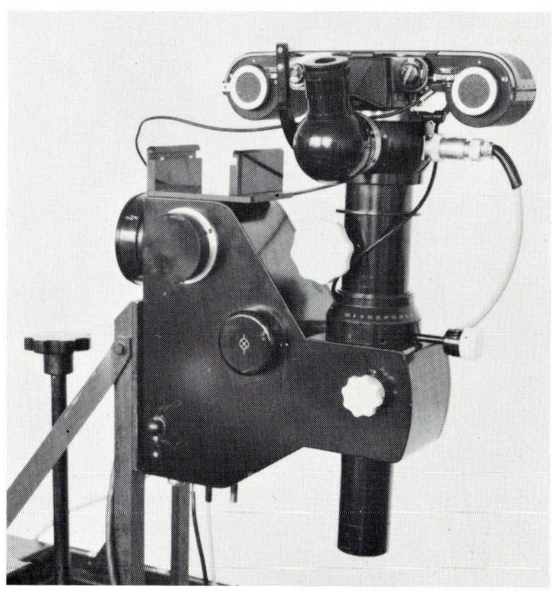

The injection should be given rapidly to keep the slug of dye as compact as possible. An automatic injector is helpful but not essential.

It is possible to view the fundus between exposures but a more evenly timed set of pictures can be obtained by allowing the equipment to fire automatically while the dye is filling the arteries and capillaries. Usually three or four injections are given to study several different areas of the retina at one session. If there is leakage of dye, as is seen in a diabetic patient with extensive new vessel systems, the second and subsequent injections may give poor-quality results.

A technique of inserting a small plastic catheter in the innominate artery by a percutaneous method has been described by Dollery.[5] This method requires special skill with intravascular catheterization and improvements in filter design now permit satisfactory results in most patients by the venous route.

Poor results may be attributable to many factors but if photographic conditions are satisfactory the most probable explanation is a long circulation time in a patient with borderline congestive heart failure. The dye is much more dispersed when it reaches the eye in these patients and the low peak concentration makes image density inadequate. The arterial route does not suffer from this disadvantage because the injection is made much closer to the eye.

CINE-FLUORESCEIN PHOTOGRAPHY

For most purposes fluorescein pictures taken at a rate of one to two frames per second give satisfactory data about the filling and emptying of the vascular structures in the retina. However, they are much too slow to measure the velocity of flow in the retinal arterioles. For this purpose cinephotography at a rate of 30 to 60 frames per second is required. It is possible to film cineangiograms directly[4,7,12,18,21] but a very bright light source is needed, and the image density falls off at framing rates above 12 to 15 per second. An alternative approach is to use an image-intensifying system. Such systems give light gains of up to a million times with a resolution of up to 50 line pairs per millimeter. At present the equipment is expensive and bulky but further development may see it brought into wider use.[4] Cine-fluorescein angiography has proved satisfactory in animals for measuring flow velocities under different circumstances.[6,7]

A further problem is the identification of the leading edge of the dye front in the retinal arteries. After a venous injection the first tongue of dye entering the retinal vessels is dilute (Fig. 9-4) and hard to locate accurately on cine-film frames. In animals where an arterial injection is used routinely the dye front is much sharper and can be measured without difficulty (Fig. 9-5).

CLINICAL PHARMACOLOGY OF FLUORESCEIN

Sodium fluorescein is the salt of a complex organic molecule whose molecular weight is 376 (Fig. 9-6). The excitation and emission spectrum of the molecule in aqueous solution have been studied by Hodge and Clemett[15] and by Wessing.[35] The peak frequencies for excitation lie between 485 and 500 mμ and for emission between 520 and 530 mμ (Fig. 9-7). The intensity of fluorescence depends upon the pH and the concentration of the dye. Physiologic changes in pH are not large enough to cause significant alterations in fluorescence. If fluorescein concentration is being recorded quantitatively to construct dye dilution curves it is important not to exceed a concentration of

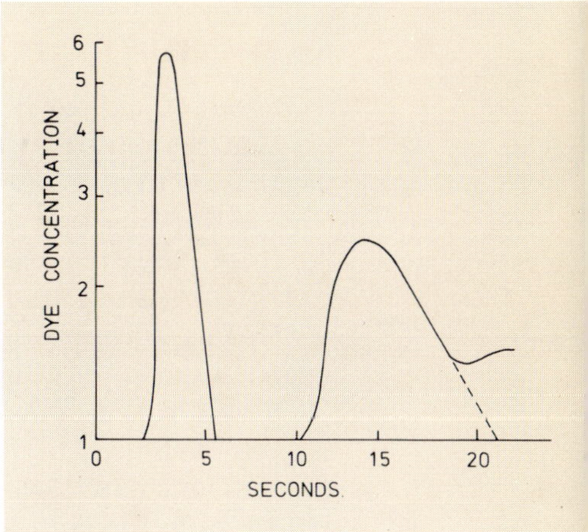

Fig. 9-4. *Top right.* Schematic diagram of dilution curves in the retinal arteries after dye injection into a peripheral vein or the carotid artery. Arterial injection gives a compact slug of dye, which arrives quickly and the initial front entering the retinal vessels is sharp. In contrast the rate of rise of dye concentration after a peripheral vein injection is less abrupt and the slug of dye is more dispersed. The curves are not to scale as the same amount of dye injected into the carotid artery as into the peripheral vein would give a 10- to 20-times higher peak concentration.

Fig. 9-5. *Middle right. A,* Fluorescein angiogram following intracarotid injection of 0.3 ml of 10% sodium fluorescein in a pig. The dye front can be identified **(arrow).** *Bottom right. B,* The next frame shows movement of the dye front down the vessel **(arrow).**

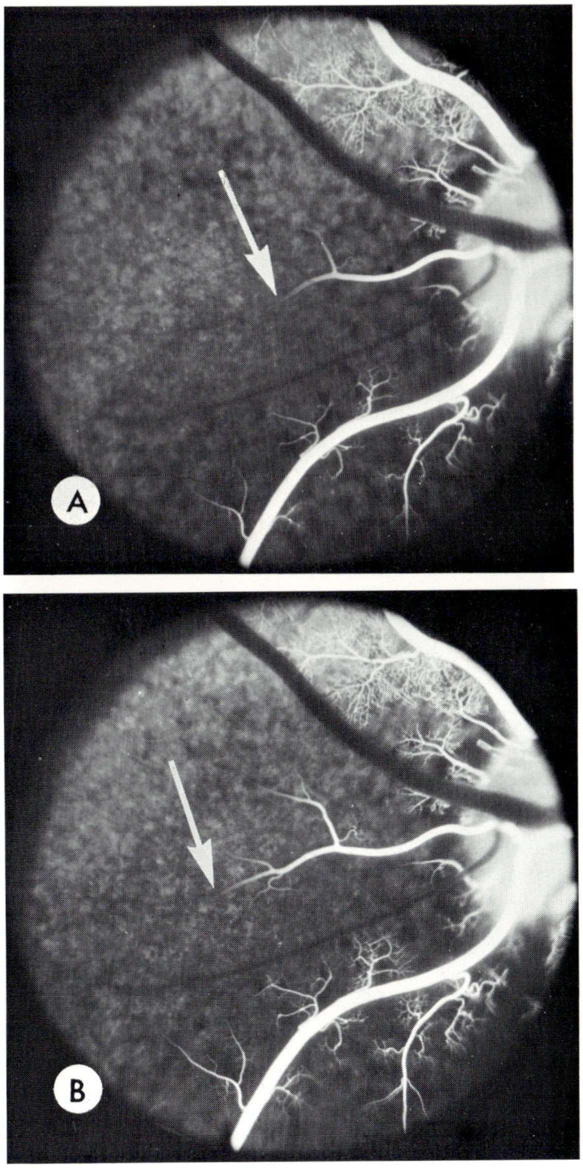

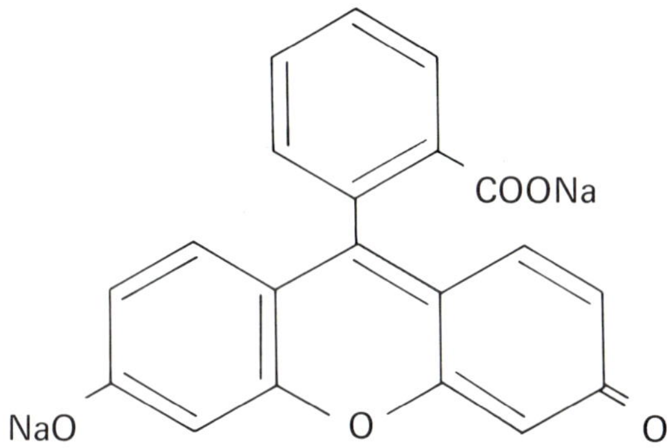

Fluorescein Sodium
mol. wt. 376-27

Fig. 9-6. Structural formula of fluorescein sodium (molecular weight 376.27), the dye used in retinal fluorescein photography.

Fig. 9-7. Excitation and emission spectrum of fluorescein in blood. The first **(1)** peak shows the optimal exciting frequency and the second **(2)** and third **(3)** the main emission peaks in arterial and venous blood. (From Hodge and Clemett.[14])

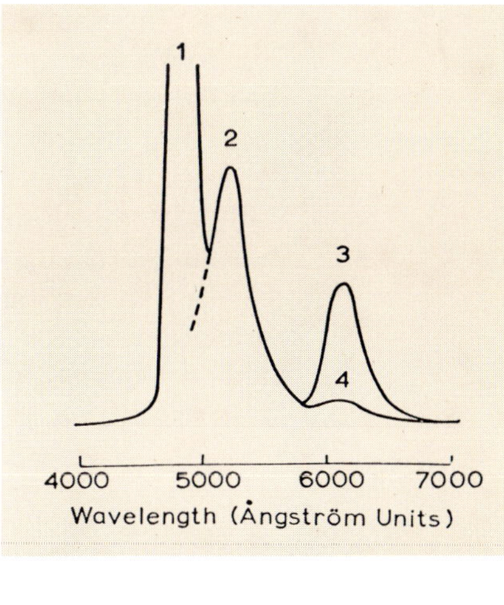

about 10 mg per liter. Above this concentration the emitted light is no longer linearly related to dye concentration.

After injection the dye is rapidly cleared from the plasma. Dollery, Hodge, and Engel[8] have found that the plasma concentration 10 minutes after injection was only one-quarter of that of radioiodine-labeled albumin which had been mixed with it in the syringe. The dye passes readily across systemic capillaries and enters the tissues, staining the skin and mucous membranes a yellow green tint. It is excreted rapidly by the kidney and the clearance exceeds the glomerular filtration rate. Usually the skin-staining fades within 4 hours and the urine ceases to be obviously colored after about 36 hours (Fig. 9-8). It is important to warn patients of the coloring of skin and urine and its probable duration. Almost all the dye is excreted unchanged in the urine although in rats a small proportion is conjugated with glucuronide.[34] Fluorescein, in common with many other weakly acidic drugs, is extensively bound to serum albumin. Equilibrium dialysis measurements showed binding varying from 50 to 84 per cent but this was readily reversible and all the dye could be dialyzed off the protein. The main importance of protein binding is that only the proportion that is free in plasma can diffuse across cell membranes. However, in the renal tubule the dye is transported by the weak organic acid transport system and as the free concentration falls more of the dye-protein complex will dissociate so that bound dye can also be cleared. In aqueous solution fluorescein emits approximately 80 per cent of the incident light as fluorescence. When bound to protein the efficiency falls to about 26 per cent.[20] Thus, the majority of the fluorescent light probably comes from free fluorescein in plasma although more than half is bound to protein.

Physiologic changes can modify the duration and intensity of fluorescence in retinal vessels. The oxyhemoglobin molecule has absorption peaks at 445 and 577 mμ and reduced hemoglobin at 555 mμ so that appreciable absorption takes place at the frequencies between 500 and 560 mμ at which the fluorescent light is emitted.[35] One result is that the intensity of fluorescence is much greater in patients with severe anemia. As these patients also have a short circulation time, particularly good results can be obtained. Fluorescein is not metabolized to any important extent and in consequence the dye may persist for long periods in the plasma and tissues of patients with severe renal failure. We have observed patients with uremia and hypertension who still had skin staining with the dye 3 days after injection.

The intensity of fluorescence and the optimum exciting frequency vary with different circumstances. Thus intravascular fluorescein is largely bound to plasma proteins which reduces the fluorescence and the emitted light is strongly absorbed by hemoglobin. Extravascular fluorescein will have a higher proportion of free dye not bound to protein which is not screened by hemoglobin. Thus leaking points on vessels may fluoresce more intensely than the blood vessels in the vascular phase.

TOXICITY

Fluorescein has been used in both ophthalmology and plastic surgery for many years and has proved to be relatively safe. Acute toxicity studies in animals show that the lethal dose is 2 to 3 gm per kilogram,[10] more than 100 times the usual clinical dose. No chronic toxicity studies with fluorescein have been reported.

No deaths, and only a small number of serious reactions, have been reported following the use of fluorescein in retinal angiography. One patient investigated at Hammersmith Hospital in London suffered vasomotor collapse with wheezing. The patient rapidly improved after treatment with 100 mg of intravenous hydrocortisone and 250 mg of aminophylline. She had a past history of allergy and had never received fluorescein before.[29] Recovery was rapid and complete. Another patient developed urticaria on two occasions following fluorescein studies. An anaphylactic reaction with nausea, pruritus, and laryngeal edema has been reported in one patient. Recovery was rapid following injection of 1:1000 epinephrine.[19] For the past 4 years we have used a test dose of 0.5 ml of 5% sodium fluorescein injected 2 minutes before the main bolus, but during more than 500 studies there has been no reaction to the test dose nor a severe reaction to the main injection.

INTERPRETATION OF FLUORESCEIN ANGIOGRAMS

It is not possible to give an account of all the numerous features of retinal disease revealed by fluorescein angiography. Recently, Shikano and Shimizu[30] and Wessing[35] have published atlases of fluorescein fundus photography which illustrate many of the typical features. It is possible to give some guidance about the interpretation of fluorescein angiograms and draw attention to some of the pitfalls.

The whole sequence of fluorescein pictures should be available for study either as prints or by using a film-strip projector. We find it helpful to project the color photographs and fluorescein negatives alongside one another at the same magnification using two projectors.

Accurate quantitative data is needed, and should always be sought. The projectors can be used to throw the image onto a table so that lesions can be traced or mapped. A planimeter or graticule can be used to measure the size of the lesions. This method has been used to measure the area of cotton-wool spots and zones of capillary closure and so establish their life cycle.[15] The turnover of microaneurysms can be determined by plotting their position on fluorescein angiograms taken at intervals of a few months. The result can be expressed as the half-life of aneurysms in months (Fig. 9-9), or as the new aneurysm formation rate, measured in aneurysms per square millimeter of retina per month.[16] A Joyce-Loebl scanning microdensitometer* can be used to measure the amount of fluorescein in vessels[3] or quantitate the amount of residual fluorescein in areas of leakage.[9]

* Joyce-Loebl & Co. Ltd., Electron House, Princesway Team Valley, Gateshead-on-Tyne, 11, England.

Fig. 9-8. Fluorescein content of blood and urine following a 1-gm intravenous dose in a normal man. The initial fall in plasma concentration is rapid as the dye diffuses into the extracellular fluid. Fluorescein is a weakly acidic substance which is heavily bound to plasma proteins, but it is cleared from the kidney at a rate 2 to 3 times higher than the glomerular filtration rate because it is transported into the tubule by the weak organic anion transport system and the dye-protein complex in the peritubular blood dissociates as the free concentration falls. (From Dollery, Hodge, and Engel[8]: *British Medical Journal* *2:*1210, 1962.)

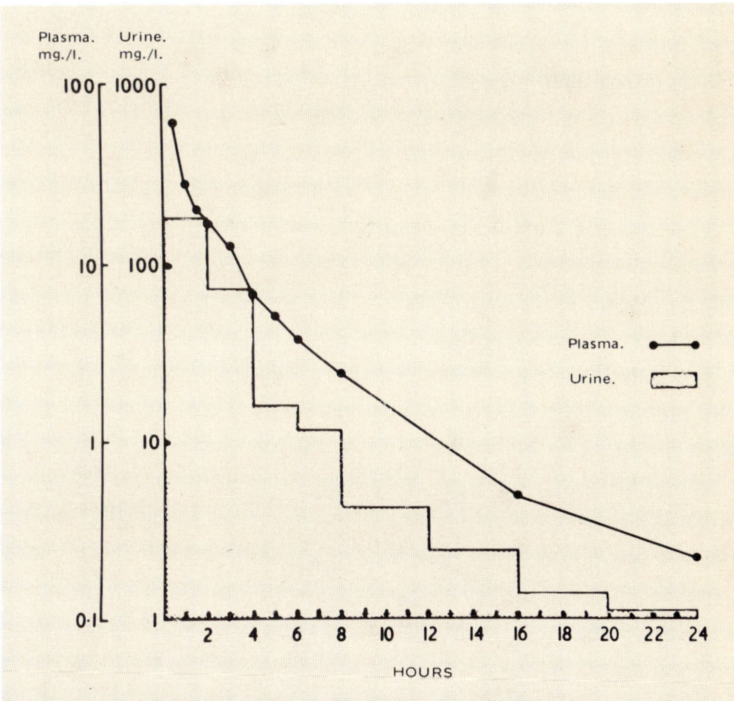

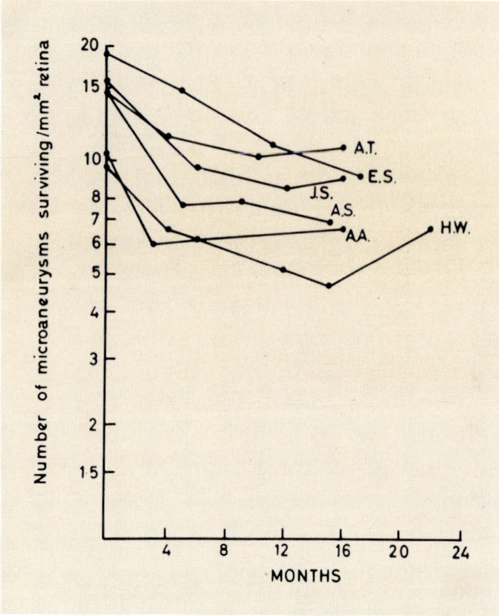

Fig. 9-9. Plot of the number of microaneurysms surviving from those originally present in patients with diabetic retinopathy. The data is derived by carefully mapping the position of each member of a group of aneurysms on a series of fluorescence angiograms of the same area of retina over a period of months or years. (From Kohner and Dollery[16]: *European J. Clin. Invest. 1:*167, 1970.)

ARTERIES

The dye front usually appears first as an axial stream in the arteries. This pattern occurs because the velocity of blood flow is highest in the center of the vessel so this blood is the first to contain dye injected at a distant point. However at a dichotomous branch the streams divide and the previous axial stream becomes the marginal stream on the inner aspect of each of the branches (Fig. 9-10). This pattern is the reverse of that seen at a dichotomous venous branch when the two adjacent marginal streams join to form the axial stream beyond the junction. One result of this branching and streamlining pattern is that capillaries fed from small arterial branches on the inner aspect of a dichotomous branch of a large artery near the disc may be the first to carry the dye. It is more difficult to measure the velocity of the axial stream following a junction of this kind but it can be done so long as the speed of the central stream of dye in the vessel is measured.

First note the pattern of arterial filling and whether the major vessels arising from the disc fill synchronously. Sometimes filling of one vessel may be delayed (Fig. 9-11). If the central retinal artery is obstructed only a cilioretinal vessel may fill (Fig. 9-12). Cilioretinal vessels generally fill before the branches of the central retinal artery. Look for irregularities of the lumen of the artery, especially at the origin of side-branches (Fig. 9-13). Identify any abnormal vessels that arise from the arteries as it is easier to trace their connection before the capillaries and veins have filled.

Fig. 9-10. *A*, Schematic diagram of flow in a retinal artery. Blood enters in the axial stream but at the dichotomous branch the axial stream becomes the marginal stream on the inner aspect of the two branches. Capillaries fed from small branches on this aspect fill first. *B*, Schematic diagram of flow in a large retinal vein. The pathway between artery and vein, and therefore the transit time, is shortened near the optic disc. In consequence small tributory veins near the disc are the first to carry dye giving the well-known marginal streams or tramline appearance. At a dichotomous branch the two marginal streams merge and form the axial stream from this point.

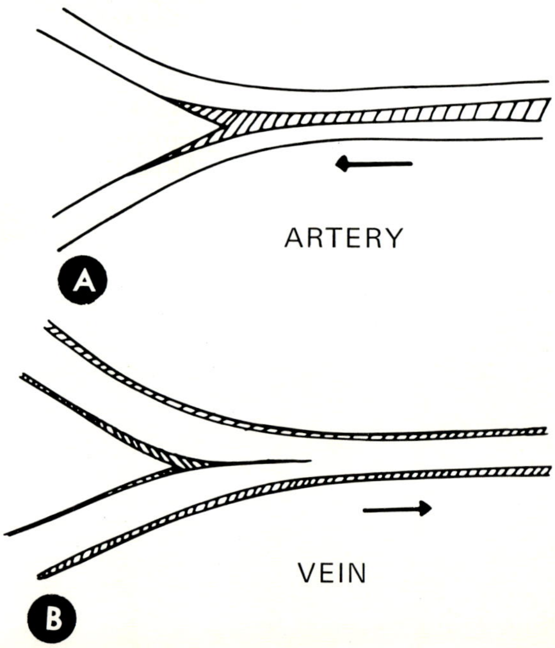

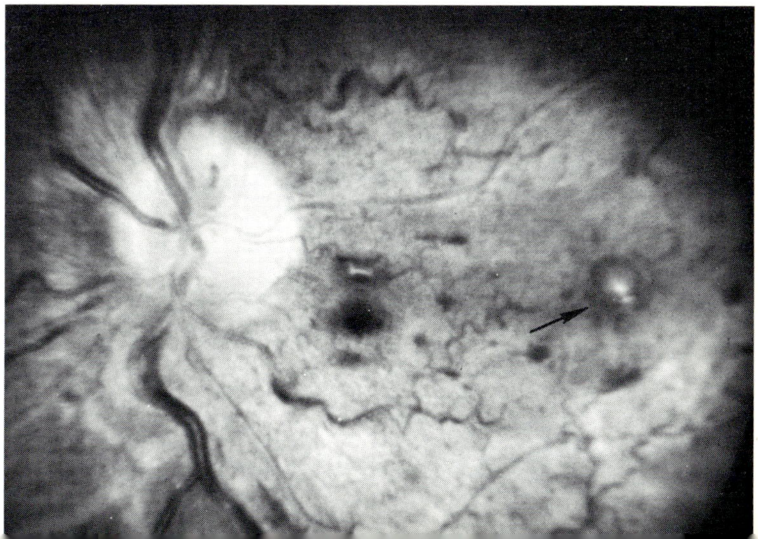

magnitude and rapidity of cell death. In central retinal artery obstruction, some bipolar cells and retinal layers external to this are spared, deriving their nourishment from the choriocapillaris. Dead cellular material of the inner retinal layers is absorbed or ingested by phagocytes and mild glial proliferation, not clinically visible, takes place. Usually within 2 weeks all opacity is gone and the retina returns to its preedematous state. Except in transient ischemic episodes, scotomas always persist following arterial obstruction.

PAPILLEDEMA

Papilledema has been defined as a noninflammatory swelling of the optic nerve head which develops when the normal pressure relationships on either side of the lamina cribrosa are disturbed. It may be due to many causes, increased intracranial pressure being the most common one.

Papilledema may also occur following sudden lowering of the intraocular pressure by filtering operations for glaucoma or globe perforations due to trauma. It can also occur in cases of chronic, severe, globe hypotony. If the onset is sudden the disc may be hyperemic and present flame-shaped hemorrhages. The chronic variety usually shows a pale edema of the disc without hemorrhages. In neither case is the disc often elevated more than 2 or 3 diopters (D). Disc elevations due to this cause may be present for years without progression of visual field defects.

Orbital tumors, aneurysms, or cysts may produce papilledema, in which case other overriding signs of the basic disease process usually lead to the proper diagnosis. Orbital abscesses, especially those secondary to sinus disease, are much more likely to produce an inflammatory papillitis than a noninflammatory papilledema.

Certain general diseases of sufficient severity may produce papilledema. Hypertension is the best example of this, but it may also occur in severe anemias and in some collagen diseases. The associated hypertension in this last group may well be the exciting factor. There has been some disagreement as to whether all patients with malignant hypertension and papilledema have a raised cerebrospinal fluid pressure.[119] Papilledema has been observed also in emphysema and chronic pulmonary insufficiency[40,52,107] where it is probably due to carbon dioxide retention with its effect on the central nervous system, producing elevated intracranial pressure. Differing from the ocular and orbital varieties which are usually monocular, papilledema associated with general diseases is binocular and usually about equal in the two eyes. The associated retinal edema and other retinal pathology of the systemic disease aid in the differential diagnosis.

Intracranial causes of papilledema are the most common. The increased intracranial pressure can be due to increased content of the cranial cavity by neoplasm, cerebral edema due to local or general causes, an increase in the cerebrospinal fluid as in meningitis, the blockage of spinal fluid passage, or a lack of normal cranial capacity as in oxycephaly. Of all these, brain tumor is the most common by far. About 59 per cent of all brain tumors are ultimately associated with choked disc.[71] This manifestation is early and severe in cerebellar tumors. It is found more frequently in parietal, temperoparietal, and midbrain tumors than in the subcortical and medullary ones because of the greater distance of the latter two from the ventricular drainage system. Papilledema is often late in frontal lobe tumors for this same reason.

Because of the importance of papilledema

due to increased intracranial pressure, the remainder of the discussion will be devoted to this.

CLINICAL DEVELOPMENT AND FLUORESCEIN FINDINGS

The reports of Glew and his colleagues,[48,49] who first documented experimental papilledema, Hayreh,[59] and Hedges [61] have clarified to some extent and redirected attention toward the mechanism of papilledema due to increased intracranial pressure. Certain clinical features and fluorescein findings still require explanation.

Prior to any disc elevation, papilledema starts with fullness of the retinal veins, disappearance of any previously present venous pulsation, and disc hyperemia. The venous pulse has been shown to disappear when the intracranial pressure reaches about 204 mm of water.[148] When disc capillaries start to leak, true disc elevation begins. It starts at the nasal disc edge, usually in the upper quadrant, and begins with a gentle arching of the nerve fibers over this border. Viewed with the ophthalmoscope, this stage presents white streaking from the rim of the disc to the retina immediately adjacent, and obscures in varying degree the previously sharp disc margin. The hazy whiteness of these streaks viewed against the red fundus background appears to start at the immediate disc border. The identical white streaking over the peripheral disc substance blends with the whitish disc background color and, due to this lack of contrast, it is not easily seen with the ophthalmoscope. However, it is readily apparent when viewed with the slit lamp and contact lens. This streaking with increasing opacity and elevation spreads along the nasal disc border extending both toward the physiologic cup and into the immediately adjacent retina. As an increasing number of disc capillaries become dilated and visible, they appear more numerous and present a highly irregular pattern, often showing hairpin loops which can be mistaken for microaneurysms. The edema then spreads around the temporal border of the disc in a similar manner and only then encroaches upon the physiologic cup. In fact, the disc can be elevated 2 D and still have an easily discernible cup. Flame-shaped hemorrhages may appear with early capillary dilatation but are more common with the onset of disc elevation and multiply throughout its development. Cotton-wool spots commonly appear a little later. It is then a matter of several days until the complete picture of an elevated, congested, edematous disc, with its prominent network of dilated, tortuous, knobbed capillaries, filled-in physiologic cup, flame-shaped hemorrhages and cotton-wool spots ensues (Fig. 10-19). While edema may spread to surrounding retina, all significant pathologic change seems limited to the disc and the zone of retina immediately adjacent. The retina abutting on the disc is often mechanically pushed aside and fine retinal folds concentric with the disc may be seen. Zimmerman [165] demonstrated three mechanical mechanisms producing enlargement of the blind spot in papilledema: (*1*) displacement of the retina by the increasing disc edema, (*2*) separation of the peripapillary retina as fluid from the edematous disc seeps beneath it, and (*3*) compression of the retina bordering the disc by a swollen, overhanging disc edge. In some cases retinal edema may spread further into the surrounding areas ultimately reaching the macula. If edema persists at the macula long enough, as it recedes, a macular wing or star of fatty exudate often may temporarily appear (see section on Fatty Exudates).

The fluorescein test shows the beginning of dye leakage with the onset of disc elevation (Fig. 10-20). Dye leakage appears to go hand in hand with edematous fluid leakage from the dilated disc capillaries, and is first apparent nasally over the more periph-

Fig. 10-19. *A*, Early papilledema showing blurred disc margins most marked superonasally (**arrow**). *B*, Advanced papilledema. Disc margin not visible, veins are dilated, and multiple superficial hemorrhages can be seen.

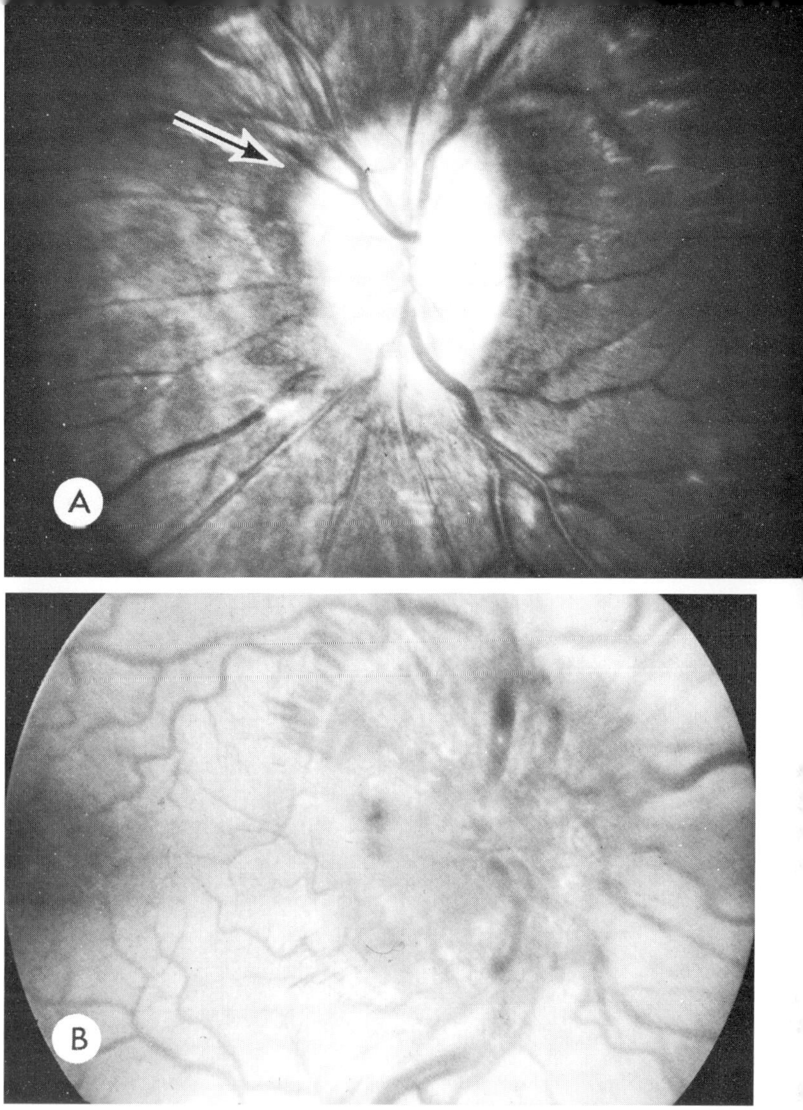

Fig. 10-20. *A*, Early papilledema right eye. *B*, Venous-phase fluorescein angiogram shows multiple capillary leaks at the disc border.

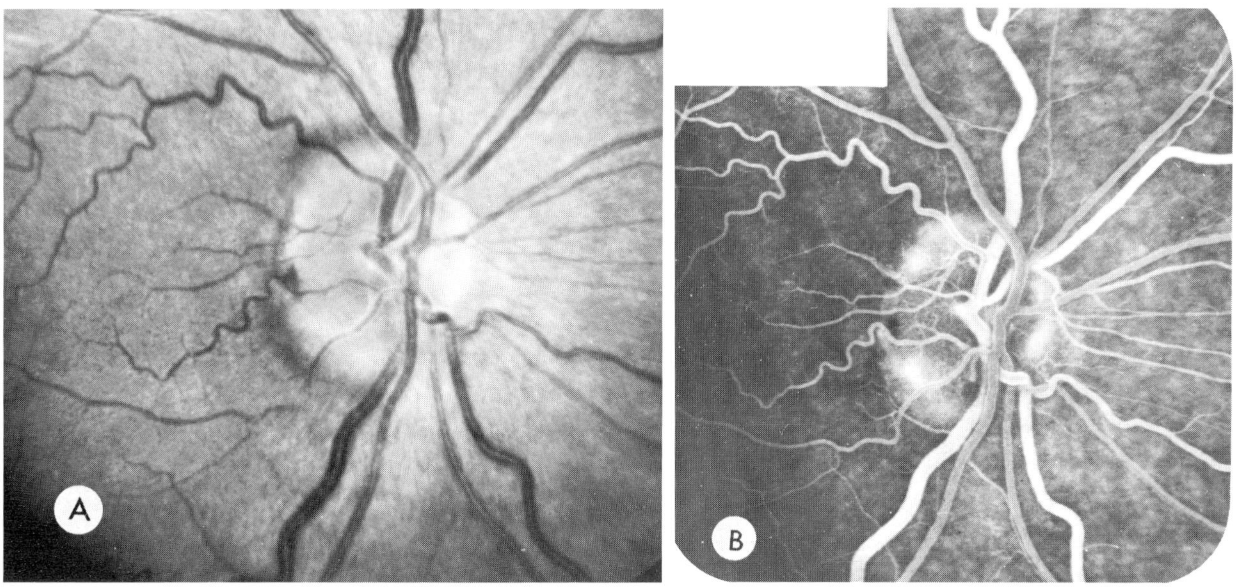

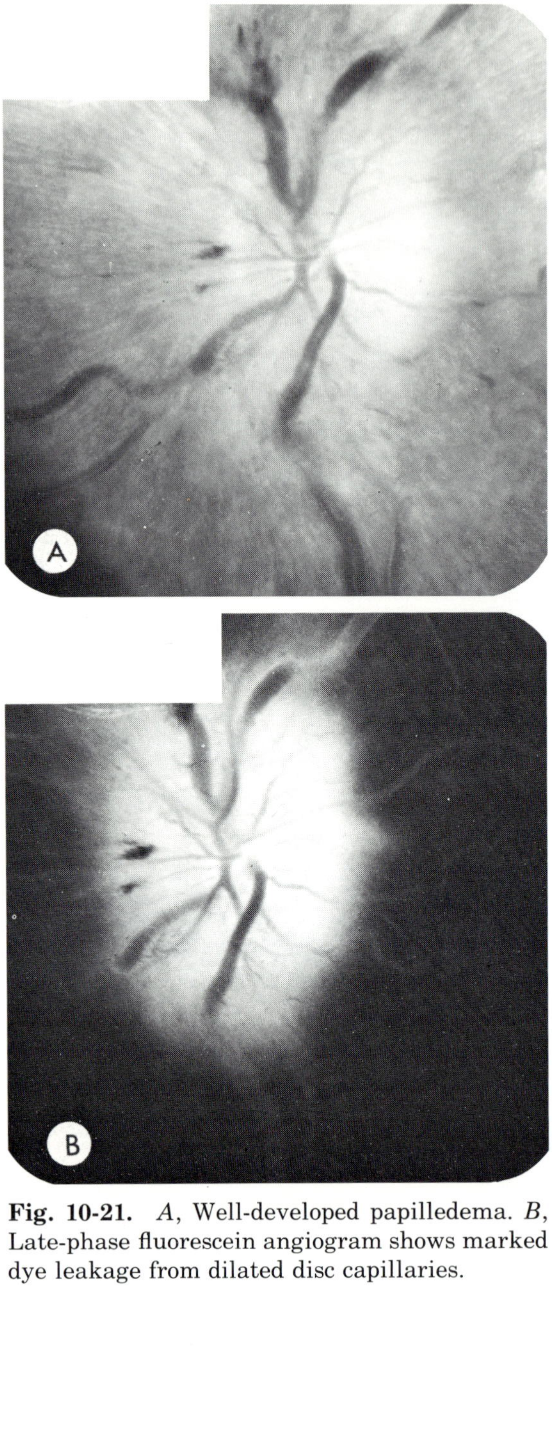

Fig. 10-21. *A*, Well-developed papilledema. *B*, Late-phase fluorescein angiogram shows marked dye leakage from dilated disc capillaries.

eral disc areas. In well-developed papilledema, dye leakage is prompt and profuse, the fluorescein spreading rapidly into the vitreous (Fig. 10-21).

MECHANISM

As increased intracranial pressure is transmitted along the optic nerves, the rise in intervaginal pressure exerts its influence on the central retinal veins as they leave the nerves and cross these intervaginal spaces. The venous outflow impedance resulting from this increased pressure on the central retinal veins accounts for the fullness of the retinal veins and the disappearance of any spontaneous venous pulse previously present. These are the only effects produced by pressure on the retinal veins. All other changes at the disc are due to the effect of the raised intervaginal pressure on the independent circulation of the disc substance itself. It has been demonstrated clearly with fluorescein that the disc and retinal circulations are independent.[32]

Two factors suggest strongly that the transmitted intervaginal pressure is not exerted on the disc arterial blood supply at the circle of Zinn:

1. The circle of Zinn lies within the rigid scleral coat which is undoubtedly strong enough to withstand increased intervaginal pressure, thus protecting these intrascleral vessels from its effect.

2. Cases of papilledema with a visible lamina cribrosa show no change of this structure during the early development of disc elevation. Each trabecula of the lamina cribrosa contains a capillary channel directly supplied from the circle of Zinn. The absence of any fluid or dye leakage upon fluorescein testing from these capillary walls is strong evidence that the deleterious effect is not on the arterial side of the disc blood supply. The clinical features of papilledema, its onset at the disc margin and the early fluorescein leakage all suggest that the raised intervaginal pressure exerts its influence by interference with the venous drainage of the disc vascular network.

Primrose[120] explains papilledema by a shunt mechanism of the arterial blood supply to the optic disc. The shunting of blood is dependent upon the interrelationships of the arterial blood pressure, the intraocular pressure, and the intracranial pressure. He believes that in papilledema due to raised intracranial pressure, blood is shunted into the circle of Zinn due to the increased resistance to flow in the pial plexus. The increased flow to the circle of Zinn floods the optic nerve head and produces the papilledema. A lowered intraocular pressure would facilitate this development while an atrophic disc, because of its closed vascular bed, would not perfuse and thus would fail to develop edema. He suggests that a raised systemic arterial pressure, as in malignant hypertension without increased intracranial pressure, produces papilledema by selectively flooding the disc vessels. Papilledema due to lowered intraocular pressure would be due to a decreased tension at the disc thereby diverting blood from the extraocular territory of the ophthalmic artery to the circle of Zinn and thence to the disc itself.

Rather than active arterial flooding as the mechanism of its development, we believe papilledema is more likely to be due to obstruction of venous drainage from the disc. Only a slight rise in the central retinal vein pressure could impede drainage of the capillary bed of the disc via its smaller-caliber connections with the central vein (see Chapter 4, Angioarchitecture of the Papilla). The rise in intracranial pressure would be transmitted along the optic nerve in the intervaginal spaces and have a compression effect on each central retinal vein as it left the optic nerve and crossed this space. This rise in intervaginal pressure would also exert an equal force acting from without upon the posterior sclero-optic nerve area. At this site it would impede venous drainage of any small pial channels emptying the capillary bed of the disc peripherally, if such venous drainage of the disc actually exists. Paton and Holmes,[115] in a microscopic study of papilledema, have found more nerve edema in the subpial region, congestion of pial veins of the nerve, and dilated capillaries in the septa—all findings suggesting such a peripheral venous drainage of the disc. They also have reported as a later feature, marked endothelial cell proliferation, even to the point of lumen closure, in many small vessels of the edematous disc. This finding also is suggestive of a basic venous drainage impedance in the mechanism of papilledema.

DIFFERENTIAL DIAGNOSIS

At times widespread superficial retinal edema will cause blurring of the disc margin and suggest an erroneous diagnosis of early papilledema. This is especially likely to occur in severe hypertensive retinopathy. Such cases lack the arched elevation of the disc border seen in early papilledema. In papilledema the disc capillaries are affected selectively, with retinal capillaries retaining their integrity. Thus edema exudes into the disc itself and simply spills over into the immediately adjacent retina. This produces a selective disc elevation above the level of the surrounding involved retina. In the widespread superficial retinal edema associated with hypertension, the capillaries of both disc and retina are involved and the minimal edematous elevation of both is always at the same level. As indicated previously, the differences in background color of disc and retina make it difficult to detect this level variation with the ophthalmoscope, but it is readily apparent with the contact lens and slit lamp.

Papillitis may resemble papilledema so closely that differentiation on the basis of ophthalmoscopic observation alone is impossible. Persistent unilaterality, a lesser degree of elevation with more extensive spread into surrounding retina and prepapillary inflammatory elements in the posterior vitreous are all indicative of papillitis. As the fluorescein picture of both papilledema and papillitis is the same, differentiation must be based on the case history and other clinical findings. Sudden loss of vision, pain on rotation of the eye, and central or centrocecal scotoma all indicate papillitis. Absence of pain, normal vision, and an enlarged blind spot only, all indicate papilledema.

Deep-lying colloid bodies (drusen) in the disc substance, while anterior to the lamina cribrosa, may be clinically invisible or very hard to see (Fig. 10-22). Such discs may be elevated 4 D and strongly suggest papilledema, although there is no disc edema, hemorrhage, nor exudates. Both conditions usually show enlarged blind spots, and arcuate or sector defects are not uncommon with disc colloid bodies. The latter appear most commonly on the nasal side of the disc, and when bilateral may be readily apparent in only one eye. A scalloped, irregular shape of the elevated disc, or a lumpy surface are suggestive of colloid bodies. The latter are seen best by retroillumination with the contact lens and slit lamp. In this manner the edges of colloid bodies may be noted at times peeking out from the edge of the disc elevation at its base. These appear smoothly rounded and often are mildly refractile. Persistent unilaterality, failure of short-term progression, and a negative fluorescein test all suggest the presence of colloid bodies.

Pseudopapilledema or a structurally full disc can be mistaken for papilledema. This condition has been described as a congenital disc formation occurring in hyperopic eyes. The discs are small, have indistinct margins, may be slightly raised, appear hyperemic, and have no physiologic cup. This type of disc is not limited only to hyperopic eyes but has been seen in eyes with insignificant refractive error. Nor do all such discs show normal blind spots on field examination. Patients with enlarged blind spots should be suspected of harboring hidden colloid bodies. This type may slowly change in appearance over a period of months. One such patient who developed colloid bodies while under observation, showed normal discs in the beginning. One year later one disc was noted to have every appearance of a structurally full disc. Eighteen months later colloid

TABLE 10-1
Differential Diagnosis

	Papilledema	Optic neuritis	Drusen of the disc
Vision	Normal	Decreased	Usually normal
Fields	Enlarged blind spot	Central or centrocecal scotoma	Enlarged blind spot, arcuate defects, inferior nasal field defects, etc.
Disc elevation	Usually more than 2 D, central pit may be preserved	Usually less then 2 D	Irregular swelling of disc and absent physiologic pit
CRV Pulse *	Often absent and hard to elicit	Present or easily elicited	Present or easily elicited
Fluorescein	Leakage of dye from disc	Leakage of dye from disc	No leakage. The disc fluoresces irregularly

* Central retinal vein pulsation

bodies became visible for the first time deep in the disc substance. Thus, some structurally full discs may actually be due to deep and hidden colloid bodies.

A markedly tilted disc with papilledema will show changes only on its high side.

An atrophic disc will not develop papilledema. Excluding those patients unable to develop papilledema from increased intracranial pressure because of a mechanical block of the intervaginal pathway about the optic nerve,[59] uniocular papilledema of this etiology becomes binocular within 2 weeks.

PROGNOSIS AND LATE APPEARANCE

Papilledema due to hypotony of the globe is usually of short duration, but may persist for years. In one of our own patients it lasted 4 years having developed after filtration surgery for glaucoma. Edema of the disc due to hypotony produces enlargement of the blind spot but no other field defect as

Fig. 10-22. *A*, Deep colloid bodies (drusen) of the disc. The **arrow** points to several barely visible colloid bodies at the upper nasal disc border. *B*, Histologic appearance of disc colloid bodies (drusen). Note position anterior to the lamina cribrosa **(LC)**.

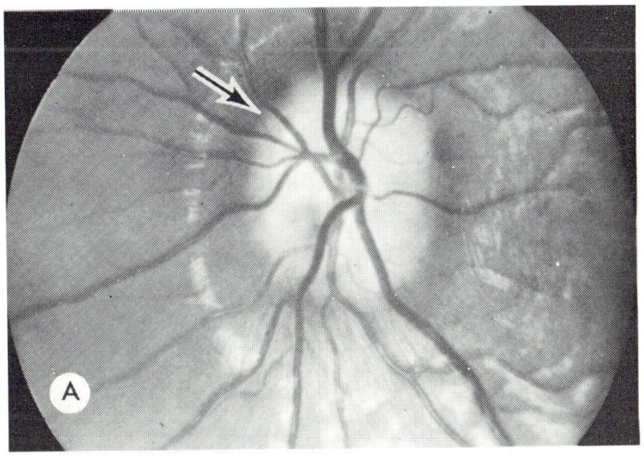

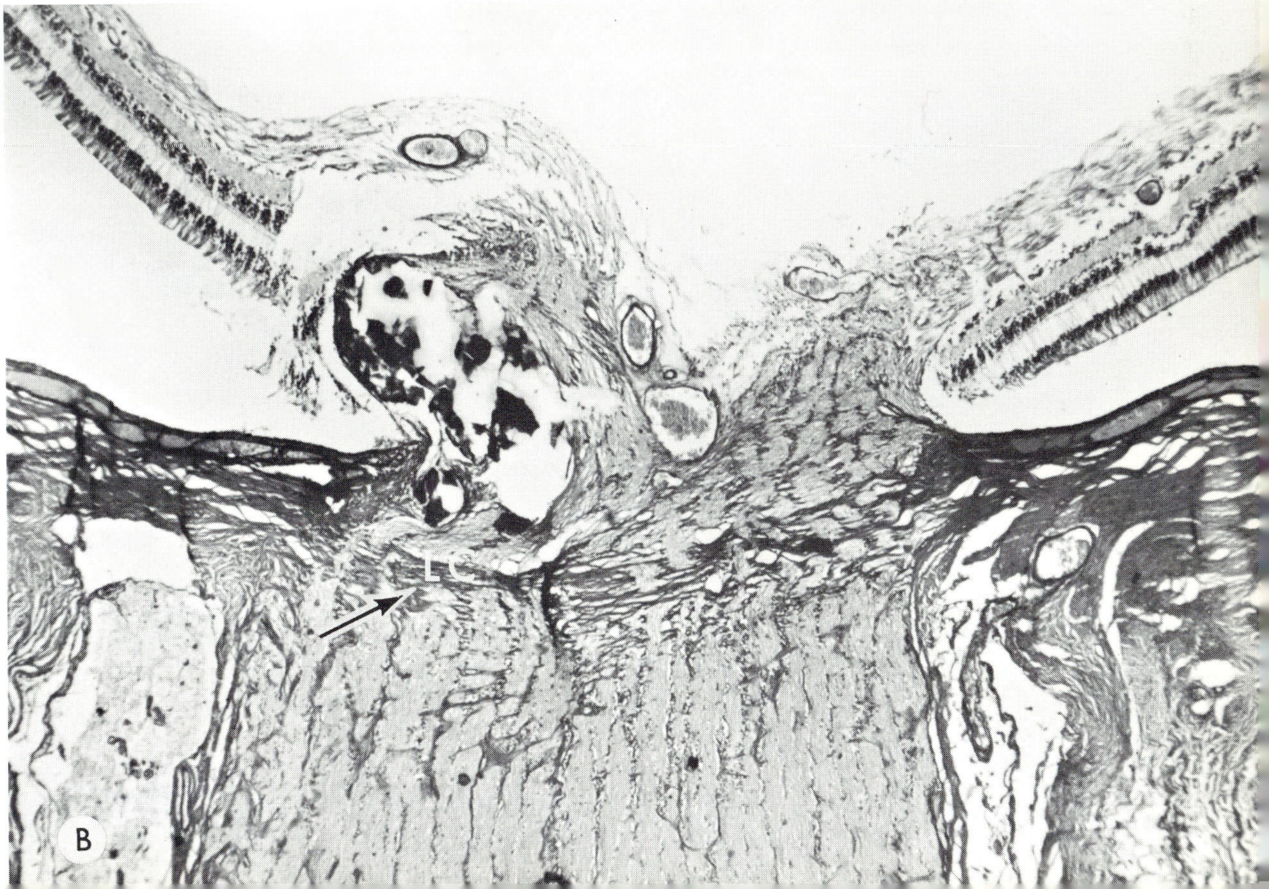

a rule. That due to pseudotumor cerebri (benign intracranial hypertension) is also often well tolerated by the eye. Rabinowicz and others [121] have reported eight patients observed from 3 to 6 years with no loss of vision and insignificant field alteration.

Prolonged papilledema due to increased intracranial pressure eventually produces peripheral field changes. There is a general depression of the visual field with increasing peripheral loss usually more marked nasally.

If papilledema is resolved promptly, the disc may return to its former appearance without any residual stigmata. A more severe and persistent papilledema almost invariably leaves some mark. Concentric retinal folds at the border of the elevated disc may persist indefinitely after the disc is again flat. Arteries and veins may show a similar white sheathing, heaviest on the disc, tapering, and disappearing within a short distance from the disc, but usually persisting on the veins for the greater distance. The disc may appear pale, its borders ragged and its physiologic cup filled in, all due to secondary gliosis. Such an appearance can equally well follow papillitis and, in either case, is often mistakenly called secondary optic atrophy. Unless there is functional loss, this picture should not be called optic atrophy. The visual function cannot be accurately judged from the disc appearance, for rather pale and gliotic discs may have no associated optic atrophy.

Any surrounding retinal edema or macular wing of fatty exudates eventually disappears after the disc flattens. Of the two, the exudates are the last to disappear, and they often increase transiently as the edema first begins to recede.

The papilledema associated with central retinal vein obstruction, acute angle closure glaucoma, and that occurring with ischemic optic neuropathy are discussed subsequently with each individual disease.

RETINAL EXUDATES

The term retinal exudate, although no longer truly descriptive, is fixed so firmly in the literature that no attempt will be made to change it. Recent study has clarified greatly the understanding of one exudate, the cotton-wool spot, and suggested that basically there are probably relatively few others. Careful analysis of their type, morphology, and distribution patterns often permits prompt categorization into one or another general disease group which thereby facilitates proper diagnosis.

COTTON-WOOL SPOTS

Cotton-wool spots result from ischemia in the nerve fiber layer. Their pathogenesis is discussed in detail elsewhere (see Chapter 17, in section on Extravascular Changes).

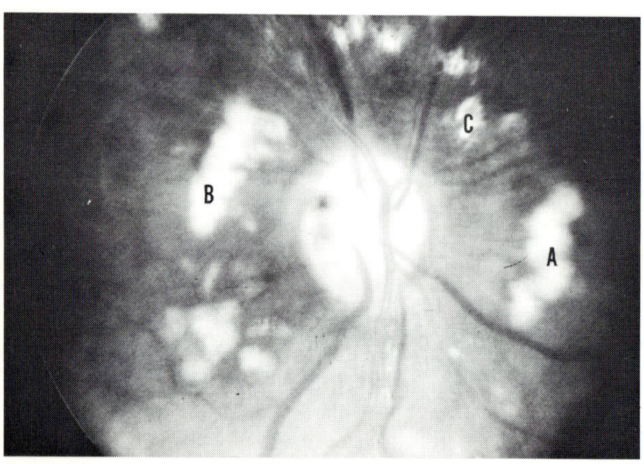

Fig. 10-23. Cotton-wool patches in dermatomyositis: **(A)** fresh; **(B)** older; and **(C)** resolving lesions.

The distribution of cotton-wool spots at the posterior pole usually corresponds to the area covered by the superficial peripapillary capillary bed. Rarely, they will occur directly on the disc, more commonly elsewhere in the distribution of the major superficial capillary bed. They do not occur in the immediate foveal region nor in the mid- nor peripheral retina. Most are limited to an area of 3 dd in radius about the optic nerve head. They occur singly or in clusters, developing fully in a matter of hours. Well-developed fresh lesions have a dense, bluish white color and a fuzzy, rather narrow, transitional border zone (Fig. 10-23). They are irregular in shape and may be either discrete or coalescent. If sufficiently dense they produce a transient local scotoma but never an arcuate defect and this vanishes with the disappearance of the exudate. Cotton-wool spots in diabetic retinopathy may have more persistent scotomas. Others may be less dense at onset, and some are filmy, vague, and easily overlooked. Although coalescent spots may be larger than the disc this is seldom true of a single lesion. Individual patches or crops of spots usually fade and disappear in 5 to 7 weeks. They lose their fuzzy borders, fade to a dirty gray color, fragment, become granular, and are completely absorbed. No clinical evidence of their previous position can be seen once absorption is complete. New spots may develop as older ones disappear, therefore spots of varying ages may be seen in the fundus at any one time. Typical white, fluffy cotton-wool spots are relatively rare in diabetic retinopathy without hypertension, but atypical ones are quite common (Fig. 10-24). These have a faint gray color, are much less obvious and much more persistent, lasting as long as 2 years. Their chronicity and different appearance suggests that they may represent local patches of capillary closure as occurs elsewhere in the retina in diabetes, rather than the acute closure seen in hypertension. As the white, fluffy cotton-wool spots are caused by a derangement of the

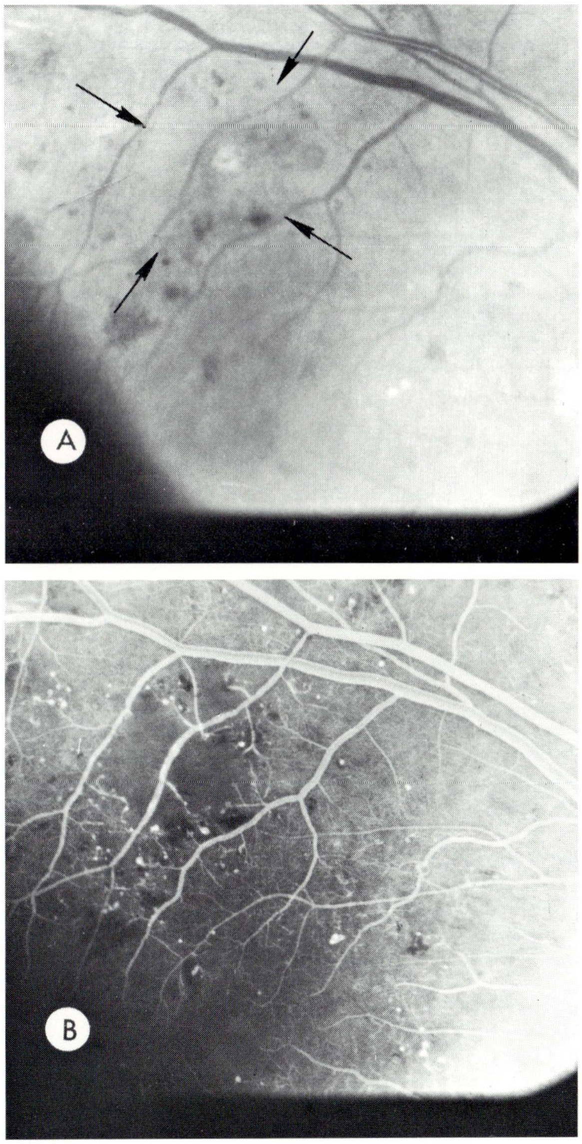

Fig. 10-24. *A*, A type of cotton-wool patch seen in diabetic retinopathy. The **arrows** outline the faintly gray area of the lesion. *B*, Fluorescein angiogram showing nonperfusion of the involved capillary bed.

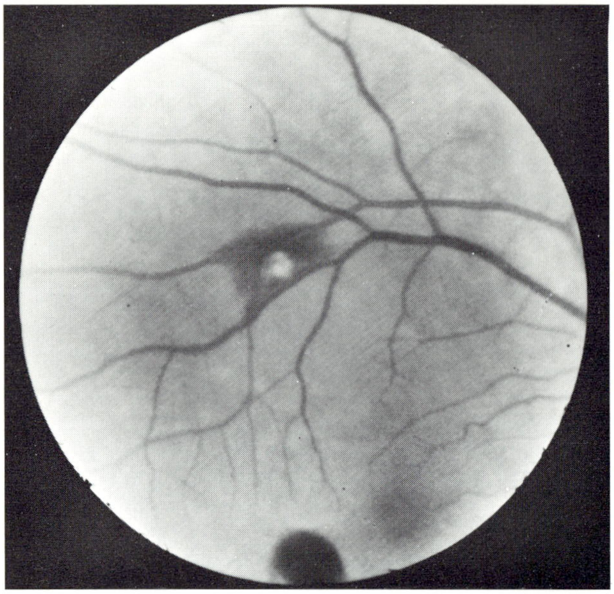

Fig. 10-25. Roth's spot in bacterial endocarditis.

Fig. 10-26. Roth's spots **(arrows)** in multiple myeloma.

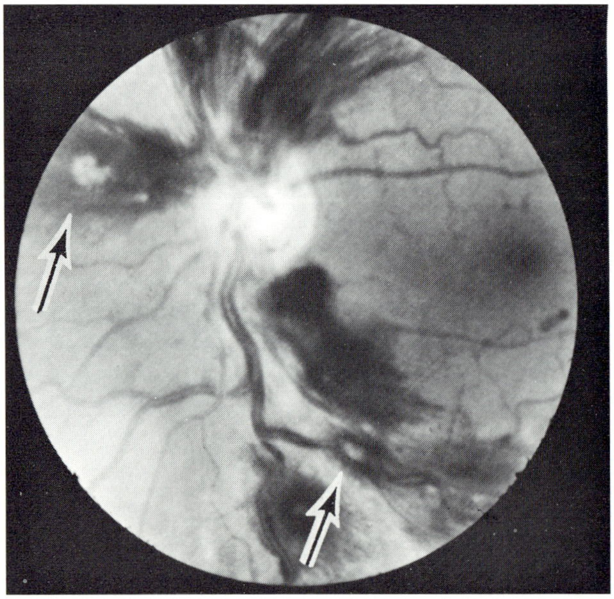

precapillary arterioles supplying the superficial capillary bed, they always lie in the nerve fiber layer of the retina. Microscopically they are composed of a central cluster of cell-like bodies (Cajal's nodes) in a zone of retinal edema. These nodes are commonly called "cytoid bodies" in ophthalmic literature but more correctly, and in conformity with general neuropathology, they should be labeled terminal swellings of Cajal, or Cajal's nodes. They represent the swollen ends of fragmented axones, occurring on the ganglion cell side of the break. They contain a central core of clumped mitochondria surrounded by a clearer outer zone.[138] The visibility of cotton-wool spots is due to the local tissue swelling and opacity, the Cajal's nodes not being clinically apparent.

Cotton-wool spots are nonspecific and common in such diseases as hypertension, disseminated lupus erythematosus, dermatomyositis, scleroderma, Purtscher's retinopathy, anemias, leukemias, septicemias, dysproteinemias, ischemic retinopathy, and severe gastrointestinal hemorrhages. They are less common in the usual vein obstructions and rare in those branch obstructions well away from the disc. Occasionally, in vein obstruction especially if it is severe and acute, they are profuse. Cotton-wool spots

Fig. 10-27. Roth's spots **(arrow)** in chronic myelogenous leukemia.

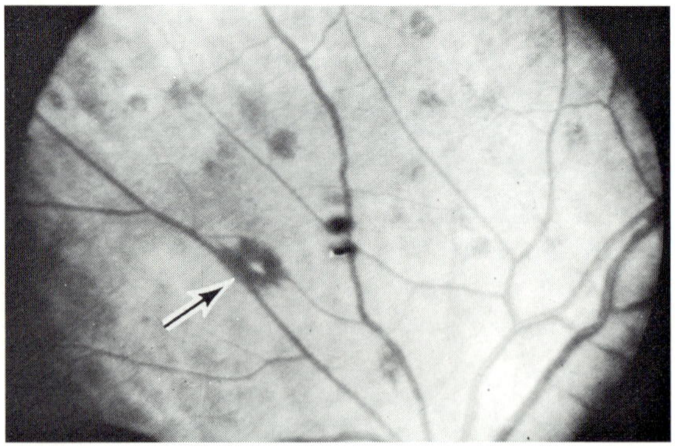

are commonly found on and near the disc in both papilledema and papillitis. They have been repeatedly reported as occurring in carcinomatosis, although no recent study of them in patients with disseminated cancer has been made. A review of these earlier reports [12,80,118,141] and our own experience suggest that the cotton-wool spots occurring in these patients are actually a result of the accompanying anemia or other factors and bear no relation to carcinoma.

ROTH'S SPOTS

In 1872, Roth [128,129] described retinal white spots as well as hemorrhages in cases of asepsis, but he did not relate the two. Six years later Litten [98] first described white-centered, retinal hemorrhages in endocarditis and he was the first to call them Roth's spots. The term has now been expanded to denote any white-centered hemorrhage.

The clinical appearance of a white spot surrounded by hemorrhage is associated with four different microscopic pictures:

1. Focal accumulations of polymorphonuclear cells in acute lesions, or mononuclear and small round cells in older lesions produce the irregularly shaped, fuzzy, white centers seen in bacterial endocarditis (Fig. 10-25).[29,31,78] Hemorrhage about such cell clusters completes the picture of a Roth's spot.

2. Some cotton-wool spots may have a surrounding zone of hemorrhage as in disseminated lupus erythematosus or dysproteinemia (Fig. 10-26).

3. In the retinopathy of leukemia, leukemic cell foci with hemorrhage about them produce the clinical picture of Roth's spots (Fig. 10-27).[1,24]

4. Wong and Bodey [161] have described a central collection of fibrin with surrounding hemorrhage in a case of fatal aplastic anemia. The lesion had the clinical appearance of a Roth's spot.

These four lesions taken alone cannot be differentiated clinically. The white centers are usually small, seldom being more than 0.5 dd in size. The surrounding hemorrhage is highly variable, sometimes only a fringe; at other times quite overshadowing the central white spots. Roth's spots are commonly seen in the superficial retina, representing thereby focal damage to the superficial precapillary arterioles and the superficial capillary bed. They are transient in nature and, in nonfatal diseases, produce little damage. They absorb without leaving clinically detectable residues.

Clearly identifiable cotton-wool spots with an incomplete fringe of hemorrhage should be called cotton-wool and not Roth's spots.

FATTY EXUDATES

The term fatty exudate (hard, waxy exudate, chronic edema residue) is used here to denote those retinal exudates composed of abnormal material free within the retina and containing a fatty component together with the fatty granular cells (microglia), which phagocytize this material. Both these cells and the free material take the usual fat stains in varying degree. Although it is not known whether all fatty exudates are basically identical, nor what their chemical nature or origin is, they are, however, similar clinically and have similar distribution patterns. They occur in certain retinal disorders and not in others. Excluding vascular tumors, they are seen much more commonly in diseases attacking capillaries and veins than in those primarily affecting arteries. For instance they are common in diabetic retinopathy, retinal vein obstruction, and Coats's disease, but are not seen in the collagenoses or in arterial or arteriolar obstructions.

Fatty exudates have three main patterns of distribution: (*1*) as a ring of exudates in nonspecific circinate retinopathy;[70] (*2*) scattered in the deeper retinal layers of the posterior fundus in impending or partially compensated central retinal vein obstruction;[89] and (3) as a star figure at the macula. Other less common patterns include: fatty exudate scattered in the deeper retina posteriorly around the disc in the later stages of hypertensive retinopathy; deep spots about the macula in the predisciform stage of disciform macular degeneration; and scattered exudate in the deep retina about the disc, heaped into a macular mound and forming a posterior arc around a temporal retinal angioma.[157] Rarely, deep retinal exudates develop subsequent to, and over some choroidal hemorrhages, or as small clusters in the retinal periphery associated with peripheral retinal vascular lesions.

It is notable that all of these distributions except the macular star lie in the deep retina with an affinity for the outer plexiform layer. Henle's layer, among whose fibers the star figure forms, is comparable anatomically to the outer plexiform layer although it has a superficial retinal position about the fovea.

It has been thought, after consideration of their characteristic pattern in circinate retinopathy, that these exudates represent fats liberated from dead retinal cells at the center of the lesion. Phagocytic cells were thought to ingest the fat, migrate to the border of the lesion and aggregate there, forming an exudative ring prior to their eventual absorption.[70]

There are, however, strong arguments against this hypothesis. In branch retinal artery obstruction in an otherwise normal retina where there is death and disintegration of the involved inner retinal cells with considerable liberation of fats, no fatty exudates are seen. Phagocytic cells do engulf this necrotic material in clearing the debris[42] but they do not give the clinical picture of fatty exudation. Indeed, where the local ischemia is of a more transient nature, with minimal cellular disruption and death, and where phagocytic cells are sparse, as in the cotton-wool spot, fatty exudates are not present. In Coats's disease the probable origin of a lipid-containing material from dilated capillaries and defective vein walls adjacent to areas of retinal cell death has been demonstrated.[156] Reese[122] has demonstrated entrapment of this material in some retinal venous walls of Coats's disease, further suggesting its intravascular origin. It has been also postulated that the basic material of the diabetic exudate seeps through the defective walls of some diabetic microaneurysms.[104]

Whether the fatty component of this material arises from the vascular lumen and seeps through defective venous and capillary walls accumulating as selective absorption proceeds, or whether it represents a more slowly absorbed by-product of the altered metabolism of viable but subnormally oxygenated retinal cells is unknown. The intimate relation of the fatty exudates to viable but hypoxic retinal cells, their presence in diseases with circulatory impedance due to capillary or vein obstruction, and their absence in diseases of arterial blockage and infarction make this general concept a more likely explanation of their pathogenesis. It also serves as a better explanation of their retinal distribution patterns in the diverse diseases in which they occur.

Typically, fatty exudates lie in the deep retina with an affinity for the outer plexiform layer (Fig. 10-28). If small, they may be localized in this vicinity or if larger, they may extend from the internal limiting membrane to the outer nuclear layer. When massive as in Coats's disease or angiomatosis retinae, they may break retinal boundaries and extend subretinally detaching the retina in mounds (Fig. 10-29). In heavy exudation this subretinal direction or extension is characteristic. Except in early juvenile diabetes and early hypertension where beginning exudates may be truly white, all have a yellowish color of highly similar character irrespective of the disease in which they occur. They are dense, even, small accumulations hiding deeper structures from view. While they may be discrete in the very early phases, they often coalesce to form irregular masses with slightly hazy borders. In massive exudations, aggregates or exudative tongues have an archipelago-like configuration at their edges. Whenever these masses accumulate in the nerve fiber layer they tend to hug retinal veins in an irregular distribution well out in the retina beyond the exudative mass border. Accumulations can be seen at the walls of capillaries and veins where absorption into the circulation probably takes place, but no intramural material or transfer through the wall has as yet been demonstrated. No similar affinity for arteries has been seen. Other than this they bear no topographical relation to visible retinal vessels.

Microscopically the material, whether free or within phagocytes, tends to push retinal elements aside. Retinal cells which appear completely normal, may lie adjacent to masses of exudate. Fatty exudates are commonly associated with both deep retinal hemorrhages and deep retinal edema, further indicating their relation to disease affecting the deep retinal capillary bed. When both hemorrhage and exudation are extensive they may become mixed, giving rise to retinal discolorations having variable values of both yellow and red. Cholesterin clefts may be seen microscopically in larger and older exudates and cholesterin crystals are often visible within exudates seen clinically (Fig. 10-30).

The fatty exudates of diabetic retinopathy (hard waxy exudates) at times bear a definite relationship to microaneurysms and patches of obliterated capillaries. Microaneurysms are often more profuse at the borders of obliterated capillary foci and fatty exudates may form an arc or ring just beyond them. Such rings of exudate appear most strikingly surrounding the macula. In

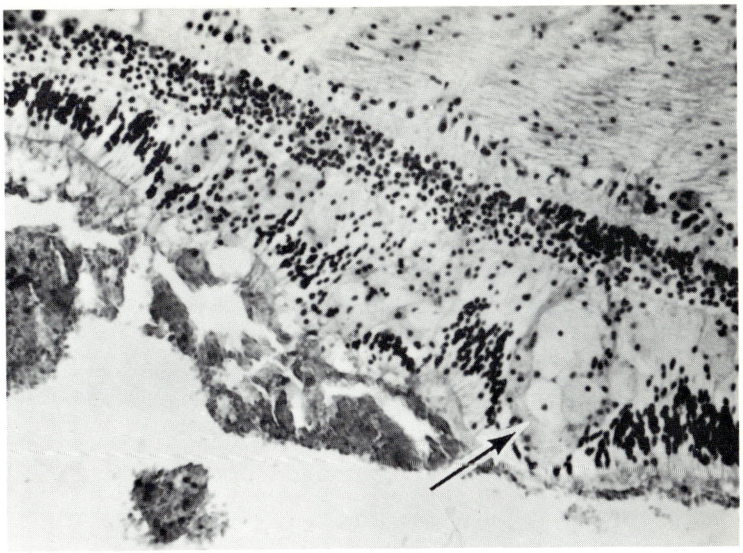

Fig. 10-28. Histologic appearance of fatty exudate ring around mound of disciform macular degeneration. The **arrow** points to a group of fatty granular cells in the outer plexiform layer (Courtesy of the Armed Forces Institute of Pathology, Washington, D.C.)

Fig. 10-29. Histologic appearance of subretinal fatty exudation in Coats's disease. Both foamy fatty granular cells and cholesterin clefts are visible. The former are clustered around a neovascular downgrowth **(arrow).** (Courtesy of the Armed Forces Institute of Pathology, Washington, D.C.)

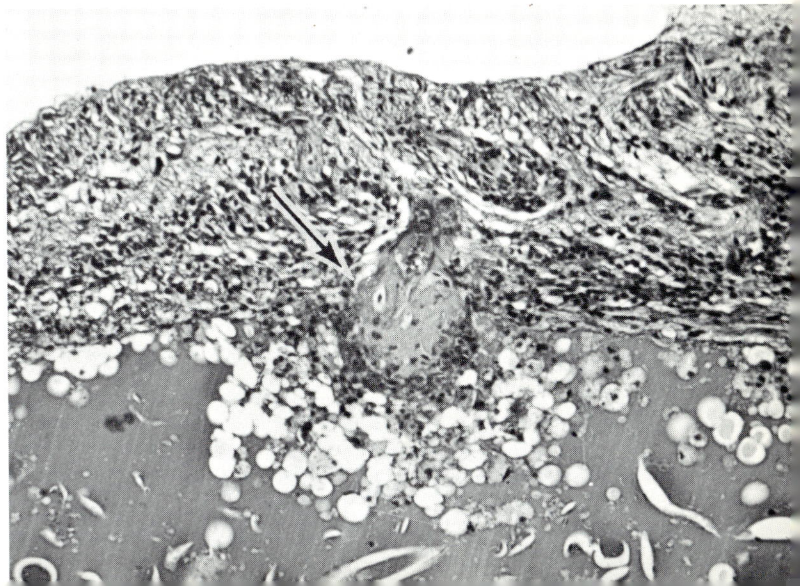

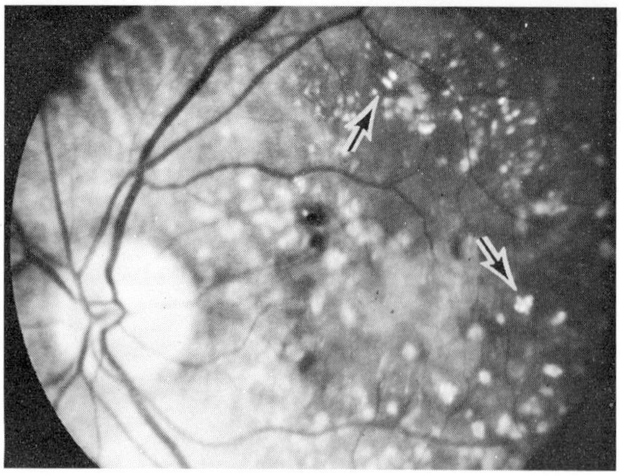

Fig. 10-30. Crystals **(arrows)** in fatty exudates in early disciform macular degeneration.

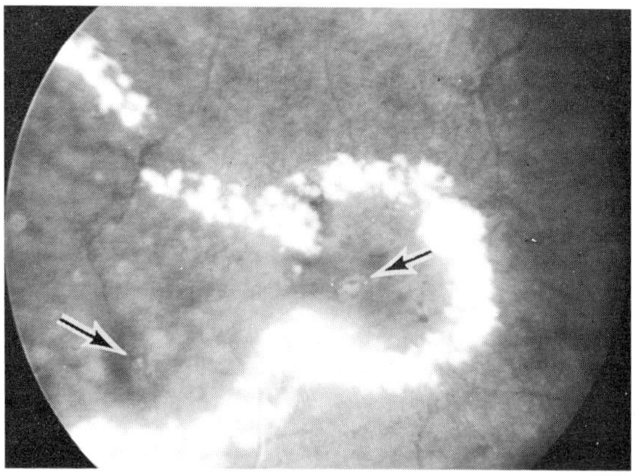

Fig. 10-31. Circinate exudates around large aneurysms **(arrows)** at posterior pole, following central retinal vein obstruction. (From Wise.[151])

Fig. 10-32. Macular star of fatty exudates in hypertensive retinopathy.

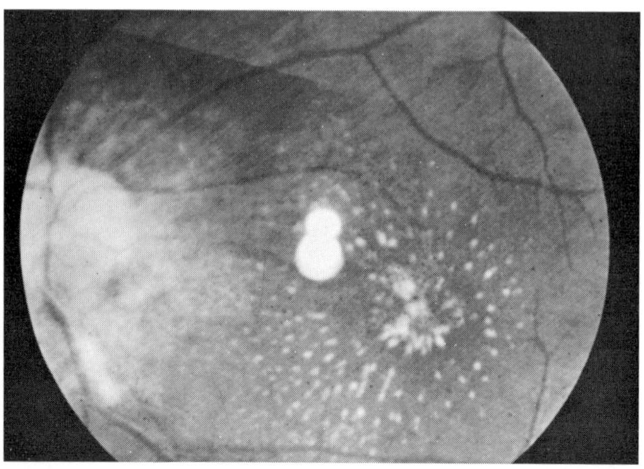

the past this has led to the faulty conception of a "circinate phase" of diabetic retinopathy. Careful clinical examination of those cases of diabetic retinopathy with widespread exudation demonstrates clearly, though less graphically, this same circinate pattern throughout the posterior retina (Fig. 15-2). Although short arcs or incomplete rings predominate, complete well-demarcated rings of exudate with large central microaneurysms are not unusual.[151]

In impending or partially compensated vein obstruction the normally red fundus reflex may assume a yellowish hue. Small droplets of fatty exudate in the deeper retinal layers at the posterior pole can be seen to account for this phenomenon. Klien and Olwin[89] first called attention to this and demonstrated the deep retinal exudates microscopically. After several months following the acute episode of vein obstruction fatty exudates may develop in the drainage area of the obstructed vein or at its border. At times they form extensive swathes with some diffuse scattering or clearly outlined rings of exudate, often with large central microaneurysms. These ring structures are identical clinically with those seen in diabetic retinopathy, and the single microscopic study of such a lesion[99] has shown it to be identical with the circinate lesion of diabetic retinopathy—central obliterated capillaries and microaneurysms surrounded by a deep retinal ring of fatty exudates. Although the mechanism of this obliteration of a patch of capillaries in the drainage area of an obstructed vein is unknown, it has been demonstrated both experimentally[92] and in man.[125,142] Thus, two separate diseases producing a patch of obliterated capillaries by different mechanisms present clinically identical pictures at the locus of capillary closures. It follows therefore that the clinical fundic picture of diabetic retinopathy is due in great part to the indirect effect of diabetes in promoting scattered clusters of obliterated capillaries.

These arc or ring lesions occuring after vein obstruction (Fig. 10-31) are more common at the posterior pole but may be seen well out toward the periphery. At times a portion of the exudative ring lies in an unobstructed area of retinal drainage abutting on the obstructed zone. The ring lesions themselves may persist for months, one having been followed for 4 years prior to its complete absorption and disappearance.

In Coats's disease great arcs or rings of fatty exudate may be seen either around exudative mounds or about flatter areas containing large microaneurysmal dilatations and bizarre vascular malformations. Such lesions are so extensive that they are seen best when viewed by indirect ophthalmoscopy. These rings are massive when compared to those of diabetes or vein obstruction. Except for size, they are highly similar clinically to other circinate lesions and from the information available, their microscopic composition is somewhat comparable.[70]

The macular star varies from discrete and confluent dots radiating in all directions from the fovea to heavier diverging streaks of exudate. Rarely when heavy exudation occurs, a macular mound may appear in which the diagnostic streak pattern is visible only at the mound border. The star figure has the color, consistency, staining characteristics, and microscopic elements of other fatty exudates. The material collects between the fibers of Henle's layer. Unless mound formation occurs, the fovea is spared and vision is little involved. Star formations are associated very rarely with foveal cysts.

Most macular stars are featured with diseases producing superficial retinal edema, and the appearance of edema at the macula is a prerequisite for their development (Fig. 10-32). They may develop slowly after the edema has been present for some time, or come on more rapidly as the edema recedes. Macular stars are not a feature of diseases producing deep retinal edema, a factor which may explain the rarity of associated foveal cysts.

Only that sector of the macula involved in superficial edema develops radiating lines of exudate. Thus if only the nasal half of the macula becomes edematous, as in some cases of papillitis or papilledema, a half-star or macular wing (Fig. 10-14) will subsequently appear nasally. Similarly, a subsiding small focus of chorioretinitis above the macula may develop radiating lines of exudate only among the upper Henle fibers.

The true explanation of star formation is as yet unknown and there is insufficient data so far to suggest a mechanism similar to that proposed for circinate patterns, although both of these fatty exudations are highly comparable.

As with circinate exudates, macular stars are absorbed eventually as the disease subsides. They differ from circinate lesions at the macula in that usually no permanent visual defect remains.

In the later stages of hypertensive retinopathy fatty exudates develop in the deep retina posteriorly, especially around the disc. These vary from minute discrete dots in clusters to coalescent sheets of variable density or conglomerate masses. Early discrete dots may seem white and do not show microscopic evidence of fat[3,137] but older and larger exudates are yellowish and histologically contain lipid. The yellow value is often paler or gray yellow, being modified by the pallor of the overlying edema and the whites and grays of cotton-wool spots in various stages of resolution.

Microscopically, these older fatty exudates of hypertensive disease have the same composition and staining characteristics described before, and the same predilection for the outer plexiform layer. As with the macular star, they become apparent more rapidly in an improving retinopathy as the edema recedes. For this reason they have been called "chronic edema residues" or "hard exudates." A heavy distribution of these exudates can disappear completely with successful hypertensive therapy and leave no discernible residue or effect on vision.

Like the macular star with which they are often associated, their pathogenesis is unknown. However, both bear the same relationship to prior retinal edema. The venous outflow impedance secondary to the effect of the arterial disease on the veins at crossings and at the lamina cribrosa, which is so common at this stage of hypertensive retinopathy could play some part in their development.

In the early phase of senile disciform macular degeneration, fatty exudates in the deep retina or subretinal zones about the macula are commonly the first indication of this disease (Fig. 10-30). They have in the past been mistakenly called drusen. Starting as discrete spots, they increase slowly in number and size and may fuse into one another. Eventually they form either a heavy or diaphanous sheet at the base of the central mound. At a later stage of this disease, and in some other disciform macular lesions (see Chapter 16, Disciform Macular Diseases) a girdle of fatty exudates commonly develops around the central mound (Fig. 10-33). These rings start as discrete dots in the outer plexiform layer at the border of the retinal elevation. While often described in the literature as being white, these exudates have the distinctly yellowish hue of other fatty exudates. As the exudative ring increases, it becomes thicker and its borders extend into the adjacent retina peripherally and upon the edge of the mound centrally. The ring may be either broken or complete, and denser in some sectors than others. In very exudative lesions it may appear to blend with mound exudates centrally and extend peripherally, even encompassing the disc. Rarely a tongue of exudate from the girdle reaches the far periphery like "the tail of a kite."[75]

In rare instances exudation may be so extensive as to develop a late clinical picture indistinguishable from Coats's disease (Type I). The transition from exudative senile disciform macular degeneration to the picture of Type I Coats's disease may take over 2 years (personal observation). In the usual case, the ring of exudates progresses with the development of the mound and recedes as the mound settles, disappearing well ahead of complete mound quiescence. The total time sequence may take from 4 to 5 years.

Fatty exudation is a regular component of both Leber's multiple miliary aneurysms with retinal degeneration (Fig. 10-34) and von Hippel's angiomatosis retinae. In the first, exudates are always preceded by both microaneurysms and vascular abnormalities, and appear peppered in such areas. In more advanced disease, they characteristically form arcs or rings around one or more large microaneurysms. These ring lesions are similar clinically to those of diabetic retinopathy or following vein obstruction, except that at least one of the central aneurysms in Leber's disease is obviously arterial.

The fatty exudation of retinal angioma also occurs after the vascular lesions have appeared. At first it is scattered irregularly in the region of vascular abnormality, and later tends to form a ring about the developing angioma, or a posterior arc if the angioma is near the ora serrata. As the disease progresses, exudation increases until it is the predominant clinical feature. A well-developed temporal angioma often demonstrates a characteristic pattern of fatty exudation—discrete and confluent, scattered, deep clumps situated posteriorly about the disc, a large mound at the macula, an exudate-free zone lying temporally to this, and a far temporal arc of exudates just posterior and to either side of the angioma itself (Fig. 10-35).

Choroidal hemorrhages may be followed in 2 or 3 weeks by the deposition of fatty ex-

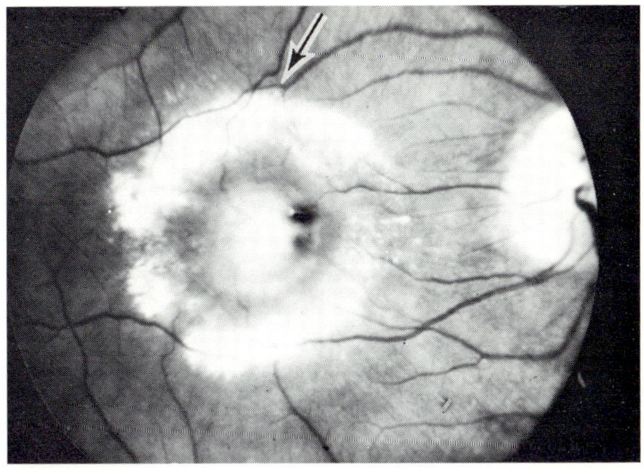

Fig. 10-33. *Top right.* Fatty exudate ring (**arrow**) around a disciform mound at the macula.

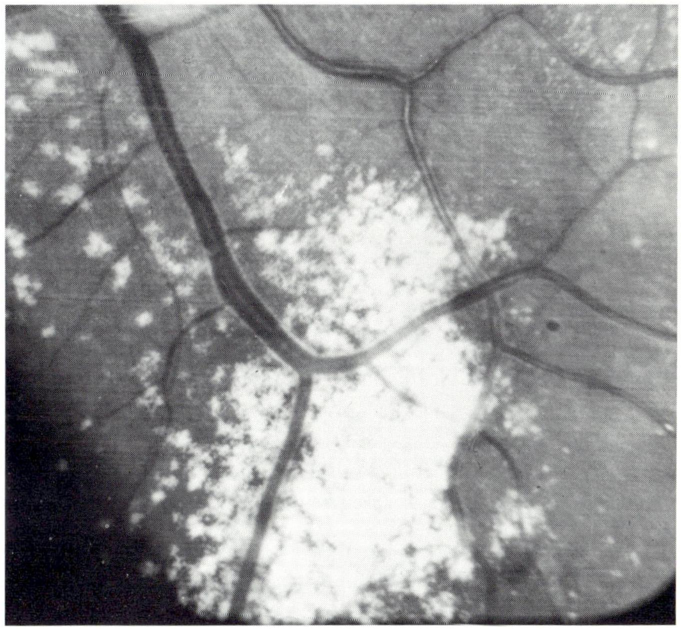

Fig. 10-34. *Right.* Fatty exudates at the border of an area of vascular malformation in Leber's multiple miliary aneurysms with retinal degeneration. (For a description of the ring lesions of this disease see Chapter 11.)

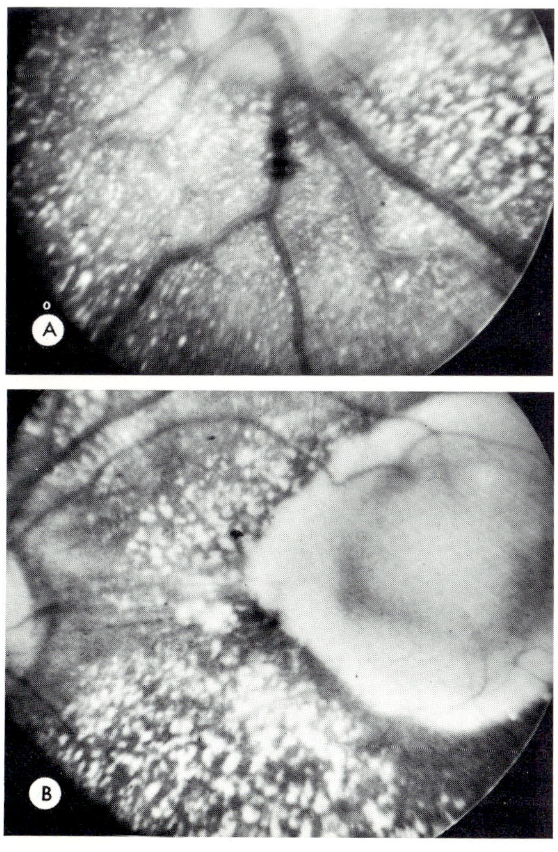

Fig. 10-35. *Left. A*, Fatty exudates scattered at the posterior pole in a case of tempororetinal angioma. *B*, Same eye shows fatty exudate mound at the macula.

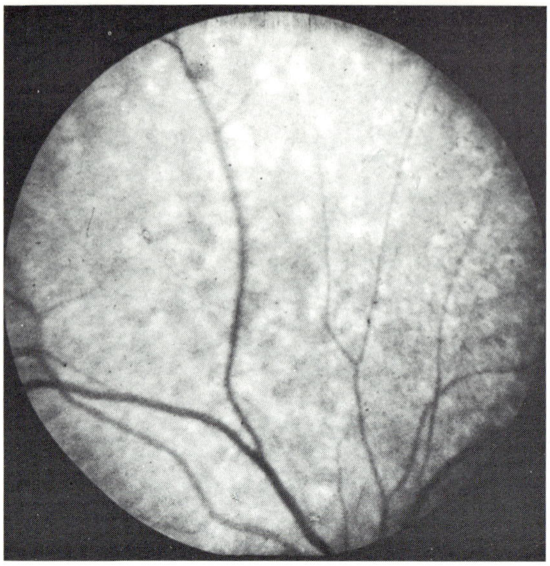

Fig. 10-36. Fundus flavimaculatus (Courtesy of Dr. R. E. Carr).

udates in the deep overlying retina (Fig 10-12). Hemorrhages beneath the pigment epithelium usually follow a similar course (see Chapter 16, Senile Disciform Macular Degeneration). Rarely, in its early stages, a malignant melanoma of the choroid may be accompanied by a small cluster of discrete, deep retinal exudates overlying its border. More than this mild degree of exudation would refute such a diagnosis. Fatty exudates tend to disappear early and are not a feature of more advanced melanomas. Occasionally a few fatty exudates appear in the vicinity of peripheral retinal vascular lesions, among a cluster of microaneurysms for instance; but here they are minute incidental findings which do not influence diagnosis.

In the flecked retina syndrome (fundus flavimaculatus), yellowish white spots with coalescent tendencies may be seen scattered over the retina from the disc to the periphery (Fig. 10-36). These lesions are not exudates, but they can be confused with fatty exudation. They may be localized to a sector, denser in some areas than others, or completely absent in broad regions. Often they demonstrate a preference for the midperiphery, tend to avoid the macula, show a fish-tail configuration, and sometimes show a rather symmetrical distribution in the two eyes. All lie at the same very deep level in the pigment epithelial cells.[88]

On retroillumination they commonly show dark fringes suggesting mild border pigment proliferation as is seen in drusen, but overlying pigment is not seen. They glow brightly on fluorescein angiography but do not leak, indicating a rarefaction or loss of pigment. They may slowly progress or they may persist for years with little change. They never show cholesterin crystals as would be expected in fatty exudates of this degree and duration.

DYSPROTEINEMIC EXUDATES

In dysproteinemic states of sufficient severity to produce exudative retinopathy, hazy, grayish white exudates, irregular and of varying sizes with poorly defined limits may appear occasionally in the superficial and commonly in the deeper retinal layers. Microscopically,[6,17] extravascular proteinemic serum is seen pooled extracellularly in the deep retinal layers. Particularly in the deep capillary bed, tremendously dilated, thin-walled vascular channels may be seen containing this same material. The source of these exudates is the capillary bed. Most of this material within or outside of the vascular lumens takes the periodic acid-Schiff (PAS) stain.

VASCULAR SHEATHING

The retinal vascular walls are normally transparent and not visible on clinical examination. The structure one sees is the column of red blood cells within the vascular lumen. When pathologic changes take place in the vessel wall, it often becomes thickened and less translucent. The blood column is partly, or completely obscured by the wall which appears as a whitish sheath around it.

No single subject in clinical ophthalmology is more confusing than that of vascular sheathing. Inexact descriptions often fail to convey to the reader an author's picture of what he has visualized. Several varieties of vascular wall pathology may be denoted simply as sheathing, or entirely different lesions on arteries and veins may be included under the general and ambiguous term "vascular sheathing." Careful clinical study reveals a number of distinct vascular wall changes, some arterial, some venous, the exact description of which is a great aid in differential diagnosis. Correlative clinicomicroscopic study will lead eventually to a more appropriate nomenclature for these individual lesions. Until such time as this is accomplished, the term vascular sheathing should be replaced by a more exact description of the specific wall change under consideration.

Retinal arterial and venous walls have different structures (see Chapter 3, Structure of Retinal Vessels), different functions, carry blood at different pressures, and contain blood constituents having different oxygen saturation values, glucose levels, etc.; so it is not surprising that they show different pathologic lesions. In only a few instances are the wall changes of arteries and veins so similar microscopically and clinically that differentiation is impossible.

THE NORMAL VESSEL WALL

The normal vessel wall is transparent and the "vessel" is actually the red cell column within it. The vast majority of major arteriovenous vessel crossings occur in the temporal retina.[72] At these crossing sites, by far the greater proportion of arteries overlie the veins. On careful observation of such crossings, the darker venous column of blood can be seen through the arterial blood column, neither of which shows caliber change or deviation. At crossings the outer wall layer of both vessels is communal and continuous with the adventitia of each vessel extending to either side of the crossing. Although not visible it is essential to remember that a similar arrangement obtains at the lamina cribrosa.

In clinical observation of a retinal vessel, one views only a single wall thickness overlying the blood column and approximately twice this wall thickness to either side. This is due to the fact that the line of observation over the blood column is radial and perpendicular, therefore transecting the shortest possible wall thickness (Fig. 10-37). To

Fig. 10-37. Diagram shows that wall thickness overlying the vessel blood column **(A)** is less than the wall thickness to each side of the blood column **(B)**.

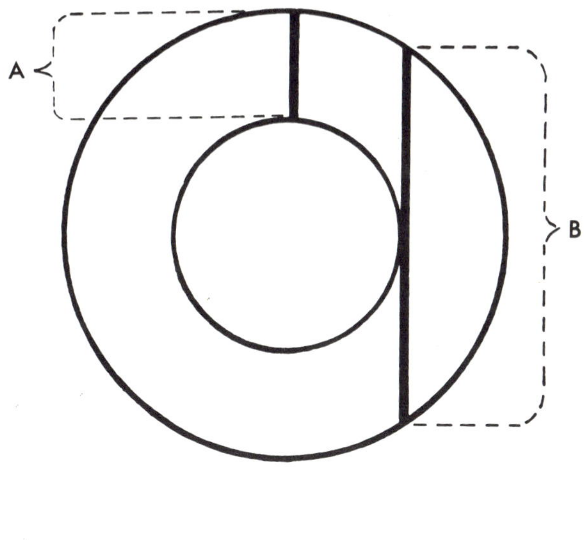

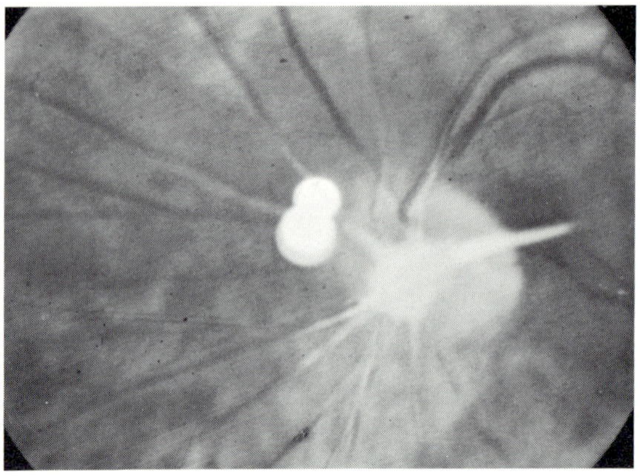

Fig. 10-38. Congenital sheathing of the vessels at the disc due to hyaloid vascular remnants.

Fig. 10-39. Epipapillary membrane showing its more common position over the nasal portion of the disc.

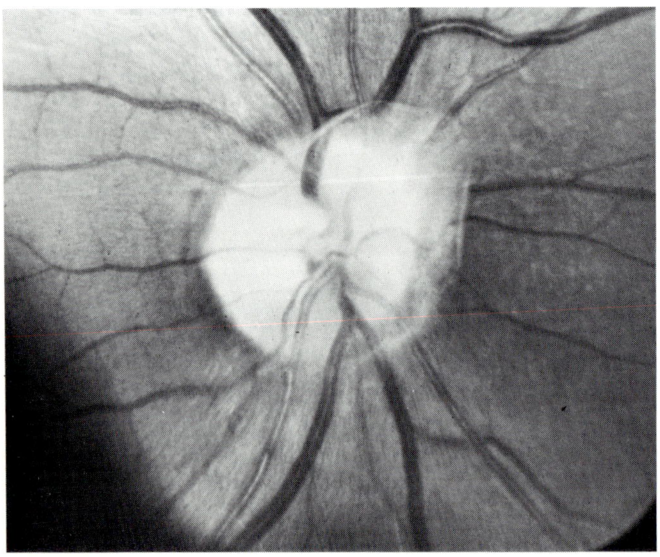

either side of the blood column the line of observation is tangential, therefore transecting a much thicker wall segment (Fig. 10-37). Any uniform wall change of either artery or vein for this technical reason is therefore always more apparent at the sides of the blood column than overlying it.

CONGENITAL SHEATHING

Smooth, white sheathing similar on artery and vein may be seen at the disc and in its immediate environment (Fig. 10-38). This occurs more often when some hyaloid vascular remnants persist but may be seen with complete involution of the latter. It is densest on the disc, where it may hide blood columns from view, and tapers gently from the disc where it seldom extends more than 1 or 2 dd into the retina. As a rule, the sheathing ends on arteries before veins, and is lost to view overlying the blood column prior to its disappearance on one or both sides of the latter. While it may appear filmy over the blood columns its edges have no hint of the fuzziness suggesting inflammatory activity. Congenital sheathing is usually most prominent and easy to diagnose when associated with a well-developed hyaloid remnant (Bergmeister's papilla). Epipapillary (prepapillary) membranes which are simply variations of this congenital papilla, may hide any vascular sheathing present (Fig. 10-39). Those cases with a complete absence of hyaloid remnant and a well-developed physiologic cup offer the most difficulty in diagnosis but here the connective tissue is usually limited to the vascular walls and the disc outline is sharply defined. This congenital sheathing, clinically, and probably microscopically, identical on artery and vein, is undoubtedly made up of the same connective tissue forming the hyaloid remnant.

POSTINFLAMMATORY VASCULAR SHEATHING AT THE DISC

Sheathing following papillitis and papilledema is sometimes termed postinflammatory. If either papillitis or papilledema is of sufficient severity and duration, white sheathing of arteries and veins similar to that of congenital sheathing may be seen at the disc and its immediate vicinity. Here, however, any significant degree of vascular sheathing is often less uniform than the congenital type and is commonly associated with a filled-in physiologic cup, hidden disc details and ragged disc borders due to gliosis. The disc may be pale as in atrophy, even in the presence of completely normal visual function. Fine retinal folds, concentric with and adjacent to the disc which are mechanically formed at the height of the disc edema, may persist permanently. While the residua of the papillitis and papilledema may not be differentiated by visualization alone, loss of disc substance especially in the region of the papillomacular bundle is strong evidence of prior papillitis.

In both of these postinflammatory sheathings, and in congenital sheathing, all changes occur only at the disc and its immediate environs. Vascular change elsewhere in the retina is not seen.

VENOUS SHEATHING

Venous sheathing is a general term used here to cover all changes involving the vein wall. Some such alterations are limited to the wall as in halo sheathing, while others may spill over into the immediately adjacent perivascular retina as in some periphlebitic foci. Collections of materials such as fatty exudates and pigment outside the walls in the perivascular retina do not represent true sheathing and are not included under this term.

Dense masses of fatty exudate may reach into the superficial retinal layers coursed by vessels and here tend to cluster in an irregular fashion along vein walls well out beyond the exudative mass itself (Fig. 10-40). When overlying the vein they give a yellowish discoloration to its blood column, or even hide the latter from view. In time these usually disappear entirely, leaving no permanent effect on the vein. Fatty exudates have no such affinity for arterial walls. Rarely, following the slow absorption of massive exudation as in Coats's disease, the halo sheathing of a previously obstructed vein may have a yellowish value suggesting some retention of lipid exudate within the vein wall. Except for the difference in color, this sheath is quite like halo sheathing.

Pigment epithelium or granules of pigment within phagocytic cells may migrate through the retina and collect along vein walls (Fig. 10-41). Although primarily a venous phenomenon, such collections may rarely be seen along arteries.[169] This change is seen typically in pigmentary degeneration of the retina where segments of veins are hugged by pigment, fitting bifurcations like a pair of tight pants. Microscopically, pigment particles adherent to the venular and capillary walls probably accounts for the "bone corpuscle" configurations seen clinically in retinitis pigmentosa.[50,158] The evidence suggesting that scattered, retinal capillary closure is a common feature of advanced retinitis pigmentosa (see under Arterial Sheathing in Pigmentary Degenerations) could explain Cogan's unwillingness to accept the occluded hyalinized clumps and strings with pigment about them as obliterated small retinal vessels.[20] This same affinity of pigment for capillary and vein wall is also seen in myopic degeneration, choroidal sclerosis, uveitis, and trauma.

It is probable that both fatty exudates and pigment collect along capillary and vein

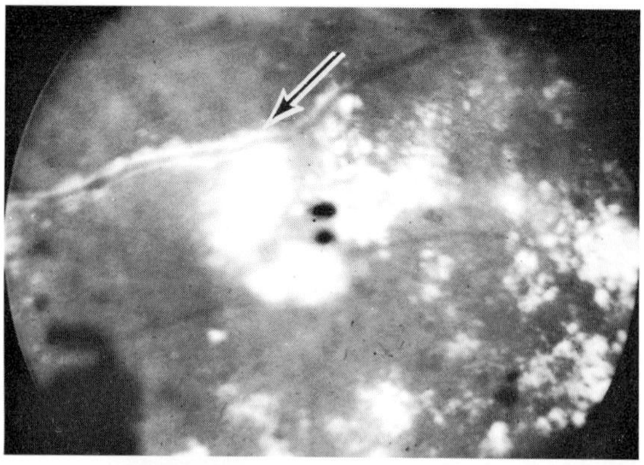

Fig. 10-40. Diabetic retinopathy demonstrating the affinity of fatty exudates for venous walls **(arrow).**

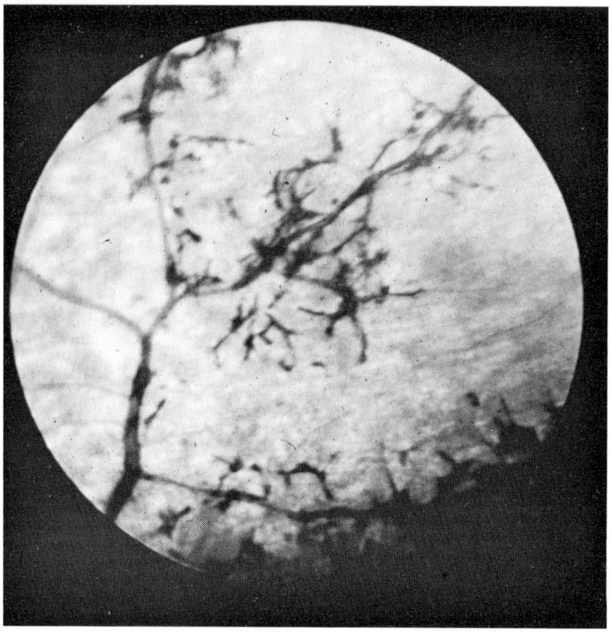

Fig. 10-41. Pigment collecting around retinal veins and capillaries in retinitis pigmentosa (Courtesy of Dr. R. E. Carr).

Fig. 10-42. Ghost vein **(A)** following branch vein obstruction at an arteriovenous crossing. Severe arteriosclerosis **(B)** which developed subsequent to the vein obstruction.

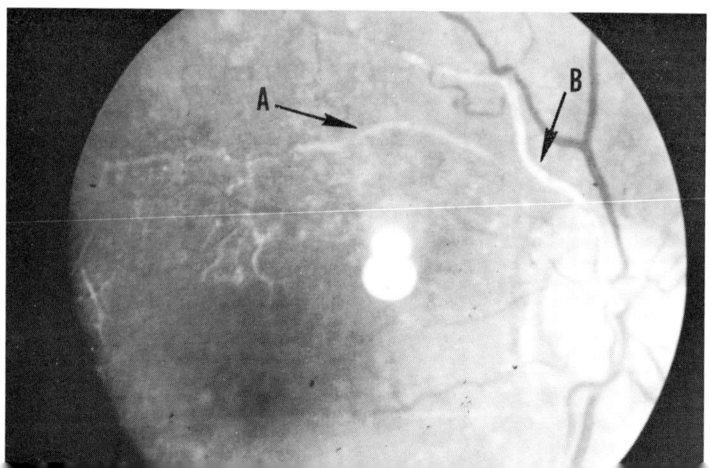

walls in the course of their absorption although neither has ever been demonstrated within the wall itself, nor has transfer through the wall been proved.

We prefer not to use the term "sheathing" for obliterated ghost veins. A ghost vein usually has a permanently closed lumen and on clinical examination not even a red thread is visible (Fig. 10-42). The heaviest halo sheathing will only rarely obscure the finest patent and functioning lumen. Where the vein is permanently occluded, its ghost appearance extends in both directions along the venous segment to the next *patent* tributary. Such a ghost vein may extend to the disc where the patent tributary is a collateral deep in the disc substance and not actually visible. These ghost veins usually have a gray white color and may be either very prominent and readily visible or quite faint, even invisible in segments. The gray white stripe with its arborizations may be mildly undulating in its course or show more bizarre twisting. The width of the stripe may show considerable variation along its course. Veins with blood columns hidden by gliosis or periphlebitic foci, whose lumen patency is readily visible on either side of the hidden locus are not true ghost vessels. Apparent ghost vessels may rarely transport fluorescein on angiography.

Halo Sheathing

This term, coined by Ballantyne,[10] denotes a relatively uniform alteration of the venous wall clinically visible as a hazy white discoloration over the venous blood column and denser white stripes to either side of it. It does not cause irregularity in the venous blood column. The only clinicopathologic studies of halo sheathing show that the change is limited to the wall itself. This factor probably accounts for its smooth contour and relatively even stripe width.

Halo sheathing tends to be uniform along the vein segments (Fig. 10-43). Depending upon the viewing angle, it may seem more apparent on one side of the blood column than on the other. Although most apparent on larger veins, it may be seen on small venous radicals, especially in the periphery. Ballantyne attributed halo sheathing to microscopically visualized lipohyalin change in the vein wall, although he also found an increase in adventitial collagen.

An example of pure halo sheathing in a nondiabetic patient viewed clinically and examined microscopically in our laboratories revealed no lipid component, only intense collagenous thickening of the outer vein wall.[79] The lumen was uniformly narrowed due to a shunt which was carrying blood formerly coursing through the venous channel. The haloed vein was fully patent, with a normal endothelial lining and the only wall abnormality was its increase in collagen (Fig. 10-44). The white color of halo sheathing, its smooth uniformity, and the absence of any yellow color value or crystalline content (both associated with lipid infiltration) make it likely that this appearance is attributed solely to the increased adventitial collagen.

Halo sheathing is of primary importance as a sign of prior venous flow impedance or vein obstruction. Impedance of flow and the associated raised venous pressure necessary to produce halo sheathing must be of some duration. Excellent collateral formation and good flow recovery after vein obstruction are deterrents to halo sheathing and in such cases it may not even be visible.

Good examples of pure halo sheathing without confusing extraneous pathology are seen best in old central or branch retinal vein obstructions. Once clearly seen, lesser degrees of this valuable sign may be viewed in any of the venous obstructive diseases.

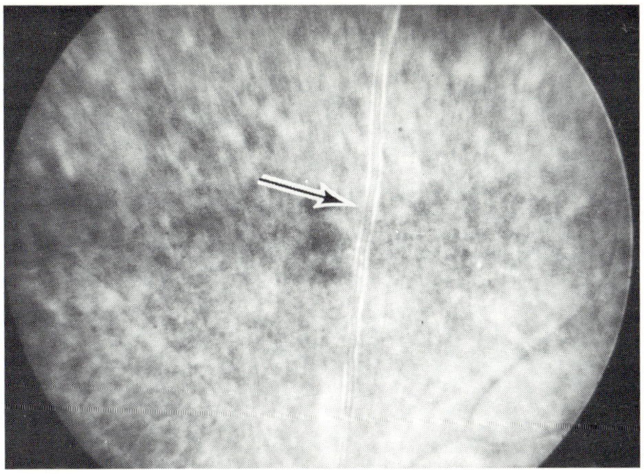

Fig. 10-43. Halo sheathing **(arrow)** of a retinal vein.

Venous Sheathing in Multiple Sclerosis

Venous sheathing in multiple sclerosis was first described by Rucker.[130–133] His findings have been repeatedly confirmed by others,[23,39,74,103,108,116,135,162,164a] and Haarr [56,57] has made a particular study of them.

These venous lesions occur in 10 per cent [132] to 23 per cent [56] of patients with multiple sclerosis. Most are seen from 5 to 10 years after symptoms start but they have been seen at any disease stage and at any patient age.[133] They appear in the absence of other retinal pathology, and attack the venous tree anywhere beyond 3 mm from the disc. Two different lesions may be seen. The first appears as an active periphlebitis, a fuzzy, white, perivenous cuffing (Fig. 10-45*A*). (This is described more fully in the section on "Periphlebitis.") Such lesions may come and go, attacking the veins in different places, and either disappearing or entering a quiescent stage as a faint or heavy halo-type sheathing (Fig. 10-45*B*) extending for some distance along the vein and tapering at either extremity as it disappears. This halo may also disappear, but usually takes longer to do so. Narrowing of the venous blood col-

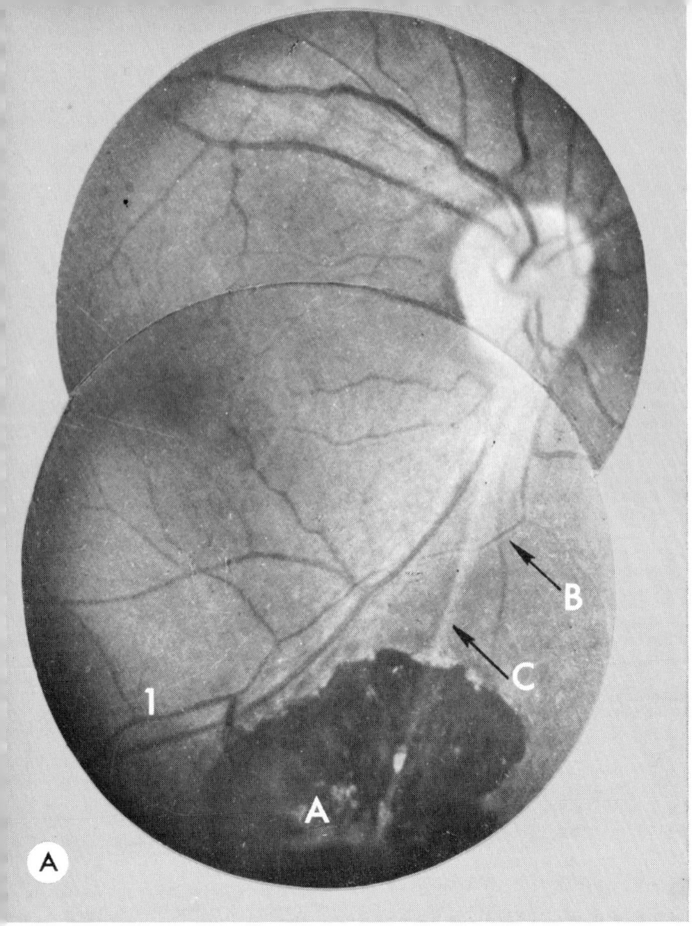

Fig. 10-44. *A*, Toxoplasmic retinochoroiditis demonstrating a retinochoroidal venous anastomosis **(A)** a halo-sheathed vein **(B)**, and a preretinal tissue strand arising from the disc **(C)**.

B, Diagram of *A*.

C, Histologic appearance of the retinochoroidal venous anastomosis **(A)** and Bruch's membrane **(B)**.

D, Histologic appearance of nonhalo-sheathed vein (see **1** in Fig. 44**A**) showing the normal wall.

E, Histologic appearance of halo-sheathed vein showing increased collagen in the wall.

(From Kennedy and Wise.[79])

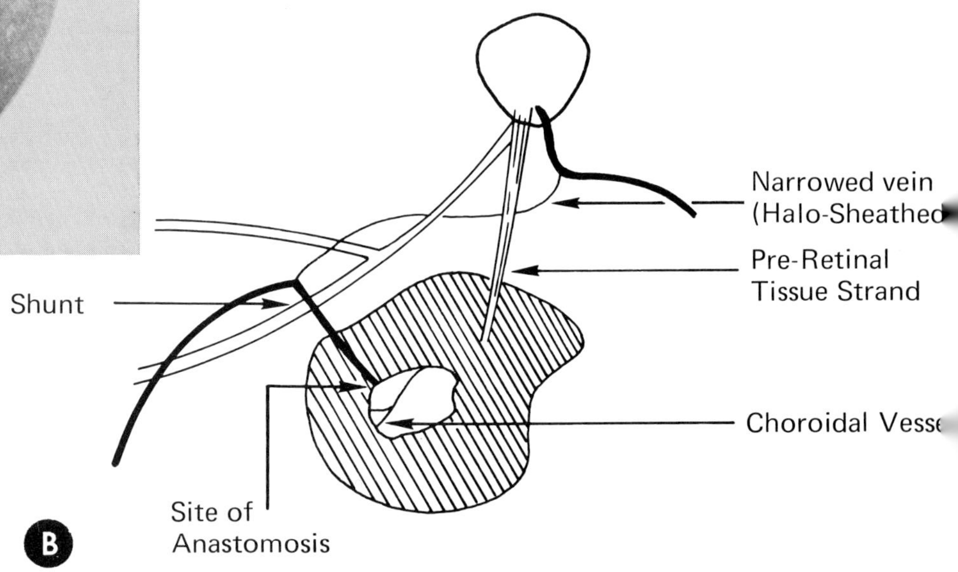

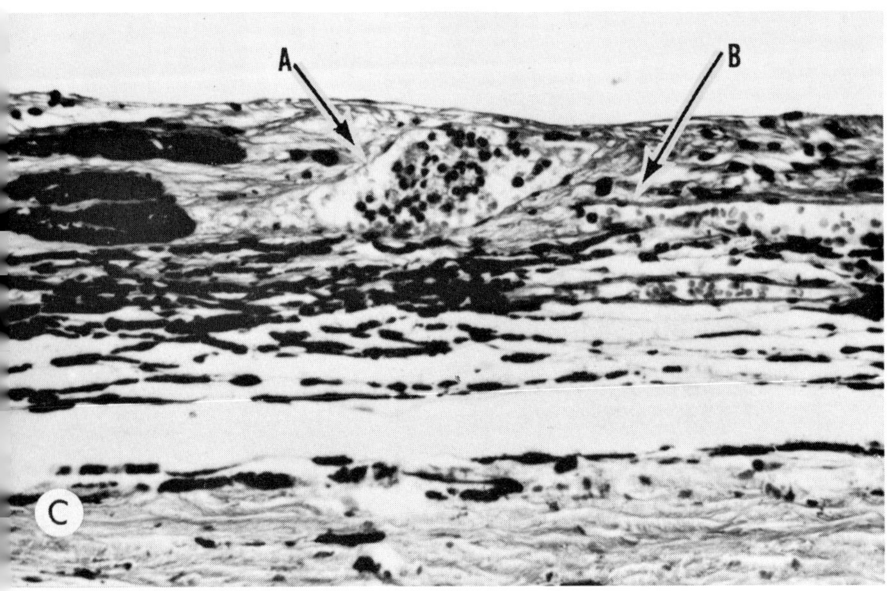

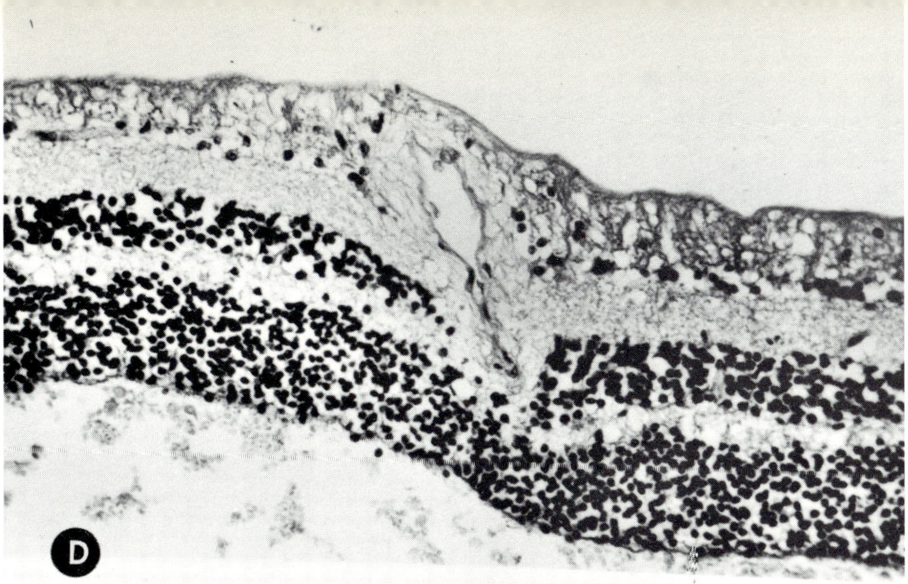

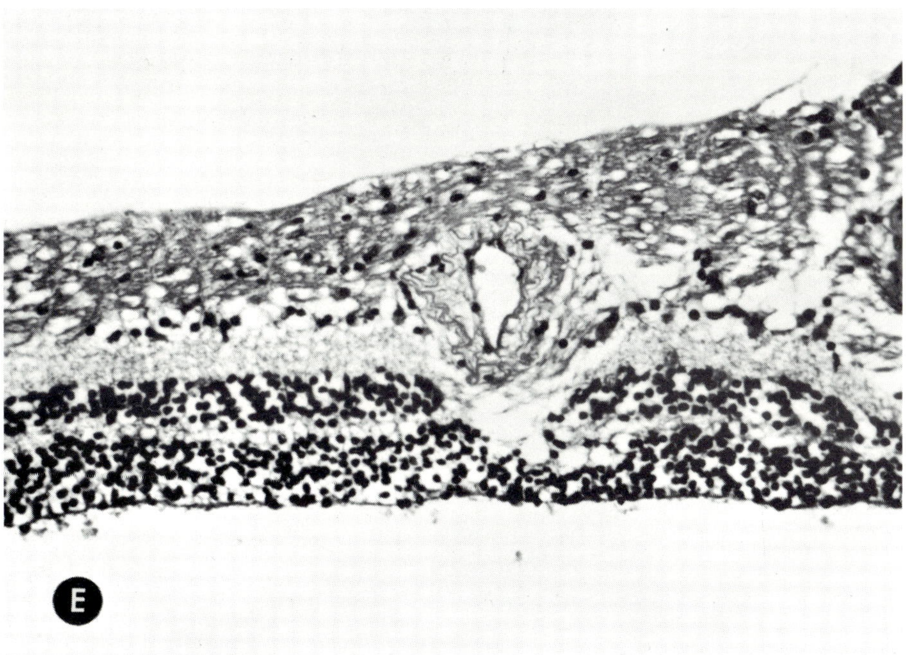

umn, both prior to the onset of a periphlebitic cuff and at a more distant place on the vein, have been reported.[56] Dilatation of the vein and several hemorrhages peripheral to an acute periphlebitic lesion have been described, and Haarr showed one obstructed vein segment with a collateral venous channel around it. Some active periphlebitic foci have fine vitreous floaters in the preretinal vitreous near the site of perivenous cuffing.

There has been no microscopic study of these lesions but similar periphlebitic cuffs in other diseases have shown round cell infiltration in, and just outside, the vein wall. Clinical evidence suggests that this leads to some blockage in the vein producing the later halo-type sheathing, resulting from increased collagen in the venous wall.

Haarr's data[56] suggested that active periphlebitic foci might be associated with ac-

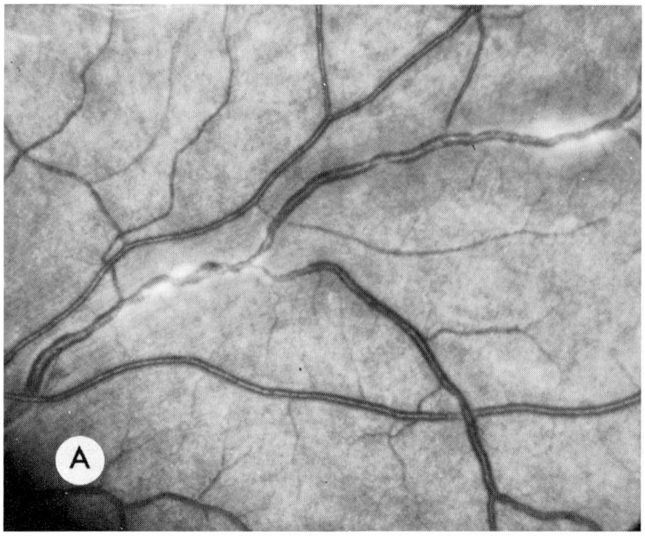

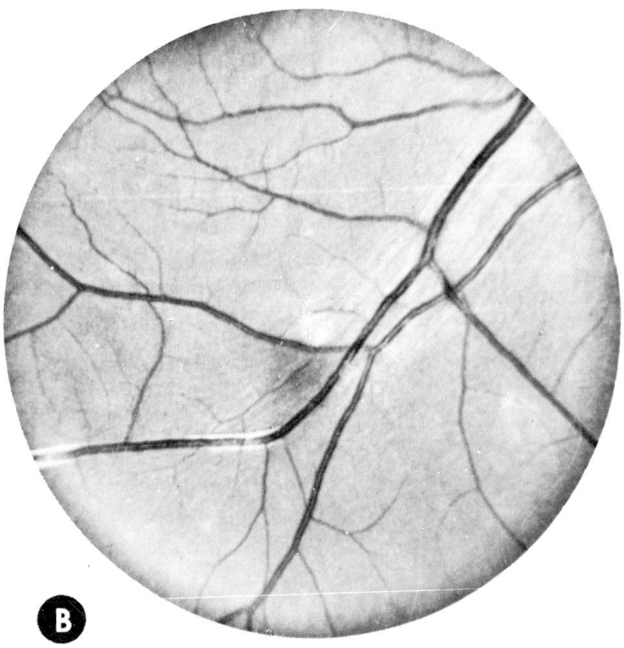

Fig. 10-45. *A*, Periphlebitic venous sheathing in a patient with multiple sclerosis.
B, Halo sheathing of a vein in a patient with multiple sclerosis. (Courtesy of Dr. C. W. Rucker.)

tive central nervous system disease, and quiescent retinal lesions with remissions.

Periphlebitis

Fuzzy, white, irregularly spotty sheathing of retinal veins represents an inflammation of the venous wall, often spoken of as "venous cuffing." It varies greatly in density, completely hiding the blood column in places and appearing only as a thin haze in others. At times it extends into the perivenous retinal tissues presenting a ragged border along the vein, not in any way restricted by the outer limit of the vein wall. Periphlebitic sheathing may occur on any vein from disc to periphery and has been demonstrated microscopically about the vein at the lamina cribrosa.[83,89,100] Inflammatory foci may occur anywhere along a vein segment being uninfluenced either by venous branchings or arteriovenous crossings (Fig. 10-46). When one occurs at such a crossing it may be seen to extend for a short distance along the arterial wall to either side. Other than this, arteries are singularly free of involvement. Those lesions, which have been observed from onset, start with a darkening, dilatation, and irregularity of the involved vein. This is followed by retinal edema in its drainage area and a few hemorrhages near its more peripheral fine tributaries. Several days later a large cuff of exudate appeared about the vein, hiding it from view and extending well out into the adjacent retina. Hazy whiteness, apparently limited to the vein wall extended to either side of this focus. Hemorrhages in the venous drainage area peripheral to the inflammatory site became more profuse, in some cases of sufficient degree to warrant a diagnosis of vein obstruction (Fig. 14-9*A*). Those cases not developing vitreous hemorrhages at this time persisted in this state for several weeks and then began to recover. One such site completely recovered in 3 months, all retinal reaction subsiding, and the vein and its wall returning to a normal appearance without residual defect. Another improved but left a duplicated collateral beyond the segment of halo sheathing. This sequence suggests strongly that periphlebitis can start as an endophlebitis attacking the inner vein wall and impeding flow from the start. It then progresses to the picture of periphlebitis. Depending upon its degree of severity, it may or may not lead to complete vein obstruction. If not fully obstructed, the vein is likely to return to a normal appearance, while obstruction without recanalization makes sequellae inevitable (see Chapter 14, under section on Vein Obstruction Secondary to Arteriosclerosis).

Some authors[11,81] have described such an inflammation about retinal arteries as well as veins and they call this "retinal perivasculitis." Severer degrees of periphlebitis are often associated with posterior vitreous detachment. In these cases inflammatory cells float in the compartment behind the receding vitreous and form clusters both on the receding posterior vitreous face and indiscriminately on the retinal surface.[86] Such nests overlying the arteries may appear to be within the retina surrounding the artery when actually they lie on the retinal surface. Both clinical and microscopic evidence corroborate these findings.[44,48,90,134,153,164] Very severe periphlebitis is seen often with no involvement of an immediately adjacent accompanying artery. In microscopic studies arterial pathology has hardly been mentioned, although it must be admitted that some vascular walls are so involved as to preclude arterial or venous identification.

No early pathology of periphlebitis has been studied microscopically. Sections at a later stage have shown an inflammatory reaction of the vein wall and involvement of the adjacent retina.[100,134] Lymphocytic cells predominated, but epithelioid and giant cells were also found. Cellular signet-ring configurations about veins were common, corresponding to the one-sided clinical appearance of many perivascular cuffs. Hyalinization and thinning of the vein wall, narrowing and obstruction of the lumen, endothelial cell proliferation, thrombosis, and necrosis with rupture of the vein permitting seepage of red blood cells through the wall have all been found repeatedly. In Eales's disease tubercle formation about the veins has been seen rarely[82,146] and Gilbert[47] has demonstrated tuberculosis bacilli in a periphlebitic focus of a single patient.

Uveitis and chorioretinitis have been noted in some cases of periphlebitis. In such cases single rows of round cells have been demonstrated on either side of retinal capillaries, especially deeper ones.[86]

Typical retinal periphlebitis occurs in Eales's disease and in some cases of uveitis. Toxoplasmic retinochoroiditis in its acute phase commonly shows widespread periphlebitis. Low-grade peripheral chorioretinitis (pars planitis) usually shows a lesser degree of periphlebitis bilaterally in the retinal periphery. In some cases of sarcoidosis peripheral periphlebitis with lardaceous "candlewax" deposits may be seen.

Postinflammatory Sheathing

Focal chorioretinitis may leave its mark on adjacent, or directly overlying retinal veins. The ultimate effect on the vein seems

Fig. 10-46. Periphlebitis in Eales's disease.

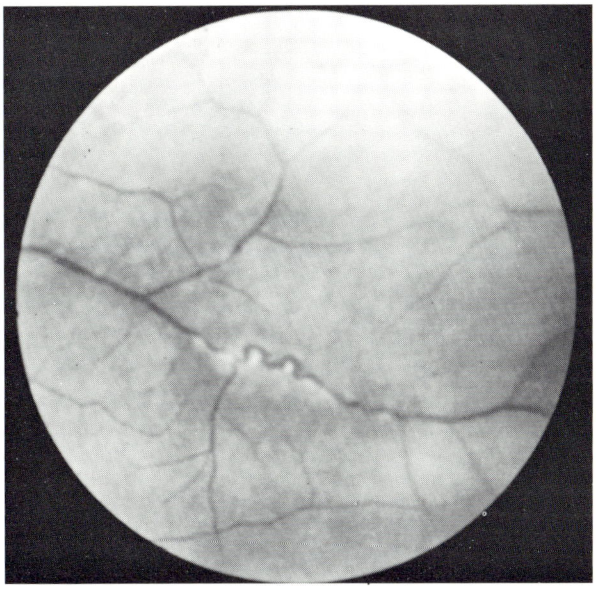

to bear no relation to the size of the chorioretinal scar. Large scars may have unaffected overlying veins, while markedly involved veins may overlie relatively small scars. An overlying artery is involved very rarely. If it is involved, it shows a milder degree of the heavier sheathing, always exaggerated on the accompanying overlying vein. There is a short stretch of halo vein sheathing to either side of a denser opaque white tissue irregularly distributed on the vein and extending often beyond the vein wall (Fig. 10-47). The latter may contain granules or clumps of proliferated pigment epithelium. The heavier tissue probably constitutes secondary gliosis. Mild degrees of this process may show only the halo vein sheathing. Old branch vein obstruction, venous collateral formations, and even retinochoroidal venous anastomoses through old chorioretinal scars are not rare in posterior uveitis, especially in retinochoroiditis due to toxoplasmosis. (Fig. 10-48).

Venous Sheathing in Retinoschisis

Narrowed, dark venous columns of blood with halo sheathing are usual on the superficial retinal layer of senile retinoschisis. With the light focused upon this layer, the blood column is red and the halo has a fine irregularity throughout its length. With the light focused upon the fundus background, the vessels are seen by retroillumination and the dark blood column may be much more difficult to appreciate. The halo sheath may be hardly discernible at the posterior edge of the retinoschisis but becomes more evident as the periphery is approached. Arteries may be slightly narrowed but show no other discernible change, except in the far periphery, where both arteries and veins may be rather abruptly converted into opaque white lines without apparent lumens. Such vessels, some of which may be ghost vessels, look so much alike that they must be traced to identifiable artery or vein to verify their nature. Shea, Schepens, and von Pirquet [139] found more white vessels in the lower temporal periphery and Byer [15] noted that many more small veins than arteries became opaque. They have thick, hyalinized walls, often devoid of nuclei and narrowed or nearly obliterated lumens.[25,168]

In juvenile retinoschisis, where the pathology is different,[163] the anterior retinal layer is missing over large regions. It tends to condense in bands about larger retinal vessels as a heavier white tissue complicating the sheathing.

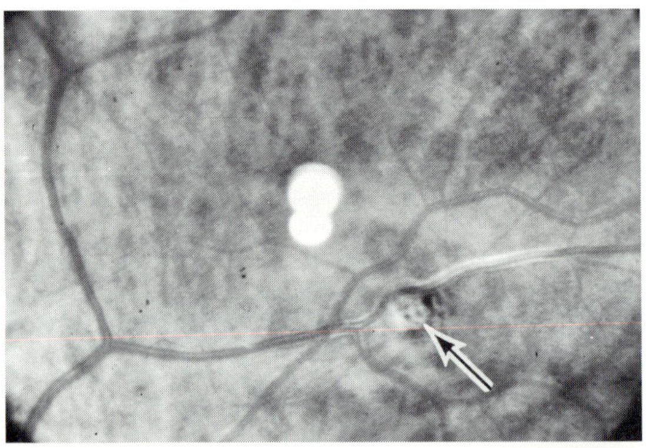

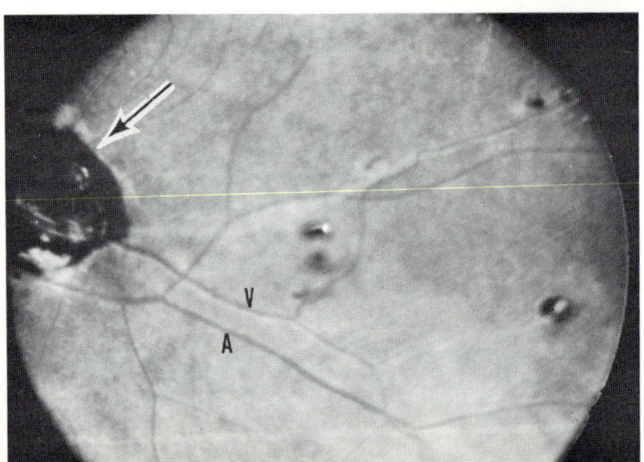

Fig. 10-47. Venous sheathing resulting from chorioretinitis **(arrow).** The adjacent artery is uninvolved.

Fig. 10-48. Toxoplasmic retinochoroiditis **(arrow)** with secondary halo sheathing of the vein and sparing of the artery. (From Wise.[153])

ARTERIAL SHEATHING (ARTERIOSCLEROSIS)

Arteriosclerosis or arterial sheathing, as in its venous counterpart, is a general term used to include all clinically visible alterations of the arterial walls in the presence of patent lumens. The retinal arteries are involved in many systemic conditions such as hypertension, diabetes, and aging, as well as local processes in the eye.

The term arteriosclerosis should be differentiated from atheroma. Atheromata consist of nodular, subendothelial, intimal lipid plaques occurring principally in large and medium-sized arteries. No one has as yet demonstrated unequivocally such a subendothelial atheroma in a retinal artery. Although unseen clinically such lesions have been identified microscopically in the central retinal artery at the lamina cribrosa. Therefore the common usage of the term atheromata or atheromatous plaques to define retinal lesions should be avoided.

Normal retinal arteries are red, gently curving and have a thin, bright reflex stripe down the center of the blood column. This is visible most readily on larger arteries. Smaller ones may demonstrate no reflex stripe. As normal arterial walls are transparent, no stripe appears beside the blood columns and where arteries cross over veins, the darker venous blood column can be seen through the lighter arterial stream. No crossing defects are present normally.

Mild Arteriosclerosis

Arteriosclerosis starts subtly and can only be noted clinically on larger arteries. Hiding of the venous blood column by increasing opacity of the overcrossing arterial wall is the first observable sign. Next, there is a broadening of the central light reflex and the development of fine white lines at the sides of the blood column, both associated with an increasing paleness of the arteries. This may be a diffuse change but it is usually more apparent on some arteries than others. So far, all changes may occur without change in arterial curvature; or an increasing sinusoidal curvature of larger arteries may begin. Increasing crossing defects (see under Arteriovenous Crossing Changes) and increasing paleness of arterial light reflexes lead ultimately to the stage of copper-wire arteries. From this point on, arteriosclerosis should be considered severe.

The changing features of arteries due solely to the aging process have never been clearly defined. Some individuals in their mid-seventies will have retinal arteries indistinguishable from those of normal youth. Others at a much younger age will begin to show changes attributable to aging, which are no different from those seen in mild arteriosclerosis. Leishman[95] has described straightening, narrowing, and paleness as signs of aging arteries. Elwyn[36] believed simple aging of arteries with their coincident loss of elasticity caused mild dilatation and lengthening, the latter producing increased, gentle, sinusoidal curvatures. He attributed the increased reflex on such vessels to their increasing wall collagen. Leishman[95] has described these same arterial changes with concomitant crossing defects and the same loss of elastic tissue and increased wall collagen in his patients with hypertension and replacement fibrosis. Normotensive patients with evidence of chronic retinal venous insufficiency (outflow impedance) will develop, over a period of time, dilated, sinusoidal, burnished arteries with increased light reflexes and crossing defects similar to the changes described by Elwyn and Leishman. These vessels are indistinguishable from those showing mild arteriosclerosis. The recognized effect of vein obstruction in promoting arteriosclerosis on its accompanying artery offers a possible explanation for this observation.[152,152a]

Mild arteriosclerosis also occurs with

chorioretinitis, Leber's multiple miliary aneurysms with retinal degeneration, angiomatosis retinae, venous outflow impedance, or venous and capillary obstructive disease, hyperviscous diseases, and diseases affecting a decreased arterial inflow. The clinical picture of arteriosclerosis in these cases is indistinguishable from that attributed to aging. When none of the other conditions is present, aging is assumed to be the causative factor.

Mild arteriosclerosis is quite innocuous in most cases. Its only direct complication is branch vein obstruction. Branch vein obstruction from this cause occurs predominantly at arteriovenous crossings, or rarely where the vessels fail to cross but lie in close proximity to one another. Branch retinal artery obstruction does not occur as a direct result of mild retinal arteriosclerosis.

Regardless of whether the process is labeled mild arteriosclerosis or aging, its complications are of practical importance, and they are the same in either case.

Severe Arteriosclerosis

As mild arteriosclerosis becomes severe, it assumes a distinctly irregular and spotty distribution. Severe arteriosclerosis may involve arteries of any size but it is more common on larger vessels. The early changes on small arteries are so subtle, that they usually go unnoticed until a severe stage is reached.

Severe arteriosclerosis is seen first at bifurcations of the larger arteries. Starting as a broadened and increased yellowish reflection from the arterial wall, it extends along one or all branches with increasing brightness and reflection. Crystalline reflections may be seen on well-developed lesions. In this phase the wall change approaches the same yellow color as that of the fatty exudate. Careful clinical observation reveals a clear zone between the border of the blood column and the yellowish opaque wall change at the ragged ends of some lesions. Although the lesion is sufficiently dense to obscure the blood column from view, fluorescein passes through uninterruptedly. The lack of any visual field change beyond many such lesions, their clinical appearance, and the passage of fluorescein all speak for an outer wall pathology not embarrassing the vascular lumen.

As arteriosclerosis increases, longer segments of arteries including small branches become involved. Long segments of irregular yellowish sheathing may fit about the blood column like a glove. As in halo sheathing, arteriosclerosis is limited to the arterial wall, never extending into the periarterial spaces or adjacent retina. Such long segments of severe arteriosclerosis have been called "pipe-stem sheathing." This is a descriptive phrase which leads to confusion and should be avoided. In this degree, arteriosclerosis is usually seen on larger vessels, and has a predilection for bends, and arteriovenous crossings as well as bifurcations. Extensive segments may have completely hidden blood columns.

With still more severe arteriosclerosis the sheath may develop crystalline areas and suggest a salted pretzel stick. Involved arteries may be narrow and straight with angular twists, or more dilated and sinusoidal with gentle curves. Short segments of smaller arteries may show very minute and bizarre twisting. The blood column may be invisible, visible as a thin thread, or patchily visible, creating a false sense of lumen irregularity. Eventually, severely involved arteries may suffer irregular narrowing of the lumen or its obliteration.[72] Such vessels may lose their irregular yellowness and become smoother, dirty gray streaks (ghost arteries).

Materials such as fatty exudation and pigment seldom accumulate around arteries, so that practically all apparent arterial sheathing truly represents some involvement of the vascular wall itself. Ghost arteries with obliterated lumens occur also, but are not seen as frequently as venous ghost vessels. Unlike veins, arterial lumen patency cannot always be judged by clinical visualization alone. Severe arteriosclerosis can so opacify walls that, in the presence of a still patent lumen, the blood column cannot be seen. When this occurs over a long arterial segment, field testing or fluorescein angiography may be necessary to determine lumen patency. Ghost arteries may have an appearance very similar to that of ghost veins, but more commonly such occluded arteries have a yellowish wall hue, with irregularly scattered yellow spots (probably lipid), some of which may harbor crystalline reflections (probably cholesterin crystals). Smaller ghost arteries may demonstrate extremely bizarre tortuosity.

Arteriosclerosis after Vein Obstruction

Following retinal vein occlusion of various etiologies, arteriosclerosis may develop in an artery lying in the zone of obstructed venous drainage. This is especially true in occlusions associated with hypertension and diabetes. In these two diseases its presence only in the artery accompanying the obstructed vein, and its absence in arteries accompanying the unobstructed veins, as is seen in cases of branch vein obstruction, conclusively demonstrates the etiologic importance of vein obstruction in its pathogenesis. In those cases where it is seen in the absence of frank vein obstruction, signs of old capillary obliteration, long-standing impedance of venous outflow, or minimal signs of old and partially hidden vein obstruction can usually be found (Fig. 10-49). Arteriosclerosis is always more obvious in the obstructed venous drainage area, being less evident or absent where the artery happens to course outside this zone. Likewise it is more apt to occur where collateral formation is poor and venous stagnation persists. In cases developing good collateral flow, it may not develop at all, or if present, may tend to clear. Indeed, slow absorption and decrease of arteriosclerosis has been observed to continue from 3 to 5 years (Fig. 10-50). Arteriosclerosis may be seen as early as 3 months after retinal vein obstruction and can become so marked as to be the dominant clinical feature in 9 months (Fig. 10-51).

One such arteriosclerotic artery, seen clinically after retinal vein obstruction, has been examined microscopically in our laboratories. Heavy lipid infiltration taking the usual fat stain was demonstrated, predominantly in the media but also in the adventitia (Fig. 10-52). Seitz[136] has also demonstrated this lesion microscopically but correlation with the clinical lesion was not recorded. Microscopic study with the usual stains has not shown the differences between mild and severe arteriosclerosis which would be expected from their clinical appearances. This is also true of choroidal sclerosis, with severe degrees of clinical sclerosis showing little microscopic evidence of it.[4] Special techniques for the demonstration of lipids have not been reported in studies of choroidal sclerosis and have only rarely been employed in the study of retinal arteriosclerosis. In both Seitz's and our own study, fat was demonstrated, and in both instances it resided primarily in the media and adventitia. Further lipid studies are necessary before such a novel pathology can be accepted. However, the yellow opacity, sharp border, and crystalline content of some lesions would fit in with a lipid etiology.

Arteriosclerosis after Arterial Obstruction

Arteriosclerosis after arterial obstruction occurs in two different clinical forms. The common type is seen more often and is usually more severe after peripheral arterial obstruction (in a branch or the central

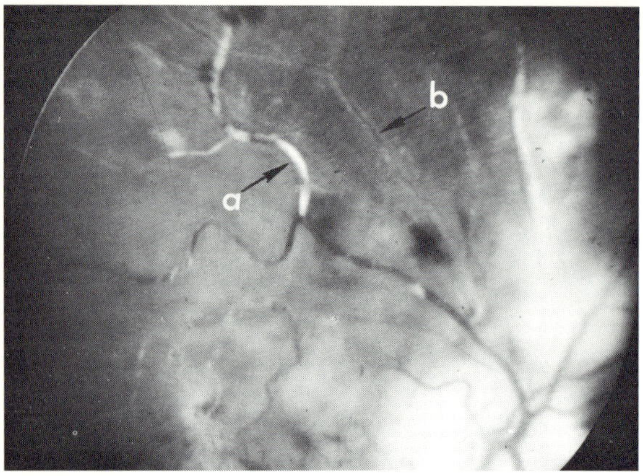

Fig. 10-49. Accelerated hypertension with severe arteriosclerosis **(a).** The signs of central retinal vein obstruction were partially hidden, but the halo-sheathed vein can be seen at (**b**). (From Wise.[152])

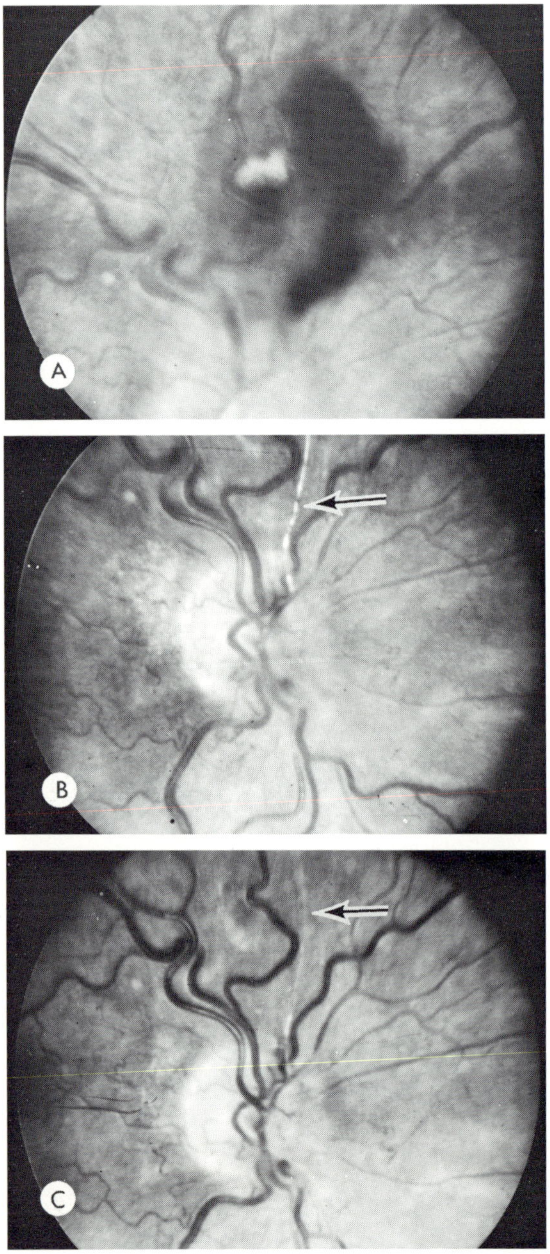

Fig. 10-50. *A*, Accelerated hypertension with obstruction of a branch vein above the disc.

B, Same eye 1 year later shows severe arteriosclerosis of the artery accompanying the obstructed vein **(arrow).** (From Wise.[152])

C, Same eye a little over 3 years after *A* showing decreased prominence of the arteriosclerosis **(arrow).**

Fig. 10-51. *Below.* Severe arteriosclerosis developing 9 months after central retinal vein obstruction.

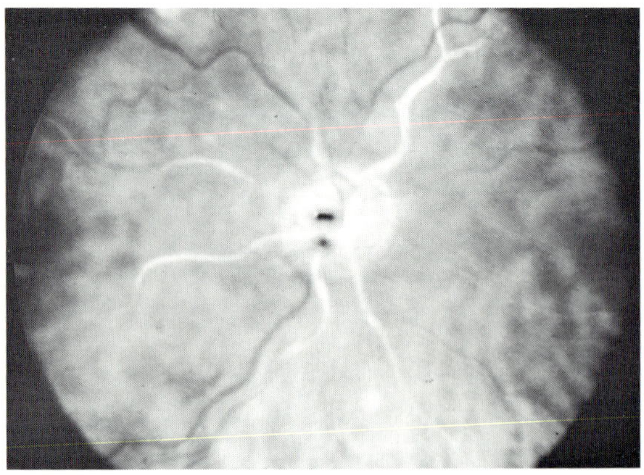

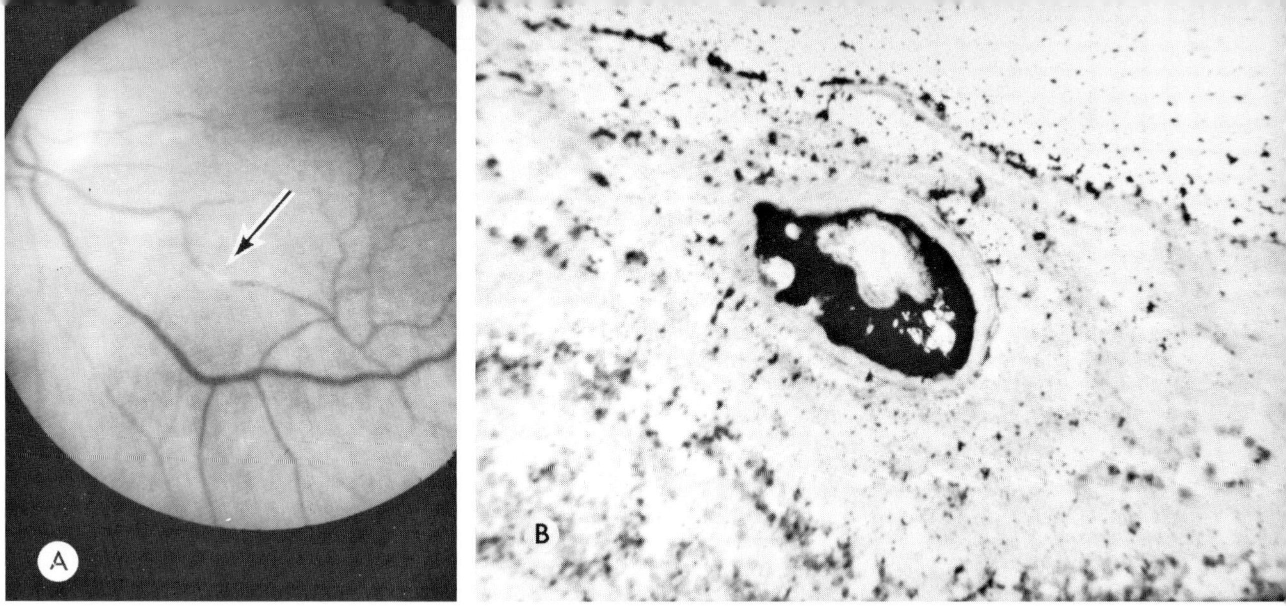

Fig. 10-52. *A*, A segment of severe arteriosclerosis of a retinal artery **(arrow)** in a 73-year-old hypertensive female. *B*, A section through the arteriosclerotic segment shown in *A*. Oil Red O stain.

Fig. 10-53. *A*, Embolus **(arrow)** obstructing inferior temporal artery at its first bifurcation. *B*, Severe arteriosclerosis developing on either side of the embolus, and on the arterial branch 4 months later. (Courtesy Dr. G. Goodman)

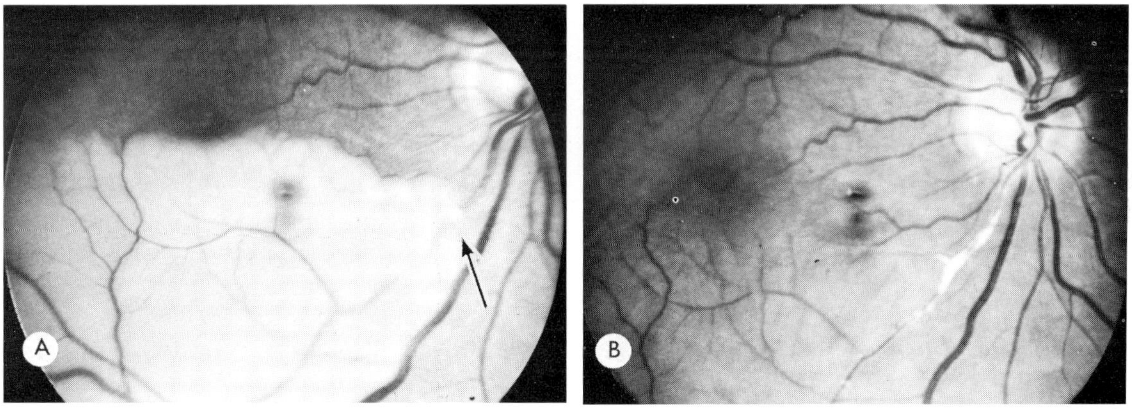

Fig. 10-54. *Below. A*, Toxoplasmic retinochoroiditis **(A)** with segmental arteriosclerosis of the inferotemporal artery **(arrows).** *B*, Similar wall changes of the inferior nasal artery **(arrows).**

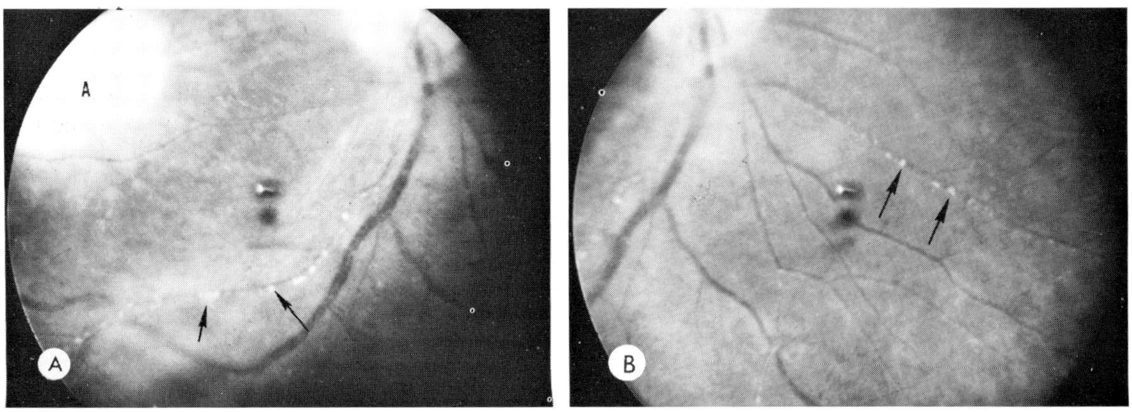

retinal artery) but does occur after obstruction of the ophthalmic or carotid artery and probably is present in the later stages of pulseless disease as well. In this type the arterial lumen is narrowed and very irregular, the lumen variability being well demonstrated by fluorescein angiography. Arterial walls are lighter in color, have a brighter reflex, appear thicker and more opaque. This change produces the white lines of irregular breadth on either side of the blood column. When very severe, the wall changes to a yellowish color with crystals in it or becomes white and opaque without a visible blood column. Some of the latter eventually lose their lumens and become ghost arteries, but lumen closure cannot be judged by clinical appearance alone. Fluorescein angiography or field testing is necessary for this diagnosis. Smaller arteries with this type of arteriosclerosis may show very bizarre contortions.

Rarely, a retinal artery will develop a clinically identical type of arteriosclerosis to that described after retinal vein obstruction. A good example of this (Fig. 10-53) followed embolic obstruction of an inferior temporal artery at its first bifurcation. The whole artery showed mild arteriosclerosis but severe change was present at the site of the embolus, in the branch artery, and in the arterial wall backward toward the disc.

Fluorescein angiography has demonstrated such a variable degree of blockage in clinically diagnosed arterial obstructions, that variable degrees of arteriosclerosis following these episodes is to be expected.

Arteriosclerosis after Uveitis

Arteriosclerosis may develop as early as 3 weeks after the onset of uveitis. It is most common with posterior uveal involvement and varies in severity with the severity of the uveal inflammation. In acute toxoplasmic retinochoroiditis scattered segmental focal lesions, clinically similar to severe arteriosclerosis, may develop on posterior retinal arteries in all quadrants irrespective of the site of inflammation. They appear first as bright spots on arteries, increase to form discrete lesions, may develop a crystalline glint, and then absorb and disappear as the inflammation subsides. Severer degrees of uveitis may cause extensive continuous sheathing of long segments of the arteries. Because of the severe vitreous clouding and the irreversibility of the uveitis in those cases observed personally, the ultimate course of these arterial lesions is unknown.

The segmental focal lesions, seen most commonly in our experience in toxoplasmosis, have been discussed rarely in the literature. As such, the arterial disease has been called periarteritis nodosa tuberculosa, retinal periarteritis, retinal arteriolitis, discontinuous reversible arteriopathy, and segmental retinal periarteritis.[153] As these names imply, many have ascribed to them an inflammatory nature. They have been confused with the focal perivenous cuffing (periphlebitis) commonly seen in this disorder. As no microscopic study is available, their true pathology must remain conjectural. However, clinical scrutiny suggests strongly their identification with arteriosclerosis because of their spotty position, yellow color, occasional crystalline glint, predilection for the bends and bifurcations of larger arteries, outer wall position without lumen interference, and indiscriminate distribution, irrespective of the site of chorioretinal inflammation (Fig. 10-54).

Arteriosclerosis in Angiomatosis Retinae and Leber's Multiple Miliary Aneurysms with Retinal Degeneration

In angiomatosis retinae the same clinical change as described above may be seen in arteries in the vicinity of the angioma. Comparable arteriosclerotic lesions may be seen in areas of marked vascular malformations, or in the circinate lesion of Leber's multiple miliary aneurysms with retinal degeneration (Fig. 10-55). Here they often persist after the exudates are gone and may remain for years in areas of beaded hyalinized arteries, beaded veins, dilated abnormal capillaries, and bulbous hyalinizing arterial aneurysms so characteristic of this disease.

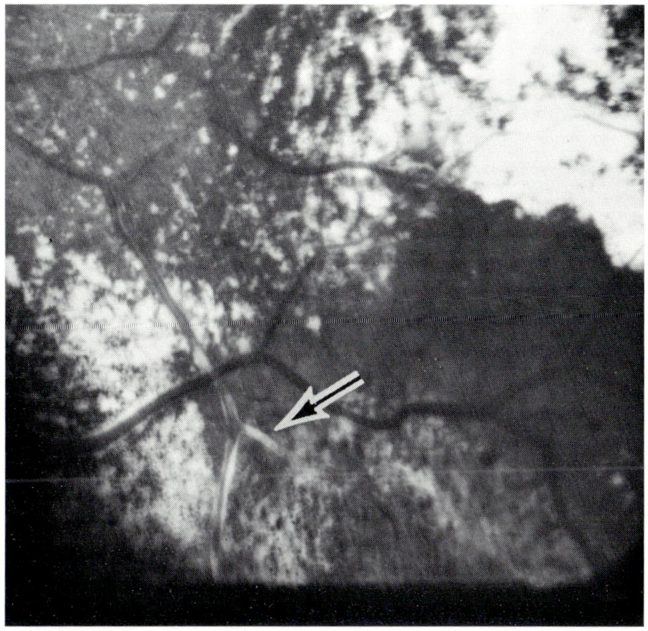

Fig. 10-55. Severe arteriosclerosis **(arrow)** in an area of vascular malformation in Leber's multiple miliary aneurysms with retinal degeneration.

Pigmentary Degeneration

In the later stages of some pigmentary degenerations, especially retinitis pigmentosa, the retinal arterial blood columns become diffusely and uniformly narrowed and pale, with white, smooth, opaque stripes on either side. This change is most obvious posteriorly in the larger vessels (Fig. 10-56) but extends well out into the retina. The striping is never wider than the arterial wall and the course of the vessels remains unaltered. The change in the arterial wall exerts no effect on retinal veins at points of crossing, and in this way differs from arteriosclerosis. When arterial narrowing is extreme, the vessels are seen with great difficulty in the far periphery. Retinal veins are usually quite normal but may sometimes appear minimally narrowed.

Microscopic study of these retinal arteries has demonstrated narrowed lumens, normal endothelium, and hyaline change in the remaining wall layers.[20,101]

Noell[113] suggested that the disappearance of outer retinal layers late in retinitis pigmentosa and the resulting approximation of retinal vessels to the choroid due to retinal thinning, could expose the retinal vessels to an altered tissue oxygen tension. This, over a prolonged period, might account for the arterial narrowing. Gerstein and Dantzker,[26,46] working with Noell, have studied hereditary visual cell degeneration in the rat, and high-intensity light and iodoacetate visual cell destruction, using both rats and cats. Histologic sections and

Fig. 10-56. Hyaline change in the arterial wall **(arrow)** of a narrowed retinal artery late in retinitis pigmentosa.

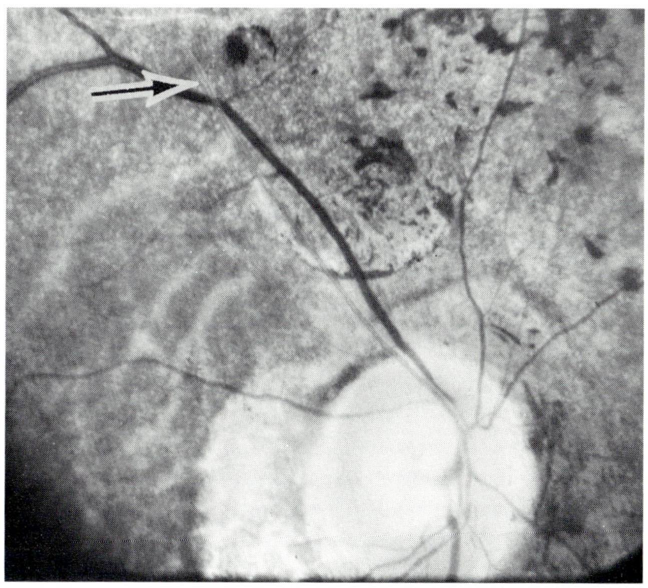

the retinal digest technique were used. Degeneration and closure of retinal capillaries was clearly demonstrated, and was equated by the authors to the visual cell loss and not to the state of the pigment epithelium or the inner nuclear layer. They concluded that the decreased retinal cell population utilizing choriocapillary oxygen and the heightened oxygen tension resulting from the increased proximity of the choroid, had a vasoconstrictive and degenerative effect on retinal capillaries. This work further supported Noell's hypothesis. The fact that iodoacetate-intoxicated cats and rats develop acellular and occluded retinal capillaries has been confirmed.[76]

The arterial narrowing and wall hyalinization of late retinitis pigmentosa are also present in late retinitis punctata albescens and are *not* seen in either choroidremia or gyrate atrophy. Wise [155] has suggested that this might be due to the coincidental choroidal degeneration in the two latter diseases. The choroidal source of increased oxygen, which could affect retinal vessels in the first two diseases, is absent in choroidremia and gyrate atrophy, and therefore unable to supply such an oxygen effect. Retinal arteries therefore retain their normal appearance, even late, in these two diseases.

ARTERIAL AND VENOUS SHEATHING

Lattice Degeneration

This uncommon degeneration usually starts in the upper retinal periphery especially temporally.[140] In its earlier stage, only a local spot of ragged, moth-eaten pigment proliferation in an area of edematous, slightly thickened retina in which a few glinting, white, scattered particles may be seen. Such lesions always occur in a particular peripheral zone a short distance from the ora, just anterior to the equator according to Byer.[14] Other discrete lesions may develop in this same zone concentric with the ora. With progression, lesions coalesce and form longer arcs. In extensive cases a broken ring may form around the entire periphery parallel to the ora and even secondary arcs may be seen rarely in a second posterior zone parallel to, and separate from, the first by an interval of normal retina. It is the glinting snowflakes of early lesions which makes diagnosis at this stage possible, for at first no vessel change may be seen. Later the lesion appears punched-out and uniform, and white sheathing—identical on arteries and veins—or fine white branching cords may be seen in the center. Pigment fades centrally exposing fully the white vascular network responsible for the designation, "lattice degeneration." Artery and vein are so similar that they may be differentiated only by tracing each to an identifying patent vessel beyond the lesion. Microscopically,[114,140] hyalinized obliterated retinal ghost vessels sometimes having pigment about them have been found responsible for the lattice appearance. The inner retinal layers are absent and the vitreous is degenerated over the area. No explanation for the pathogenesis of this disease, nor the usual position of its occurrence is available.

Retinoschisis

Attention has been called already to the clinically identical sheathing of the small peripheral arteries and veins in retinoschisis when vascular changes are severe. Both vessels appear as thin white cords without visible blood columns in the peripheral retina [15,139] (see section on Venous Sheathing in Retinoschisis).

OTHER VASCULAR FEATURES

CALIBER IRREGULARITIES

As there is no sympathetic vasomotor innervation of the retinal vessels, changes in their caliber must be due either to local regulatory responses of the vascular smooth muscle, or possibly to circulating vasoactive substances. In healthy vessels a uniform response would be expected, but in disease, a spotty distribution of wall pathology could cause an irregular response. Such local factors might potentiate the constrictor effects of other stimuli, or if smooth muscle has been replaced by collagen, could prevent constriction.

Since the walls of retinal veins contain little if any smooth muscle it is difficult to explain the pathogenesis of venous irregularity. Presumably structural changes take place in a patchy fashion and lead to a beaded or irregular appearance. The possible, but unproved contractile properties of the intramural pericyte is not considered relevant to this discussion.

"Vascular beading" is a term used to describe vessel segments showing a roughly uniform alternately wide and narrow, vascular caliber. As all beading demonstrates abnormally narrowed segments, it may be produced by segmental narrowing alone, or by alternately narrowed and dilated components. Such arterial beading may be seen on the larger arteries of older patients who develop moderately severe hypertension.

Comparable though exaggerated arterial beading is seen on the arteries in the vicinity of retinal angioma, especially on the large feeding artery near the tumor. Similar beading may be seen on smaller arteries in areas of active Leber's disease (multiple miliary aneurysms with retinal degeneration). This is often exaggerated by a string of microaneurysms, some of which may demonstrate various stages of hyalinization. Similar arterial beading near vascular malformations in Coats's disease is a common occurrence. In peripheral angioma the feeding artery may show very fine and, hence, easily overlooked beading at the disc. It then assumes a more normal contour until it approaches the tumor where beading again appears in an exaggerated and readily apparent fashion.

Venous beading can be a feature of any venous obstructive disease. It is variable in occurrence, being a prominent feature in some cases and absent in others. Local venous dilatations alternate with venous constrictions creating a smoothly contoured beaded column. Often such blood columns are darker than normal. While seen most commonly on larger veins, beading may be readily apparent on small peripheral venules. It is seen characteristically in diabetes (Fig. 10-57), but occurs commonly in vein obstructions, Eales's disease and sickle-cell retinopathy. Less commonly, true venous beading may be seen in the hyperviscosity syndrome of the leukemias and dysproteinemias. Here it is usually milder and is greatly overshadowed by the sausage

Fig. 10-57. Venous beading in diabetic retinopathy.

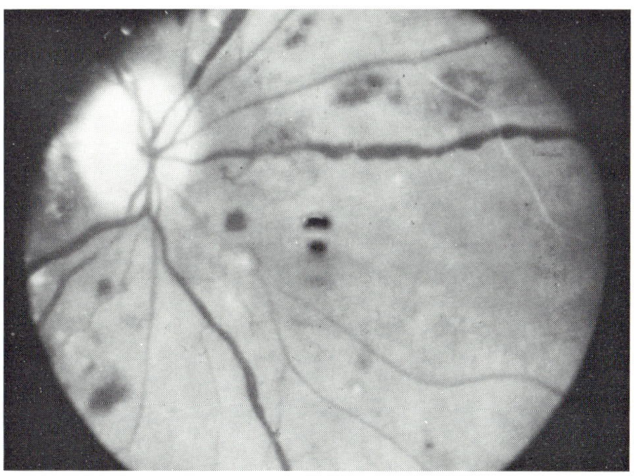

appearance created as resistant, burnished arteries crease greatly dilated, dark veins at crossings. This latter phenomenon, which is not a true beading may be seen in any condition which sufficiently dilates veins.

In the vascular malformations of Coats's disease, retinal angioma, and Leber's multiple miliary aneurysms with retinal degeneration, venous beading occurs with, and may be more prominent than, arterial beading. Both tend to occur in the same general regions.

TORTUOSITY

Normal retinal arteries and veins spread out from the disc in a gently undulating pattern. The pattern variability and undulation are usually more prominent in veins. The degree of vascular tortuosity shows so much normal variation that, taken alone it is an unreliable diagnostic criterion. Extreme degrees of tortuosity in all quadrants, with no other discernible defect is spoken of as congenital tortuosity and as such is of no significance. Congenital tortuosity is more apt to involve arteries than veins.

Tortuosity of retinal vessels in one sector, or the development of tortuosity in vessels known to have been normal previously, is of definite pathologic significance. Increasing tortuosity of vessels is almost invariably accompanied by vessel dilatation and, in the case of veins, by darkening of the blood column.

Isolated abnormal arterial tortuosity is seen more rarely but occurs in some patients with coarctation of the aorta. In older persons with nonmalignant hypertension of sufficient duration and degree, larger retinal arteries will often show an increased gentle sinusoidal tortuosity. This is best seen in temporal arteries where the vascular walls are pale and burnished due to their increased collagen. This same arterial appearance will at times be seen in the absence of hypertension.

Increased tortuosity of arteries and veins is more common. Both vessels become dilated and tortuous early in retrolental fibroplasia, and are dilated, dark, and tortuous in children with congenital heart disease. Arteries and veins are tortuous in areas of Leber's and Coats's diseases and both vessels are greatly dilated and snakelike when taking part in a racemose angioma. A draining vein becomes dilated and tortuous followed by a similar change in the feeding artery of a retinal angioma. When a paired artery and vein are more dilated and tortuous than other retinal vessels, a peripheral retinal angioma somewhere in their bed should be sought.

While exaggerated venous tortuosity often accompanies increased arterial tortuosity, it is commonly seen in its absence. Abnormal venous tortuosity is *always* accompanied by venous dilatation and frequently by darkening of the blood column. As such, it is an indication of venous stasis, impedance of flow or frank obstruction, decreased arterial inflow, retinal hypoxia, or serum hyperviscosity.

Increased vein tortuosity is seen typically, as an isolated phenomenon, peripheral to a pathologic arteriovenous crossing. Proximal to the crossing the vein has a normal color and contour and its width is normal or slightly narrowed; distally, it is dilated, dark, and tortuous (Fig. 10-58). A similar change in all retinal veins may be seen in impending obstruction of the central vein. When temporal arteries become sclerosed and affect small macular draining veins at arteriovenous crossings, these veins become very tortuous, dilated, and sometimes darkened on the foveal side of the crossings. Venous darkening, dilatation, and tortuosity seem to be roughly proportional to the acuteness and degree of vein obstruction. In frank vein obstructions from whatever cause these changes can be extreme.

In milder form this venous phenomenon occurs also in diseases of decreased arterial inflow such as pulseless disease or carotid

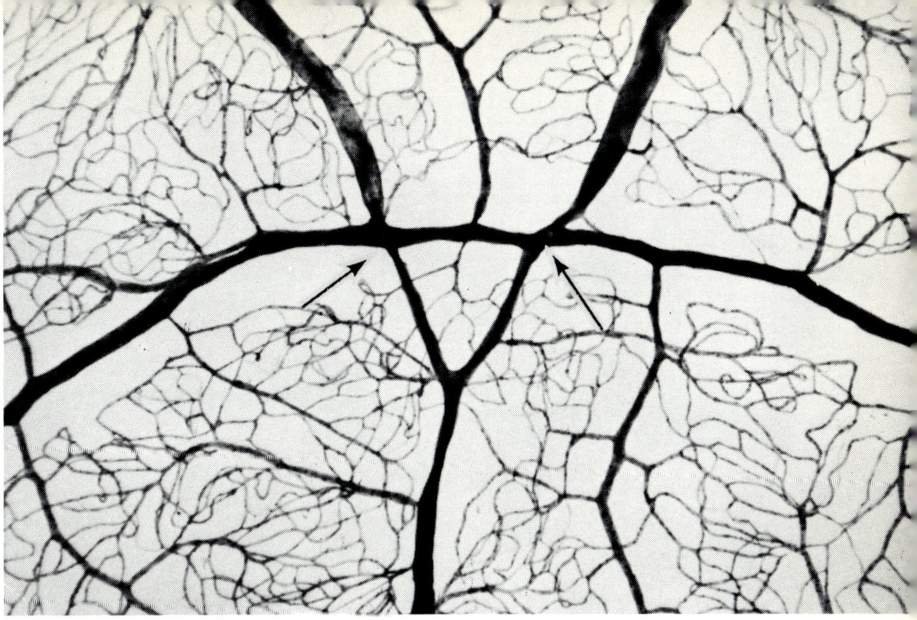

Fig. 10-58. Retinal-digest preparation of branch vein obstruction showing the dilated veins distal to the arteriovenous crossing **(arrows).** PAS, ×50.

artery occlusion. The sudden and marked venous engorgement and tortuosity photographed by Ashby et al.,[2] following a transient embolization of the central retinal artery suggests retinal hypoxia as a factor in its etiology.

This same venous alteration is common in the hyperviscosity syndrome where it may be seen in the retinopathies of the polycythemias, leukemias, and dysproteinemias. In the latter, when blood viscosity levels are markedly elevated, venous changes may reach extreme degrees.

In branch retinal vein obstructions, unobstructed collateral veins often become dilated, dark, and tortuous undoubtedly related to the increased load they are forced to carry. Unless this response is kept in mind, these abnormal veins can be construed as being located behind the venous block and the site of blockage will be misdiagnosed. If the collateral vein is small and carrying a heavy load from a larger obstructed vein, there may even be capillary leakage with edema and hemorrhages in the collateral venous bed. This leakage clears usually within several weeks but may at first be diagnostically confusing.

It is probable that venous dilatation and tortuosity are due to the stretching effect of increased luminal content and increased intraluminal venous pressure. A lengthened vein would have to become tortuous to be accommodated in its restricted retinal environment.

ARTERIOVENOUS SHUNTS

The multiple arteriovenous shunts of a racemose angioma, those in Leber's disease and angiomatosis retinae, those suspected in Coats's disease, the ultimate effects of such shunts, and their possible relation to vascular malformations are discussed in Chapter 11, under the section on Anomalous Vascular Formations.

For a discussion of de novo shunt formation in diabetes see Chapter 15 (under the section on Capillary Closure).

In pulseless disease arteriovenous shunts are seen first in the peripheral retina. As the disease progresses, new shunts form more posteriorly until finally arteriovenous loops form a rosary around the disc.[116] Both arteries and veins progressively collapse peripherally to the shunts as the latter advance toward the disc. As arterial intraluminal pressure decreases, it is insufficient to fill peripheral vascular channels. Short circuits back to the disc develop progressively through the capillary bed as the intra-arterial pressure and volume steadily decrease.

Ashton[5] has noted the similarity of this

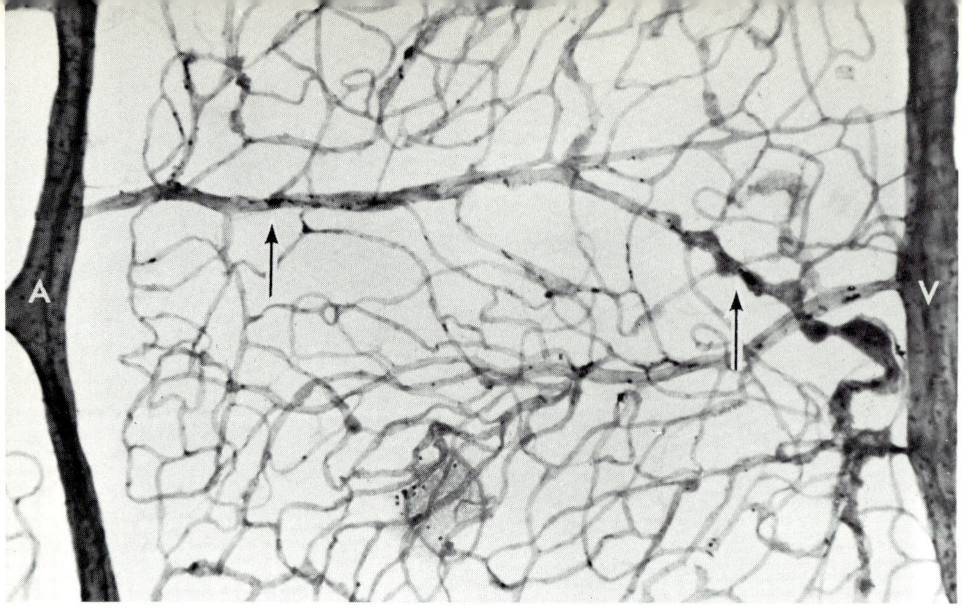

Fig. 10-59. Retinal-digest preparation of chronic glaucoma showing an irregular arteriovenous shunt **(arrows)** through the capillary bed. **(A)** artery; **(B)** vein. PAS, ×50.

arteriovenous rosary around the disc to the late stage of retinal vasoobliteration in experimental retrolental fibroplasia.

Although not seen clinically, arteriovenous shunts are commonly present in retinal digest preparations of patients having chronic glaucoma (Fig. 10-59). The impedance to retinal vascular filling of a chronically elevated intraocular pressure is an undoubted factor in their formation.

COLLATERALS

Arterial Collaterals

The development of collaterals following experimental obstruction of a precapillary arteriole is discussed elsewhere (see Chapter 17, under section on Arterial Occlusion). Passage of blood through patent capillaries, around the block to the distant arterial segment beyond the obstruction, and reversal of flow discward along this arterial segment into the ischemic area begins immediately after arterial obstruction. Dilating capillary collateral channels take on more and more flow and their walls assume an arterial structure.[62] This proceeds until one or more collateral arteries are sufficiently developed to supply the ischemic area. In obstruction of large arteries, diffusion at the edge of the blocked bed may sustain peripheral cells, but collateral flow develops too slowly to sustain cellular life in the remainder of the obstructed area and infarction with permanent field defect ensues. It seems likely under these circumstances that collateral flow develops entirely as a result of altered pressure gradients within the blocked artery and its regional capillary bed.

Collateral formation after experimental retinal vein or artery obstruction is always a vein-to-vein or artery-to-artery anastomoses although arteriovenous communications are found in areas of capillary closure following vein obstruction. Digested preparations of diabetic retinae commonly show arteriovenous shunts in areas of capillary closure.[21,93] These are more frequent in advanced retinopathies and involve vessels little larger than capillaries which may explain why they are not visible clinically.

While there have been several reports of arterial collateral formation after blockage of larger retinal arteries in man (Fig. 10-60),[9,33,73] only one has been observed during the course of development.[150] The latter developed about a site partly obstructed twice by aseptic thrombi in a case of rheumatic heart disease. The collateral became clinically apparent several months after the

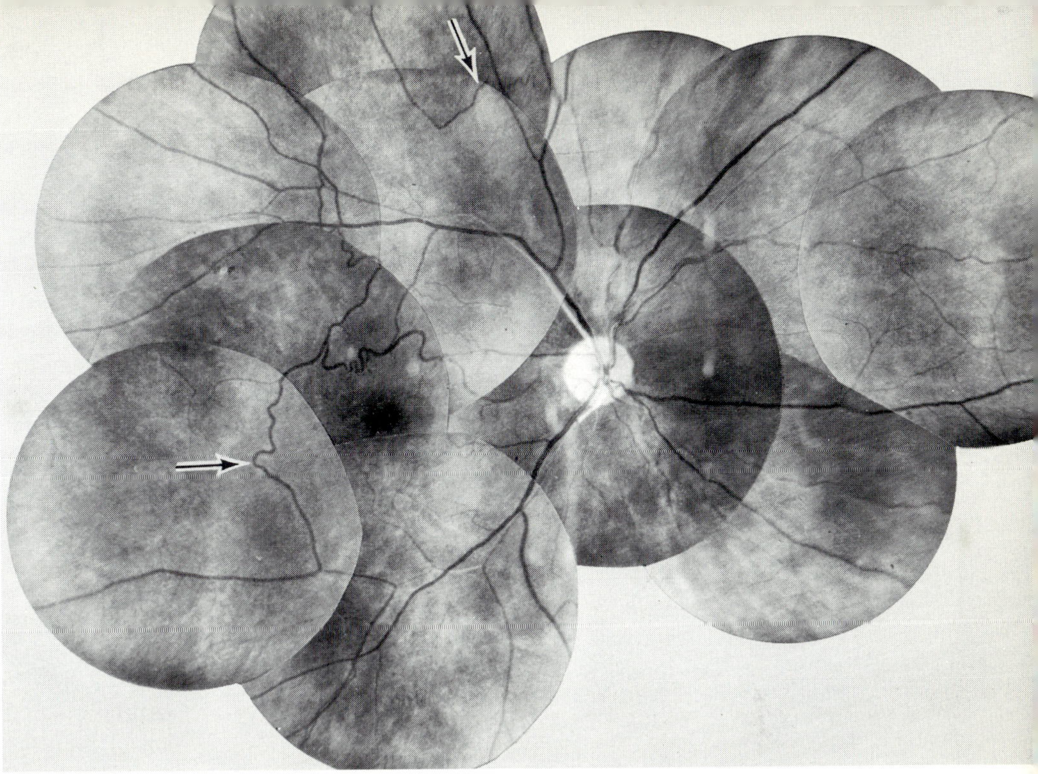

Fig. 10-60. Arterial collaterals **(arrows)** in a young man with severe hypertension. (From Ball and Henkind. *Brit. J. Ophthal. 51:* 688, 1967. By permission of the Editor and Publisher.)

second embolic episode, and developed into a loop about the first bifurcation of the inferior temporal artery, two disc diameters from the disc. Its lumen approached that of the original artery in size. Field examination showed two small relative scotomas just above fixation, indicating insignificant cell death in the obstructed sector.

Venous Collaterals

Following vein obstruction there is irregular fluorescein leakage through obstructed vein and capillary walls distal to the obstruction, but the cells of the vein wall remain viable. Patches of obliterated capillaries in obstructed venous beds have been produced experimentally[92] and patches of obliterated capillaries have been reported after vein obstruction.[99,125,151] These obliterated capillary patches occur in the territory of the blocked vein but in no way impede the formation of venous collaterals.

Collateral formation after vein obstruction from whatever cause is an extremely common occurrence (Fig. 10-61). Again, it is likely that hemodynamic factors determine largely the direction of diverted blood flow through patent capillaries to the same vein proximal to the obstruction, or to adjacent patent venules. Blood under increased pressure peripheral to the obstruction leaves the vein and enters the adjacent capillary bed of lower intraluminal pressure. Overfilling of these capillaries raises their internal pressure and in this manner the blood flow, ever moving in the direction of decreasing intraluminal pressure eventually reaches nearby unobstructed veins via the deep capillary bed. Preferential channels develop next, and, as their lumens enlarge to carry more blood, so do their walls take on more venous characteristics. This sequence has been demonstrated experimentally (see Chapter 17, under section on Collaterals). Once collateral channels are sufficiently large, they become visible clinically. From this point on their development can be traced in the human fundus. Slowly over months or even several years, some channels become obliterated and dis-

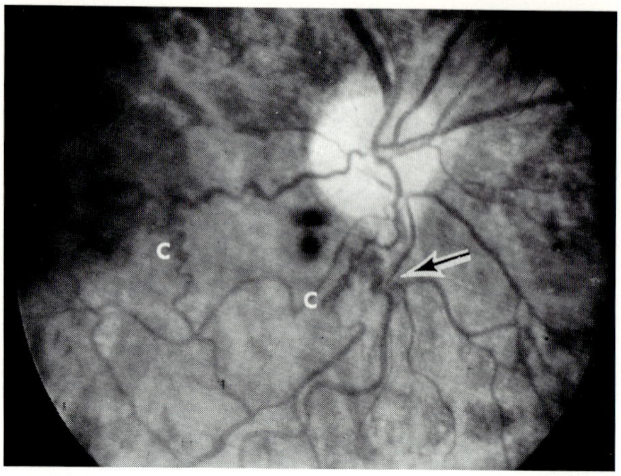

Fig. 10-61. Venous collateral formation **(c)** after vein obstruction at an arteriovenous crossing **(arrow).**

appear from view while others enlarge progressively. The number of residual channels varies, but commonly a single well-developed collateral of the approximate size of the original vein is all that is left. Except for its course, it may then have the clinical appearance of a normal vein. There is tremendous variability in the later stages of this process. The original vein obstruction may clear with restoration of lumen patency and all collaterals may disappear. This is particularly likely in Eales's disease. Often an obstructed vein will partially regain its patency and carry some of the flow, while most of the stream continues through a large collateral. In such cases the original vein segments have narrowed lumens and are halo sheathed (increased adventitial collagen). This sequence has been observed clinically and microscopically in toxoplasmic retinochoroiditis.[79]

Commonly a vein segment will become an obliterated white cord (ghost vein), or, rarely, even disappear between the point of obstruction and the next more peripheral and proximal bifurcations. In some cases peripheral flow may be regained normally down one venous branch, turn at the now sharply but smoothly curved bifurcation, flow in a reversed direction peripherally through the other branch, and eventually pass through peripheral collaterals to an adjacent patent vein and back to the disc. This phenomenon is easily overlooked unless the entire regional vascular pattern is studied. Collaterals such as these may be seen after branch vein obstructions, or in chorioretinitis.[153] On one occasion after branch vein obstruction, a segment of an arteriosclerotic artery was used as a vein in establishing collateral circulation.[152,152a] This segment carrying venous blood toward the disc had the clinical appearance of a normal vein.[152,152a] Such accommodations may be of more frequent occurrence than this single observation would suggest. Bizarre doubling of channels, and constantly changing patterns of apparent venous collateral formations are not unusual in diabetic retinopathy and Eales's disease.

Venous collateral channels either remain patent, or collapse and disappear. Except very rarely at the disc, they have not been observed to become halo sheathed, nor do they, when they disappear, leave any clinical evidence of their former position. At most, a vague, irregular fibrosis, without vascular configuration may remain.

In central retinal vein obstruction, where the obstructed site is at the lamina cribrosa and not clinically visible, collaterals form within the disc substance between the choroidal circulation and the original vein, close to, but peripheral to the obstruction site. Less commonly they occur on the disc surface and rarely loop forward from the latter. Here they are readily visible. Generally speaking, adequate collateral circulation develops quicker and better at the disc than peripherally. Rudimentary collaterals between the retinal and choroidal circulation at the disc have been considered responsible for this difference.

Since many patients are seen initially long after central retinal vein obstructions and give an inadequate history, it is essential that disc collaterals, the sine qua non of prior central vein obstruction, be recognized. Some patients never develop the full picture of acute central vein obstruction, particularly those having smouldering, long-standing uveitis or chronic glaucoma. Such patients may develop easily overlooked, "silent," central retinal vein obstructions while under regular observation for their primary disease. "Silent" is used to denote those obstructions which probably develop slowly and at no time show the apoplectic retinopathy characteristic of the more acute obstructions. In these latter cases, observation of disc collateral formation is the best and only certain way of making a diagnosis.

Collaterals may occur in all disc quadrants, on one side of the disc, or be limited to a single quadrant. They pass from the central vein, or from one or more of its branches near the physiologic cup across the disc, and dip in at its border to join the choroidal circulation. When deeper in the disc substance they may be seen best by intense retroillumination as a vague, red, wormy configuration in a disc sector (Fig. 10-62). When deeper still, their outline may be invisible, but their presence may be suspected by an otherwise unexplained intense redness of some portion of the disc. Minimal residual retinal signs of old, central vein obstruction may be helpful in reaching a proper diagnosis. Slight halo sheathing of retinal veins, arteriosclerotic arteries, a few deep retinal hemorrhages, pigment stippling at the macula, deep retinal edema, and microaneurysms about the macula are common residual retinal signs.

Retinal venous collaterals show great variability in their rapidity and profuseness of development. In diseases affecting the young, such as juvenile diabetes, Eales's disease, sickle cell disease, or chorioretinitis, such collaterals may form quickly and in many cases plentifully. In older patients with vein obstructions, as in those occurring

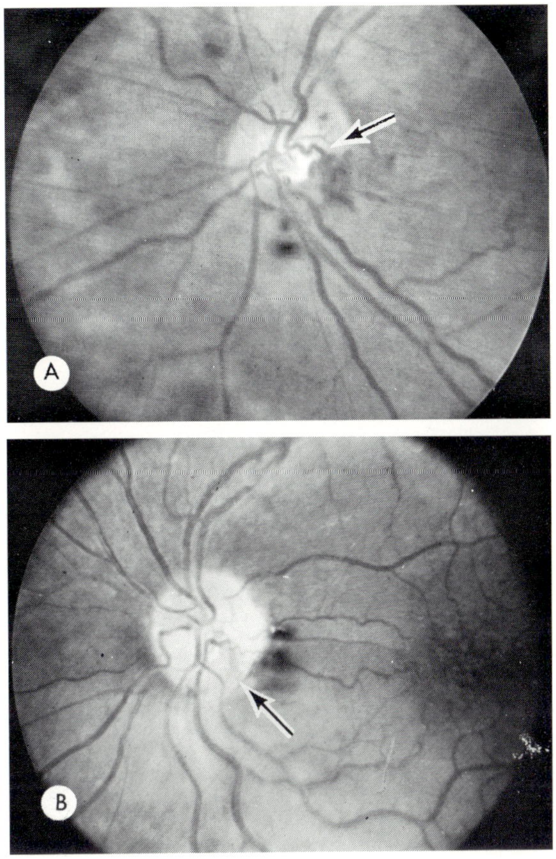

Fig. 10-62. *A*, Superficial venous collaterals on the disc **(arrow)** following vein obstruction. *B*, Deep venous collaterals within the disc substance **(arrow)** following vein obstruction.

in hypertensive retinopathy and nonhypertensive branch or central vein obstructions, venous collaterals often form sparsely and more slowly. Here no clinically visible sign of them may be seen for 2 to 6 months. In fact, if the obstructed vein drains the macular area, they may not develop well enough or quickly enough to save the macula from permanent damage. In these cases, so long as there is no macular pigment change, fibrosis, or cyst rupture, the macular pathology is reversible and visual improvement can be anticipated. The development of any of these changes heralds permanent macular visual loss.

Collateral veins may arise anywhere along the vein peripherally to the obstruction. Channels which do not form closely about the site of obstruction are often multiple and may be scattered. Collaterals are sometimes found in the far periphery running from a branch of the obstructed vein, roughly paralleling the ora, to a branch of an adjacent unobstructed vein. These develop quite commonly in experimental vein obstructions in the cat, even when the obstruction site is just off the disc.

Retinochoroidal anastomoses as a part of collateral circulation may uncommonly be seen anywhere in the fundus (Fig. 10-44). Arterial connections of this type are indeed a rarity[87] but we have observed venous types in hypertension, chorioretinitis, Coats's disease, and near the macula in disciform macular degeneration.

ALTERATIONS IN THE BLOOD COLUMN

Color Changes

Oxygen saturation and hemoglobin concentrations are the major determinants of blood column color. With humans in an oxygen environment, the retinal vascular tree narrows and venous blood columns become redder. With hypoxia, both vessels dilate and darken, with veins showing more change than arteries. A halted blood column, whether arterial or venous, becomes intensely dark almost losing its red value and often appears fragmented.

In diabetic and some other types of hyperlipemia, serum lipid concentrations increase and the serum becomes milky. This phenomenon may reach sufficient proportions to impart a yellowish, or even white color to the blood (Fig. 10-63). It is the increase of neutral triglycerides rather than the level of total serum lipids that produces the larger emulsified fat particles responsible for this lactescence.[35] Clinically the yellowish white color appears in peripheral vessels first and then extends in both arteries and veins toward the disc. In severer cases a similar yellowish white fundus discoloration may appear, due to involvement of the choroidal circulation. At its height, blood columns may appear broadened and have fuzzy irregular borders. Fat particles in the plasma zone around the red cell column are responsible for this appearance.

As the disorder is controlled, the fundus reflex returns toward the normal red color and vessels begin to clear. As clearing proceeds, a central core of red blood with lactescent margins may be seen within the vascular lumen. Lactescence at its height has no effect on vision.

Blood Sludging

If the movement of red blood cells within a vascular lumen is slowed sufficiently, red cell aggregates will form and may be clinically visible. The separation of clumps of cells by clearer serum enhances their visibility. This occurrence is known as "blood sludging" (Fig. 10-64). It is also spoken of as "cattle truck" or "box car" phenomenon. When arterial inflow is reduced, blood sludging appears first in venous channels but may be seen in arteries as well. Sometimes when not present, it may be elicited by slight pressure on the globe.

In venous obstructive diseases it is a later manifestation and may sometimes be seen as collaterals begin to develop, or as channels begin to reopen.

In severe, diabetic retinitis proliferans, it is seen commonly toward the terminal new vessel loops and is apparent less often in the large dilated venous channels from which the new vessels arise.

Blood sludging is infrequent in hyperviscosity diseases.

Its presence in the veins and then in arteries, followed shortly by complete stoppage of flow, is a sign of cessation of circulation in cardiac arrest. Subsequently, pallor of the disc as capillaries are drained and a hazy pallor of the retina develop. Timely resumption of circulation in temporary cardiac arrest reverses the appearance of the fundus to normal. For more comprehensive consideration of blood sludging see Knisely.[91]

Chalk-White Vessels

Goodman, von Sallman, and Holland[51] described chalk-white vessels in the peripheral retina of two patients with sickle cell retinopathy. One had hemoglobin C disease and the other was thought to have hemoglobin D disease. Some peripheral arteries and veins were noted to become chalk-white within several days. Clusters of red blood cells appeared as pink breaks in these chalk-white lines. Within a week the intervening capillary-like channels were converted into a white lattice work. Three months later the white material was greatly reduced, the vessels were attenuated and hardly visible except where ensheathed by pale, gray envelopes. Newly formed vessels were present in the area. The authors believed that the granular white appearance was due to sickling, hemolysis of the sickled cells, and fragmentation of the decolored, red blood cell membranes in these areas of vascular stasis.

RETINAL EMBOLI

Many extraneous materials have been reported as retinal emboli. Among these, cholesterol crystals, cholesterol esters, fat and

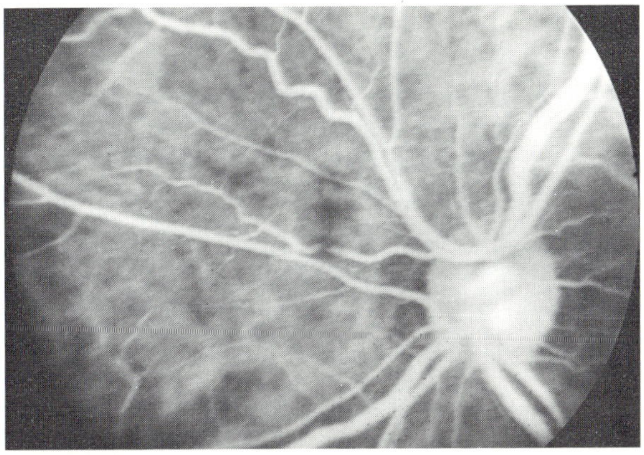

Fig. 10-63. Lipemia retinalis. Note fuzzy borders of the retinal vessels and lipemic serum in choroidal vessels.

Fig. 10-64. Obstruction of the central retinal artery with interrupted venous and arterial blood columns.

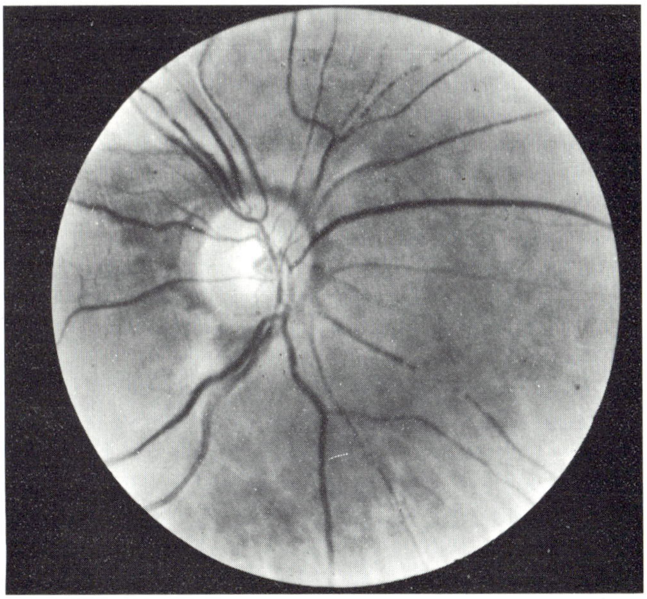

amorphous material from arteriosclerotic plaques in the great arteries to the head are most common (Fig. 10-53*A*).[8,22,27,63,65,66] Other materials include particles of septic vegetations in bacterial endocarditis, aseptic mural thrombi in auricular fibrillation, decompensation and myocardial infarction,[167] fat in crush injuries of the chest or long bones,[30,77] broken off pieces of endocardial myxoma,[102] amniotic fluid,[38] mercury,[143] and both inert paraffin used in reconstructive plastic procedures and air bubbles.[34] Embolization of retinal arteries has also followed arteriography.[54,96] In these cases the visual defect is usually less severe, sometimes transient, and as a rule, considerable recovery ensues. It is not known whether atheromatous material is broken off at the time of intraarterial needling, or whether the embolism is more directly related to the contrast medium injected.[54] Evidence suggests that platelet aggregates and calcific emboli may represent a more frequent type of embolism than thought previously.

Emboli, probably composed of cholesterol crystals, are seen more frequently in arteriosclerosis of the carotid arteries. Here they occur commonly in showers during carotid artery manipulation, in angiography, and arterial surgery. The vast majority are transient and while they often rest temporarily at arterial bifurcations, they usually fail to produce sufficient obstruction to cause retinal infarction. Clinically they appear as highly refractile, glinting spots always within the dimensions of the blood column. At times the reflection is so brilliant or so broad that it makes the embolus appear to extend beyond the width of the blood column. However, this is seen only to one side of the blood column and by altering the direction of observation and thereby reducing the reflex, its true position within the vascular lumen may be determined. Such emboli are lightly attached to the endothelium and spontaneously, or by lightly tapping the globe may be freed. They then dart rapidly down an artery, only to lodge at a smaller bifurcation, or to disappear. That such emboli may occlude two-thirds of the arterial lumen without infarction has been demonstrated in Ball's clinicomicroscopic study.[8] At times such glinting spots may be seen in areas that do not contain visible vessels. Here they probably lie in capillary or precapillary channels. While these have been placed by some in the choroidal circulation,[66] the wider vascular lumens of the latter and the hiding effect of the pigment epithelium makes the clinical visualization of choroidal cholesterol emboli unlikely.

Emboli obstructing the arterial lumen sufficiently to produce infarction, present the same clinical appearance. These fuzzy white spots extend beyond the width of the blood column due to stretching of the wall over the emboli. It could well be that opacification of the arterial wall over the embolus[149] accounts for this similarity of clinical appearance and in part for the extension of the opacity beyond the blood column width.

Purtscher's traumatic retinal angiopathy has been considered to result from the escape of bone marrow fat into the circulation following severe bone injuries. Embolization is usually found in other tissues as well as the retina. It is at times so extensive as to suggest some other mechanism of development. Rather than bone marrow embolization, it has been proposed[7] that a physiochemical change in the size of chylomicrons, initiated in some way by the trauma, produces macromolecules large enough to block small vessels. In either case the clinical picture is one of scattered, multiple cotton-wool patches, superficial retinal edema, and occasional flame-shaped hemorrhages.

PLATELET EMBOLI

Some patients, especially those with a severe stenosis of an internal carotid artery, experience recurrent, episodic, transient, monocular blindness. Examination of the retinal vessels during such an attack may show the arterial branches plugged by a long length of dull, white embolic material, sometimes interspersed with segments containing blood. This material has been observed to pass through the retinal vessels and disappear during periods ranging from a few minutes to hours. If the material passes through within a few minutes, as it usually does, vision returns immediately and is unimpaired.[105,126,127]

Because of the transient nature of the attacks, it was necessary in one of our cases, to keep the patient's pupils dilated and a nurse in constant attendance in order to summon the resident immediately when an attack began. In this way the diagnosis was proved and photographs were obtained. It seems reasonable to speculate that many transient attacks of monocular blindness may have the same cause.

Though the composition of these emboli has not been proved, circumstantial evidence suggests that they are aggregated masses of platelets. Platelets are the only blood constituent known to be capable of forming such malleable white bodies which can readily break up and disperse. Artificially clumped platelets injected into the carotid artery of pigs produce a very similar transient obstruction of the retinal vascular bed by whitish plugs (see Chapter 17, in section on Reversible Arterial Obstruction with Platelets or Fibrin).

Ross Russell has suggested that platelet emboli may be responsible for many transient neurological disturbances in patients with internal carotid artery disease. He reported a patient who had had recurrent attacks of monocular blindness with carotid artery stenosis. Surgical exploration revealed a long, white, friable mass attached to the stenosed section of the artery. Histologically this was made up of platelets.[126]

CALCIFIC EMBOLI

Surgical procedures, particularly closed aortic valvotomy performed to correct calcific aortic stenosis, may release small pieces of calcified material into the carotid circulation. These can embolize the retinal vessels. They appear as small, irregular, white or yellow white chunks lodged in a retinal artery branch. They do not scintillate and usually obstruct the flow through the vessels in which they lie. Collaterals may develop around them in time, but not soon enough to prevent necrosis of the tissue downstream.[64,68,69,117]

ARTERIOVENOUS CROSSING CHANGES

At a normal retinal arteriovenous crossing there is no deflection nor change in caliber of either blood column. Both vessel walls are invisible at the crossing and one may see only occasionally the slightest detour in the venous column above or below the artery. When the vein lies beneath the artery as it does at most crossings, the darker venous blood column may be visualized as undeviated through the arterial blood. The earliest abnormality of the arterial wall decreases its mural lucency and hides the venous blood column from view. This phenomenon of hiding of the vein by the artery was described by Gunn[55] and is still recognized as the first clinical sign of arterial wall pathology. The visibility of the venous blood column through the arterial wall may persist into very late life in some individuals.

Anatomically, at visible vessel crossings and at the lamina cribrosa both artery and vein have a common outer wall coat. Disease of the arterial wall therefore exerts its influence on the vein at crossings, and at the lamina cribrosa where portions of these wall sheaths are held in common. Clinically, crossing changes are visible most readily at major vessel crossings and where temporal arterial branches cross fine macular veins. Similar changes, however, may occur at any retinal arteriovenous crossing, be the artery above or below the vein, and even at points where the vessels lie in close proximity and do not actually cross (Fig. 10-65). Mild medullation of nerve fibers, congenital gliosis on and near the disc, and the bends in vessels as they loop up toward the retinal surface from the nasal side of the physiologic cup and dip often deeply into the retina before assuming a final, more uniform level in the nerve fiber layer, all make arteriovenous crossing defects at, or adjacent to the disc very difficult to evaluate. A marked, normal tapering of veins as they enter the disc substance adds further difficulty to such judgments. One must therefore use great caution in diagnosing pathology at the lamina cribrosa from apparent vascular changes just peripheral to, on, or near the disc.

As arterial walls lose transparency through pathologic change, an increasing effect is exerted on the veins at crossings (Fig. 10-66). Following hiding of the venous blood column by the artery, the venous column is seen to taper on either side of the crossing. Associated with this there may be an apparent depression of the venous column deeper into the retinal substance. As the arterial wall becomes sufficiently dense, it hides the venous column from view on either side of the arterial channel. At this stage the vein tapers and then disappears, leaving a narrow "vacant" zone to either side of the artery. Further opacity of the arterial wall produces a white stripe in this previously vacant zone, which tapers and disappears shortly to either side of the crossing. The latter is undoubtedly due to the doubled wall thickness viewed at the crossing where artery and vein, with their common sheath, overlie one another.

As the effect of the artery upon the vein increases, three other changes may occur: (*1*) deflection or displacement of the vein; (*2*) change in the venous flow or the column itself; and (*3*) retinal changes about the vein just distal to the crossing.

Deflection of the vein increases its crossing angle from the normal acute toward a more perpendicular angulation. Not uncommonly, where the crossing is more nearly perpendicular, the vein appears to be dragged peripherally at the crossing so that the venous bend is directed away from the disc. More rarely, the direction of this bend is discward. If it develops, an increasingly sinusoidal configuration of the larger arteries plays its part in crossing patterns. Finally, deflections may also take a vertical direction where the vein is humped up over the artery, or displaced deeply into the retina beneath it.

The venous flow, both by visual appearance and fluorescein study may be quite normal in the presence of obvious crossing change. The first change in flow as detected by fluorescein is the conversion of a laminated pattern distal to the crossing to solid luminal filling on its disc side—an indication of turbulence at the crossing. Later the vein may be seen to dilate and even darken on the distal side of the crossing—a phenomenon known as "venous banking." At this stage the vein usually shows an increasing peripheral tortuosity as well.

From this stage to clinical obstruction at the crossing site, clues as to the severity of venous impedance must come from changes in the retinal regions drained by the involved vein. These appear earliest in the region around the vein just peripheral to the crossing. One or more small superficial hemorrhages, a white halo about the vein and a pale transudate in the area constitute Bonnet's prethrombosis sign.[13] Such signs are of no value in prophesying when the obstruction will actually occur, for in Bonnet's eight cases, one occurred after a month and an-

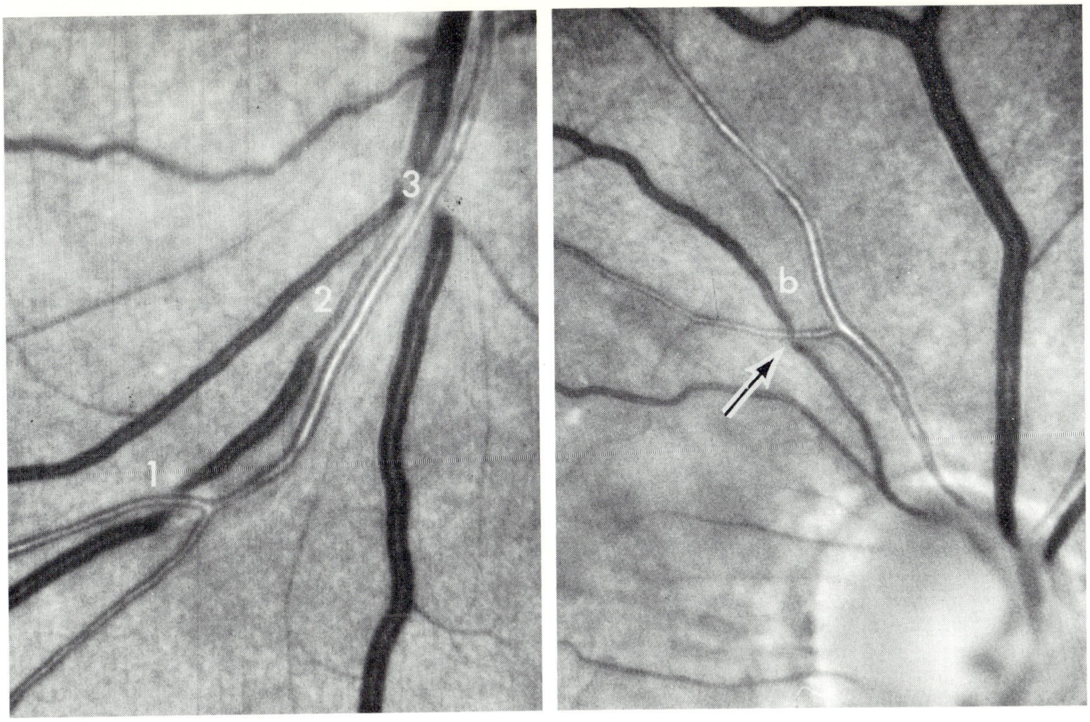

Fig. 10-65. *A*, The effect of arteriosclerosis on the vein at an arteriovenous crossing **(1)** and where the vein lies adjacent to, but does not cross the artery **(2)**; **(3)** designates an unusual trifurcation. *B*, Same eye showing similar effect on an overcrossing vein **(arrow).** Note venous banking **(b).**

Fig. 10-66. Retinal arteriosclerosis illustrating copper-wire arteries. Arteriovenous crossing defect **(arrow).**

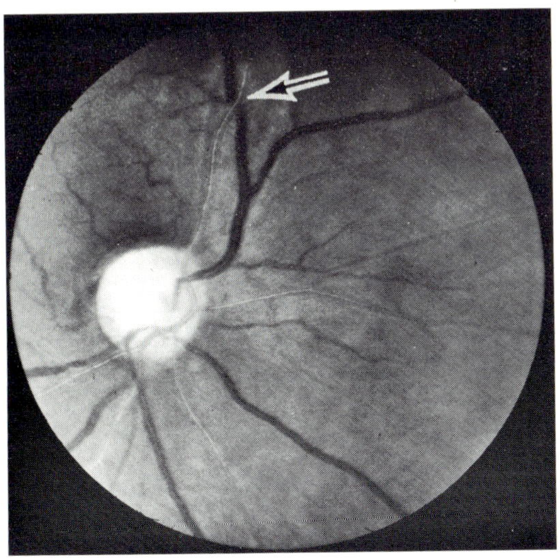

other after 14 years. Our own observations confirm this view. Small blot hemorrhages occurring about venous twigs in the far periphery of the drainage area are easily overlooked. The retina between these and the area of crossing is often clinically uninvolved. As they constitute an early clinical sign of venous failure, their presence is of considerable practical importance. With increasing embarrassment of venous flow, microaneurysms, either attached to small venous twigs, or appearing clinically isolated in the retina just beyond the crossing may be seen. In the same region, dilated, anastomosing, small, vascular channels not previously visible become clinically apparent. In rarer instances these may increase slowly to form collaterals around the crossing in the absence of a retinal picture of frank vein obstruction. Associated with the retinal hemorrhages, transudate, microaneurysms, and capillary dilatation, a small cotton-wool patch may rarely develop. Beyond this stage the typical picture of branch vein obstruction ensues.

All variations of crossing phenomena may be seen in nonhypertensive fundi, usually in older individuals who show large, pale arteries with a broadened light reflex at the center of the blood column, and pale stripes to either side. Such arteries may be relatively straight, or have graceful sinusoidal curves. While the arterial changes themselves are most visible on larger vessels, their effect on small veins at crossings may be quite apparent. Small veins draining the macular areas seem especially vulnerable to crossing defects when traversed by a sclerotic main temporal artery. Proximal to the crossing they remain straight and normal in appearance; distally they become dilated, tortuous, and often darker in color. Such changes, if mild, have no effect on vision but more severe ones impeding venous flow may be deleterious (see Chapter 14, under section on Preretinal Macular Fibrosis).

Crossing defects are seen almost always after uveitis. These can be of variable degree of severity, to and including vein obstruction but are commonly much milder. Even long after the uveitis is quiescent, enough arterial wall pathology remains to hide the vein at crossings. This effect must be taken into consideration for instance, when evaluating early hypertensive retinopathy in the presence of old, healed chorioretinitis.

Crossing defects are responsible for the venous sausage-link phenomenon occurring in hyperviscosity diseases. The early presence of crossing defects in Leber's multiple miliary aneurysms with retinal degeneration and angiomatosis retinae in young individuals may be of diagnostic importance (see Chapter 11, under section on Anomalous Vascular Formations).

Crossing defects are common in such diverse conditions as sickle cell retinopathy, Coats's disease, some cases of preretinal macular fibrosis, and severe collagen retinopathies although other features of the disease are much more prominent. Clinical branch vein obstruction may occur at any stage during the development of crossing pathology. While this is much more common with severe defects, frank obstruction may develop at the point of mild ones. Rare cases progress through a "silent" obstructive phase, developing collaterals without ever presenting the typical clinical picture of vein obstruction. Prognostication of the time of vein obstruction based on clinical appearances of the crossing is therefore hazardous.

CAPILLARY BED CHANGES

In an ophthalmoscopic view of the fundus, normal retinal arteries and veins may be traced to vessels of very small size, but there are extensive intervening retinal areas totally free of clinically visible vasculature. Such regions are seen as readily posteriorly about the disc and macula as they are in the mid- or peripheral retina. In certain disease states fine anastomosing vessels often with small knobs or wall irregularities become visible in such areas. These vessels are dilated capillaries. The retinal position of this capillary dilatation is often of diagnostic importance.

In papillitis or papilledema the dilated capillary bed of the elevated disc is readily visible. It is these dilated capillaries that in part intensify the red color of the disc and leak the edematous serum and fluorescein so characteristic of both conditions. They decrease in size and pass from view as each entity recedes and in disc atrophy, their closure increases the disc pallor.

In impending vein occlusion, dilated capillaries are seen readily in sectors behind the venous blockage. They are not present uniformly throughout this zone but appear in a patchy distribution. With the passage of time microaneurysms increase among them. The appearance of dilated capillaries peripheral to an arteriovenous crossing defect is one reliable sign of embarrassed venous flow at that point. Some time after a central or temporal vein occlusion, usually in an individual under 45 years of age, and in one who has had an excellent recovery, a few microaneurysms and dilated capillaries above or below the fovea may be the only remaining clinical sign of the obstructive episode. Patches of dilated capillaries and microaneurysms may be seen also in old areas of obstructed venous drainage, where most pathology has cleared but mild decompensation persists. Increased prominence of this fine vascularity is seen also in the far periphery between terminal venous tributaries in impending vein occlusion. The latter are common in all quadrants if the central retinal vein is attacked, but are seen only in a single quadrant with embarrassment of a single major branch vein. Such dilated and visible patches of capillaries are common also in sickle cell retinopathy, diabetes, and Eales's disease.

A patch of dilated and clinically visible capillaries may be one of the earliest signs of Leber's multiple miliary aneurysms with retinal degeneration or angiomatosis retinae. While these may occur in any retinal position, they are common in the far periphery especially temporally. At times they become very prominent and have even demonstrated a clinically visible periarterial capillary-free zone as is usually seen only in digested or injected retinal laboratory preparations.[70]

Dilated and visible capillaries in the retinal periphery of all quadrants are an early manifestation of pulseless disease. Aneurysms and small peripheral arteriovenous anastomoses may be associated with these dilated capillaries.

Following obstruction of the central retinal artery or one of its major branches at the disc, total or sector disc atrophy ensues. With this, involved capillary channels become obliterated and fail to carry red blood cells, thereby adding to the disc pallor. Although a similar change occurs in the capillary bed of affected zones throughout the retina, it does not practically affect the color of the fundus reflex which is determined largely by choroidal blood.

TELANGIECTASIA

The word "telangiectasia" has been used indiscriminately in retinal disease to describe bizarre, dilated, anastomosing vascular formations seen in Coats's disease, the vascular alterations of angiomatosis retinae and Leber's disease, collateral formations in venous obstruction, Eales's disease and sickle cell retinopathy, and has also been used erroneously to describe some immediately preretinal neovascular formations. Possibly of some use descriptively, it represents neither an entity nor adds to an understanding of the basic pathophysiology at hand, and for these reasons, should be eliminated.

TOPOGRAPHICAL DISTRIBUTION OF RETINAL PATHOLOGY

The distribution of some retinal lesions such as cotton-wool spots and flame-shaped hemorrhages is primarily determined by anatomic factors such as the position of the radial peripapillary capillary bed and the direction of the nerve fiber distribution. The reason for the topographical localization of other types of lesion that have a predilection for the posterior pole, the macula, or the periphery is not obvious.

MACULAR AND PERIPHERAL RETINAL ALLIANCE

Certain peripheral retinal lesions are not uncommonly associated with pathologic changes at the macula, while other lesions fail to show any relationship between the two. The macular pathology will occasionally so predominate that, unless this kinship be kept in mind, less obvious peripheral disease may be overlooked. Explanation as to why some peripheral lesions are associated with macular pathology and others are not is unknown at present.

The vascular patterns at the fovea and ora serrata are both terminal. Their vessel-free zones are about the same width and both are bordered by direct arteriovenous loops without intervening capillary beds. Any noxious factor which would attack selectively such terminal zones of circulation conceivably could affect both locales.

The functions of the two regions, their cellular constituents, the increased choroidal vascularity beneath the macula and the double-layered capillary network with its finer mesh about the macula all suggest its more active metabolism. Fluorescein evidence is accumulating to show that the retinal circulation time to the macula is short, intimating a high flow to this area, even taking into consideration its short conduit. This lends further support to the concept of a heightened macular metabolic activity. It is therefore conceivable that a peripheral retinal lesion, exerting its influence on the entire retina could produce minimal or subclinical pathology elsewhere, and an exaggerated and clinically obvious response at the macula (see section on Exaggerated Macular Response to Retinal Disease).

While the absence of intervening pathology between associated macular and peripheral lesions makes unlikely any directly extending influence of one upon the other, their link-up via the retinal vascular system makes the latter a possible pathway for such associations. The predominant incidence of the macular and peripheral retinal alliance in retinal vascular tumors, vascular malformations, and venous and capillary obstructive diseases lends support to a vascular intermediary in associated diseases of the two regions.

Present knowledge makes some combination of the latter two factors a most attractive explanation for the simultaneous disease of these two disparate retinal areas. However, some completely unknown mechanism is still a distinct possibility.

Two macular lesions are associated most frequently with peripheral retinal pathology: (*1*) deep retinal edema associated with cystic maculopathy, i.e., microcystic macular edema; and (*2*) a macular mound of fatty exudation (see Chapter 11, under section on Cerebrovascular Anomalies and Retinal Angioma).

Low-grade, nonspecific chorioretinitis (pars planitis) is associated commonly with microcystic maculae. Often the latter is responsible for the initial complaint of reduced vision. Due to the bilaterality of the disease, bilateral macular lesions are common, although unequal in degree. The more involved macula is associated with the more involved peripheral inflammation. A relatively quiet periphery may show no macular activity. During the usual waxing and waning of the peripheral inflammation, microcystic maculae may come and go with full return of vision, disappearance of all microcystic change, and reappearance of a normal foveal reflex. Microcystic maculae similarly have been observed to return to normal appearance and function following the eradication of peripheral activity by light coagulation or freezing. Other peripheral chorioretinitic lesions can behave in this same manner.

Similar microcystic maculae have been reported in cases of peripheral melanoma of the choroid [43] and have been seen personally with peripheral retinal holes. Upper peripheral holes are likely to proceed to retinal detachment but those in the lower periphery may persist for some time with only a local flat detachment. It is these latter which may be missed when associated with an obvious microcystic macula. Successful repair of the peripheral hole is associated almost invariably with disappearance of the macular lesion and full functional recovery. One patient observed personally with several peripheral holes, all apparently sealed by pigment proliferation and no local detachment, responded similarly to peripheral treatment with complete disappearance of the macular cysts.

Peripheral senile retinoschisis extends directly to involve the macula in very rare cases but in the juvenile variety, an intervening uninvolved retinal zone is often present between the peripheral and macular lesions. Microcystic macular pathology sometimes distorted by fine retinal folds or wrinkles is the posterior lesion seen most commonly.

Microcystic maculae are common in more advanced sickle cell retinopathy, but may be present when the peripheral lesions are early but active. The peripheral disease is predominantly temporal in such cases.

Considerable interest has been shown in the microcystic macular lesion with or without disc edema seen following cataract extraction.[45,112,124] Its etiology is still an enigma but several cases have been associated with peripheral retinal hemorrhages toward the six o'clock meridian. The question of trauma to this global region in cataract expression has been raised as a possible etiologic mechanism.[154] Although this contention is by no means proved, careful study of the retinal periphery in such lesions is indicated.

The microcystic maculae of chorioretinitis, central retinal vein obstruction, and those occurring after cataract extraction are clinically identical; their undistorted macular star patterns, seen on fluorescein angiography are similar. Even the mode of star development is the same in each. An associated, diffuse deep retinal edema is present in the two former conditions and suggested strongly in the microcystic macula following cataract extraction. Reduced magnification after lens extraction makes its visualization difficult, but this deep retinal edema has been seen throughout the posterior retina in several severe cases. Such identical findings in three separate diseases suggests the activity of a common vascular mechanism.

Not all microcystic maculae associated with peripheral lesions recover. They are potentially reversible until rupture of the larger central cyst occurs (see section on Deep Retinal Edema).

The vascular malformations of Coats's disease and peripheral angioma, if in the temporal retina and of sufficiently large size, are succeeded commonly by massive fatty exudation in the macula. The latter develops usually in Henle's layer but loses the star configuration as it increases in size. Ultimately, a large oval mass of yellowish exudation appears. It may reach 3 or 4 D elevation and be three times a disc diameter across. Eradication of the vascular malformation or angioma is followed by slow absorption of exudate over several years (see Chapter 11, under section on Cerebrovascular Anomalies and Retinal Angioma). These macular mounds are so striking that two of ours have been misdiagnosed as disciform macular degeneration, their peripheral cause having been overlooked.

A disciform exudative and hemorrhagic macular mound assumed to be of histoplasmic etiology commonly show quiescent, ragged, pigment-bordered, gray white or yellowish, centered peripheral lesions usually about 1/3 dd in size and called "histo" spots. Such spots are not limited to the periphery but may be seen in the midretina, or at the posterior pole. In the fellow eye some patients show histo spots without macular pathology.

Other peripheral retinal lesions show no associated macular disease. Among these are peripheral cystic degeneration, peripheral paving-stone degeneration, peripheral pigmentary degeneration, and lattice degeneration. Similarly, repeated search has failed to reveal any single, regularly occurring, peripheral retinopathy in disciform macular degeneration, senile macular degeneration, or central areolar choroidal sclerosis. Likewise there are cases of microcystic maculae, some with central ruptured cysts which show no clinically demonstrable peripheral retinal disease.

TEMPORAL PERIPHERAL PREFERENCE

Several retinal diseases have a predilection for the peripheral temporal retina. The preference for the inferotemporal periphery followed in frequency by the superotemporal periphery of retinoschisis and the common symmetrical bilaterality of this disease is unexplained. Also unknown is the affinity of angioma for the tempororetinal periphery. Two other diseases showing a preference for the temporal peripheral retina are retrolental fibroplasia and sickle cell disease. In the former, the dependence of the disease upon prior oxygen capillary obliteration, the delay in embryologic vascularization of the more distant temporal periphery, and the preponderance of oxygen-sensitive, immature retinal vessels at this site in premature and even mature infants (see Chapter 1, Development of Retinal Vessels) probably explains the preferential site of disease onset. In sickle cell disease the increased tendency to sickle at lower oxygen tensions [110] and the suggested delay in circulation time of the more remote tempororetinal periphery are likely factors. The vascular path from the central retinal artery to the tempororetinal periphery is the longest in the retina. The length of the conduit is of likely significance in both diseases.

EXAGGERATED MACULAR RESPONSE TO RETINAL DISEASE

For reasons at present unknown, the macula shows an exaggerated pathologic response in some generalized, and other localized retinal disorders.[157] An appreciation of this phenomenon is helpful in understanding the clinical morphology of pathology seen in certain retinal diseases. The readily apparent macular lesion often suggests a careful search of the peripheral retina when some posterior explanation is absent.

During the course of the retinal response to central vein occlusion, there occurs a collection of fluid in the outer plexiform layer. At the macula this accumulation appears in Henle's layer (comparable to the outer plexiform layer) and is two or three times greater than elsewhere. Clinically it produces an elevated, microcystic, honeycomb appearance of the macula which is best seen by retroillumination. The fibers of Henle's layer normally have a slanting, almost horizontal position, while in microcystic edema they assume an alignment vertical to the retina. This alteration could permit the increased fluid collection at the macula. Verhoeff[144] demonstrated microscopically this exaggerated cystic edema of the macula. Fluorescein angiography shows dye leakage from perimacular retinal capillaries with slow permeation into the microcystic spaces. Ultimately the classic macular fluorescein star pattern is formed. Although Verhoeff also demonstrated a lesser degree of this deep edema throughout the remaining retina, other than at the macula, it is insufficient in degree to create clinically visible retinal "cysts," or to demonstrate fluorescein dye leakage with present techniques. Occasionally after collateral circulation has become established, a low-grade cystic edema will persist only at the macula as one indication of mild, persisting venous insufficiency.

Late proliferation or atrophy of the pigment epithelium after central vein obstruction is almost an exclusive macular reaction. On only one occasion has such pigment change personally been seen near the ora serrata, but at no time in any intervening retinal area. Other late exaggerated macular changes are preretinal fibrosis, often with fine visible retinal folds, small retinal hemorrhages, increased fine vascularity, and microaneurysms.[151] In younger patients making a good recovery from central retinal vein obstruction, the disc collaterals and residual pathologic findings at the macula may be the sole clinical evidence of a prior obstruction.

Retinal damage as demonstrated by visual field examination following moderately severe central vein obstructions also emphasizes this macular sensitivity. While the peripheral field shows only relative depression, the central field shows a denser, or an absolute scotoma.

Certain cases of uveitis demonstrate a diffuse secondary retinal involvement clinically showing many features commonly seen in central retinal vein obstruction.[153] The macular reaction to uveitis is out of proportion to that seen throughout the remaining retina. Microcystic macular edema, macular cysts which may rupture, and the late mottling of pigment epithelium are the usual phenomena seen. Less commonly some central field defect may remain permanently. Fluorescein angiography demonstrates an identical macular star pattern to that described following central retinal vein obstruction. All of these changes, which are mild or absent elsewhere throughout the retina, demonstrate again this exaggerated macular response.

Cases of hypertensive retinopathy with a waxing and waning retinal edema may show scattered, small fatty exudates in the posterior retina, but their deposition at the macula is always exaggerated. Here they collect and coalesce in Henle's layer to form a macular star. Except in severe, late hypertensive retinopathy, where other complicating factors intervene, the fatty exudate of the macular star makes up a total mass greater than the sum of all other fatty retinal exudates.

Angioid streaks are most prominent around the disc and fade toward the fundus periphery. It seems likely that the tug of everyday ocular rotations on the optic nerve attachments at the disc might account for this distribution and in this sense, be analogous to the increased skin changes evident at flexion areas in pseudoxanthoma elasticum. These streaks may have a uniform reddish color, a granular appearance, or even be gray white if gliosis is present. Their borders show varying degrees of pigment proliferation. In this disorder the macular lesions, when present, show four to five times more retinal elevation than other areas, an increased amount of deep connective tissue, and much heavier pigment proliferation. At times fatty exudation appears within the macular mound, or in a circinate distribution around it. Such exudation is not found elsewhere in the fundus. Hemorrhages may be seen about angioid streaks but again, are much more prominent in the macula. Thus once the macula has become involved in this generalized retinal disease of angioid streaks, it demonstrates graphically the locally exaggerated pathologic response.

The macula shows this exaggeration of pathology, not only where the entire retina is involved in a disease process, but also when the disorder involves only a limited retinal area, so long as the macular zone is included.

In diabetic retinopathy a circinate lesion centered upon the macula is larger, has more fatty exudate and shows more central retinal thickening due to microcystic edema than circinate lesions centered extramacularly. When resolved, the macular ring lesion commonly leaves a clump of subfoveal proliferated pigment epithelium, or a ruptured macular cyst, both of which are associated with central scotomas. Extramacular circinate lesions may disappear completely in months without clinical evidence of their prior position.

Any nonspecific circinate retinopathy, as may be seen in diabetic retinopathy, following retinal vein obstruction, or in Leber's multiple miliary aneurysms with retinal degeneration, will show a heaping of fatty exudates at the macula if the lesion is so situated that the ring of exudates passes through the macula. Such a ring will be asymmetric and signet-ring in appearance. Indeed, this may explain the clump of exudate often seen at the macula in diabetic retinopathy, for with the passage of time and the slow absorption of the exudate, the thinner portion of the ring will disappear first.

When temporal retinal angioma becomes sufficiently large, often the fundus will present a rather characteristic pathology. There is a band of heavy fatty exudation and cystic retinal degeneration about the peripheral tumor, a relatively normal intermediate zone, scattered fatty exudates about the disc, and a mound of fatty exudate at the macula. The latter may reach 4 D in height and be so striking that the causative peripheral angioma is overlooked.

There are, therefore, many examples of this exaggerated macular response. Although an explanation for it is lacking, an appreciation of its frequency is clinically helpful.

REFERENCES

1. Allen, R. A., and Straatsma, B. R.: Ocular involvement in leukemia and allied disorders. *Arch. Ophthal. 66:*490, 1961.
2. Ashby, M., Oakley, N., Larentz, I., and Scott, D.: Recurrent transient monocular blindness. *Brit. Med. J. 2:*894, 1963.
3. Ashton, N.: Retinal micro-aneurysms in the non-diabetic subject. *Brit. J. Ophthal. 35:* 189, 1951.
4. Ashton, N.: Central areolar choroidal sclerosis. *Brit. J. Ophthal. 37:*140, 1953.
5. Ashton, N.: Pulseless disease and oxygen studies (letter). *Amer. J. Ophthal. 38:*418, 1954.
6. Ashton, N., Kok, D'A., and Foulds, W. S.: Occular pathology in macroglobulinemia. *J. Path. Bact. 86:*453, 1963.
7. Aufranc, O. E., Jones, W. N., and Harris, W. H.: Fat emboli: discussion by Hermann, J. *JAMA 178:*1187, 1961.
8. Ball, C. J.: Atheromatous embolism to the brain, retina and choroid. *Arch. Ophthal. 76:*690, 1966.
9. Ball, C. J., and Henkind, P.: Retinal arteriolar collaterals in man. *Brit. J. Ophthal. 51:*688, 1967.
10. Ballantyne. A. J.: The state of the retina in diabetes mellitus. *Trans. Ophthal. Soc. U.K. 66:*503, 1946.
11. Ballantyne, A. J., and Michaelson, I. C. *Textbook of the Fundus of the Eye.* Baltimore, Md., Williams & Wilkins, 1962.
12. Bonamour, J., Bonnet, L., and Buovolo: La Retinopathie dysorique. *Bull. Soc. Franc. Opthal. 63:*126, 1950.
13. Bonnet, P.: The prethrombosis sign observed in retinal vessels in arterial hypertension: Its semiologic value. *Arch. Ophtal. 11:*12, 1951.
14. Byer, N. E.: Clinical study of lattice degeneration of the retina. *Trans. Amer. Acad. Ophthal. Otolaryng. 69:*1064, 1965.
15. Byer, N. E.: Clinical study of senile retinoschisis. *Arch. Ophthal. 79:*36, 1968.
16. Caccamise, W. C., and Okuda, K.: Takayasu's or pulseless disease. *Amer. J. Ophthal. 37:*784, 1954.
17. Carr, R. E., and Henkind, P.: Retinal findings associated with serum hyperviscosity. *Amer. J. Ophthal. 56:*23, 1963.
18. Coats, G.: Thrombosis of the central vein of the retina. *Roy. London Ophthal. Hosp. Rep. 16:*62, Part I, 1904.
19. Coats, G.: Further cases of thrombosis of the central vein. *Roy. London Ophthal. Hosp. Rep. 16:*516, Part IV, 1906.
20. Cogan, D. G.: Symposium: Primary chorioretinal aberrations with night blindness.

Pathology. *Trans. Amer. Acad. Ophthal. Otolaryng. 54:*629, 1949.

21. Cogan, D. G., and Kuwabara, T.: Capillary shunts in the pathogenesis of diabetic retinopathy. *Diabetes 12:*293, 1963.
22. Cogan, D. G., Kuwabara, T., and Moser, H.: Fat emboli in the retina following angiography. *Arch. Ophthal. 71:*308, 1964.
23. Croll, K.: The ocular manifestations of multiple sclerosis. *Amer. J. Ophthal. 60:*822, 1965.
24. Culler, A. M.: Fundus changes in leukemia. *Trans. Amer. Ophthal. Soc. 49:*445, 1951.
25. Curtin, V. T., Norton, E. W. D., and Smith, T. R.: Pathological confirmation of retinochisis. *Arch. Ophthal. 63:*978, 1960.
26. Dantzker, D. R., and Gerstin, D. D.: Retinal vascular changes following toxic effects on visual cells and pigment epithelium. *Arch. Ophthal. 81:*106, 1969.
27. David, N. J., Klintworth, G. K., Friedberg, S. J., and Dillon, M.: Fatal atheromatous cerebral embolism associated with bright plaques in the retinal arterioles. *Neurology 13:*708, 1963.
28. Davis, M. D.: Vitreous contraction in proliferative diabetic retinopathy. *Arch. Ophthal. 74:*741, 1965.
29. Dellmann, F. L.: Metastatische Prozesse am Auge bei Endocarditis lenta. *Klin. Mbl. Augenheilk. 63:*661, 1919.
30. DeVoe, A. G.: Ocular fat embolism. *Arch. Ophthal. 43:*857, 1950.
31. Dienot, E. C., and Gartner, S.: Pathologic changes in the eye with subacute bacterial endocarditis. *Arch. Ophthal. 31:*198, 1944.
32. Dollery, C. T., Henkind, P., Kohner, E. M., and Paterson, J. W.: Effect of raised intraocular pressure on the retinal and choroidal circulation. *Invest. Ophthal. 7:*191, 1968.
33. Dollery, C. T., Hill, D. W., Paterson, J. W., Ramalho, P. S., and Kohner, E. M.: Collateral blood flow after branch arteriolar occlusion in the human retina. *Brit. J. Ophthal. 51:*249, 1967.
34. Duke-Elder, S.: *System of Ophthalmology: Diseases of the Retina.* London, Kimpton, 1967, vol. X, pp. 82–87.
35. Duke-Elder, S.: *System of Ophthalmology: Diseases of the Retina.* London, Kimpton, 1967, vol. X, pp. 152–153.
36. Elwyn, H.: *Diseases of the Retina,* 2nd ed. New York, Blakiston, 1953.
37. Fahmy, J. A., Knudsen, V., and Andersen, S. R.: Intraocular hemorrhage following subarachnoid hemorrhage. *Acta Ophthal. 47:*550, 1969.
38. Fischbein, F. I.: Ischemic retinopathy following amniotic fluid embolization. *Amer. J. Ophthal. 67:*351, 1969.
39. François, J., and Neetens, A.: L'engainement des veines rétiniennes dans la sclérose en plaques. *Ophthalmologica 138:* 322, 1959.
40. Freedman, B. J.: Papilloedema, optic atrophy and blindness due to emphysema and chronic bronchitis. *Brit. J. Ophthal. 47:*290, 1963.
41. Friedenwald, J. S., Wilder, H. C., Maumenee, A. E., Sanders, T. E., Keyes, J. E. L., Hogan, M. J., Owens, W. C., and Owens, E. U.: *Ophthalmic Pathology,* Philadelphia, Saunders, 1952, p. 313.
42. Friedman, E., Smith, T. R., and Kuwabara, T.: Senile choroidal vascular patterns and drusen. *Arch. Ophthal. 69:*220, 1963.
43. Fry, W. E., and McDonald, P. R.: Malignant melanoma in the temporal periphery associated with macular symptoms as an initial finding. *Trans. Amer. Acad. Ophthal. Otolaryng. 61:*397, 1957.
44. Fuchs, E.: Ueber Veranderungen des Schnerven bei extogener interokularer Entzundung. *Arch. Ophth. 91:*1, 1915.
45. Gass, J. D. M., and Norton, E. W. D.: Fluorescein studies of patients with macular edema and papilledema following cataract extraction. *Trans. Amer. Ophthal. Soc. 64:*232, 1966.
46. Gerstein, D. D., and Dantzker, D. R.: Retinal vascular changes in hereditary visual cell degeneration. *Arch. Ophthal. 81:*99, 1969.
47. Gilbert, W.: Concerning periphlebitis and endovasculitis of the retinal vessels, also remarks on sclerotic, tuberculous and septicemic choroidal disease. *Klin. Mbl. Augenheilk. 94:*335, 1935.
48. Glew, W. B.: "An Experimental Study of the Pathogenesis of Papilledema." Thesis, University of Minnesota, 1957.
49. Glew, W. B., Kearns, T. P., Rucker, C. W., and Essex, H. E.: The experimental production of papilledema. *Arch. Ophthal. 60:* 1074, 1958.
50. Gold, D. H., Henkind, P., Sturner, W. Q., and Baden, M.: Oculodermal melanocytosis

and retinitis pigmentosa. *Amer. J. Ophthal. 63:*271, 1967.

51. Goodman, G., Sallmann, L. von, and Holland, M. G.: Ocular manifestations of sickle-cell disease. *Arch. Ophthal. 58:*655, 1957.
52. Greaves, D. P.: Discussion on the swollen optic disc. *Trans. Ophthal. Soc. U.K. 79:* 109, 1959.
53. Guerry, D., III: Personal communication.
54. Guerry, D., III, and Wiesinger, H.: Ocular complications in carotid angiography. *Amer. J. Ophthal. 55:*241, 1963.
55. Gunn, R. M.: Ophthalmoscopic evidence of (1) arterial changes associated with chronic renal disease, and (2) of increased arterial tension. *Trans. Ophthal. Soc. U.K. 8:*356, 1897–98.
56. Haarr, I. M.: Periphlebitis retinae in association with multiple sclerosis. *Acta Psychiat. Scand. 28:*175, 1953.
57. Haarr, I. M.: Retinal periphlebitis in multiple sclerosis. *Acta Neurol. Scand.* (*Suppl. 4*) *39:*270, 1963.
58. Hagedoorn, A.: Angioid streaks. *Arch. Ophthal. 21:*746, 935, 1939.
59. Hayreh, S. S.: Pathogenesis of oedema of the optic disc (papilloedema) a preliminary report. *Brit. J. Ophthal. 48:*522, 1964.
60. Heath, P.: Pathology of the retinopathy of prematurity: Retrolental fibroplasia. *Amer. J. Ophthal. 34:*1249, 1951.
61. Hedges, T. R.: A correlative study of orbital vascular and intracranial pressure in the rhesus monkey. *Trans. Amer. Ophthal. Soc. 61:*589, 1963.
62. Henkind, P.: Ballotini occlusion of retinal arteries. Collateral vessels. *Brit. J. Ophthal. 50:*482, 1966.
63. Hollenhorst, R. W.: The ocular manifestations of internal carotid thrombosis. *Med. Clin. N. Amer. 44:*897, 1960.
64. Hollenhorst, R. W.: Significance of bright plaques in the retinal arterioles. *Trans. Amer. Ophthal. Soc. 59:*252, 1961.
65. Hollenhorst, R. W.: Vascular status of patients who have cholesterol emboli in the retina. *Amer. J. Ophthal. 61:*1159/219, 1966.
66. Hollenhorst, R. W., Lensink, E. R., and Whisnant, J. P.: Experimental embolization of the retinal arterioles. *Trans. Amer. Ophthal. Soc. 60:*316, 1962.
67. Hollenhorst, R. W., and Stein, H. A.: Ocular signs and prognosis in subdural and subarachnoid bleeding in young children. *Arch. Ophthal. 60:*187, 1958.
68. Holley, K. E., Bahn, R. S., McGoon, D. C., and Mankin, H. T.: Spontaneous calcific embolization associated with calcific aortic stenosis. *Circulation 27:*197, 1963.
69. Holley, K. E., Bahn, R. C., McGoon, D. C., and Mankin, H. T.: Calcific embolization associated with valvotomy for calcific aortic stenosis. *Circulation 28:*175, 1963.
70. Houston, W. R., and Wise, G. N.: Circinate retinopathy. *Arch. Ophthal. 58:*777, 1957.
71. Huber, A.: *Eye Symptoms in Brain Tumors.* (Translated by S. Van Wien.) St. Louis, Mo., Mosby, 1961, p. 93.
72. Jensen, V. A.: Clinical studies of tributory thrombosis in the central retinal vein. *Acta Ophthal.* (*Suppl. 10*)*:*1, 1936.
73. Jensen, V. A.: Anastomosis formation after embolism of the central retinal artery. *Acta Ophthal. 16:*485, 1938.
74. Johnson, H. C.: Retinal venous sheathing in multiple sclerosis. *Amer. J. Ophthal. 29:* 1150, 1946.
75. Kakler, A. R., and O'Brien, C. S.: Disciform degeneration of the macula. *Arch. Ophthal. 13:*937, 1935.
76. Kandori, F., Kurimoto, S., and Fukumaga, K.: "Retinal Vascular Patterns after Experimental Vascular Intoxication of the Retina of Rats and Cats." in *Proceedings of the XX International Congress of Ophthalmology.* Nijmegen, MacDonald, 1967, p. 278.
77. Kearns, T. P.: Fat embolism of the retina. *Amer. J. Ophthal. 41:*1, 1956.
78. Kennedy, J. E., and Wise, G. N.: Clinicopathological correlation of retinal lesions: Subacute bacterial endocarditis. *Arch. Ophthal. 74:*658, 1965.
79. Kennedy, J. E., and Wise, G. N.: Clinicopathological correlation of retinal lesions. 2. Retinochoroidal vascular anastomosis in uveitis. *Amer. J. Ophthal. 71:*1221, 1971.
80. Kiewe, P. L., and Hart, F. D.: Cytoid bodies in the retina in a case of malignant disease. *Trans. Ophthal. Soc. U.K. 71:*309, 1951.
81. Kimura, S. J., Carriker, F. R., and Hogan, M. J.: Retinal vasculitis with intraocular hemorrhage. *Arch. Ophthal. 56:*361, 1956.
82. Klien, B. A.: Anticoagulant therapy of occlusion of central vein of retina in relation to pathogenesis and differential diagnosis. *Arch. Ophthal. 29:*699, 1943.

83. Klien, B. A.: Obstruction of the central retinal vein. *Amer. J. Ophthal. 27:*1339, 1944.

84. Klien, B. A.: Clinical and histopathologic aspects of angioid streaks. *Amer. J. Ophthal. 30:*955, 1947.

85. Klien, B. A.: Prevention of retinal venous occlusion. *Amer. J. Ophthal. 33:*175, 1950.

86. Klien, B. A.: Retinal lesions associated with uveal disease. Part I. *Amer. J. Ophthal. 42:*831, 1956.

87. Klien, B. A.: Spontaneous vascular repair. Arteriolar and venous cilioretinal communications. *Amer. J. Ophthal. 50:*691, 1960.

88. Klien, B. A., and Krill, A. E.: Fundus flavimaculatus: Clinical function and histopathologic observation. *Amer. J. Ophthal. 64:*3, 1967.

89. Klien, B. A., and Olwin, J. H.: A survey of the pathogenesis of retinal venous occlusion. *Arch. Ophthal. 56:*207, 1956.

90. Knapp, A.: Retinal periphlebitis in the course of acute exudative choroiditis. *Arch. Ophthal. 26:*750, 1941.

91. Knisely, M. H.: Intravascular Erythrocyte Aggregation (Blood Sludge) in *Handbook of Physiology. Section 2: Circulation.* Baltimore, Md., Waverly Press, 1965, vol. III, pp. 2249–2292.

92. Kohner, E. M., Dollery, C. T., Shakib, M., Henkind, P., Paterson, J. W., de Oliveira, L. F. N., and Bulpitt, C.: Experimental retinal branch vein occlusion. *Amer. J. Ophthal. 69:*778, 1970.

93. Kohner, E. M., Dollery, C. T., Paterson, J. W., and Oakley, N. W.: Arterial fluorescein studies in diabetic retinopathy. *Diabetes 16:*1, 1967.

94. Kroll, A. J.: Experimental central retinal artery occlusion. *Arch. Ophthal. 79:*453, 1968.

95. Leishman, R.: The eye in general vascular disease. Hypertension and arteriosclerosis. *Brit. J. Ophthal. 41:*641, 1957.

96. Levine, R. A., and Henry, M. D.: Ischemic infarction of the retina following carotid angiography. *Amer. J. Ophthal. 55:*365, 1963.

97. Lieb, W. A., Geeraets, W. J., and Guerry, D.: Sickle-cell retinopathy. *Acta Ophthal. (Suppl. 58)* 1959.

98. Litten, M.: Ueber akute maligne Endocarditis und die dabei vorkommenden Retinalveränderungen. *Charité-Am. 3:*135, 1878.

99. Loewenstein, A., and Garrow, A.: A contribution to the anatomy of circinate retinopathy. *Trans. Ophthal. Soc. U.K. 63:*120, 1943.

100. Loewenstein, A., Michaelson, I. C., and Hill, J.: Retinal vasculitis in the young. A pathological report. *Trans. Ophthal. Soc. U.K. 66:*211, 1946.

101. Lucas, D. R.: Retinitis pigmentosa pathological findings in two cases. *Brit. J. Ophthal. 40:*14, 1956.

102. Manschot, W. A.: Embolism of the central retinal artery. *Amer. J. Ophthal. 48:*381, 1959.

103. Marshall, D.: Ocular manifestations of multiple sclerosis and relationship to retrobulbar neuritis. *Trans. Amer. Ophthal. Soc. 48:*487, 1950.

104. Maumenee, A. E.: Fluorescein angiography in the diagnosis and treatment of lesions of the ocular fundus. *Trans. Ophthal. Soc. U.K. 88:*529, 1968.

105. McBrien, D. J., Bradley, R. D., and Ashton, N.: The nature of retinal emboli in stenosis of the internal carotid artery. *Lancet 1:* 697, 1963.

106. McKeown, H. S.: Retinal hemorrhages in the newborn. *Trans. Amer. Ophthal. Soc. 38:*510, 1940.

107. Meadows, S. P.: Discussion on the swollen optic disc. *Trans. Ophthal. Soc. U.K. 79:* 121, 1959.

108. Moller, P. M., and Hammerberg, P. E.: Retinal periphlebitis in multiple sclerosis. *Acta Neurol. Scand. (Suppl. 4) 39:*263, 1963.

109. Morris, D. M., and Henkind, P.: Relationship of intracranial, optic nerve sheath and retinal hemorrhage. *Amer. J. Ophthal. 64:* 853, 1967.

110. Murphy, R. C., Jr., and Shapiro, J.: The pathology of sickle-cell disease. *Amer. Intern. Med. 23:*396, 1945.

111. Naunton, W. J., and Forester, R. M.: Severe vitreous hemorrhage in a premature infant. *Brit. J. Ophthal. 39:*563, 1955.

112. Nicholls, J. V. V.: Concurrence of macular edema with cataract extraction. *Arch. Ophthal. 55:*595, 1956.

113. Noell, W. K.: Differentiation, metabolic organization and viability of the visual cell. *Arch. Ophthal. 60:*702, 1958.

114. Okun, E.: Gross and microscopic pathology in autopsy eyes: Part III. Retinal breaks

without detachment. *Amer. J. Ophthal. 51:*369, 1961.

115. Paton, L., and Holmes, G.: The pathology of papilledema. *Trans. Ophthal. Soc. U.K. 31:*117, 1911.
116. Paufique, L., and Etienne, R.: Un signe peu connu de la sclerose en plaques: la periphlebite des veines retiniennes. *Ann. Oculist. 188:*701, 1955.
117. Penner, R., and Font, R. L.: Retinal embolism from calcified vegetations of aortic valve. *Arch. Ophthal. 81:*565, 1969.
118. Pick, L.: Netzhautveranderungen bei chronischen Anamieen. *Klin. Mbl. Augenheilk. 39:*177, 1901.
119. Pickering, G. W.: *High Blood Pressure.* New York, Grune & Stratton, 1955.
120. Primrose, J.: Mechanism of production of papilloedema. *Brit. J. Ophthal. 48:*15, 1964.
121. Rabinowicz, I. M., Ben-Sira, I., and Zauberman, H.: Preservation of visual function in papilledema. *Brit. J. Ophthal. 52:*236, 1968.
122. Reese, A. B.: Telangiectasis of the retina and Coats' disease. *Amer. J. Ophthal. 42:* 1, 1956.
123. Reese, A. B., and Jones, I. S.: Hematomas under the retinal pigment epithelium. *Amer. J. Ophthal. 53:*897, 1962.
124. Reese, A. B., Jones, I. S., and Cooper, W. C.: Macular changes secondary to vitreous traction. *Trans. Amer. Ophthal. Soc. 64:* 123, 1966.
125. Ricci, A., and Déruaz, J. P.: Pronostic et séquelles des thromboses veineuses retiniennes. *Ophthalmologica 156:*325, 1968.
126. Ross Russell, R. W.: Observations on the retinal blood vessels in monocular blindness. *Lancet 2:*1422, 1961.
127. Ross Russell, R. W.: The source of retinal emboli. *Lancet 2:*789, 1968.
128. Roth, M.: Ueber Netzhautaffectionen bei Wundfiebern. *Deutsch. Z. Chir. 1:*471, 1872.
129. Roth, M.: Beiträge zur Kenntnis der varicosen Hypertrophie der Nervenfasern. *Virchow Arch. Path. Anat. 55:*197, 1872.
130. Rucker, C. W.: Sheathing of the retinal veins in multiple sclerosis. *Mayo Clin. Proc. 19:*176, 1944.
131. Rucker, C. W.: Sheathing of the retinal veins in multiple sclerosis. *JAMA 127:* 970, 1945.
132. Rucker, C. W.: Retinopathy of multiple sclerosis. *Trans. Amer. Ophthal. Soc. 45:* 564, 1947.
133. Rucker, C. W.: "Sheathing of the Retinal Veins in Multiple Sclerosis," in *Multiple Sclerosis and the Demyelinating Diseases. Proceedings of the Association for Research in Nervous and Mental Diseases.* Baltimore, Md., Williams & Wilkins 1950, pp. 396–402.
134. Samuels, B.: Chronic postoperative or posttraumatic retinitis (Retinitis serosa). *Amer. J. Ophthal. 19:*493, 1936.
135. Scott, G. I.: Ophthalmic aspects of demyelinating disease. *Proc. Roy. Soc. Med. 54:* 38, 1961.
136. Seitz, R.: *The Retinal Vessels.* (Translated by Blodi, F. C.) St. Louis, Mo., Mosby, 1964.
137. Semple, N. M.: Some questions concerning the method of development and the pathology of the retinitis of Bright's disease. *Trans. Amer. Ophthal. Soc. 12:*817, 1911.
138. Shakib, M., and Ashton, N.: Part II. Ultrastructural changes in focal retinal ischaemia. *Brit. J. Ophthal. 50:*325, 1966.
139. Shea, M., Schepens, C. L., and Von Pirquet, S. R.: Retinoschisis: I. Senile type: A clinical report of one hundred seven cases. *Arch. Ophthal. 63:*1, 1960.
140. Straatsma, B. R., and Allen, R. A.: Lattice degeneration of the retina. *Trans. Amer. Acad. Ophthal. Otolaryng. 66:*600, 1962.
141. Streiff, E. B., Bischler, V.: Retinopathie dysorique dans deux cas de carcinoma du foie. *Ophthalmologica 105:*229, 1943.
142. Sugi, K.: Studies on the pathological changes in the retinal vessels of human eyes using the trypsin digestion method. *Jap. J. Ophthal. 10:*252, 1966.
143. Vallotton, W. W., and Stokes, H. R.: Mercury embolism of the central retinal artery. *Amer. J. Ophthal. 57:*476, 1964.
144. Verhoeff, F. H.: Obstruction of the central retinal vein. *Arch. Ophthal. 36:*1, 1907.
145. Verhoeff, F. H., and Grossman, H. P.: Pathogenesis of disciform degeneration of the macula. *Arch. Ophthal. 18:*561, 1937.
146. Verhoeff, F. H., and Simpson, G. V.: Tubercle within central vein. *Arch. Ophthal. 24:*645, 1940.
147. Walsh, F. B., and Hedges, T. R., Jr.: Optic nerve sheath hemorrhage. *Amer. J. Ophthal. 34:*509, 1951.
148. Walsh, T. J., Garden, J., and Gallasher, B.:

Neuro-Ophthalmology. Ed. by Smith, J. L. St. Louis, Mo., Mosby, 1968, vol. IV, p. 288.

149. Werner, L.: On vascular and other retinal changes associated with general disease. *Trans. Ophthal. Soc. U.K. 33:*9, 1913.

150. Wise, G. N.: Retinal neovascularization. *Trans. Amer. Ophthal. Soc. 54:*729, 1956.

151. Wise, G. N.: Macular changes after venous obstruction. *Arch. Ophthal. 58:*544, 1957.

152. Wise, G. N.: Arteriosclerosis secondary to retinal vein obstruction. *Trans. Amer. Ophthal. Soc. 56:*361, 1959.

152a. Wise, G. N.: Arteriosclerosis secondary to retinal vein obstruction. *Arch. Ophthal. 61:*766, 1959.

153. Wise, G. N.: Uveitis with secondary retinal arteriosclerosis. *Trans. Amer. Ophthal. Soc. 58:*263, 1960; or *Amer. J. Ophthal. 51:* 797, 1961.

154. Wise, G. N.: Discussion of Gass, J. D. M., and Norton, E. W. D.[45]

155. Wise, G. N.: Discussion of McCulloch, C.: Choroideremia – a clinical and pathologic review. *Trans. Amer. Ophthal. Soc. 67:*191, 1969.

156. Wise, G. N., and Horava, A.: Coats' disease. *Amer. J. Ophthal. 56:*17, 1963.

157. Wise, G. N., and Wangvivat, Y.: The exaggerated macular response to retinal disease. Part II. *Amer. J. Ophthal. 61:*1359, 1966.

158. Wolter, J. R.: Retinitis pigmentosa a histopathologic study with a new technique. *Arch. Ophthal. 57:*539, 1957.

159. Wolter, J. R., Goldsmith, R. I., and Phillips, R. L.: Histopathology of the star-figure of the macular area in diabetic and angiospastic retinopathy. *Arch. Ophthal. 57:* 376, 1957.

160. Wolter, J. R., Phillips, R. L., and Butler, R. G.: The star-figure of the macular area. *Arch. Ophthal. 60:*49, 1958.

161. Wong, V. G., and Bodey, G. P.: Hemorrhagic retinoschisis due to aplastic anemia. *Arch. Ophthal. 80:*433, 1968.

162. Wybar, K. G.: The ocular manifestations of disseminated sclerosis. *Proc. Roy. Soc. Med. 45:*315, 1952.

163. Yanoff, M., Rahn, E. K., and Zimmerman, L. E.: Histopathology of juvenile retinoschisis. *Arch. Ophthal. 79:*49, 1968.

164. Zeeman, W. P. C.: Ueber Netzhaut und Schnervenleiden bei Iridocyclitis. *Arch. Ophth. 112:*152, 1923.

164a. Zeller, R. W.: Ocular findings in the remission phase of multiple sclerosis. *Amer. J. Ophthal. 64:*767, 1967.

165. Zimmerman, L. E.: Histology and general pathology of the optic nerve. *Trans. Amer. Acad. Ophthal. Otolaryng. 60:*14, 1956.

166. Zimmerman, L. E.: Personal communication. March 1960.

167. Zimmerman, L. E.: Embolism of the central retinal artery. *Arch. Ophthal. 73:*822, 1965.

168. Zimmerman, L. E., and Spencer, W. H.: The pathologic anatomy of retinoschisis. *Arch. Ophthal. 63:*11, 1960.

169. Ziv, V., and Dunphy, E. B.: Pigmented retinal arteries. *Amer. J. Ophthal. 57:*132, 1964.

chapter 11

Anomalous Vascular Formations, Neovascularization, and Microaneurysms

It seemed appropriate to include neovascularization in the chapter with anomalous vascular formations, although the two bear no fundamental relation to one another. New vessels do develop in some diseases with anomalous vascular formations, but their presence in such cases is secondary, and due to factors other than those producing the primary disease.

Significant numbers of retinal microaneurysms regularly occur in those conditions having associated neovascularization. They are usually sparse or even absent in other retinal vascular diseases. Indeed, the etiologies of retinal microaneurysms and neovascular formations have been considered by some [5,58,81,97] to be intimately related. Therefore, a section devoted to them follows the discussion of neovascularization.

ANOMALOUS VASCULAR FORMATIONS

Four rare retinal vascular diseases are included under the title anomalous vascular formations: (*1*) angiomatosis retinae; (*2*) Leber's multiple miliary aneurysms with retinal degeneration; (*3*) Coats's disease; and (*4*) racemose aneurysm. The last of these and rarest of the four presents a characteristic fundus appearance and is not readily confused with the others.

There has been considerable confusion and discussion in the literature regarding the first three of these vascular anomalies. Angiomatosis retinae was at first described as a third type of massive retinal exudation (Type III Coats's disease) by Coats in his original article.[16] Leber's multiple miliary aneurysms with retinal degeneration was originally considered by Leber to be a specific entity.[46,47] Reese [66] first labeled this same lesion a capillary hemangioma and later thought it a form of telangiectasia.[67] Wise [80] first called it an early form of Type II Coats's disease but more recently [87] has considered it to be an early form of angiomatosis retinae.

Long-term observation of a number of these cases, inquiry into the mechanisms of the disease processes, the application to the retinal angioma of knowledge gained through study of its associated cerebellar angioma and other cerebral vascular malformations, and retinal fluorescein angiography have all increased the understanding of these diseases. Following a description of the four anomalous vascular formations, a section will be devoted to their interrelationships.

ANGIOMATOSIS RETINAE

Clinical, Microscopic, and Fluorescein Findings

Angiomatosis retinae, or retinal angioma was first separated from Coats's disease by von Hippel [77] and the lesion has subsequently borne his name. Later, Lindau [48] noted the association of retinal and cerebellar angioma and the combined lesions have been called von Hippel-Lindau disease and classified by Van der Hoeve [38] as a member of the phakomatoses.

Retinal angioma has an autosomal dominant inheritance with incomplete penetrance and a varying expressivity.[25] Although the retinal lesion has been considered to arise from an "activated congenital rest," a recent study of very early lesions using the retinal digest technique has suggested that the retinal tumors arise from previously normal retinal vessels.[39] Retinal angiomas are more frequently seen in early life but may first appear in the older age groups. The disease may occur in one or both eyes, approximately one-third being bilateral,[76] and one-fourth of the ocular cases also having intracranial lesions.[48]

The retinal angioma starts most commonly in the retinal periphery especially temporally, but it also may develop posteriorly, or at the disc. Early lesions show an area of dilated, small vascular channels with associated retinal edema, microaneurysms, a few minute fatty exudates and often small arteriovenous communications. An occasional intraretinal blot hemorrhage may be seen at this stage. A retinal digest preparation of an early angioma showed a nest of proliferating endothelial cells, enlarged draining venule and two capillary feeders of normal size.[39] As the arteriovenous communication enlarges, the lesion takes on more and more of its own mature features (Fig. 11-1). The angioma with its arteriovenous shunt becomes apparent and the draining vein enlarges, followed by enlargement of the feeding artery. With an angioma 0.5 dd in size, all of its typical features may be seen except the arteriovenous shunt, which at this stage may be hidden by the associated pathology and is hard to locate. The tumor may be red, or a yellowish white, oval mound, with adjacent lateral or peripheral cystic retinal degeneration. The cystic change may be inconspicuous, but occasionally an adjacent cyst may be larger than the angioma. Retinal vessels are usually not visible peripherally to the angioma and may be thread-like or invisible peripherally to the cystic retina. An arc of heavy, fatty exudation is common just posterior to the angioma, extending peripherally on either side. The draining vein is enlarged, beaded, and may show segments of white halo sheathing. Near the angioma the latter may be difficult to differentiate from the feeding artery, for it now contains arterial blood and both artery and vein have burnished, thickened walls (Fig. 11-2). Microaneurysms and small retinal hemorrhages in the vicinity of the lesion are common. In rare instances where the pigment epithelium is disturbed, a migrated clump of proliferated pigment may be present. When

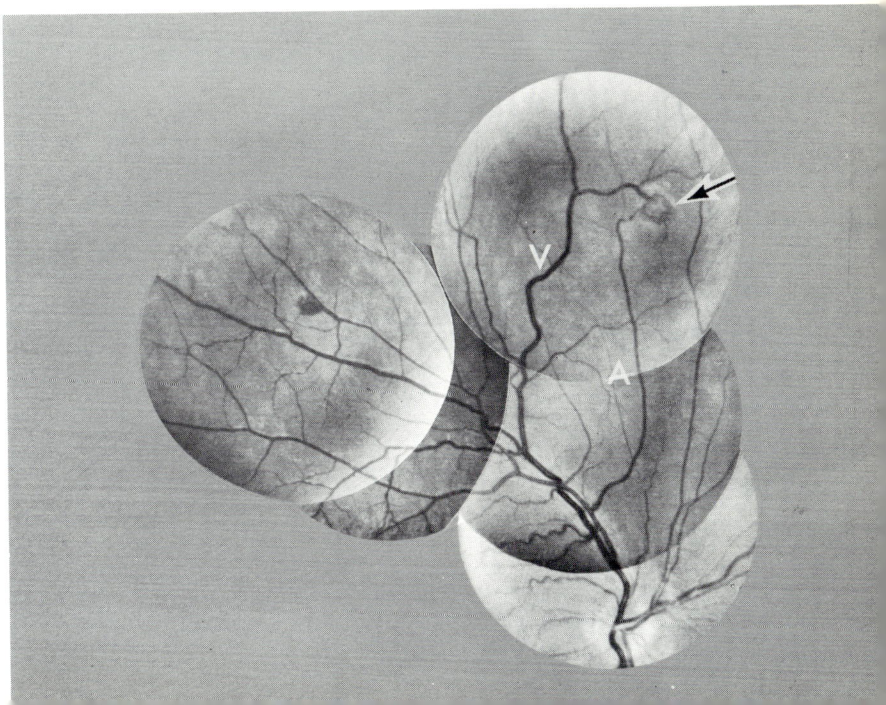

Fig. 11-1. Early retinal angioma (**arrow**). Note that the vein (**V**) enlarges before the feeding artery (**A**).

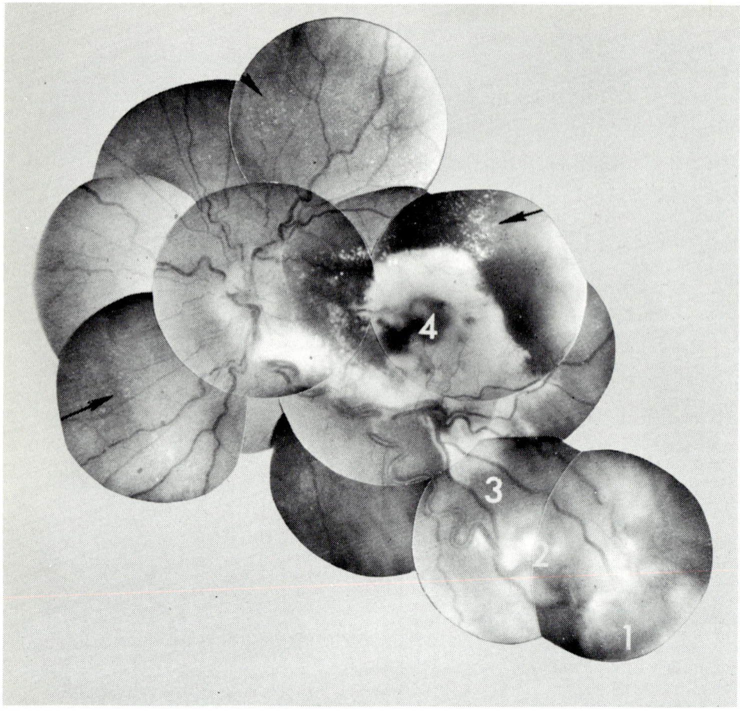

Fig. 11-2. Well-developed retinal angioma **(1)**. Note fatty exudates about angioma **(2)**; zone free of exudates **(3)**; exudative mound at macula **(4)**; scattered small fatty exudates posteriorly **(arrows)**.

the angioma is of sufficient size, the paired feeding and draining vessels show change back to the disc. Highly burnished arteries with early crossing defects posteriorly, occurring in a young, nonhypertensive individual, should alert one to the possibility of early angiomatosis retinae. Later, the feeding and draining vessels become more tortuous and dilated than vessels in other sectors, and the feeding artery may show fine beading at, or near the disc, then become smooth only to resume an exaggerated beading near the angioma.

The pinkish color of some retinoblastomas and their enlarged feeding and draining vessels have occasionally led to mistaken diagnoses because of their similarity to retinal angioma.[14]

Large temporal angiomas commonly show a scattering of fatty exudates at the posterior pole and an exaggerated mound of exudate at the macula (Fig. 11-2). Exudate at the macula starts as a star figure but progresses to an oval, elevated, yellowish mass with smoothly rounded borders. Such macular mounds have been mistaken for disciform macular degenerations, the peripheral angiomas having been overlooked. With increasing exudation, a retinal angioma becomes difficult to differentiate clinically from Coats's disease. Progressive cystic change and exudation, retinal detachment, retinal and subretinal hemorrhage, vitreous hemorrhage, rubeosis iridis, secondary glaucoma, and loss of the globe may ensue.

By no means are all retinal angiomas solitary. They may be multiple, of different sizes, and occur in various locations. In some cases all peripheral retinal quadrants may be involved.

Goldberg and Duke[34] microscopically have demonstrated proliferation of the vascular endothelium within the feeding artery just proximal to the angioma. The cells were piled into irregular nests, considerably narrowing the lumen where they were most numerous. The significance of this finding is not yet apparent.

Fluorescein angiography in this disease is techically difficult because of the peripheral location of the pathology. The angioma fills rapidly and leaks profusely. Rapid filling of the draining vein with some leakage through its wall near the angioma can be demonstrated. Norton[57] has demonstrated angiographically, an arteriovenous fistula at the site of the angioma and shown that its shunting effect causes underfilling of the regional capillary bed.

Cerebrovascular Anomalies and Retinal Angioma

Cerebellar angiomas have had more study than retinal angiomas and cerebral angiography has had a longer history than retinal fluorescein angiography. As cerebellar and retinal angiomas are each a part of the same disease process and can be assumed to have a common pathogenesis, findings in the cerebellar disease may well have a retinal application.

In the brain, cerebellar angiomas are grouped with other angiomatous malformations whose major feature is that of a localized arteriovenous shunt. Potter[65] has suggested that a small arteriovenous shunt may be of sufficient size to syphon off a critical flow of arterial blood from the regional capillary bed. At first, local cellular metabolic requirements would still be met and tissue alterations about the shunt would not occur. Persistence of this state is presumed to account for their prolonged periods of inactivity. If a quiescent arteriovenous shunt enlarges, a point is reached at which sufficient blood is diverted through this low resistance channel to affect adversely the neighboring vascular bed and the tissues which it supplies. Potter[65] called such a shunt a "parasite on the circulation."

Shenkin and his co-workers,[70] in a proved case of a large brain arteriovenous malformation, have demonstrated a three to five times increased blood flow through the lesion, and Luessenhop and Spence[50] and Robles and Carrazco[68] successfully have utilized this high-flow shunt concept to obliterate such a human vascular malformation by arterial embolization.

Norlén[56] has demonstrated by cerebral angiography the rapid circulation through such a vascular anomaly and poor contrast filling of the adjacent vascular bed. Following surgical removal of the lesion, the previously underfilled vascular bed filled well and was seen clearly. He called attention to the anoxemia of the brain areas adjacent to an angiomatous malformation due to this circulatory alteration.

Olivecrona and Riives[59] have noted this regional anoxemia due to shunting of blood through the low resistance arteriovenous communication and have spoken of the resulting regional brain atrophy. Not only atrophy but also cystic brain changes[18] have been demonstrated as a result of cerebral anoxia from various causes.

The application of these principles to retinal angiomas makes the associated retinal pathology more understandable. The arteriovenous shunt of a retinal angioma may be present in its earliest stages,[39] has been demonstrated by fluorescein angiography, and certain clinical findings make its presence indisputable. Only an arteriovenous shunt would permit the presence of lightly colored, oxygenated blood in the draining vein of a retinal angioma. The enlarging supply artery and draining vein also constitute indirect evidence of a functioning high-flow fistula. That the vessel growth is secondary to the enlarging vascular malformation has been demonstrated in cerebral lesions,[56] can be observed clinically in retinal angioma and has been suggested as well from their microscopic study.[39,40] The return of these vessels to a more normal size following obliteration of the angioma has been proved angiographically in the brain,[56] and is readily visible in the retina following light coagulation of the tumor. Decreased blood flow and underfilling of the regional vascular bed about an angiomatous malformation, and more normal filling of this same bed following shunt eradication has been shown angiographically in the brain. Although not yet demonstrated in retinal angioma, this same circulatory improvement may occur.

In both brain and eye, deprivation of blood flow about the tumor would lead to a relative anoxia in this same area with subsequent cystic degeneration. A large angioma might shunt sufficient flow to cause ischemia posteriorly and account for the fatty exudation scattered about the posterior pole. A heightened macular sensitivity would then account for the formation of a mound of exudate in its vicinity (see Chapter 10, under the Exaggerated Macular Response to Retinal Disease). Such a concept would explain the common distribution of retinal pathology seen in the course of retinal angioma.

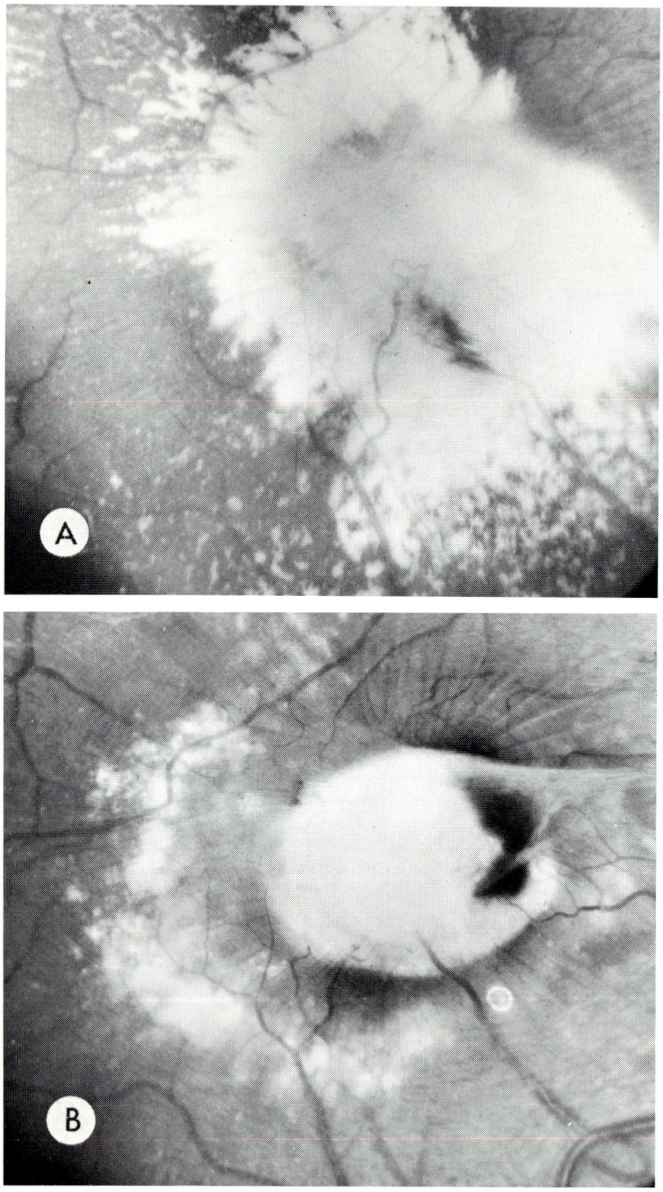

Fig. 11-3. *A*, Exudative macular mound in a 16-year-old girl with a temporal angioma. *B*, Ten months after eradication of the tumor by photocoagulation. Note decreasing exudate and retinal traction lines produced by the contracting macular scar.

Treatment

Treatment of a retinal angioma should be undertaken as soon as the diagnosis is made in those tumors of moderate size. If they are very small, and do not threaten the macula, a period of observation is permissible. A large temporal angioma with a mound of exudate at the macula should always be treated. Successful eradication of such an angioma will be followed by slow absorption of the macular exudate over succeeding months or years with sometimes surprising visual recovery (Fig. 11-3). Angiomas of the optic disc are at present best left untreated. Those near the macula should be treated promptly, especially if there are exudates involving the fovea. We have not observed spontaneous resolution of a retinal angioma.

Retinal angioma are best treated by the xenon arc photocoagulator. The initial treatment of angiomas of moderate size must be cautious. Overzealous treatment can result in hemorrhage, massive exudation, and retinal detachment. Subsequent coagulations are less likely to produce complications.

LEBER'S MULTIPLE MILIARY ANEURYSMS WITH RETINAL DEGENERATION

Clinical, Microscopic, and Fluorescein Findings

Leber's multiple miliary aneurysms with retinal degeneration [46,47] is more common in the young, but has been observed in middle age, and in one patient at age 65. It occurs more frequently in one eye but both may be involved. In the latter instances, the disease of the second eye is often minimal. The retinal lesions may be peripheral, midretinal, at or near the macula and very near the disc, but a lesion on the disc has not been seen.

Fig. 11-4. Leber's multiple miliary aneurysms with retinal degeneration in a 44-year-old man with a blood pressure of 120/80. Note burnished arteries with arteriovenous crossing defects **(1)** and arterial beading near the disc **(2)**.

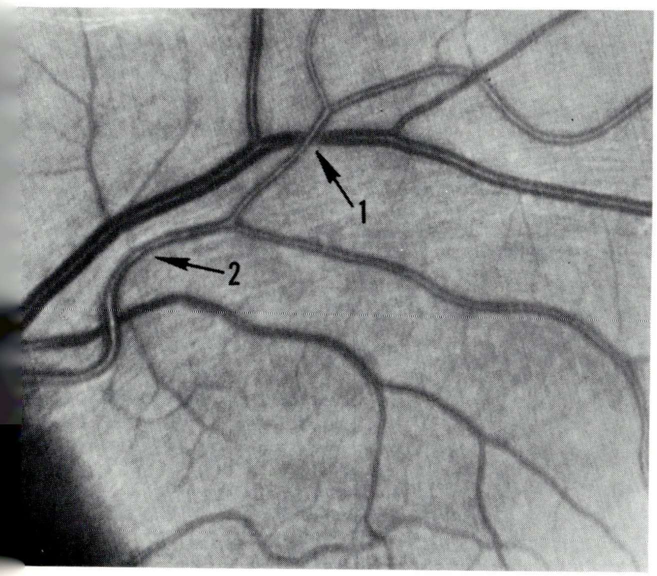

Very burnished brilliant arteries and mild arteriovenous nicking seen posteriorly in a young or middle-aged, nonhypertensive individual, (Fig. 11-4) suggests either this disease, or a retinal angioma. In both instances, the posterior fundus has the same appearance.

Rings of fatty exudates with central microaneurysms are common in Leber's disease (Fig. 11-5). Increased brilliance of the light reflex, whitening and thickening of a short segment of a major, secondary, or tertiary artery is first noted. A few microaneurysms may be seen nearby, and sometimes, small retinal hemorrhages. Next, yellow fatty exudates begin to form in a ring centered on the arterial lesion and 1 or 2 dd from it. As the arterial segment continues to enlarge and whiten, deep edema thickens the retina within the ring and aneurysms hyalinize, becoming first a lighter red, then a yellowish white color. The exudative ring thickens, and the bulbous segment of the artery becomes two or three times its normal width—a brilliant, whitish, aneurysmal dilatation likened by Guerry [35] to an electric light bulb.

Over a period of time such a ring lesion may completely disappear with absorption of edema, exudate, hemorrhages, and aneurysms. The change in the arterial wall recedes and eventually returns to normal, leaving no residual sign of its prior position. From start to finish, this process may take 3 to 4 years (Fig. 11-6).

Ring lesions which involve the fovea, may leave a residual macular cyst, a ruptured cyst, some pigment proliferation, or white gliosis at the fovea, producing a permanent scotoma and variable visual loss (Fig. 11-7).

While typical of this disease, these circinate lesions are not always present. Other areas of involvement will first show dilated capillaries and scattered microaneurysms, some of which are connected to small venous radicals, and others in which no vascular connection is visible (Fig. 11-8). These vas-

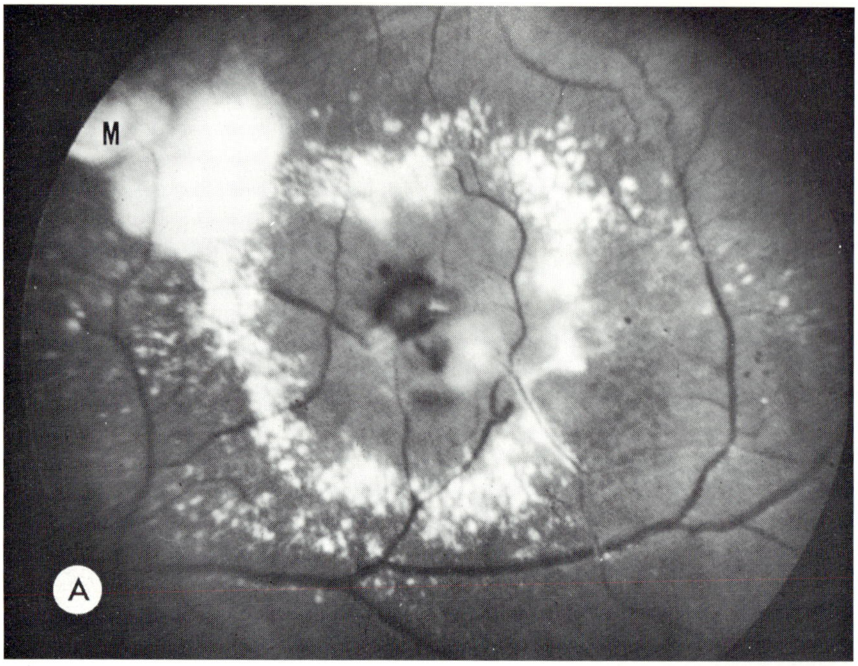

Fig. 11-5. *A*, Leber's multiple miliary aneurysms with retinal degeneration. Note ring of fatty exudates around central arterial aneurysm. The signet effect at the macula **(M)** is produced when the ring passes near or through it.

B, A similar ring lesion in another patient. Note that the vein **(V)** near the arterial aneurysm **(arrow)** is uninvolved.

C, Fluorescein angiogram of this same lesion in the early venous phase showing unimpeded flow through the aneurysm.

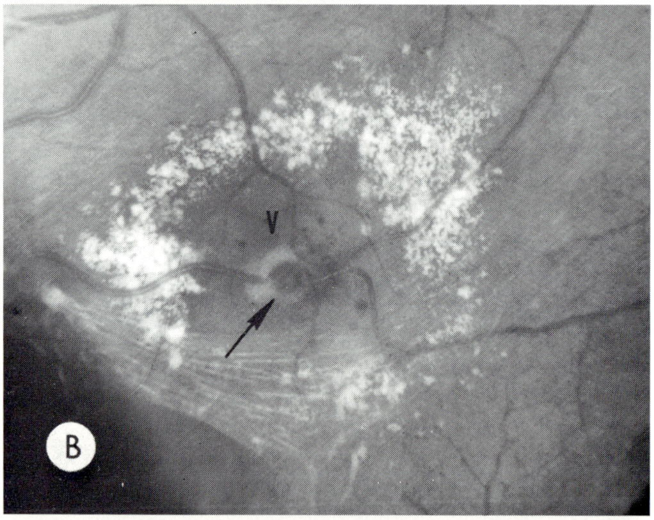

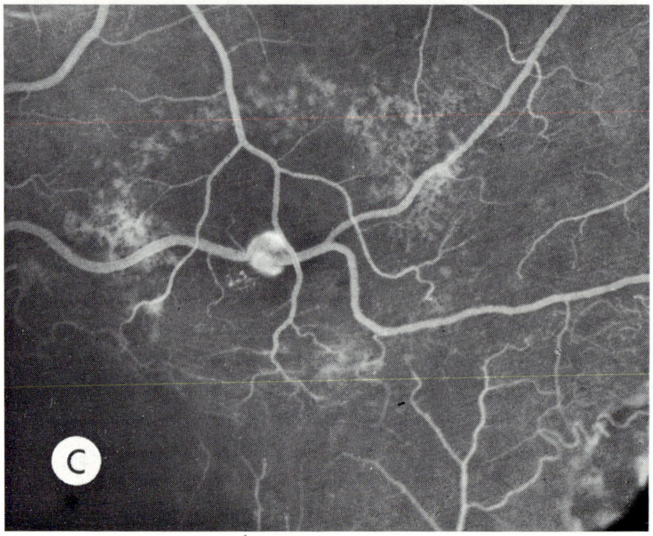

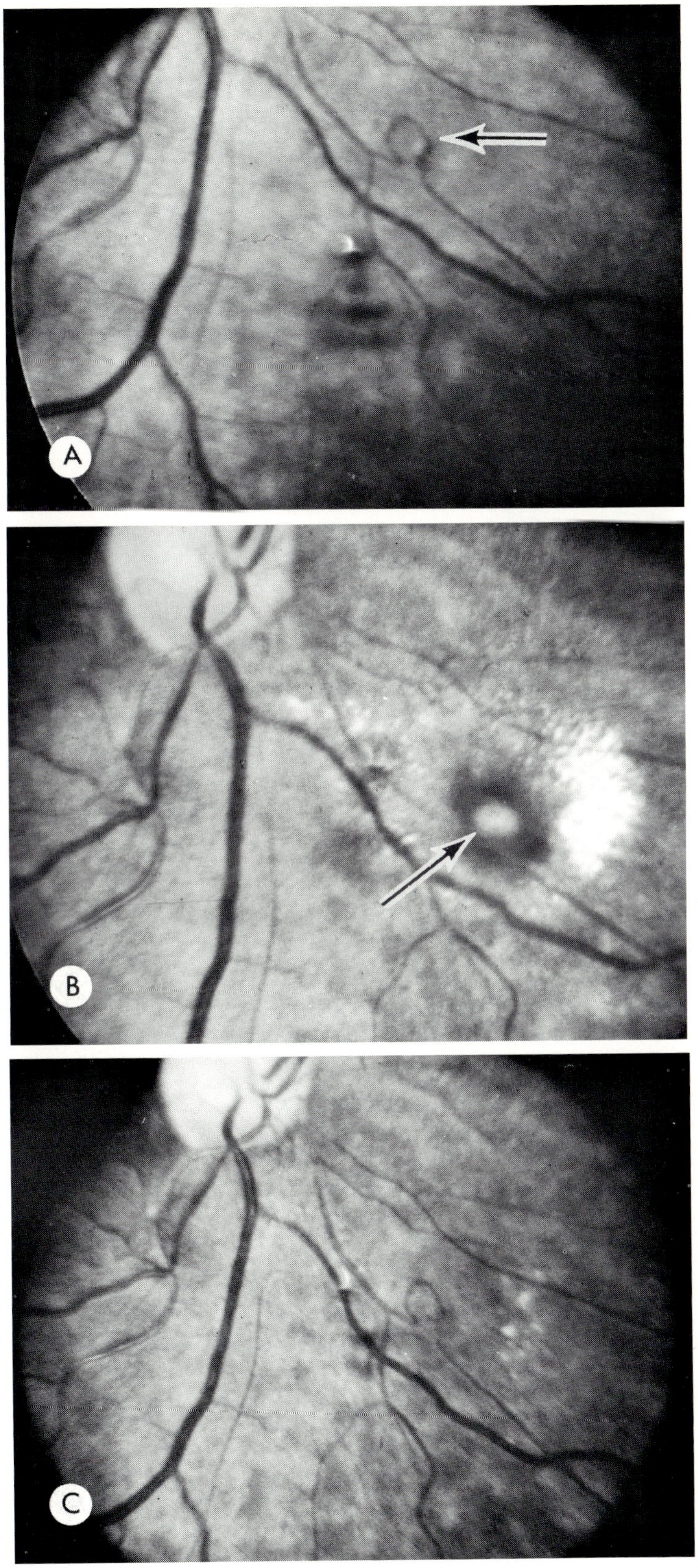

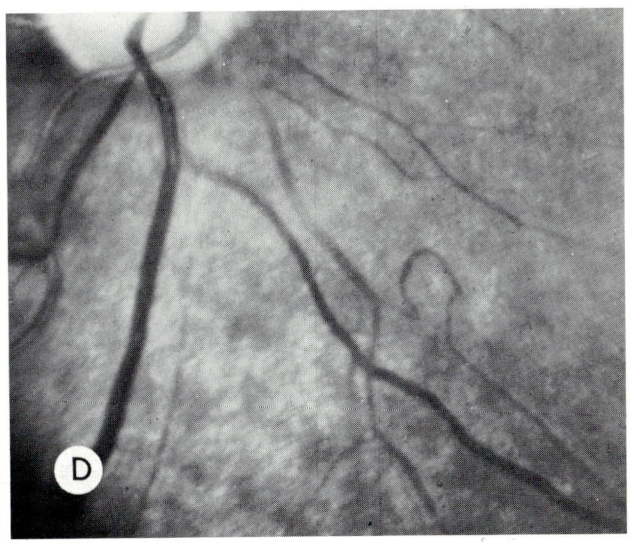

Fig. 11-6. The spontaneous development and regression of a Leber's ring lesion in a 56-year-old hypertensive female.

A, November 1957: unusual, slightly irregular arterial loop **(arrow)** without surrounding reaction. Subsequently, several places on the arterial loop became highly burnished with wall thickening and a few fatty exudates developed a short distance temporally.

B, March 1959: note arterial aneurysm **(arrow)** with surrounding ring of fatty exudates and retinal hemorrhages.

C, April 1960: regression of exudates and hemorrhages, and disappearance of the aneurysm.

D, November 1969: the lesion cleared completely shortly after that shown in *C* and has remained quiescent.

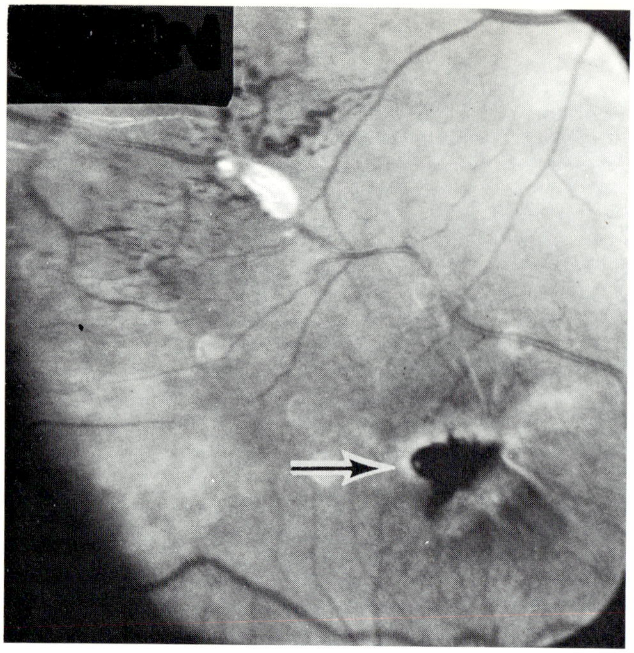

Fig. 11-7. *Above.* Late macular scarring **(arrow)** secondary to Leber's ring lesion involving the macula. The vascular abnormalities of this disease can be seen at the upper left-hand corner.

Fig. 11-8. *Below.* Fluorescein angiogram of an area of vascular abnormality in Leber's multiple miliary aneurysms with retinal degeneration. Note disappearance of or underfilling of some capillaries and dilatation of others.

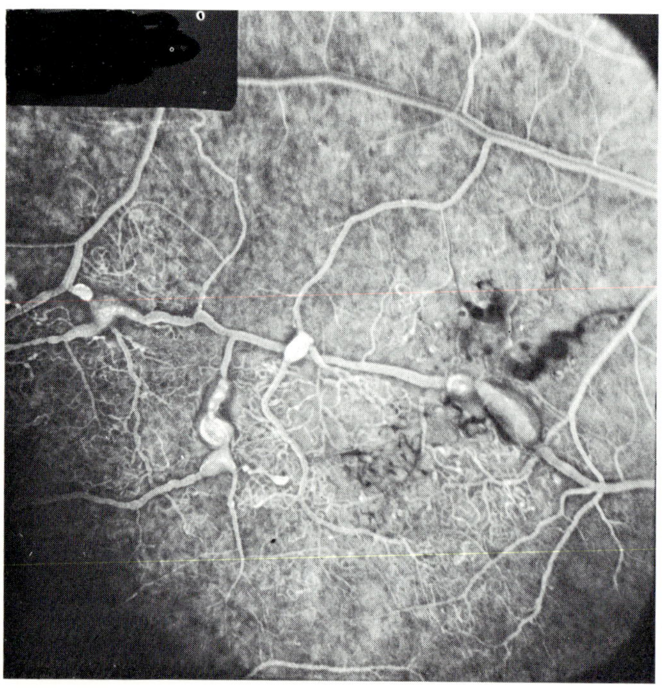

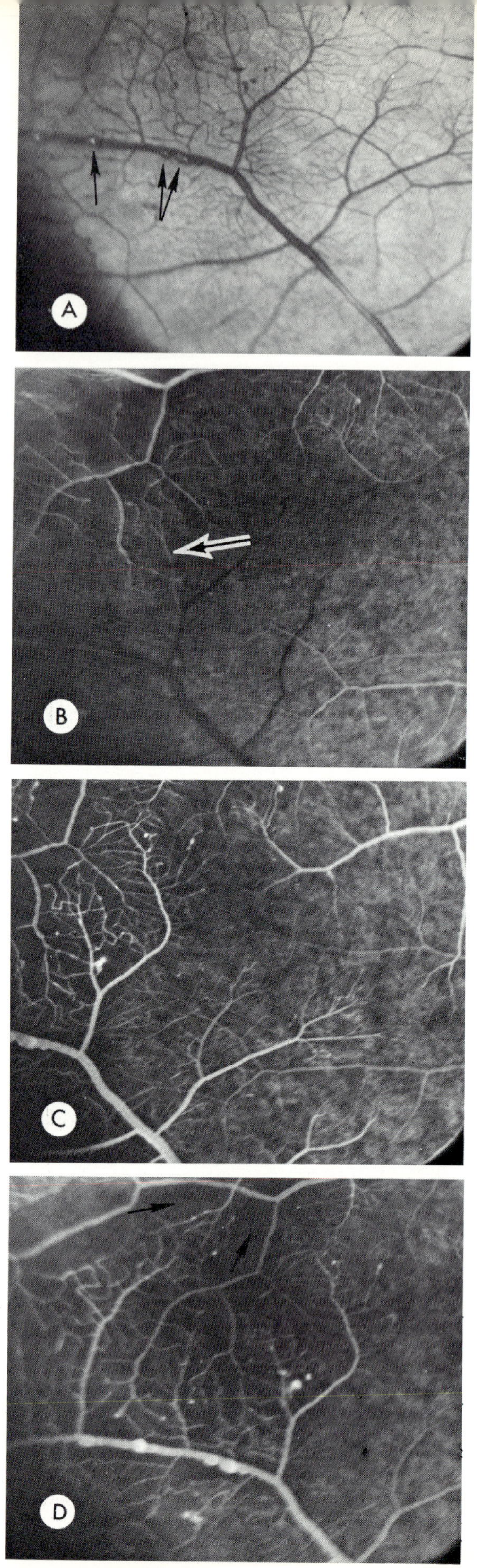

Fig. 11-9. *Opposite page.* Leber's multiple miliary aneurysms with retinal degeneration.

A, An area of vascular abnormality without exudation. Some retinal capillaries are abnormally prominent. Capillary microaneurysms and aneurysmal dilatations **(arrows)** of a vein are present.

B, Fluorescein angiogram of *A* showing capillary arteriovenous shunt **(arrow).**

C, Arteriovenous phase showing preferential filling of abnormal capillaries.

D, A later phase showing filling of the venous aneurysmal dilatations and nonperfusion of many capillaries, especially around the arteries **(arrows).**

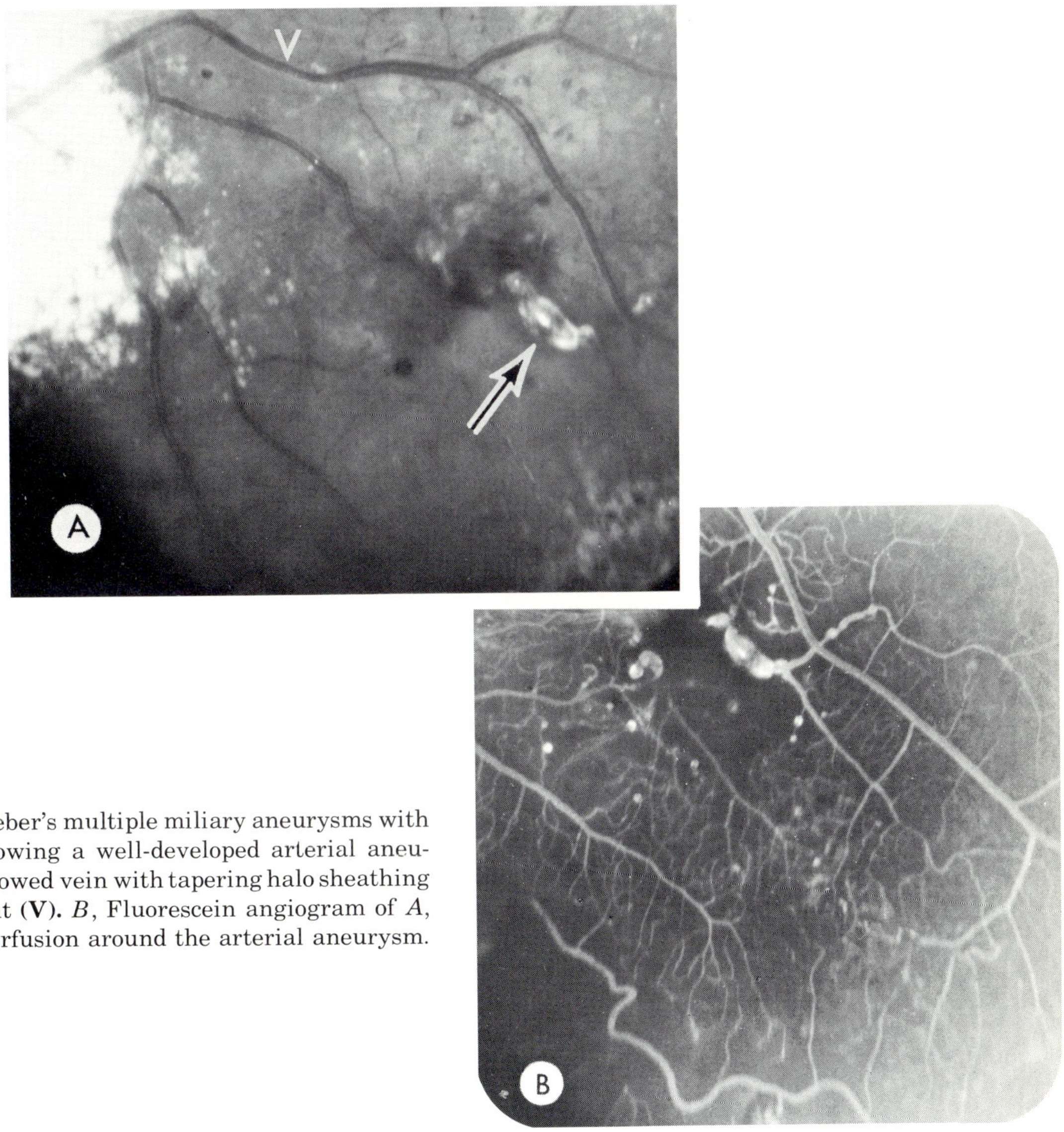

Fig. 11-10. *Right. A*, Leber's multiple miliary aneurysms with retinal degeneration showing a well-developed arterial aneurysm **(arrow)** and a narrowed vein with tapering halo sheathing of the narrowed segment **(V).** *B*, Fluorescein angiogram of *A*, showing capillary nonperfusion around the arterial aneurysm.

cular changes always precede fatty exudation. The latter develop as small clumps or arcs around or among the aneurysms. A few retinal hemorrhages and deep retinal edema can both be seen. Occasionally in such regions, arteriovenous communications may be visible, but it is often hard to be certain of this observation. One or two small arterial branches in this zone are often very burnished and sclerosed, and may show a string of arterial "aneurysms." Similarly, small venous radicals may show marked beading, highly irregular halo sheathing, and considerable variability in lumen caliber (Fig. 11-10*A*. A narrowed segment of vein, with dense halo sheathing at the point of narrowing is not uncommon.

Rarely, extreme capillary dilatation and microaneurysms will appear over a broad region with so little other pathology that the changes in this area of the microcirculation can be well seen. In the two cases like this which we have observed, the periarterial capillary-free zone of a trespassing artery was as readily visible by slit-lamp examination as that in a retinal digest specimen under the dissecting microscope. Much of the capillary network was invisible, the dilated, obvious capillaries representing only a portion of the entire bed. Several arteriovenous communications were easily seen and some of these appeared to be joined via an irregular, widely dilated, capillary channel (Fig. 11-9).

In the nonexudative vascular lesions some areas show little change over periods of months. Others show periodic activity with developing exudates, hemorrhages, aneurysms, and vessel changes. Still others slowly regress. New zones of previously uninvolved retina at the border of the diseased areas may themselves become involved, or new areas of active disease may develop at a distance.

Three cases, originally diagnosed as Leber's multiple miliary aneurysms with retinal degeneration, have been observed to progress with ultimate formation of typical retinal angioma.

Fluorescein angiography of the more markedly diseased areas has shown arteriovenous shunts, leakage from involved capillaries and veins, delayed emptying from other involved vessels, nonfilling of many capillaries in the areas of shunts, and some patches of unfilled capillaries (Fig. 11-9). The bulbous arterial "aneurysms" usually lie in one of these nonperfused capillary regions (Fig. 11-10). The lumens of such "aneurysms" are smooth and of normal or slightly irregular bore, thus these lesions are not true aneurysms. There is no leak of fluorescein from their walls and no slowing of its passage through them.

Treatment

Only those lesions near the macula and those progressing to actual angiomas require treatment. Macula-centered lesions are obviously untreatable, but those off-center whose circinate exudates pass through the fovea should be treated early (Figs. 11-11 and 11-12). If the center of such ring lesions is destroyed by photocoagulation, the exudative ring will absorb and this result can be obtained before permanent macular damage ensues.

COATS'S DISEASE

Clinical and Microscopic Findings

Coats [16] originally described three types of this disease: Type I, massive subretinal exudation without vascular change; Type II, massive subretinal exudation with vascular changes; and Type III, massive subretinal exudation with arteriovenous communications.

Von Hippel [77] later showed that Coats's Type III was actually a retinal angioma and

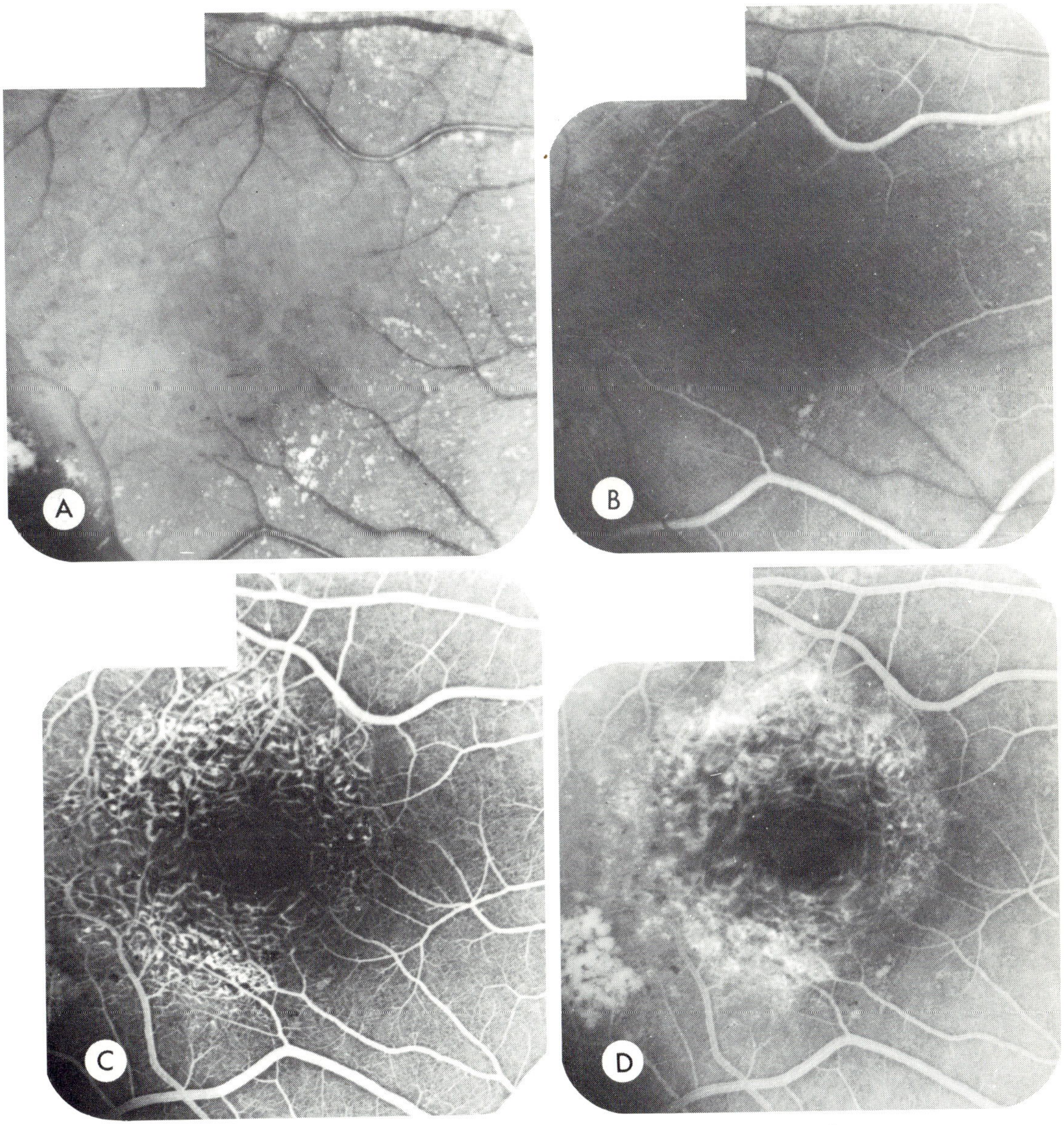

Fig. 11-11. Leber's multiple miliary aneurysms with retinal degeneration. Marked vascular abnormalities in the entire temporal periphery and a ring of fatty exudates around the macular. *A,* Retinal microaneurysms and intraretinal macular edema. *B,* Arterial-phase fluorescein angiogram. *C,* Arteriovenous phase showing marked dilatation of the perimacular capillaries. *D,* Late phase showing leakage from capillaries producing the intraretinal edema.

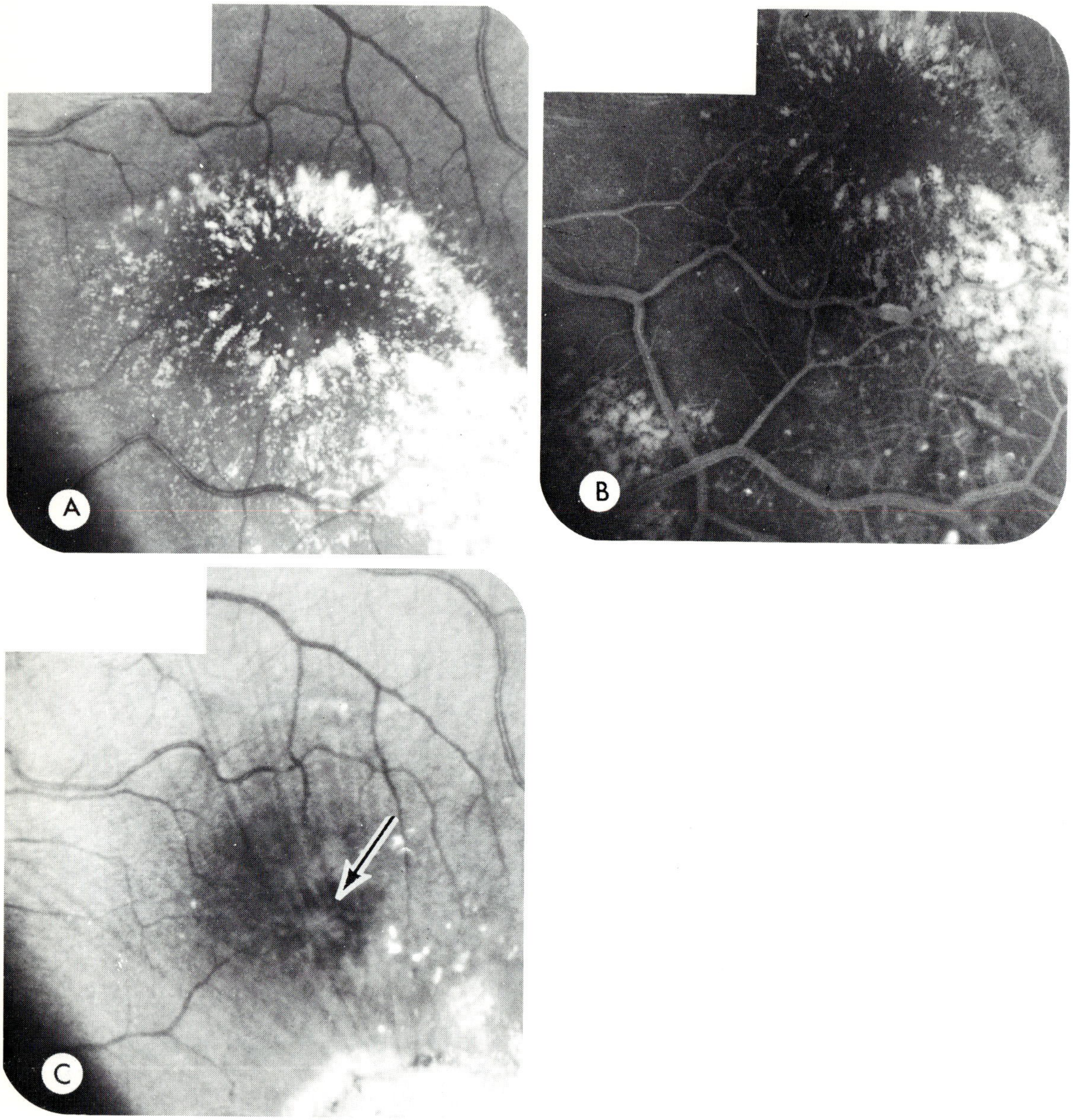

Fig. 11-12. Leber's multiple miliary aneurysms with retinal degeneration in a 44-year-old male. *A,* Fatty exudation collects in Henle's layer around the fovea secondary to a large ring lesion around abnormal vessels below the macula. Only a portion of this ring is shown. *B,* Fluorescein angiogram showing vascular abnormalities. *C,* twenty-five weeks after the second photocoagulation of the area of vascular abnormalities. The perifoveal exudates have disappeared and retinal traction lines have developed through the fovea **(arrow).** Vision improved from 20/40 to 20/25.

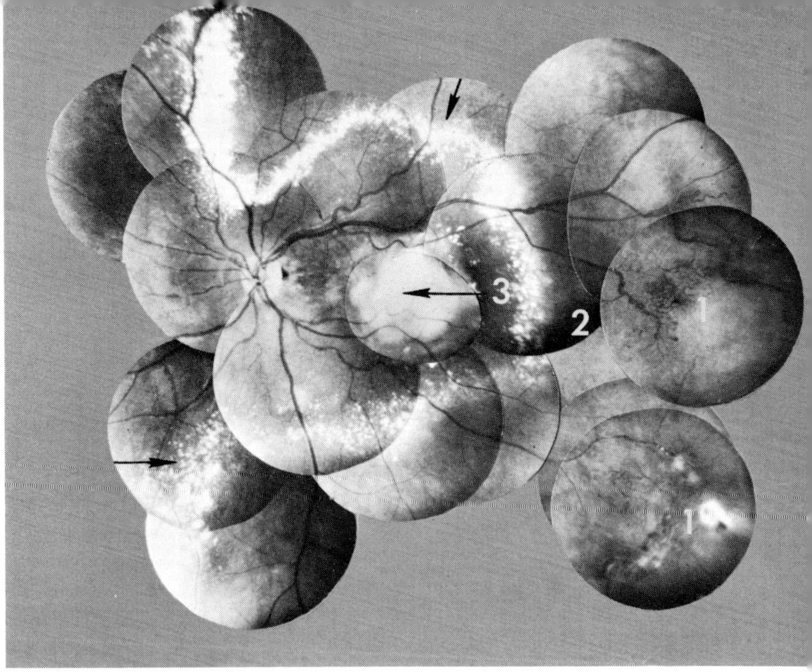

Fig. 11-13. Coats's disease in a child. Note areas of vascular malformation **(1)**; exudate free zone **(2)**; macular mound of exudation **(3)**; scattered fatty exudates posteriorly **(arrows)**. Compare with Fig. 11-2.

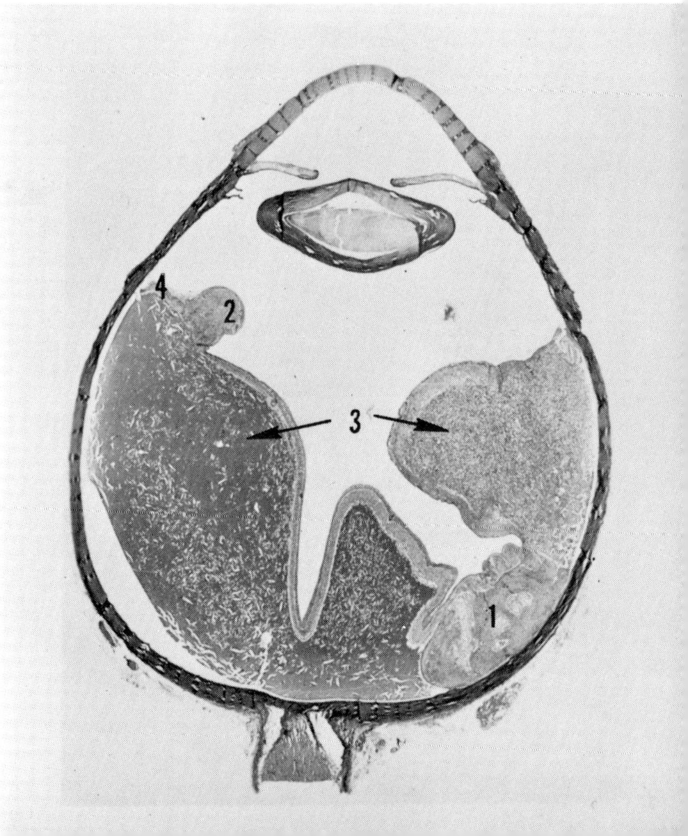

Fig. 11-14. Cross section of a globe with Coats's disease shows mounds of diseased retina of various ages. The oldest contracted mound **(1)** shows the typical pathology of late disease and includes a subretinal choroidal vascular connection through Bruch's membrane. The next oldest mound **(2)** shows subretinal neovascular fibrosis from the retina as do the more recent mounds **(3)**. There is preretinal neovascular fibrosis from superficial retinal capillaries at the ora **(4)** and in other sections, from the disc area. There was no preretinal nor subretinal hemorrhage in this patient (Courtesy of the Armed Forces Institute of Pathology, Washington, D.C. From Wise. *Amer J. Ophthal. 52*:637, 1961.)

this concept has retained universal acceptance since that time.

Both Types I and II occur primarily in the young and are almost invariably uniocular. Occurrence in older individuals, although more rare, has been reported.[22,37,73,80,95]

Type I is characterized by widespread, subretinal fatty exudation, normal retinal vasculature, the absence of hemorrhage and aneurysms, and a better ultimate prognosis. Marshall and Michaelson[52] have described five such cases. Microscopically the choroid, pigment epithelium, and inner retina were well preserved but there was a subretinal layer of fatty exudation and fatty granular cells approximately twice the retinal thickness. Type I is rarer than Type II and we have only observed it in older individuals. Two of the latter developed from highly exudative senile disciform macular degenerations. In both, only those areas which remained free of exudation retained retinal function. In one, when the exudate finally absorbed from the lower half of the retina, there remained a scattered pigment migration and proliferation suggesting healed, disseminated chorioretinitis.[80] In addition, there were foci of subretinal gliosis and some inspissated, yellowish clumps of old fatty exudate. Both arteries and veins showed a dirty, yellowish white uniform sheathing. The disc showed no atrophy.

Type II Coats's disease is more common and may start in the periphery, or posteriorly. It is characterized by sheets or mounds of subretinal exudation and foci of irregularly dilated capillaries, large microaneurysms, and bizarre configurations of twisted, sausage-like, hugely dilated vascular channels (Fig. 11-13). Clinically these have the appearance of veins, although microscopically it is, at times, hard to differentiate artery from vein. Subretinal hemorrhage, at times extensive, is mixed with exudate and gives a dirty, dark color. Mounds of detached retina, solidly elevated by massive, subretinal, fatty exudation and hemorrhage, have developed at different stages in the disease and microscopically appear of varying ages (Fig. 11-14). Sometimes heavy exudation will surround a zone of bizarre vessels and microaneurysms, or ring a dome-shaped mound darkened by a mixture of subretinal blood and exudation. At other times a heavy tongue of exudate with its archipelago-like borders will jut out into an otherwise normal retinal area, bearing no apparent relation to the retinal vessels (Fig. 11-15).

This type of Coats's disease may reach a certain stage and spontaneously regress with settling and contracture of the mounds by subretinal neovascular fibrosis, or the disease may proceed to rubeosis iridis, secondary glaucoma, and eventual loss of the globe.

Useful information of the early pathology has been derived from those eyes removed early in the disease process with the mistaken diagnosis of retinoblastoma.[87] Retinoblastoma may be mistaken for Coats's disease when exudate is present, for rarely it has the yellowish color and appearance of the fatty exudation seen in Coats's disease. New areas of retinal elevation show normal choroid and pigment epithelium. Between the latter and the retina there are massive PAS-positive fatty exudation, fatty granular cells, and occasional cholesterin clefts. The rods and cones are degenerated and there is early degeneration of dilated, deep retinal capillaries. Exudate appears to leak from these damaged retinal vessels and streams through outer retinal elements and subretinally (Fig. 11-16). A little later, tufts of new vessels with delicate associated fibrosis grow down through the retina and extend along its undersurface (Fig. 11-17). Most of these arise from dilated capillaries of the superficial bed, the deep bed having been largely destroyed. By this time most of the outer nuclear layer has been lost but inner retinal layers remain relatively well preserved.

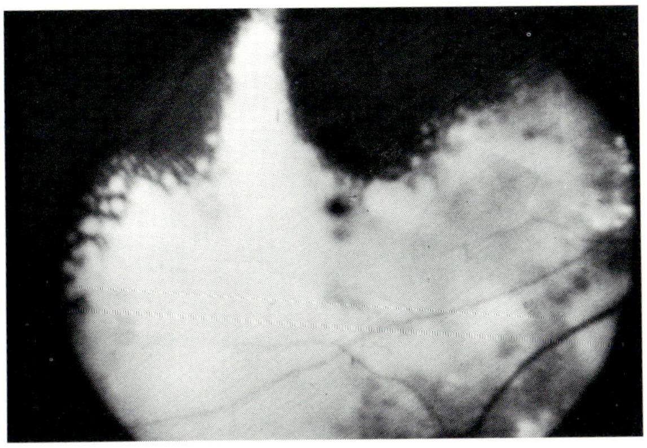

Fig. 11-15. Coats's disease. Massive exudation showing archipelago-like borders (From Wise.[80])

Fig. 11-16. *Left.* Histologic appearance of early Coats's disease. Exudate **(arrow)** streams from the deep retinal capillary bed through the disorganized outer retina and subretinally **(SR)** (Courtesy of the Armed Forces Institute of Pathology, Washington, D.C.)

Fig. 11-17. *Right.* Neovascular tuft arises from the superficial capillary bed and extends subretinally beneath the mound **(2)** shown in Fig. 11-14. (Courtesy of the Armed Forces Institute of Pathology, Washington, D.C. From Wise. *Amer. J. Ophthal. 52:*637, 1961.)

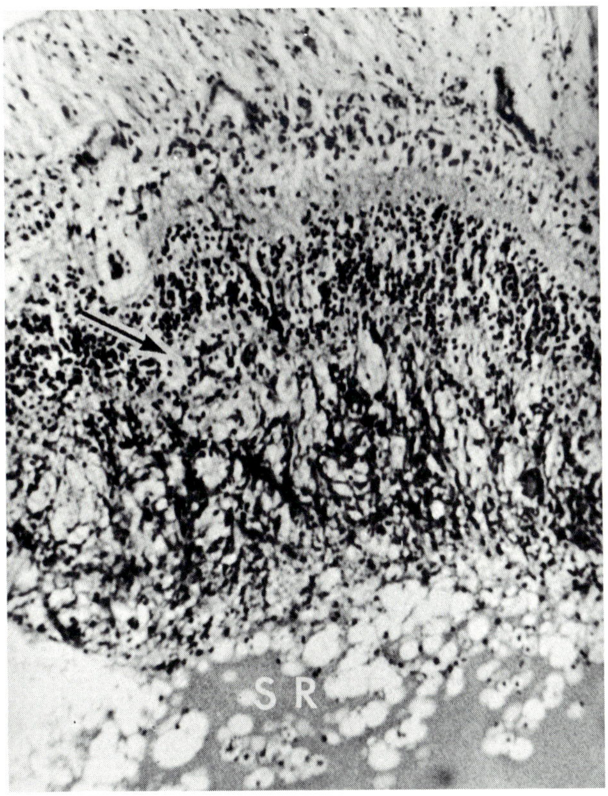

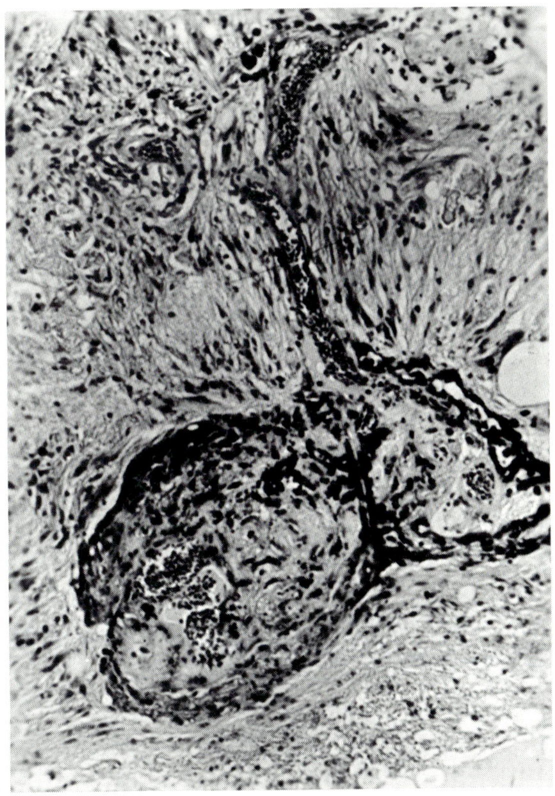

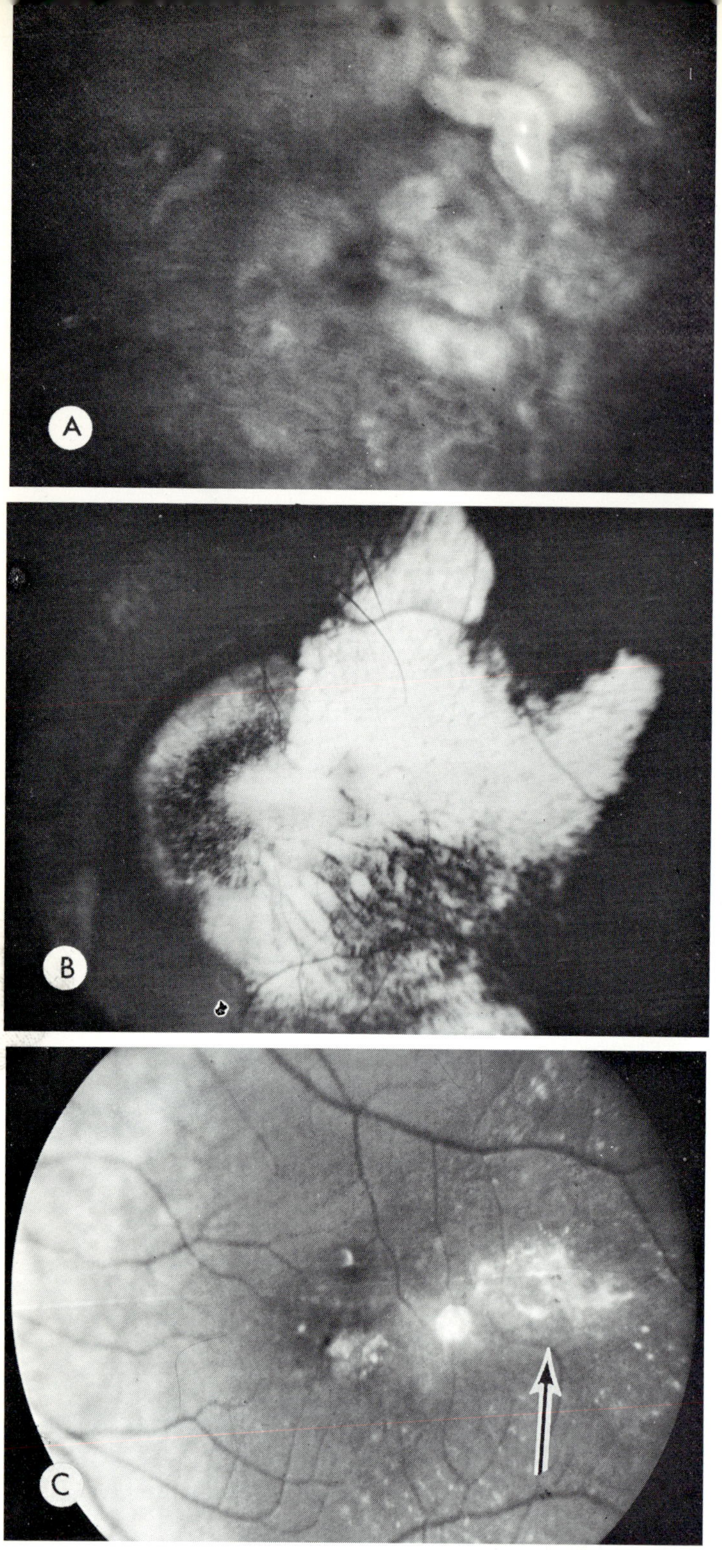

Fig. 11-18. Coats's disease in left eye of a 6-year-old boy. *A,* Vascular malformation in the far temporal periphery. *B,* Macular mound of exudation. Vision 14/200. *C,* Macular area of left eye, 5½ years after diathermic destruction of vascular malformation. Inspissated fatty exudates **(arrow)** persist. Following treatment, the left eye was amblyopic until the vision in right eye was destroyed several years later by an injury. Vision in left eye then improved to 20/40+. (Courtesy of Dr. M. Charlap.)

From this point on, the subretinal neovascularization is associated with an increasing fibrosis until eventually, the latter is predominant. Slowly, subretinal hemorrhages and exudates are absorbed, pigment proliferates and migrates, and the mound settles against the choroid as a contracted, fibrosed, pigmented retinal scar (Fig. 11-14 (1)). Later, ruptures of Bruch's membrane with an ingrowth of neovascular fibrosis beneath the mound may contribute to the subretinal scar tissue.

Treatment

The early successes reported [75] in the treatment of Coats's disease by photocoagulation of anomalous vascular formations suggests that this form of treatment has considerable merit and should be undertaken at the earliest possible moment, for it is well-known that untreated Coats's disease has a very poor visual prognosis (Fig. 11-18).

RACEMOSE ANGIOMA

The racemose angioma (arteriovenous aneurysm of the retina, retinal arteriovenous fistula, racemose hemangioma, cirscoid aneurysm) is very rare. The disease, in its full form, involves the retina, optic nerve, and midbrain. According to Wyburn-Mason [96] over 75 per cent of the patients have both retinal and midbrain lesions.

The retinal lesion usually involves one or more retinal sectors including the optic disc. Extreme degrees of worm-like, dilated, twisting vessels are characteristic of the anomaly. Numerous involved veins develop arterialized walls and contain arterial blood due to many small and larger arteriovenous shunts. This makes differentiation of artery from vein clinically difficult at times. Involved vessels are usually evenly contoured and smoothly graded (Fig. 11-19).

When the retinal lesions are quiescent, as is the usual case, they may persist unchanged for years. The retina usually shows almost no clinical reaction, no hemorrhages, edema or exudation; and these bizarre vessels may very closely approach the macula without interference with visual acuity. Uninvolved retinal areas appear normal.

Fluorescein angiography is very helpful in demonstrating the abnormal arteriovenous connections. Quiescent cases show no vascular fluorescein leakage (Fig. 11-19).

Krug and Samuels [42] have reported the microscopic findings in an involved eye. Huge vessels monopolized the retinal thickness and the optic nerve. The retinal tissue among the abnormal vessels showed cystic degeneration. Cameron and Greer [15a] have described the microscopic findings in a similar case involving the right retina, optic nerve, optic tract, geniculate body and midbrain.

The racemous angioma is not easily mistaken clinically and bears so little relation to the other anomalous vascular formations that it is not included in the following discussion.

INTERRELATIONSHIPS OF ANOMALOUS VASCULAR FORMATIONS

Both Leber's multiple miliary aneurysms with retinal degeneration and angiomatosis retinae demonstrate many of the same features; brilliant arteries hiding the veins at crossings, retinal microaneurysms, larger arterial "aneurysms," severe arteriosclerosis and beading in the more involved areas, arteriovenous communications, fatty exudates, and an identical type of venous sheathing and beading. Both diseases may be bilateral.

On the other hand, there are striking differences between the two. Leber's disease appears to involve primarily the smaller retinal vessels, is milder but often more wide-

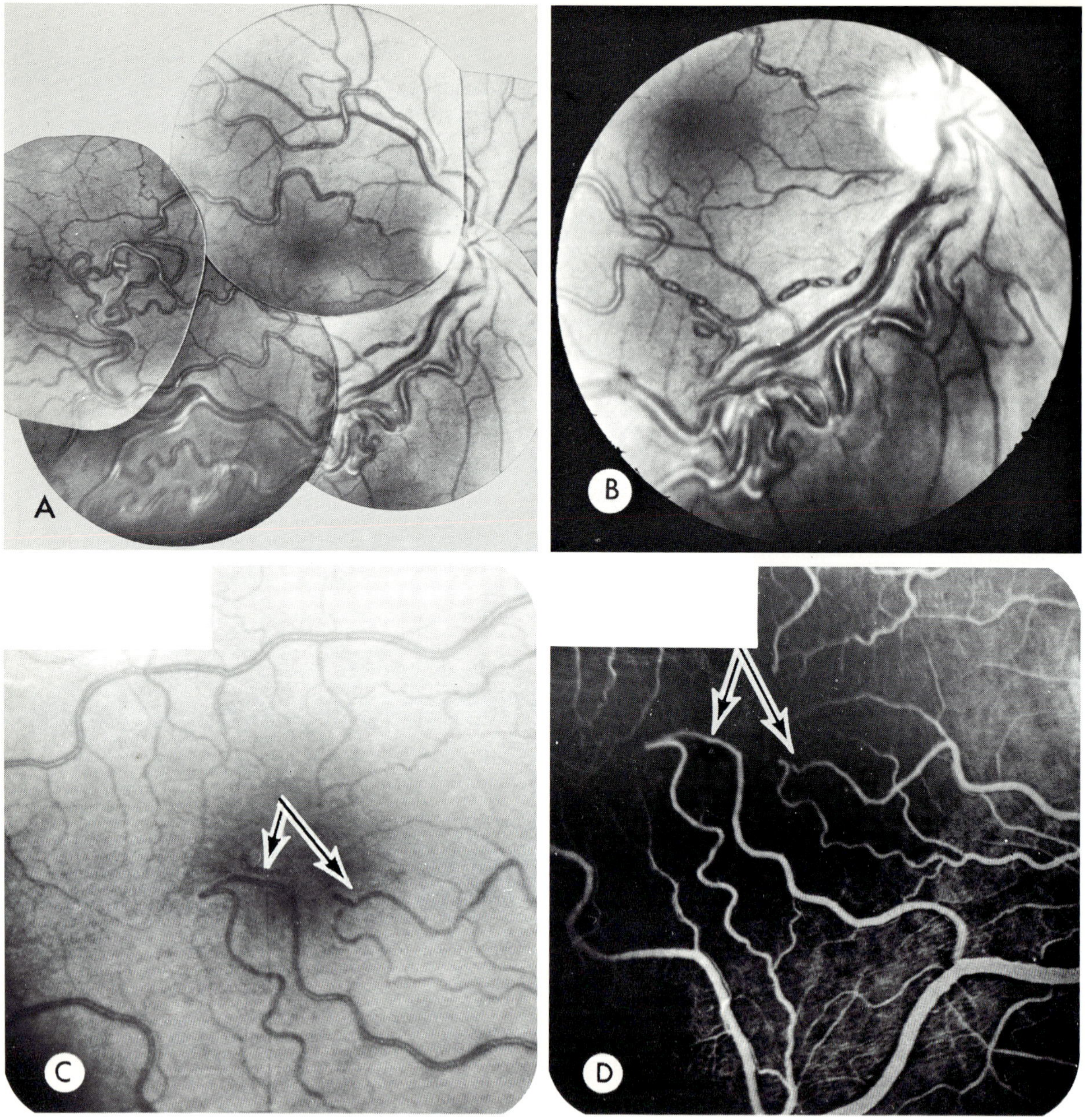

Fig. 11-19. *A*, Racemose angioma in right eye. Vision 20/20. *B*, Enlargement of a segment of *A* showing abnormal vessels. *C*, Another case of racemose angioma with two arteriovenous communications (**arrows**) near the macula. Vision 20/20. *D*, Fluorescein angiogram of *C* in arteriovenous phase.

spread in its retinal distribution, and individual areas of involvement have a strong tendency to spontaneously regress. Because of the latter, an involved retina will often show several localities of disease in different phases of evolution or resolution. Unlike angiomatosis retinae, no systemic manifestations have been reported in Leber's disease and no genetic study of it has been made.

Retinal angioma is an ocular manifestation of a genetically determined systemic disease. The tumors may be single or multiple and of varying sizes but all are steadily progressive in development, although haltingly so in some cases. In their early stages retinal angioma and Leber's disease have similarities, but as the angiomas enlarge they develop their typical enlarged draining and feeding vessels. During this stage they have their most characteristic features and are most easily diagnosed. Three patients with Leber's disease have eventually developed such retinal angiomas.

With further angiomatous development and increasing exudation the clinical features tend to merge with those of Type II Coats's disease. Type II Coats's disease with a cluster of malformed, dilated vessels in the temporal periphery may show the same distribution of retinal exudates as is seen in the large temporal angioma (Fig. 11-2), i.e., scattered exudates at the posterior pole, a massive mound of exudation at the macula, and both exudation and cystic changes about the site of the abnormal vessels (see Fig. 11-13). Retinal arteries and veins toward this area may be dilated, but they do not show the tremendously dilated paired artery and vein seen in a typical angioma. Except for this latter feature, and the clusters of malformed vessels instead of the solitary angioma, the vascular changes and exudation of one disease are little different from the other. Coats's disease does differ from retinal angioma in that it is almost invariably uniocular and is not genetically determined.

As vascular malformations and angioma are not considered separately in cerebrovascular disease and both have arteriovenous shunts as their salient feature, should one not suspect that they are comparable in the retina? Obviously, the retinal pathology of Type II Coats's disease is dependent on something occurring in the region of vascular malformation, for eradication of this area is attended with healing of the disease process (Fig. 11-18). In all likelihood multiple, small arteriovenous communications may be discovered in these angiomatous malformations of Type II Coats's disease and it will rejoin angiomatosis retinae as a simple variant of a similar disease process.

In this connection, Henkind and Morgan's finding of unsuspected angiomatous malformations hidden by exudate and not seen clinically in three of their patients[37] suggests that some cases clinically diagnosed as Type I Coats's disease may in actuality be Type II Coats's disease.

RETINAL NEOVASCULARIZATION

For the purposes of this discussion new vessels are defined as those growing inside the internal limiting membrane or anywhere between the deep retinal capillary bed and the choriocapillaris. Both of these zones are normally avascular, so that any vessels in either must therefore be newly formed. The formation of new vessels within the normally vascular areas of the retina is much more difficult to assess. While they probably do form, and certain fluorescein patterns suggest their presence, it is still impossible, either clinically or microscopically, to identify any except those at the borders of normally vascularized retina directly continuous with obvious neovascularization. Most of the abnormal vascular channels seen between the deep retinal capillary bed and the internal limiting membrane are probably modifications of preexistent vessels and are therefore not considered true neovascular formations.

The associated proliferation of fibrous connective tissue must be considered in any discussion of retinal neovascularization. While new retinal vessel formations may at times appear clinically to be devoid of an associated fibrosis, naked neovascular growths without an accompanying fibrous scaffold have never been demonstrated microscopically. Similarly, preretinal fibrosis having no clinically visible new vessels, may show microscopic fine neovascular channels hidden in the connective tissue.

Retinitis proliferans was the term originally used to describe the growth of new vessels and their accompanying connective tissue into the vitreous. Coats [16] was the first to suggest that subretinal proliferation of fibrovascular tissue might be an example of this same phenomena and that both might prove to have a common etiology. Both were at that time considered to result from the organization of preexistent hemorrhage.

The idea that retinitis proliferans resulted from the organization of preexistent hemorrhage was firmly held until about 1940 when it was first challenged by Klien,[41] Salzmann,[69] and Ballantyne.[10]

Ballantyne [10] divided retinitis proliferans into two types, reté and fibrotic. In the reté form the proliferation was predominantly vascular. Delicate new vessels of capillary structure having wide lumens, and their associated, scarcely visible, fibrous scaffolding grew on the inner retinal surface. Clinically, Ballantyne saw that these vessels were attached to small veins and he demonstrated their microscopic connections with both retinal veins and capillaries. In fibrotic retinitis proliferans, the fibrotic connective tissue predominated and vessels when present were often larger, but fewer in number. The late stages of this type could appear avascular. The vessels of fibrotic proliferans have also been shown histologically to be connected to retinal veins.[41] Ballantyne [10] believed that his reté proliferans developed without antecedent hemorrhage but still attributed the fibrotic type to the organization of preexistent hemorrhage.

HYPOTHESIS OF ETIOLOGY

In a study of retinitis proliferans in various retinal diseases, Wise [82] has noted the similarities of the neovascularization in each. He also traced the development of reté into fibrotic proliferans and showed that in most cases reté proliferans represented an early phase and fibrotic proliferans a late stage in the normal life history of retinitis proliferans. Retinal capillary or vein disease commonly preceded preretinal neovascular formations while new vessels failed to develop following retinal artery obstructions. The only arterial obstructive disease followed by preretinal neovascularization was pulseless disease, a condition in which the site of arterial obstruction was at the aortic arch, some distance from the eye.

Any hypothesis to explain retinitis proliferans must be compatible with the following clinical observations:

1. Viable retinal tissue is essential for the development of retinitis proliferans. It does not occur in a completely infarcted retina or retinal area.

2. When proliferative retinopathy occurs subsequent to vein obstruction, it may develop anywhere in the obstructed region. A strand may bridge unobstructed retina and be attached at the disc, or rarely be connected to adjacent unobstructed retina.

3. In severe, acute vein obstructions heavy fibrovascular proliferans may occur initially without a reté phase.

4. Following retinal vein obstruction,

rapidly developing and adequate intraretinal collateral circulation, or early recanalization of the obstructed vein are both deterrents to the vasoproliferative response.

5. In the presence of retinitis proliferans signs of improved retinal circulation are often associated with a decrease in the proliferating fibrous and vascular tissues.

6. Retinitis proliferans associated with the aortic arch syndrome usually starts in the peripheral retina.

7. A young retina is more reactive than an elderly retina.

As a working hypothesis Wise [82] has proposed that, following retinal capillary or vein obstruction, involved retinal cells become hypoxic but not necrotic. If recanalization of an obstructed vein or collateral circulation developed promptly, normal tissue nutrition was restored and no vasoproliferative response ensued. If, however, retinal cells remained viable and critically hypoxic, they produced a vasoproliferative stimulus and neovascularization developed primarily from preexistent retinal veins and capillaries and grew through the internal limiting membrane and along the inner retinal surface. In retinal artery obstructions, cell death prevented the elaboration of a vasoformative stimulus and no vasoproliferation followed. In pulseless disease, which produces a slowly decreasing arterial inflow to the eye, some retinal cells die but others remain viable and sufficiently hypoxic to produce a vasoformative stimulant. As this slowly decreasing arterial inflow first fails peripherally, the vasoproliferation of this disease is first seen in these peripheral regions.

This same hypothesis was used to explain the subretinal fibrovascular proliferation of Coats's disease and retrolental fibroplasia.[80, 83] In its further support, Baum and Wise [13] experimentally produced subretinal fibrovascular proliferation in the adult cat by obstructing the retinal veins and injecting subretinal fluorosilicone to block choriocapillary nutrition of outer retinal elements. They showed its microscopic similarity to that of human Coats's disease.[85]

The complete hypothesis may be summarized as follows. In the normal human eye, the retina lies against the choroid and its outer avascular zone is supplied by the choroidal circulation; the inner vascularized retina is supplied by retinal vessels. Following retinal capillary or vein obstruction, or during the course of pulseless disease, involved retinal cells become hypoxic but do not die. They elaborate a vasoproliferative stimulus and fibrovascular proliferation develops in response along the inner retinal surface and toward the vitreous (Fig. 11-20). Outer retinal cells are adequately nourished by the intact and adjacent choroidal circulation, no vasoformative stimulus develops in these cells and here neovascularization does not occur.

Simple detachment of the embryonic reactive retina or detachment plus the blocking effect of subretinal exudation in the less

Fig. 11-20. Schematic representation of the hypothesis of preretinal and subretinal neovascular formations (see text for details). (From Wise. *Amer. J. Ophthal. 52:*637, 1961.)

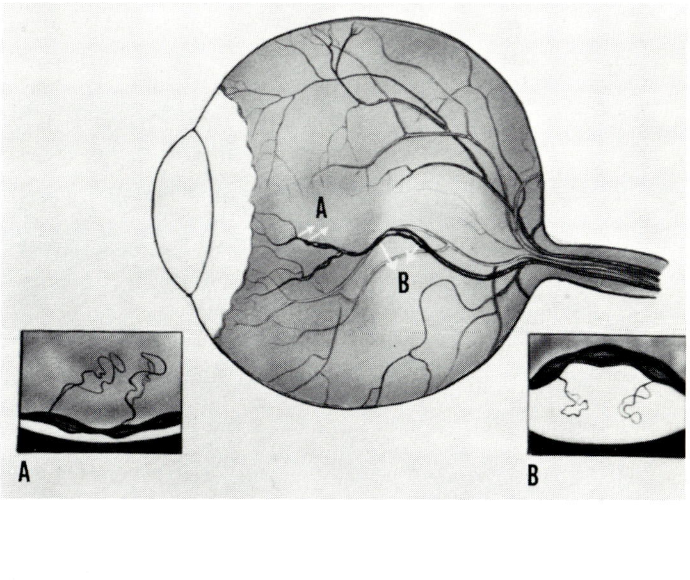

reactive adult retina, in conjunction with retinal capillary or vein obstruction, produces hypoxic inner retinal cells but much more hypoxic outer retinal cells. The latter are now removed from their choriocapillary blood supply, partially blocked from it by the subretinal exudation, and thereby dependent on diffusion from an already embarrassed retinal circulation. In these circumstances the vasoproliferative stimulus will be greater in outer retinal cells and neovascular development will proceed downward and extend along the undersurface of the retina (Fig. 11-20). Simple retinal detachment in the presence of a normal adult choroidal and retinal circulation produces insufficient cellular hypoxia to elaborate any vasoformative stimulus and neovascularization under these circumstances does not occur.

The actual vasoformative stimulant or stimulants is unknown. While retinal metabolism is normally predominantly oxidative, it is fully capable of conversion in part to a less efficient anaerobic metabolism.[26] Hypoxic retinal cells would be expected to undergo such conversion and the altered metabolic pathways or any of the byproducts of such altered metabolism could represent the vasoformative factor. That the vasoformative factor is not produced by degenerating retinal cells[60] is shown by the absence of preretinal proliferans in arterial obstructions and neovascular growth beneath the macula in central areolar choroidal sclerosis.[1] In the former, dead retinal cells are replaced by a mild intraretinal gliosis, and in the latter even gliosis is absent, the inner nuclear retinal layer lying directly against Bruch's membrane. In neither does vasoproliferation take place. The long-held concept that preexistent blood acted as a vasoproliferative stimulant is slowly being discarded as increasing evidence of neovascularization in the absence of hemorrhage accumulates.[2,19,23,45,82] Although the actual vasostimulating factor is unknown, it is closely related to cellular hypoxia. It seems appropriate therefore to use the term "hypoxia," which is both short and descriptive of the cellular milieu from which the stimulant arises, until the actual factor is identified.

MORPHOLOGY AND NATURAL HISTORY

Retinal neovascularization appears to originate and develop in the same manner regardless of the disease in which it occurs. In human retrolental fibroplasia, where its early stages have been studied, multiplication of endothelial cells in patent superficial retinal capillaries is the earliest visible evidence of new vessel formation[83] (Fig. 11-21). In experimental subretinal neovascularization[13] a cell with a large, elongated, pale, ovoid nucleus and thin, strand-like cytoplasm is first seen penetrating the mid- or external retina (Fig. 11-22). The origin of this cell has not been determined. Early, it has both glial and mesenchymal staining characteristics but later it has more of the morphological and staining features of a fibroblast. It is probably derived from the endothelium of retinal capillaries and is at this stage undifferentiated. The potential ability of endothelial cells to differentiate into fibroblasts supports the mesoblastic origin of neovascular channels.

The fibroblastic component of new vessel formations has a marked tendency to drag adjacent retinal tissues along with it as it grows and contracts. Preretinal neovascularization usually grows along the retinal surface or posterior face of the hyaloid. Subretinal new vessels prefer the undersurface of the retina but at times are attached to Bruch's membrane. As growth extends and fibrous strands contract, the more rigid Bruch's membrane retains its normal configuration but the retina is thrown into ridges and folds – short unattached stretches of retina buckling inward to create a scal-

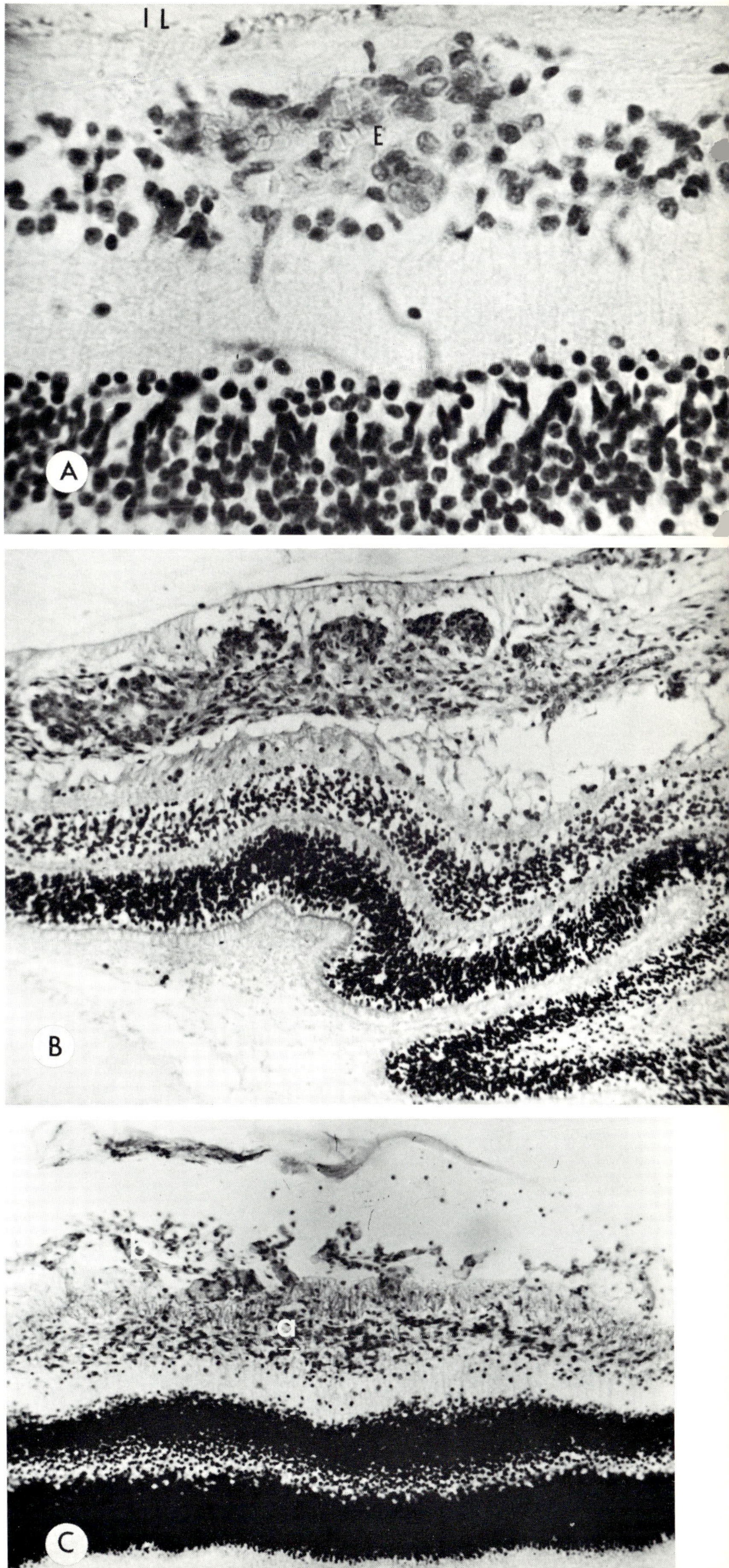

Fig. 11-21. Early human retrolental fibroplasia.

A, A nest of proliferating endothelial cells **(E)** in the nerve fiber layer. Internal limiting membrane **(IL).** This is the initial evidence of vascular proliferation. (Courtesy of the Armed Forces Institute of Pathology, Washington, D.C.)

B, Multiple nests of proliferating intraretinal endothelial cells simulating the preretinal glomerular tufts seen at a slightly later stage. (Courtesy of the Armed Forces Institute of Pathology, Washington, D.C.)

C, Endothelial cell proliferation in the inner retinal layers **(a)** and neovascular formation on the inner retinal surface. (From Wise. *Amer. J. Ophthal. 52:*637, 1961.)

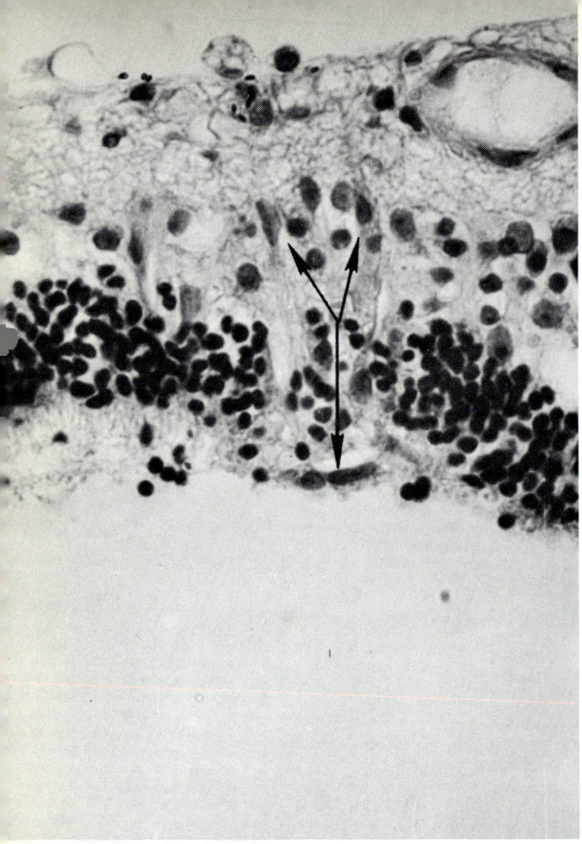

Fig. 11-22. *Left.* Experimental subretinal neovascularization in the adult cat. The earliest subretinal cellular proliferation are indicated by **arrows.** (From Baum and Wise. *Amer. J. Ophthal. 61:*528, 1966.)

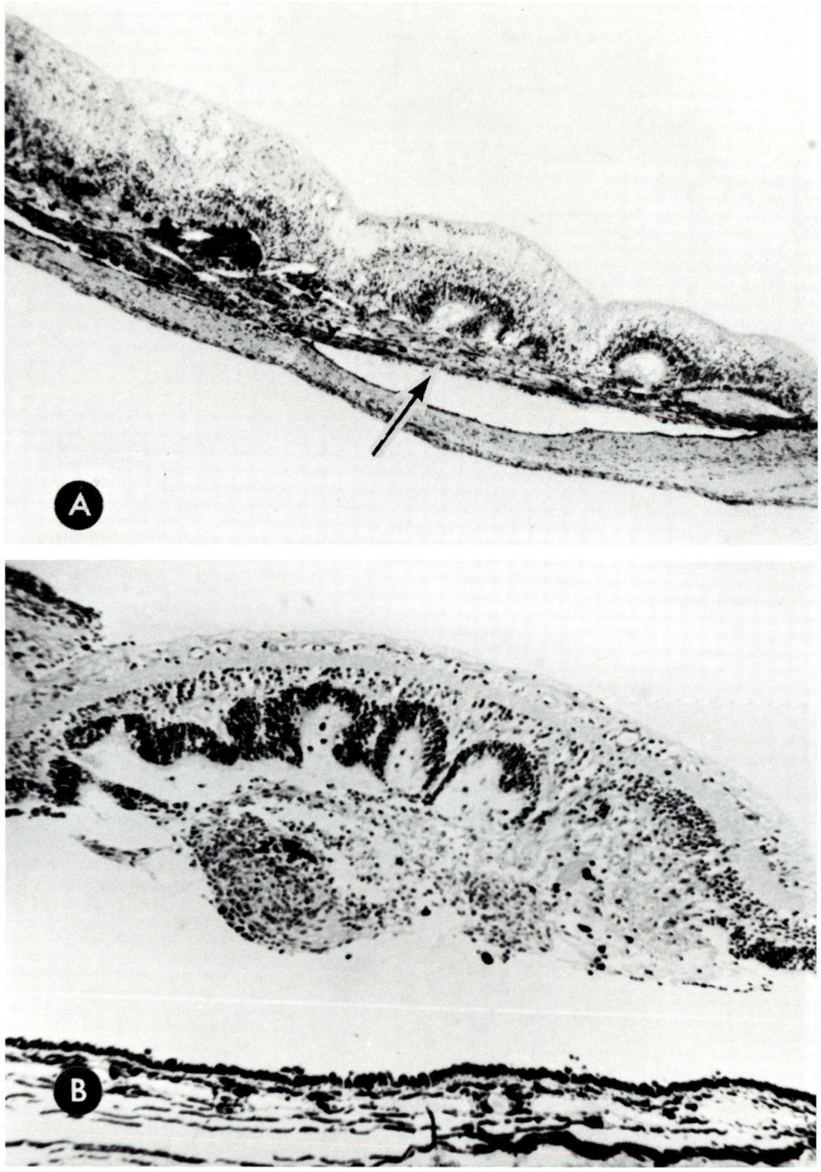

Fig. 11-23. *A*, Human Coats's disease showing subretinal fibrosis (**arrow**) contracting and drawing the retina into scalloped folds. (Courtesy of the Armed Forces Institute of Pathology, Washington, D.C.) *B*, Similar appearance of the subretinal fibrosis and its effect on the retina from experimental subretinal neovascularization in the adult cat.

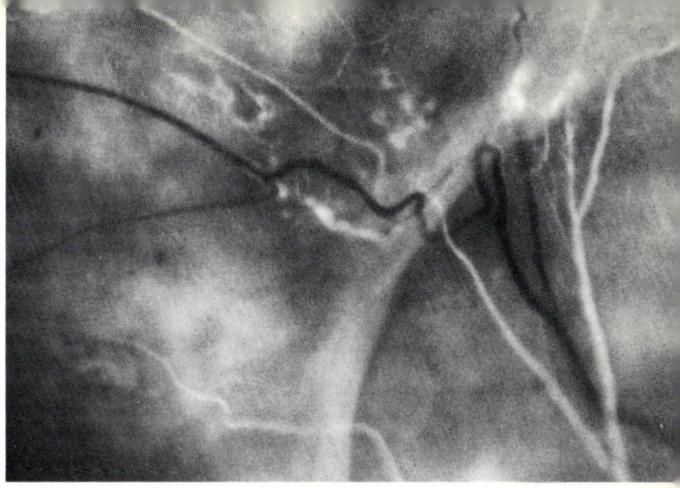

Fig. 11-24. Fluorescein angiogram of diabetic retinitis proliferans showing contracting scar tissue tenting the retina.

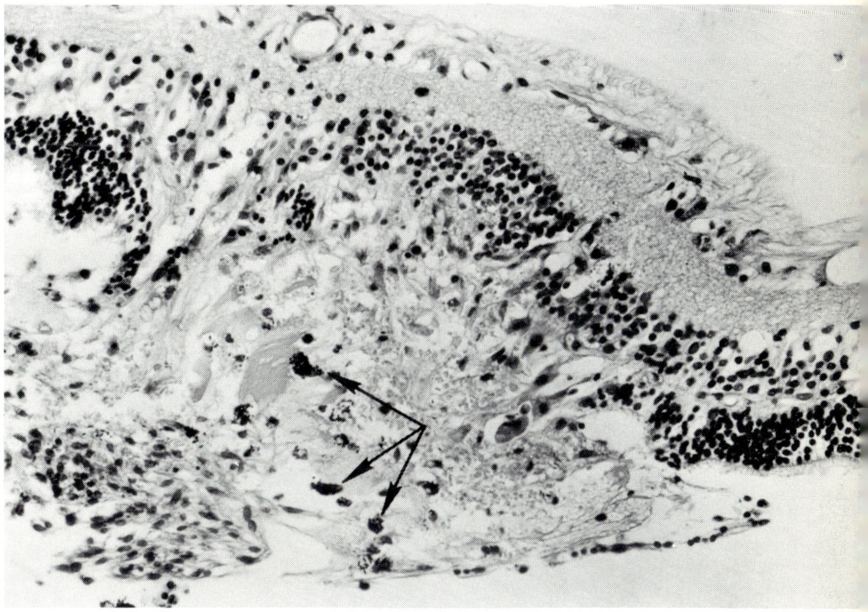

Fig. 11-25. Experimental subretinal neovascularization in the adult cat showing affinity of pigment **(arrows)** for subretinal new vessels.

loped appearance in cross-sectional view (Fig. 11-23). Retinal folds and tented retinal elevations are common with preretinal proliferans, the nonresistant posterior hyaloid becoming entangled with the retina (Fig. 11-24).

There is a marked affinity of pigment granules or clumps of ingested or proliferated pigment epithelium for the walls of subretinal neovascular channels. This has been seen in human retrolental fibroplasia and Coats's disease [83] (Fig. 11-17) and was equally obvious in experimental subretinal neovascularization [13] (Fig. 11-25). This finding is unusual in preretinal new vessel formations.

Clinically, new vessels seem to arise predominantly from capillaries and veins and microscopic connections with these vessels have been demonstrated (Fig. 11-26).[83] Arterial connections are harder to see but sometimes can be identified, especially in the more advanced new vessel formations. Some neovascular formations have two vein or capillary connections and no direct arterial supply. With fluorescein angiography some very early proliferating vessels fill during the arterial phase showing a clinically unsuspected arterial supply, while other more extensive formations fill only during the venous phase.

By light microscopy normal retinal capil-

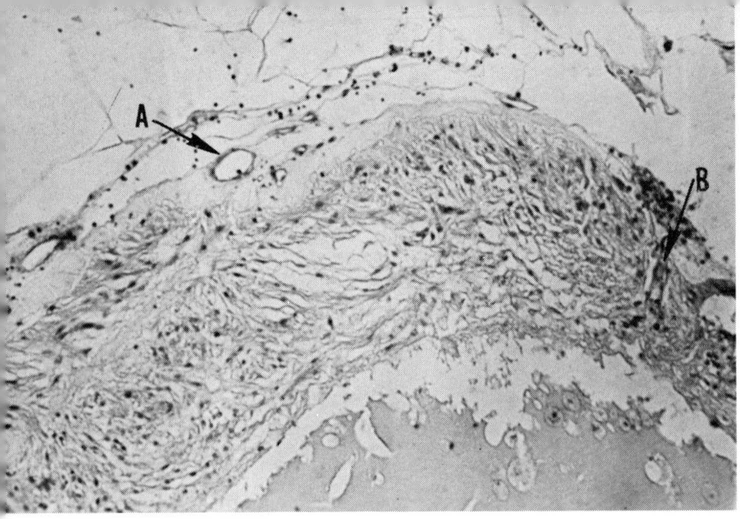

Fig. 11-26. Human Coats's disease. Preretinal neovascularization **(A)** arising from a superficial retinal capillary **(B)** near the ora. (See also Fig. 11-14, point **4.**)

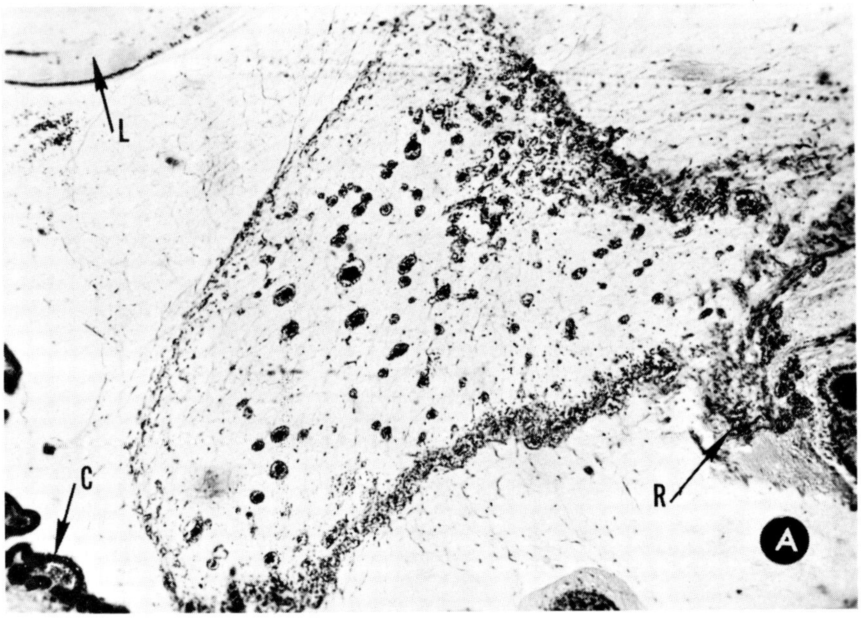

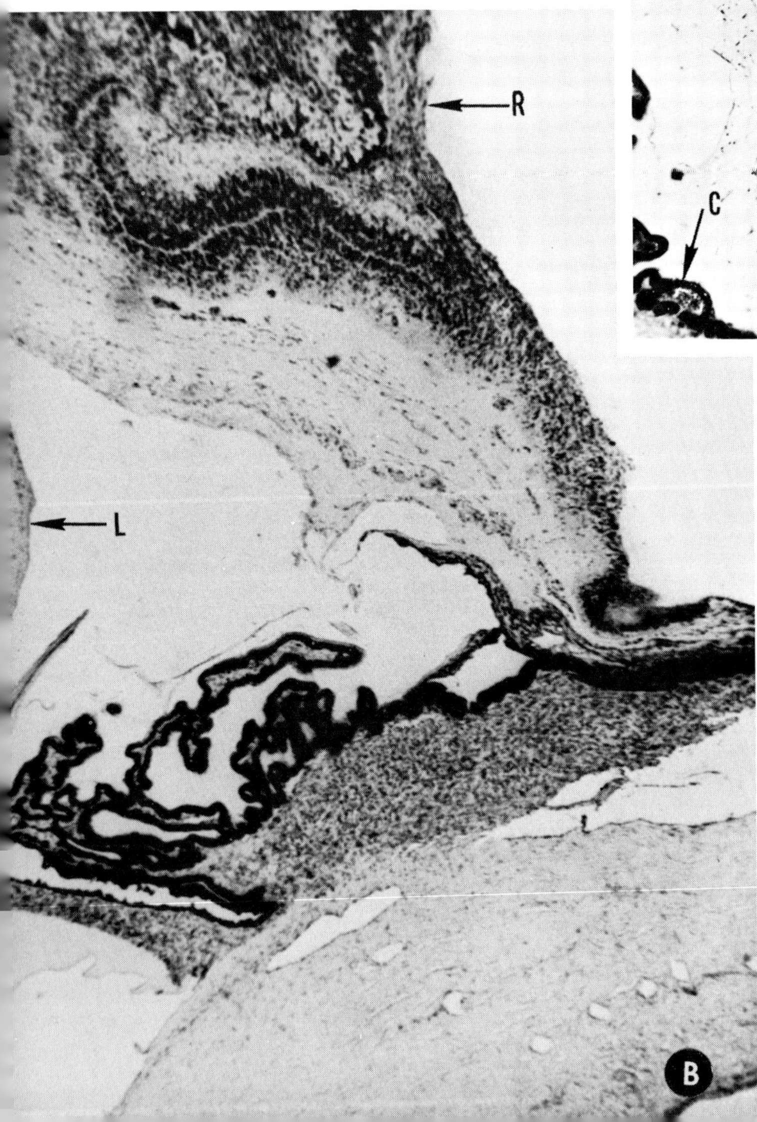

Fig. 11-27. Human retrolental fibroplasia.

A, Early highly vascular proliferans detaching the retina **(R)** behind the lens **(L).** Note the thin-walled vessels with large lumens. The ciliary body is at **(C).**

B, Late fibrotic stage of the proliferans in another patient. Note fibrotic scar detaching the retina **(R)** behind the lens **(L)** and the relative avascularity.

(Courtesy of the Armed Forces Institute of Pathology, Washington, D.C.)

lary and neovascular walls resemble one another. They differ physiologically in the profuse leakage of fluorescein from even the smallest neovascular formations. Thus, fluorescein angiography provides an easy means of identifying early new vessel sites.

The lumen size of neovascular formations varies tremendously. The bore is always wider than that of a normal retinal capillary and much more variable along the vessel course. Channels may be wide enough to accommodate 8 to 10 red blood cells abreast (Fig. 11-27).

Early neovascular formations tend to be reté in form and are most common in the posterior fundus, especially at the disc. Large, highly vascular reté formations at the disc have been called reté mirabile (Fig. 11-28). As new vessel formations age, they become more fibrotic and less vascular. The natural progression of early vascular to late fibrotic retinitis proliferans in the course of retrolental fibroplasia is a good example of this[83] (Fig. 11-27). In some retinal vein obstructions no reté phase occurs and from the beginning the proliferation is mainly fibrotic (Fig. 11-29). In other instances a slowly developing preretinal fibrosis with fine retinal folds and no clinically visible vessels may occur. Such cases give the clinical impression of following a protracted impedance of venous outflow rather than a frank vein obstruction[84] (see Chapter 14 under section on Preretinal Macular Fibrosis).

Both new vessel formations and their associated fibrosis can spontaneously disappear if not too far advanced. This has been reported in diabetic retinopathy[19,82] and Eales's disease,[29,61,82] and is usually associated with an improvement in other features of the retinal pathology. On the other hand, vessel proliferations more often proceed inexorably.

In preretinal proliferans new vessels are always retinal in origin except for rare instances at the ora in Coats's disease where they have been seen to arise from the cho-

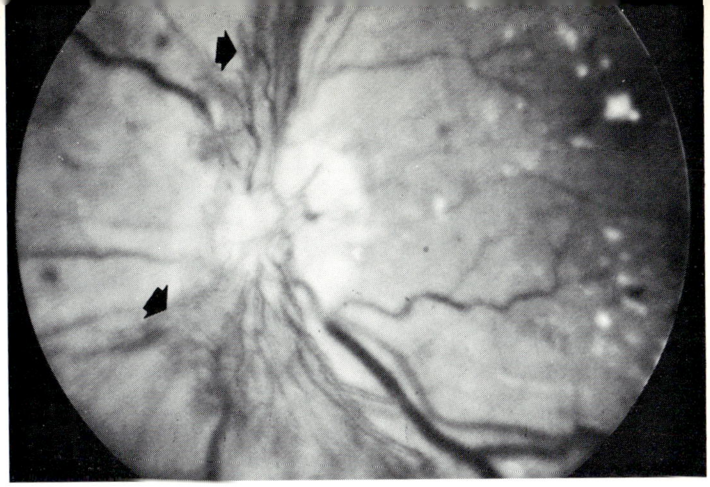

Fig. 11-28. Diabetic retinopathy. Reté mirabile from the disc area.

Fig. 11-29. Diabetic retinopathy. *A,* Dilated and tortuous superior vein **(V).** *B,* Fibrotic proliferans **(arrow)** from the disc preretinally toward the area of venous abnormality. This developed 8 months after *A* and in the absence of any vitreous hemorrhage. (From Wise. *Amer. J. Ophthal. 52:*637, 1961.)

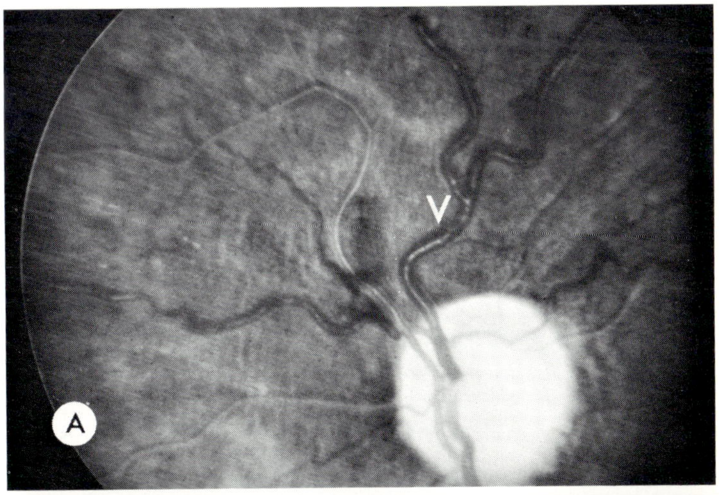

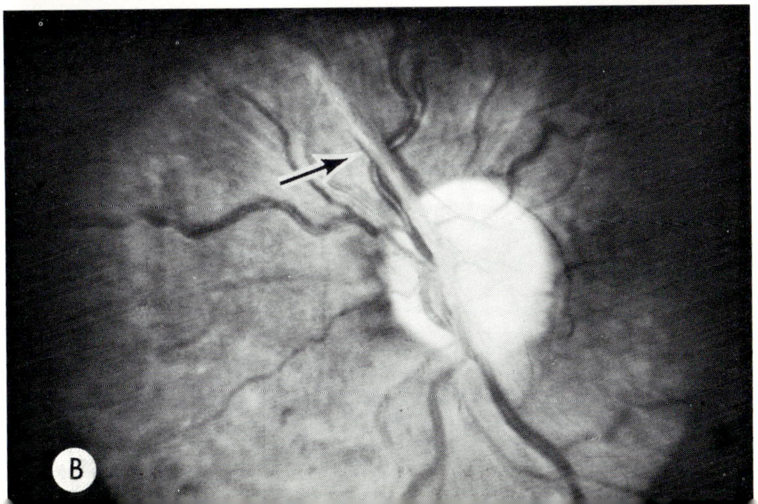

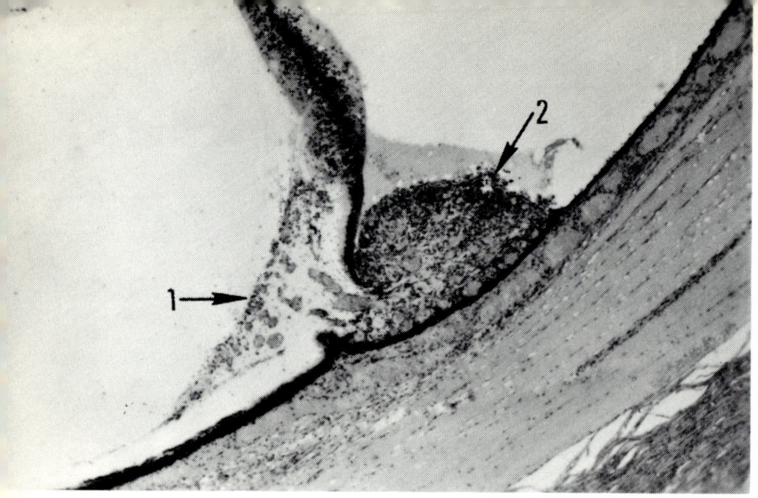

Fig. 11-30. Human Coats's disease. Subretinal neovascular formation **(2)** at the ora breaking through the retina and extending preretinally **(1).** (Courtesy of the Armed Forces Institute of Pathology, Washington, D.C.)

roid, pass through the thinned peripheral retina, and extend along the inner retinal surface (Fig. 11-30). Subretinal proliferans may take origin from either retinal or choroidal vessels (see Chapter 16, under section on Senile Disciform Macular Degeneration). A fibrovascular proliferation always originating from the choroid and following trauma, especially through and through penetrating injuries of the globe, is called chorioretinitis proliferans. It forms along the path of the injury and usually contains some proliferated pigment epithelium.[24,44,53,54] The factors effecting the development of chorioretinitis proliferans are unknown and have not been considered in the preceding discussion.

Although preretinal proliferans has an affinity for the retinal surface or the posterior face of the hyaloid, it may at times break through into the formed vitreous and grow forward. Growths into the vitreous most commonly arise from the disc, at the center of which there is no true internal limiting membrane[88,89] to act as a barrier. As these growths proceed, they often have a number of forward projections like the spread fingers of an outstretched hand. A few larger vascular channels and the heavier fibrosis lie closer to the disc. A delicate fibrosis and more numerous finer vessels occupy the growing tips. With retroillumination and high magnification details of these growing vascular projections can be seen. The vessels end in loops often slightly bulbous at the turn and sludged red blood cells can often be seen moving within their lumens. A tapering, pointed, grayish, transparent tissue projects about 0.5 dd beyond the tip of the vascular loop. With eye movements, these fibrovascular "fingers" wave about in the vitreous.

The importance of posterior vitreous liquefaction, shrinkage, and detachment from the very onset of diabetic retinitis proliferans has been stressed by Davis.[19] The attachment of the proliferans to both the retinal surface and the posterior face of the vitreous is the cause of the retinal tenting, folding, and detachment as the vitreous recedes from the retina and as the fibrous connective tissue contracts.

RETINITIS PROLIFERANS IN VARIOUS DISEASES

Some cases of retinitis proliferans are minimal and stop early in their course; others are relentless in their progression. The picture presented in any single case is dependent upon the severity and type of underlying retinal disease.

In retrolental fibroplasia neovascular formations are usually first seen in the temporal retinal periphery. If the condition is mild the residual fibrotic proliferans may be limited to the retinal periphery. All degrees of scarring from this mildest form to complete detachment of the retina in a fibrovascular retrolental membrane may occur. The condition is always bilateral although one eye may be only minimally affected.

Neovascular proliferans in diabetes starts as a rule posteriorly, often from the region of the disc itself. Ballantyne[10] noted the ease with which retinal new vessels passed through the diabetic internal limiting membrane. He stated that the membrane seemed to melt away, as if by lysis, before the advancing neovascular growth. The apparent lack of a significant restraining influence by the internal limiting membrane in diabetic retinopathy may well be a factor in the wide spread foci and luxuriant growth of preretinal new vessels often seen in this disease (Fig. 11-31). Both eyes are usually involved in diabetic retinitis proliferans although not necessarily to the same degree nor at the same time. In the late stages of diabetic retinitis proliferans, the extensive sheets of preretinal fibrosis containing a few vessels can sometimes be mistaken for retinal detachment.

Retinitis proliferans in Eales's disease may start peripherally or posteriorly. Here, too, new vessels pass through the internal limiting membrane of the retina with apparent ease. The periphlebitis of Eales's disease involves the internal limiting membrane in many places where the veins lie adjacent to or near the retinal surface. The destruction of this barrier, often at the very site of proliferating new vessels, undoubtedly plays some part in the profusion of their preretinal growth so often seen. Retinitis proliferans is usually bilateral in Eales's disease, one eye usually following the other.

Retinitis proliferans in retinal vein obstruction is less common than in the three preceding diseases. While some vein obstructions never develop retinitis proliferans, it is profuse in others, and is always limited to the eye with the vein involvement. Here it is further limited to the retinal region drained by the obstructed vein or an area immediately adjacent to it. The internal limiting membrane appears to be a more potent barrier to neovascular penetration, for it is unaffected by the basic disease process occluding the vein.

In sickle cell disease, retinitis proliferans is usually bilateral but more advanced in one eye. It starts peripherally, temporally as a rule, and progresses posteriorly. Peripheral vascular fans are common in hemoglobin-C disease.

Preretinal neovascular formations in pulseless disease are predominantly peripheral at first and are both spotty and mild.

In uveitis and the retinopathies of sarcoidosis, malaria, polycythemia, the dysproteinemias, Behçet's disease and syphilis, the proliferative retinopathy is quite variable and primarily related to the type and degree of vein or capillary involvement.

Subretinal neovascular proliferation from the retina is common in Coats's disease and

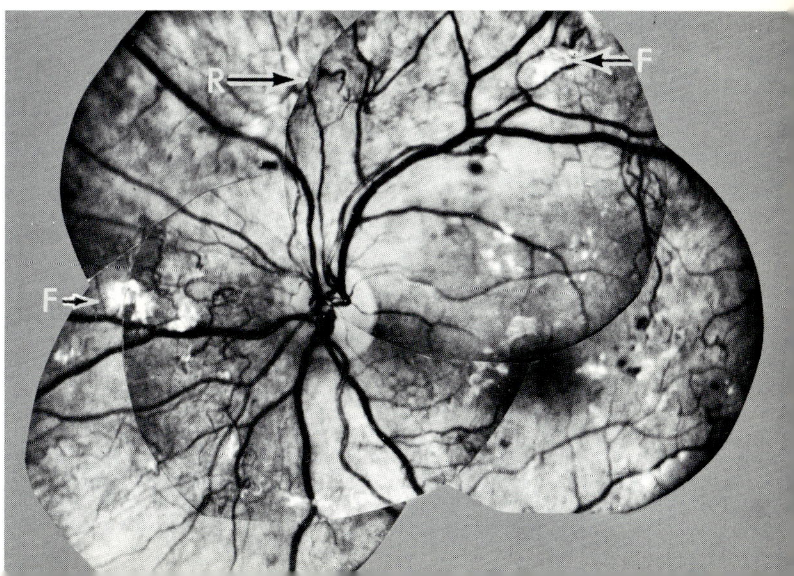

Fig. 11-31. Proliferative juvenile diabetic retinopathy showing early reté (**R**) and later fibrotic (**F**) proliferans in the same eye without antecedent vitreous hemorrhage. Vision 20/20.

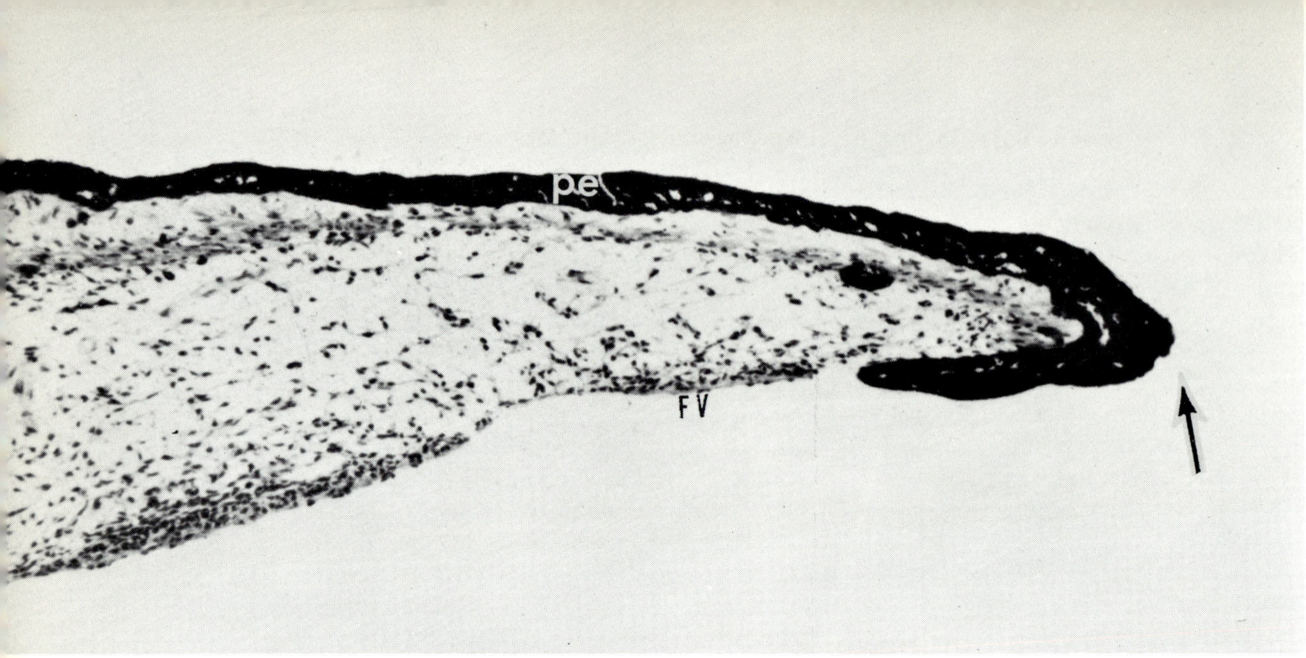

Fig. 11-32. Diabetic rubeosis iridis showing the vacuolated pigment epithelium **(pe)** drawn around the pupillary margin **(arrow)** by the contracting fibrovascular membrane **(FV)** on the anterior iris surface.

the later stages of both retrolental fibroplasia and retinal angioma. It is less frequently seen in the late stages of the disciform macular syndrome. Long-standing retinal detachments with complicating retinal vein obstructions show a subretinal fibrosis at the ora and may show a thinner subretinal fibrosis elsewhere.

Both high myopia and chronic glaucoma are deterrents to neovascularization and retinitis proliferans in such cases is often mild. In the case of glaucoma it is often predominantly fibrotic and restricted to the area of the disc.

ASSOCIATION WITH RUBEOSIS IRIDIS

Rubeosis iridis is the formation of neovascular fibrosis on the anterior surface of the iris and in the anterior chamber angle. It is commonly associated with proliferative retinopathy and most often follows central retinal vein obstruction. Rarer cases have been reported after central retinal artery obstruction,[62,93] retinoblastoma,[78] cranial arteritis,[94] carotid artery occlusion,[71] and pulseless disease.[63] Mild rubeosis has been observed to subside but progression to angle closure hemorrhagic glaucoma with pupillary distortion and fixation is the usual course.

Fine anastomosing new vessels first appear on the anterior iris surface at the collarette or in the angle. They develop progressively around the pupil and spread over the iris toward its root. For reasons unknown, new vessels do not form on the posterior iris surface. As the fibrous tissue associated with the new vessels contracts, it averts the pupillary margin bringing the dark posterior pigment epithelium of the iris into view (Fig. 11-32). In watching closely for the onset of rubeosis iridis in suspected cases, and before the appearance of new vessels, this ectropion uveae, due to fine anterior iris fibrosis, may be the first visible sign.

With progression, larger channels form on the anterior iris surface and extensive rubeosis may invade the pupil and lie on the anterior lens surface. When the blood in larger vessels is sludged and its direction of flow identified, it has always been found to move from the pupil toward the iris root.

The neovascular growth in the angle spreads over the iris root, the meshwork and the peripheral posterior cornea, drawing the iris forward and eventually closing the entire angle with a firm peripheral anterior synechia.

The pathogenesis of rubeosis iridis is unknown, but its frequent association with retinal neovascularization, their similar backgrounds of vascular insufficiency, comparable morphology and development, and their frequent occurrence in the same group of diseases suggests some common denominator for both.

PROGNOSIS AND TREATMENT

The purpose of neovascularization is unknown. It has been suggested that it may help to nourish the retina when the circulation is impaired. Its limitation to that retinal area drained by an obstructed branch vein might suggest a frustrated attempt at collateral formation. However, its sieve-like leakage of serum, fragility, and bleeding tendency, and the distorting effect of the contracting associated fibrosis make its ultimate effect on retinal integrity and function a disastrous one. Even those cases of advanced proliferans without serious hemorrhage and with a sufficiently preserved macula for good visual acuity, have a grave prognosis.

Some of the small tufts of new vessels will have serious bleeding episodes early in the development of proliferative retinopathy. In other cases the vessels do not bleed nor is the macula involved until the proliferation is extensive. All preretinal new vessel formations must be considered visually threatening.

In diabetic retinopathy, retinitis proliferans can spread out into the four quadrants from the disc and slowly over a period of several years become quiescent, fibrotic, sheetlike, and practically avascular. In these patients central vision is destroyed, but, if the central retinal artery remains patent, and rubeosis iridis does not appear, some peripheral vision may be retained. The residual vision will at times permit the patient a limited independence of movement. On the other hand, progression of diabetic proliferative retinopathy to rubeosis iridis, hemorrhagic glaucoma, and atrophy, or loss of the globe is more common.

The prognosis in Eales's disease had always been considered grave until Elliot's studies[27,28] which showed an eventually good visual recovery in about one-half of the cases.

Preretinal neovascular growths can best be eradicated by xenon arc photocoagulation. New vessel formations before the disc and involving the macula presently cannot be treated in this manner. Prepapillary new vessels over the nasal disc area have been

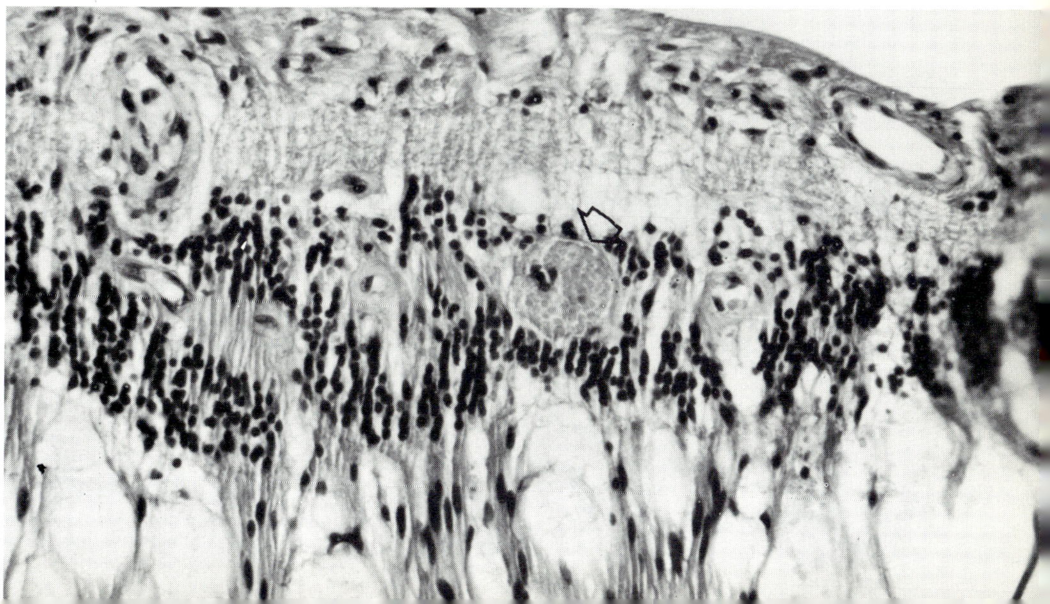

Fig. 11-33. Central retinal vein obstruction with a blood-filled microaneurysm (**arrow**) in the inner nuclear layer of the retina.

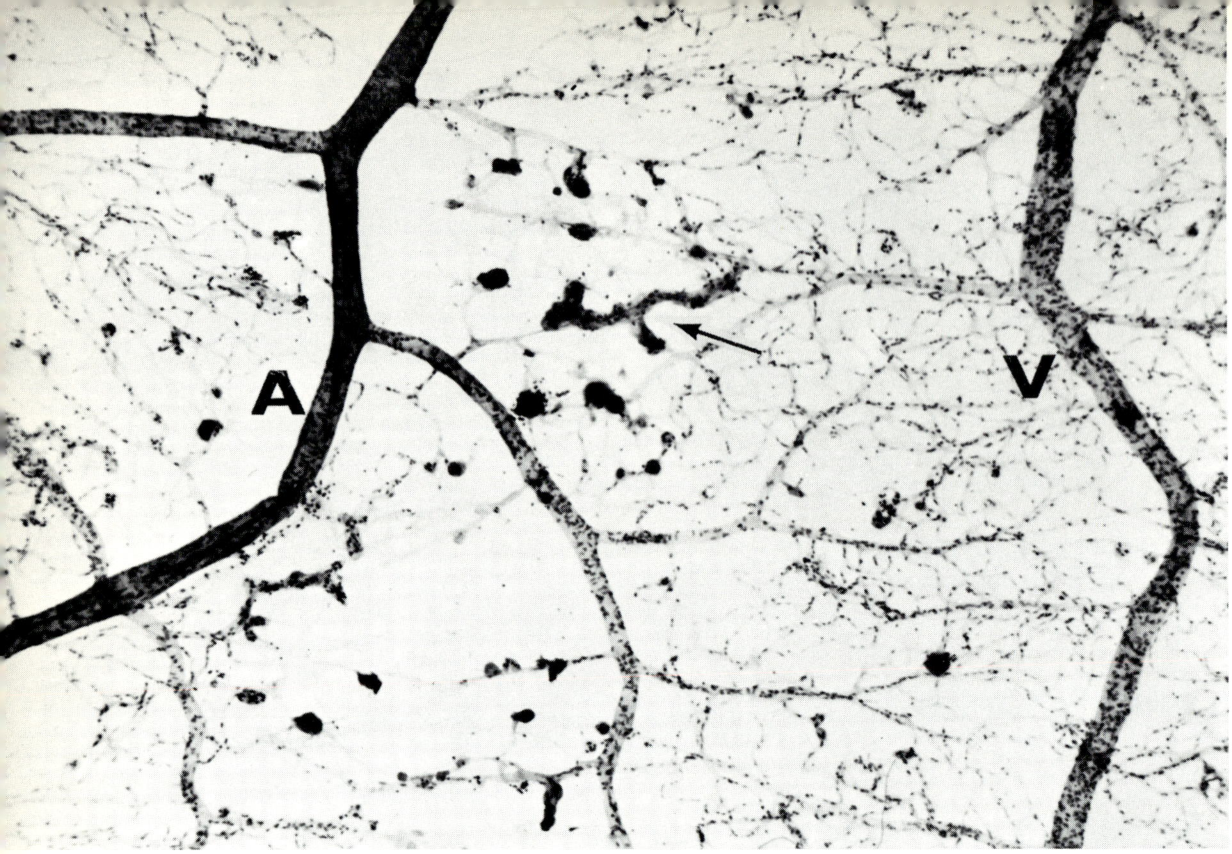

Fig. 11-34. Retinal digest of diabetic retinopathy showing capillary microaneurysms in and around areas of capillary obliteration **(A)** artery and **(V)** vein. Note the hypercellular vessel **(arrow)** in an area of capillary obliteration (see also Fig. 11-43). (PAS and Hematoxylin, ×50.)

cautiously light coagulated.[79] Formations over large retinal arteries and veins can be eradicated without serious damage to the underlying major vessels. Although it has little useful application, photocoagulation and blockage of the small artery supplying an area containing new vessels, infarcts the retinal area and neovascular channels "wither on the vine." Widespread photocoagulation with the destruction of many retinal cells may, by reducing the vasoformative stimulant, have a beneficial effect on retinal neovascularization.[86]

The major retinal complications of this treatment are bleeding at the time of photocoagulation and the formation of traction lines or denser retinal folds following excessive treatment.

RETINAL MICROANEURYSMS

OCCURRENCE

Retinal microaneurysms were first seen by Sir William Bowman [3] but were first described by MacKenzie and Nettleship [51] in a patient with diabetes mellitus. This observation was then "lost" until 1943, when Ballantyne and Loewenstein [11] rediscovered the lesion also in a patient with diabetic retinopathy. Michaelson's and Steedman's revival of the vascular injection technique [55]

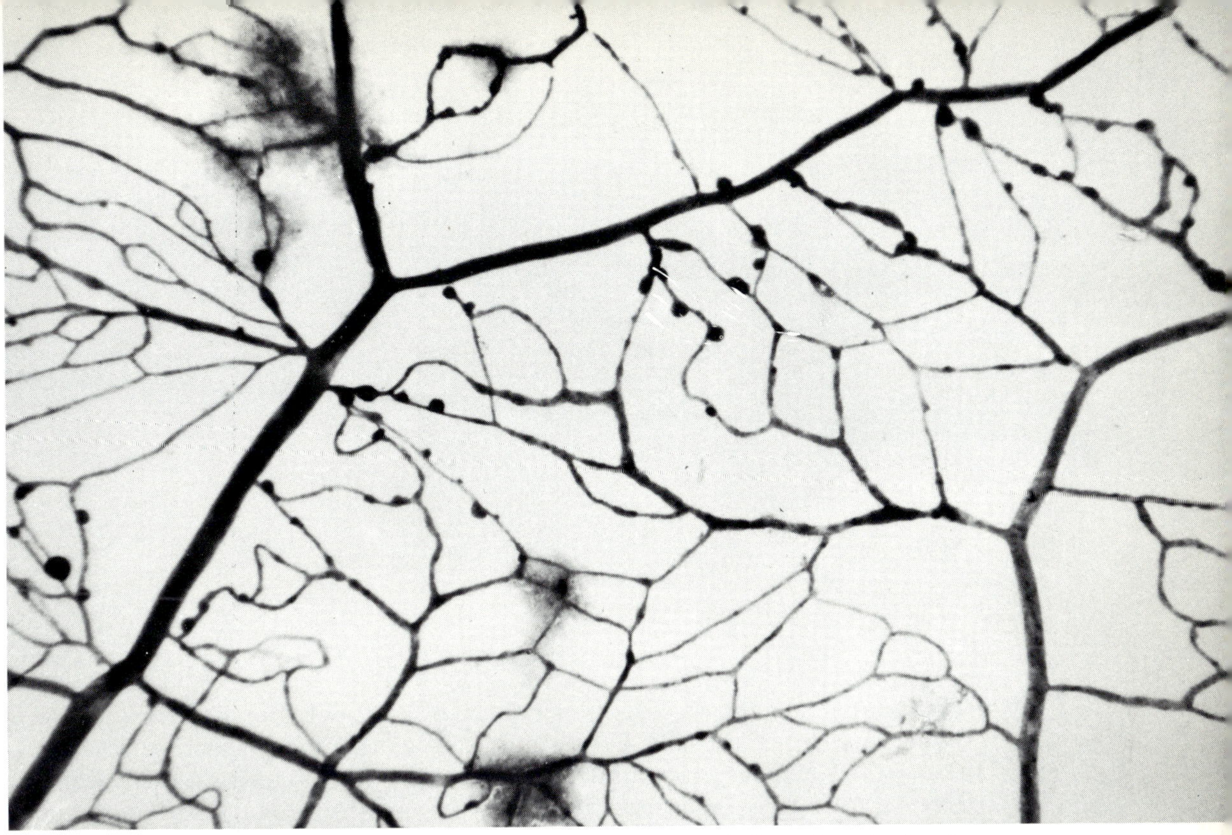

Fig. 11-35. Retinal digest showing capillary microaneurysms in branch retinal vein obstruction. (PAS and Hematoxylin, ×50.)

popularized by Ashton,[4] Friedenwald's application of the Hotchkiss-McManus stain,[30] and the retinal digest technique of Kuwabara and Cogan [43] have greatly added to our knowledge of these microaneurysms.

The capillary microaneurysm was at first considered to be a specific lesion in diabetic retinopathy. It is now generally held that all capillary microaneurysms, regardless of their varied morphology and irrespective of the disease in which they occur, are manifestations of a single pathogenic process.

Retinal microaneurysms are more frequent on the venous side of the capillary bed and have been reported on superficial, deep (Fig. 11-33), and interconnecting capillaries, but have not been specifically mentioned as occurring on the radial peripapillary capillaries. Significant numbers of lesions comparable to these microaneurysms have not been identified in other body tissues. Thus, the capillary microaneurysm seems to be a specific retinal lesion.

They have now been reported as occurring profusely in diabetic retinopathy (Fig. 11-34), venous thrombosis (Fig. 11-35), Eales's disease, sickle cell retinopathy, chorioretinitis, and severe hypertensive retinopathy—especially the malignant variety. They are found in moderate numbers in chronic glaucoma, less severe hypertensive retinopathy, the dysproteinemias (Fig. 11-36), pulseless disease, Coats's and Leber's diseases, and in retinoblastoma. A few have been reported in pernicious anemia, secondary anemias, and even in some essentially normal retinas, where they are more likely to be seen in the periphery. Ashton [8] has reported microaneu-

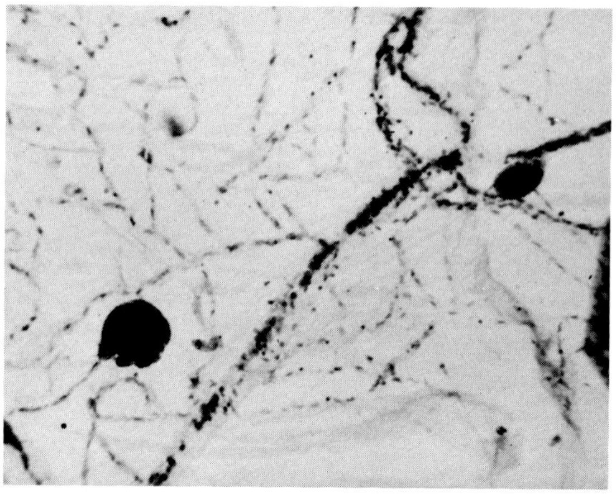

Fig. 11-36. Retinal digest showing capillary microaneurysms in multiple myeloma (dysproteinemia).

rysms around cotton-wool spots in malignant hypertension but others [17] have stated that obliterated patches of capillaries in hypertension are rarely associated with microaneurysms. They are not a clinical feature of the cotton-wool spots which occur in uncomplicated hypertensive retinopathy. Fluorescein studies suggest the presence of microaneurysms around cotton-wool spots in hypertension (see Chapter 13, under section on Clinical Features of Retinopathy in Accelerated Hypertension).

MORPHOLOGY AND NATURAL COURSE

Morphologically, retinal microaneurysms appear as bulges, saccules, elongated pouches, and bizarre forms, varying in diameter from approximately 20 μ to 100 μ. The aneurysmal wall may be normal with endothelium, basement membrane, and intramural pericyte. Several aneurysms may develop on one side of a capillary, its opposite wall being quite normal. They often occur in clusters (Fig. 11-37) oriented toward areas of obliterated capillaries and are associated at times with dilated capillary channels, sausage-shaped vessels, and loops and coils in the regional capillary network. They are commonly seen in diseases associated with retinal neovascularization except retrolental fibroplasia, and they occur in retinal areas showing endothelial proliferation. In branch vein obstruction they are found, as is any neovascular formation present, only in that retinal region drained by the obstructed vein.

They tend to occur within circinate lesions (Fig. 11-38) irrespective of the disease in which these ring lesions appear. Here, large, central microaneurysms can often be seen clinically. Microaneurysms may also occur at the borders of the more persistent cotton-wool patches occurring in diabetic retinopathy. In both of these positions they are intimately associated with areas containing obliterated capillaries. Indeed, in all cases, they are found in association with damaged, obliterated, or ghost capillaries.

Many microaneurysms have sufficiently fragile walls that red blood cells seep through them and form small regional hemorrhages. Their common intimate association with fatty exudates in diabetes has suggested that the material forming these exudates also passes from the blood stream through the aneurysmal walls.

Microaneurysms may persist with patent

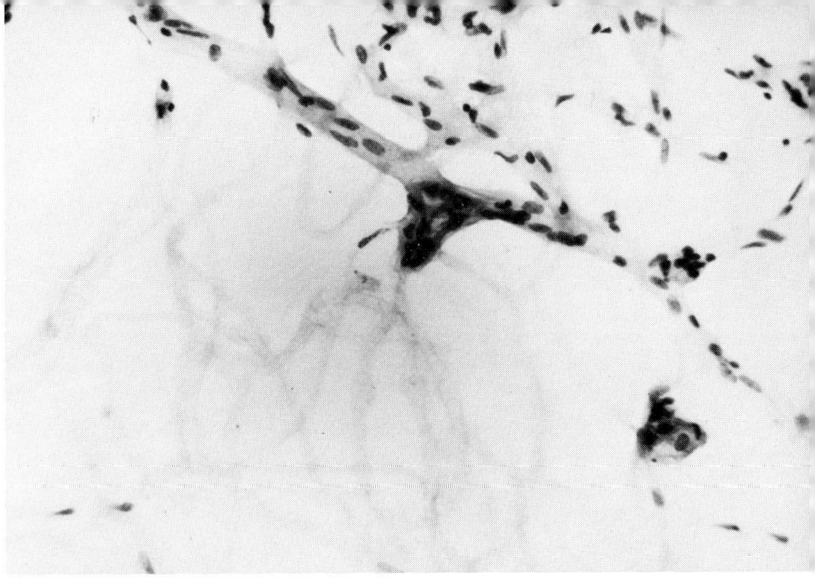

Fig. 11-37. Retinal digest in diabetic retinopathy showing endothelial cell multiplication and microaneurysms at the border of an area of capillary obliteration.

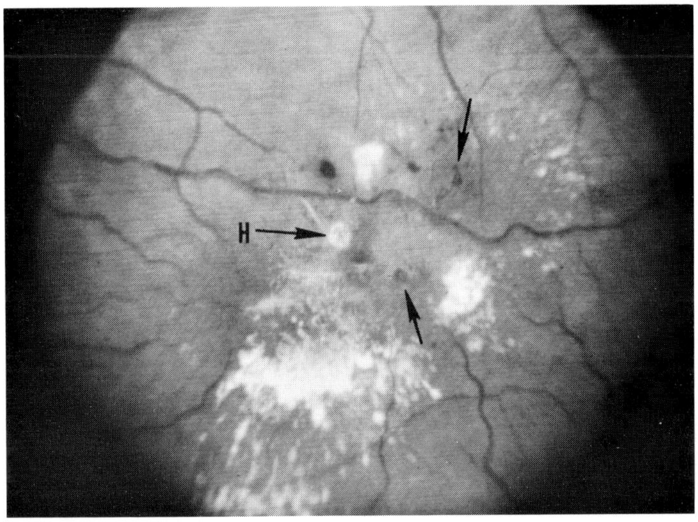

Fig. 11-38. Leber's multiple miliary aneurysms with retinal degeneration showing hyalinized **(H)** and nonhyalinized microaneurysms **(arrows),** mainly within the rings of fatty exudates.

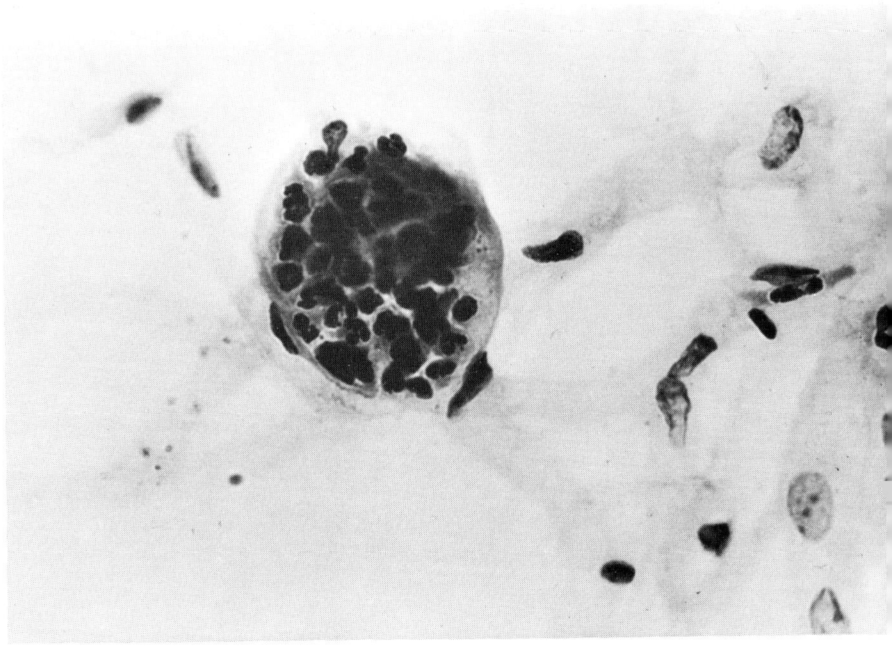

Fig. 11-39. Diabetic retinopathy. Retinal digest showing a microaneurysm filled with red and white blood cells.

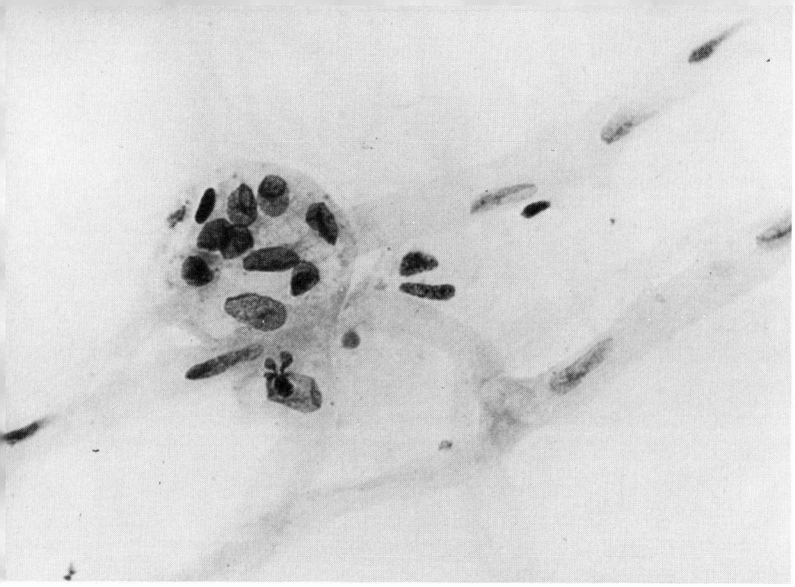

Fig. 11-40. Diabetic retinopathy. Retinal digest showing a microaneurysm containing proliferated endothelial cells. (PAS and Hematoxylin ×560.)

Fig. 11-41. Diabetic retinopathy. Retinal digest showing a hyalinized microaneurysm. (PAS and Hematoxylin ×220.)

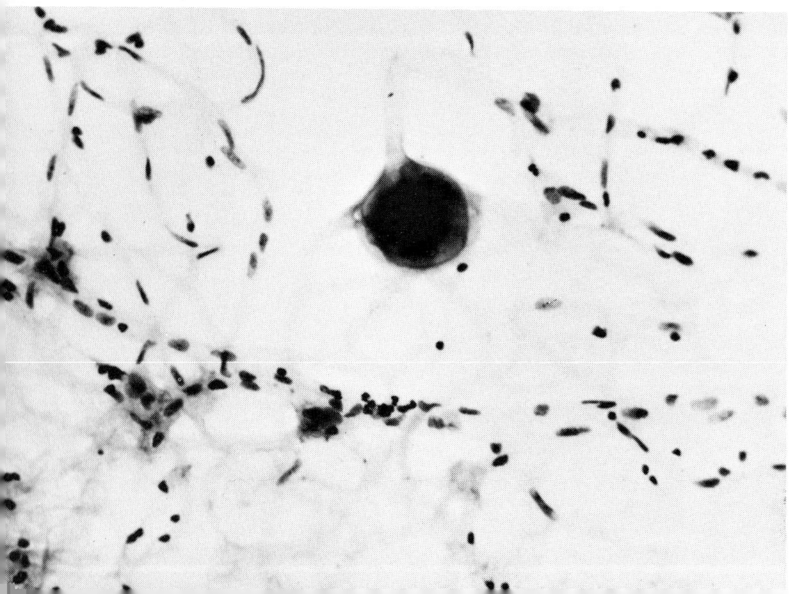

lumens for months. Others, especially those in diabetes, develop thickened basement membranes. Most microaneurysms eventually fill with packed blood cells (Fig. 11-39), proliferated endothelium (Fig. 11-40), or become thrombosed. Various combinations of these events are followed by laminar hyalinization (Fig. 11-41), obliteration, fragmentation, disintegration, and absorption.

ETIOLOGY

There is still no universally accepted explanation for the pathogenesis of retinal microaneurysms but a number of suggestions have been made.

Ballantyne and Loewenstein,[11,12,49] have found fatty infiltration of the capillary endothelium prior to aneurysm formation. They thought this fatty endothelial change led to venous and capillary stasis which was followed by aneurysm formation. Wolff[90] has subscribed to this same view and thought that ectasias of the capillary wall and aneurysms were prone to occur at points of fatty endothelial change.

Friedenwald[31,32] also believed in a wall weakness theory. He considered neither sclerosis of retinal vessels nor increase of intracapillary pressure a factor in microaneurysm formation. Hartford[36] also believed that diabetes, in time, produced a weakening of the capillary wall, and that microaneurysms were secondary to this.

Ashton[5] first proposed that microaneurysms were arrested new vessel formations, then[6] suggested a U-shaped capillary kink theory (Fig. 11-42) which he has subsequently partly discarded as not explaining all microaneurysm formation. He no longer supports the aborted new vessel concept but suggests that the microaneurysms may be due to nothing more specific than stasis and engorgement of the capillaries.[7]

Bloodworth[15] thought that neovascularization played no part in microaneurysm formation. He believed that capillary wall

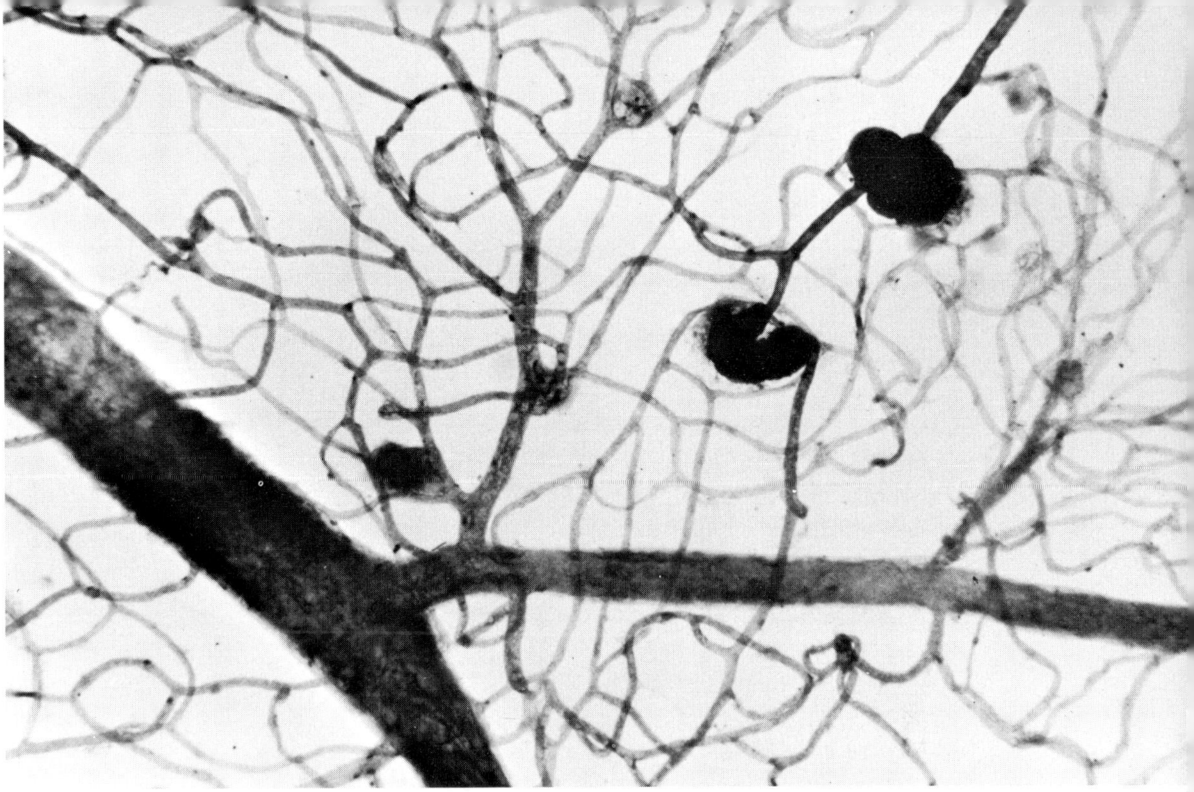

Fig. 11-42. Diabetic retinopathy. Retinal digest showing microaneurysms suggests Ashton's loop mode of formation (PAS and Hematoxylin ×125).

Fig. 11-43. An enlargement of arrowed vessel shown in Fig. 11-34. Note endothelial cell proliferation suggesting an attempted reopening of an obliterated capillary **(arrow).** (PAS and Hematoxylin ×320.)

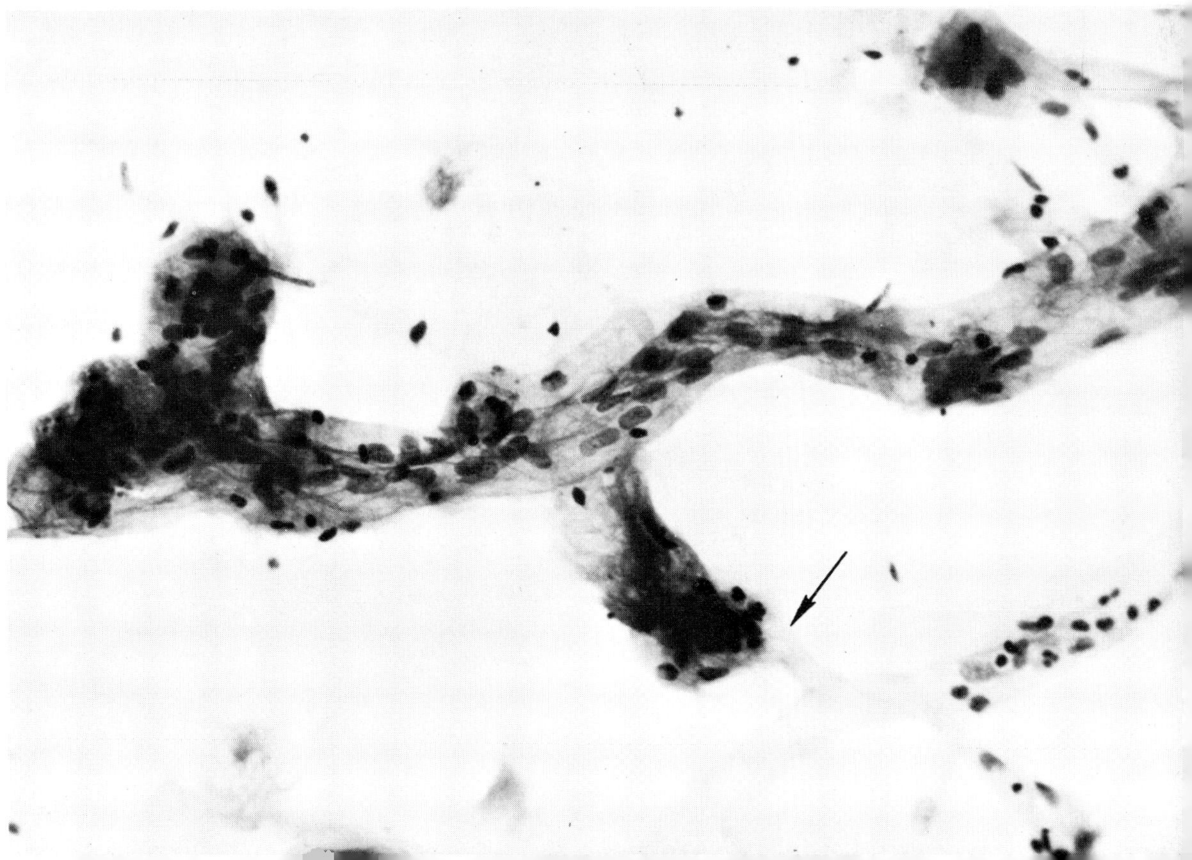

ectasia or aneurysm formation in diabetes was due to pericapillary neural cell degeneration and loss of wall support. This theory has not gained adherents and Yanoff[97] has offered strong arguments against it.

Pope[64] has suggested that fat emboli might be responsible for the development of diabetic microaneurysms. This concept is hard to correlate with the usual picture of fat embolism in the retina and seems an unlikely explanation.

Wolter[91,92] has demonstrated tissue strands extending outward from the tips of many microaneurysms in both diabetes and retinoblastoma. He has suggested that the pulling of such strands of the capillary wall could account for microaneurysm formation. These strands probably represent the remnants of obliterated ghost capillaries. Rounded aneurysm formation at such points more likely suggests an attempt to reopen obliterated channels—a frustrated revascularization. This idea is also supported by Okun and Collins[58] and Yanoff.[97]

In their study of diabetic retinopathy, Cogan, Toussaint, and Kuwabara[17] found a selective loss of intramural pericytes in posterior retinal areas, and suggested that microaneurysms formed at such sites of wall weakening that previously were occupied by the intramural pericyte. They found no support for Wolter's strand concept nor for Ashton's fusion of adjacent loops idea. Others[72,74,98] have confirmed their finding of selective posterior retinal loss of intramural pericytes in diabetes, but de Oliveira[21] disputed both this finding and their concept of microaneurysm formation. He found examples of well-preserved intramural pericytes on some microaneurysmal walls in his material. There were also areas of selectively degenerated intramural pericytes without microaneurysm formation. Nor did Sugi[74] always find aneurysms at sites previously occupied by intramural pericytes. As Yanoff[97] noted, the scattered posterior loss of intramural pericytes is not etiologically compatible with the finding of clustered microaneurysms. Furthermore, this theory would be of no value in diseases other than diabetes wherein microaneurysms are plentiful, but selective loss of the intramural pericyte does not occur.

By independent study, Wise[81,82] reached the same conclusion originally espoused by Ashton—that retinal microaneurysms represented an aborted effort at neovascularization. Gibson[33] was an early proponent of this view and the neovascular concept is also supported by Okun's and Collins' experimental study[58] and both Yanoff's[97] and Davis and his co-workers' studies[20] of human retina.

Excluding "old" microaneurysms, i.e., those with significant basement membrane thickening, thrombosis, or hyalinization, and emphasizing apparently "young" ones, there seem to be two requisites for their formation—obliterated capillaries and viable endothelial cells. Given these circumstances and a neovascular stimulus, one would expect endothelial cells to multiply with some attempt being made to reopen obliterated capillaries (Fig. 11-43). The early proliferation of endothelial cells within microaneurysms, the nearby endothelial cell proliferation in patent channels, the orientation of microaneurysms at the border of and toward obliterated patches of capillaries, and the tissue strand (very likely the obliterated capillary remnant) often seen extending from the cap of a microaneurysm, all suggest just such an effort.

The appearance of several microaneurysms in a row on only one side of a capillary, their presence in areas where the capillary wall is normal, and their absence in some zones of diseased vascular wall (thickened basement membrane and absent intramural pericyte), suggest that factors other than pathologic alterations in the vessel wall may be responsible for microaneurysm formation.

Microaneurysms are present in most diseases in which neovascularization occurs and commonly precede the formation of new vessels. However, microaneurysms have not been observed to develop into new vessels. Although the evidence is not conclusive, they could represent aborted attempts to reopen closed capillary side branches. The sparse intercapillary connections in the radial peripapillary capillary bed would explain their rarity in this layer, if further study proves this to be the case.

Although microaneurysms are not seen in human retrolental fibroplasia, in the experimental animal, as the previously obliterated capillary bed is attempting to reopen, bulbous capillary swellings somewhat suggestive of microaneurysms can be seen.[9]

REFERENCES

1. Ashton, N.: Central areolar choroidal sclerosis. A histo-pathological study. *Brit. J. Ophthal. 37:*140, 1953.
2. Ashton, N.: Oxygen and the growth and development of retinal vessels. *Amer. J. Ophthal. 62:*412, 1966.
3. Ashton, N.: The blood-retinal barrier and vaso-glial relationships in retinal disease. *Trans. Ophthal. Soc. U.K. 85:*199, 1965.
4. Ashton, N.: Injection of the retinal vascular system in the enucleated eye in diabetic retinopathy. *Brit. J. Ophthal. 34:*38, 1950.
5. Ashton, N.: Discussion on diabetic retinopathy. *Proc. Roy. Soc. Med. 44:*742, 1951.
6. Ashton, N.: Arteriolar involvement in diabetic retinopathy. *Brit. J. Ophthal. 37:*282, 1953.
7. Ashton, N.: Studies of the retinal capillaries in relation to diabetic and other retinopathies. *Brit. J. Ophthal. 47:*521, 1963.
8. Ashton, N.: Diabetic retinopathy, a new approach. *Lancet 2:*625, 1959.
9. Ashton, N., Ward, B., and Serpell, G.: Role of oxygen in the genesis of retrolental fibroplasia. *Brit. J. Ophthal. 37:*513, 1953.
10. Ballantyne, A. J.: The state of the retina in diabetes mellitus. *Trans. Ophthal. Soc. U.K. 66:*503, 1946.
11. Ballantyne, A. J., and Loewenstein, A.: The pathology of diabetic retinopathy. *Trans. Ophthal. Soc. U.K. 63:*95, 1943.
12. Ballantyne, A. J., and Loewenstein, A.: Retinal microaneurysms and punctate hemorrhages. *Brit. J. Ophthal. 28:*593, 1944.
13. Baum, J. L., and Wise, G. N.: Experimental subretinal neovascularization. *Amer. J. Ophthal. 61:*528, 1966.
14. Bedford, M. A., and MacFaul, P. A.: Retinal vascular changes in untreated retinoblastoma. Resemblance to von Hippel-Lindau disease. *Brit. J. Ophthal. 53:*382, 1969.
15. Bloodworth, J. M. B., Jr.: Diabetic retinopathy. *Diabetes 11:*1, 1962.
15a. Cameron, M. E., and Greer, C. H.: Congenital arterio-venous aneurysm of the retina. *Brit. J. Ophthal. 52:*768, 1968.
16. Coats, G.: Forms of retinal disease with massive exudation. *Roy. London Ophthal. Hosp. Rep. 17* (Pt. 3)*:*440, 1908.
17. Cogan, D., Toussaint, D., and Kuwabara, T.: Retinal vascular patterns IV. Diabetic retinopathy. *Arch. Ophthal. 66:*366, 1961.
18. Courville, C. B.: Antenatal and paranatal circulatory disorders as a cause of cerebral damage in early life. *J. Neuropath. Exper. Neurol. 18:*115, 1959.
19. Davis, M. D.: Vitreous contraction in proliferative diabetic retinopathy. *Arch. Ophthal. 74:*741, 1965.
20. Davis, M. D., Myers, F. L., Engerman, R. L., De Venecia, G., and Magli, Y. L.: *Clinical Observations Concerning the Pathogenesis of Diabetic Retinopathy. Symposium on the Treatment of Diabetic Retinopathy.* Washington, D.C., Public Health Service Publication No. 1890, 1968, p. 47.
21. De Oliveira, F.: Pericytes in diabetic retinopathy. *Brit. J. Ophthal. 50:*134, 1966.
22. De Schweinitz, G. E.: Concerning a form of retinal disease with extensive exudation; being a clinical contribution, with the report of two cases. *Trans. Amer. Ophthal. Soc. 12:*273, 1909.
23. Dobree, J. H.: Proliferative diabetic retinopathy; evolution of the retinal lesions. *Brit. J. Ophthal. 48:*637, 1964.

24. Doherty, W. B.: Some of the most important ocular and orbital wounds in war. *Amer. J. Ophthal. 25:*135, 1942.

25. Duke-Elder, S.: *System of Ophthalmology.* London, Kimpton, 1967, vol. X, p. 741.

26. Duke-Elder, S.: *System of Ophthalmology.* London, Kimpton, 1968, vol. IV, p. 398.

27. Elliot, A. J.: Recurrent intraocular haemorrhage in young adults (Eales' disease). *Trans. Amer. Ophthal. Soc. 52:*811, 1954.

28. Elliot, A. J.: Recurrent intraocular haemorrhage in young adults (Eales' disease) with continuous subconjunctival therapy with hydrocortisone. *Trans. Amer. Ophthal. Soc. 56:*383, 1958.

29. Friedenwald, H.: Über jugendliche Netzhaut und Glaskorper-blutungen durch sichtbare. Netzhautvenenhrankungen bedingt. *Centralbl. Prakt. Augenheilk. 20:*33, 1896.

30. Friedenwald, J. S.: A new approach to some problems of retinal vascular disease. *Amer. J. Ophthal. 32:*487, 1949.

31. Friedenwald, J. S.: Diabetic retinitis: the ophthalmologist's view. *Arch. Ophthal. Soc. Trans. 50:*124, 1953.

32. Friedenwald, J. S.: Diabetic retinopathy. *Amer. J. Ophthal. 33:*1187, 1950.

33. Gibson, G.: Discussion of Beetham, W. P.: Diabetic retinopathy in pregnancy. *Trans. Amer. Ophthal. Soc. 48:*205, 1950.

34. Goldberg, M. F., and Duke, J. R.: Lindau-von Hippel disease: a case report with histopathologic findings in a treated and in an untreated eye. *Trans. Amer. Ophthal. Soc. 66:*243, 1968.

35. Guerry, D.: Personal communication, 1963.

36. Hartford, J. J.: Retinal vascular changes in diabetes mellitus. *Amer. J. Ophthal. 36:*324, 1953.

37. Henkind, P., and Morgan, G.: Peripheral retinal angioma with exudative retinopathy in adults (Coats's lesion). *Brit. J. Ophthal. 50:*2, 1966.

38. Hoeve, J. Van der: Eye symptoms in phakomatoses. *Trans. Ophthal. Soc. U. K. 52:*380, 1932.

39. Jesberg, D. O., Spencer, W. H., and Hoyt, W. F.: Incipient lesions of von Hippel-Lindau disease. *Arch. Ophthal. 80:*632, 1968.

40. Joe, S., and Spencer, W. H.: von Hippel-Lindau disease. *Arch. Ophthal. 71:*508, 1964.

41. Klien, B. A.: Retinitis proliferans: clinical and histologic studies. *Arch. Ophthal. 20:* 427, 1938.

42. Krug, E. F., and Samuels, B.: Venous angioma of the retina, optic nerve, chiasma and brain. *Arch. Ophthal. 8:*871, 1932.

43. Kuwabara, T., and Cogan, D. G.: Studies of retinal vascular patterns. Part I. Normal architecture. *Arch. Ophthal. 64:*904, 1960.

44. Lagrange, F.: *Fractures of the Orbit and Injuries to the Eye in War.* London, Univer. London Press, 1918, pp. 134–139.

45. Larsen, H. W.: Diabetic retinopathy. *Acta Ophthal. (Suppl. 60):* 1960.

46. Leber, T.: Über eine durch Vorkommen multipler Miliaraneurysmen charakterisierte Form von Retinaldegeneration. *Arch. Ophth. 81:*1, 1912.

47. Leber, T.: "Die Aneurysmen der Zentralarterie und ihrer Verzweigungen. Retinaldegeneration bei Multiplen Miliaraneurysmen," in *Handbuch der gesamten Augenheilkunde,* 2nd ed. Ed. by Saemisch, T., Leipzig, Engelmann, 1915, vol. 7, p. 20.

48. Lindau, A.: Studien über Klienhirncysten, Bau, Pathogenese und Beziehungen zur Angiomatosis Retinae. *Acta Path. Microbiol. Scand. (Suppl. 1):*1, 1926.

49. Loewenstein, A.: Double staining for bulk specimens of retina and choroid. *Brit. J. Ophthal. 32:*748, 1948.

50. Luessenhop, A. J., and Spence, W. T.: Artificial embolization of cerebral arteries: Report of use in a case of arteriovenous malformation. *JAMA 172:*1153, 1960.

51. Mackenzie, S.: A case of glycosuric retinitis, with comments. *Roy. London Ophthal. Hosp. Rep. 9 (Pt. 2):*134, 1877.

52. Marshall, J., and Michaelson, I. C.: Exudative retinitis in children. *Trans. Ophthal. Soc. U.K. 53:*102, 1933.

53. Michaelson, I. C.: Traversing intraocular foreign bodies with retinal detachment. *Trans. Ophthal. Soc. U.K. 66:*193, 1946.

54. Michaelson, Major I. C., and Kraus, J.: War injuries of the eye; Traumatic proliferative choroiditis due to double penetrating foreign body. *Brit. J. Ophthal. 27:*448, 1943.

55. Michaelson, I. C., and Steedman, H. F.: Injection of the retinal vascular system in enucleated eyes. *Brit. J. Ophthal. 33:*376, 1949.

56. Norlén, G.: Arteriovenous aneurysms of the brain: Report of ten cases of total removal

of the lesion. *J. Neurosurg. 6:*475, 1949.

57. Norton, E. W. D.: Discussion of Goldberg, M. F. and Duke, J. R.: Lindau-von Hippel disease: a case report with histopathologic findings in a treated and in an untreated eye. *Trans. Amer. Ophthal. Soc. 66:*243, 1968.
58. Okun, E., and Collins, E. M.: Histopathology of experimental photocoagulation in the dog eye. Part III. Microaneurysm-like formations following branch vein occlusion. *Amer. J. Ophthal. 56:*40, 1963.
59. Olivecrona, H. and Riives, J.: Arteriovenous aneurysms of the brain: their diagnosis and treatment. *Arch. Neurol. Psychiat. 59:*567, 1948.
60. Owens, W. C.: Discussion of Baum, J. L. and Wise, G. N.: Experimental subretinal neovascularization. *Trans. Amer. Ophthal. Soc. 63:*103, 1965.
61. Paton, R. T.: Recurrent retinal and vitreous hemorrhages in the young—Eales' disease. *Arch. Ophthal. 20:*276, 1938.
62. Perraut, L. E., and Zimmerman, L. E.: The occurrence of glaucoma following occlusion of the central retinal artery. *Arch. Ophthal. 61:*845, 1959.
63. Pinkham, R. A.: The ocular manifestations of the pulseless syndrome. *Acta XVII, Concilium Ophthalmologicum 1954, 1:*348, 1955.
64. Pope, C. H., Jr: Retinal capillary microaneurysms. *Diabetes 9:*9, 1960.
65. Potter, J. M.: Angiomatous malformations of the brain: their nature and prognosis. *Ann. Roy. Coll. Surg. 16:*227, 1955.
66. Reese, A. B.: *Tumors of the Eye.* New York, Hoeber, 1951, p. 375.
67. Reese, A. B.: Telangiectasis of the retina and Coats' disease. *Amer. J. Ophthal. 42:*1, 1956.
68. Robles, C., and Carrazco, J.: Treatment of cerebral arteriovenous malformations of the brain by muscle embolization. *J. Neurosurg. 29:*603, 1968.
69. Salzmann, M.: Prepapillary proliferation of connective tissue in glaucoma and its relation to retinitis proliferans. *Arch. Ophth. 140 (Pt. 4):*629, 1939.
70. Shenkin, H. A., Spitz, E. B., Grant, F. C., and Kety, S. S.: Physiologic studies of arteriovenous anomalies of the brain. *J. Neurosurg. 5:*165, 1948.
71. Smith, J. L.: Unilateral glaucoma in carotid occlusive disease. *JAMA 182:*683, 1962.
72. Speiser, P., Gittelsohn, A. M., and Patz, A.: Studies on diabetic retinopathy III. Influence of diabetes on the intramural pericytes. *Arch. Ophthal. 80:*332, 1968.
73. Sugar, J. S.: Coats' disease: Telangiectatic or multiple vascular origin? *Amer. J. Ophthal. 45:*508, 1958.
74. Sugi, K.: Studies on the pathological changes in the retinal vessels of human eyes, using the trypsin digestion method. *Jap. J. Ophthal. 10:*252, 1966.
75. Tasman, W.: Personal communication, 1968.
76. Usher, C. H.: The Bowman Lecture. On a few hereditary eye affections. *Trans. Ophthal. Soc. U.K. 55:*164, 1935.
77. Von Hippel, E.: Die anatomische Grundlage der von mir beschriebenen "sehr seftenen Erkrankung der Netzhaut." *Arch. Ophth. 79:*350, 1911.
78. Walton, D. S., and Grant, W. M.: Retinoblastoma and iris neovascularization. *Amer. J. Ophthal. 65:*598, 1968.
79. Wetzig, P. C., and Jepson, C. N.: Treatment of diabetic retinopathy by light coagulation. *Amer. J. Ophthal. 62:*459, 1966.
80. Wise, G. N.: Coats' disease. *Arch. Ophthal. 58:*735, 1957.
81. Wise, G. N.: Retinal microaneurysms. *Arch. Ophthal. 57:*151, 1957.
82. Wise, G. N.: Retinal neovascularization. *Trans. Amer. Ophthal. Soc. 54:*729, 1956.
83. Wise, G. N.: Factors influencing retinal new vessel formation. *Amer. J. Ophthal. 52:*637, 1961.
84. Wise, G. N.: Arteriosclerosis secondary to retinal vein obstruction. *Trans. Amer. Ophthal. Soc. 56:*361, 1958.
85. Wise, G. N., and Baum, J. L.: Subretinal neovascularization in Coats' disease and the experimental animal. *Trans. A.M.A. Sect. Ophthal.* 1965, p. 69.
86. Wise, G. N., Campbell, C. J., Wendler, P. F., and Rittler, M. C.: Photocoagulation of vascular lesions of the macula. *Amer. J. Ophthal. 66:*452, 1968.
87. Wise, G. N., and Horava, A.: Coats' disease. *Amer. J. Ophthal. 56:*17, 1963.
88. Wolff, E.: The internal limiting membrane of the retina. *Trans. Ophthal. Soc. U.K. 57:* 186, 1937.
89. Wolff, E.: *The Anatomy of the Eye and Orbit,*

4th ed. New York, Blakiston, 1954, pp. 109–110.

90. Wolff, E.: *Pathology of the Eye*, 2nd ed. London, Lewis, 1944, p. 331.

91. Wolter, J. R.: Diabetic capillary microaneurysms of the retina. *Arch. Ophthal. 65:*847, 1961.

92. Wolter, J. R.: The blood vessels of retinoblastomas. *Arch. Ophthal. 66:*545, 1961.

93. Wolter, J. R., and Phillips, R. L.: Secondary glaucoma following occlusion of the central retinal artery. *Amer. J. Ophthal. 47:*335, 1959.

94. Wolter, J. R., and Phillips, R. L.: Secondary glaucoma in cranial arteritis. *Amer. J. Ophthal. 59:*625, 1965.

95. Woods, A. C., and Duke, J. R.: Coats' disease I. Review of the literature, diagnostic criteria, clinical findings and plasma lipid studies. *Brit. J. Ophthal. 47:*385, 1963.

96. Wyburn-Mason, R.: Arteriovenous aneurysms of mid-brain and retina, facial naevi and mental changes. *Brain 66* (*Pt. 3*)*:*163, 1943.

97. Yanoff, M.: Ocular pathology of diabetes mellitus. *Amer. J. Ophthal. 67:*21, 1969.

98. Yanoff, M.: Diabetic retinopathy. *New Eng. J. Med. 274:*1344, 1966.

chapter 12

Diseases of Arterial Insufficiency

The nutrition of the retina depends upon a supply of blood of the correct composition. Blood flow is chiefly determined by the level of the systemic arterial and intraocular pressures, the blood viscosity, and the state of the blood vessels supplying the eye. Alterations in the composition of the blood, of which the most important are hemoglobin concentration and oxygen saturation, determine the volume of blood flow that is required for a given value of oxygen uptake. In a normal retina these physiologic variables can fluctuate over a wide range without affecting visual function or causing retinal vascular disease. If the abnormalities are severe or sustained, or if the eye is already diseased they may cause harm.

These factors do not act in isolation. Increase in intraocular pressure decreases blood flow through both retinal and choroidal vessels. If the systemic blood pressure is high, a given increment in intraocular pressure will have less effect than if it is low. Blood pressure reduction in a patient who has systemic hypertension, with or without glaucoma, can cause a critical reduction in blood flow with the onset of visual impairment and loss of visual field.[52,69]

The level of the systemic venous pressure is less important. It only exerts an effect on the retina when the pressure exceeds the intraocular pressure, as it may in superior mediastinal obstruction or strangulation.[64]

The presence of other ocular diseases can greatly modify the expected response to vascular insufficiency. The retinas of high myopia, extensive healed chorioretinitis, and chronic glaucoma produce less obvious retinopathy than do normal retinas under similar circumstances. Central retinal artery obstruction in high myopia shows much less retinal opacity, a less vivid cherry red spot, and the later alteration in disc color with ensuing atrophy is less marked. Central retinal vein obstruction with subsequent well-developed disc collaterals is common in chronic glaucoma with the retina having at no time shown the usual apoplectic features of such an episode. Somewhat darkened and dilated retinal veins and a few deep retinal hemorrhages or no retinopathy whatsoever may have occurred during the development of such a "silent" vein occlusion. Late retinitis proliferans and clinically visible microaneurysms are usually minimal or absent. Permanent evidence of the occlusion may be limited to mildly tortuous, dark, halo-sheathed veins, collaterals at the disc and minimal prepapillary fibrotic proliferans.

RETINAL RESPONSES TO VASCULAR INSUFFICIENCY

There are a number of retinal diseases which in the course of their development present a very similar clinical appearance and fall naturally into groups. Whatever the original cause, these diseases seem to produce only a limited range of pathologic responses in the retina. Four such groups can be identified. These are arterial obstructive diseases, those obstructing capillaries and veins, hyperviscosity diseases, and the group producing disc-like macular elevations.

One of the main reasons for the differences between the clinical features of the arterial and venous obstructive diseases lies in their differing impact on the superficial and deep retinal capillary beds. The superficial capillaries are supplied directly by the precapillary arterioles. The deep bed is supplied by some precapillary arterioles and also by connections from the superficial capillary bed. Therefore, some blood flow from both superficial and deep beds drains into the numerous terminal venules of the deep bed. Thus the superficial bed is more associated with the arterial side of the circulation and the deep bed with the venous.

Signs of involvement of the superficial capillary bed include superficial retinal edema, flame-shaped or preretinal hemorrhages, cotton-wool patches, and a macular star figure. Signs of deep bed involvement include deep retinal edema, microcystic edema of the macula, macular cysts, dot-and-blot hemorrhages, fatty exudates, capillary microaneurysms, and retinitis proliferans. In diseases predominantly affecting the arterial side of the circulation the former group of lesions predominate, while venous lesions tend to produce the latter.

This division is arbitrary and there are exceptions, but these do not nullify its usefulness in understanding disease mechanisms and avoiding a repetitive catalog of features under individual disease headings.

RETINAL ARTERIAL DISEASES

This group of diseases includes those associated with arterial obstruction, diseases such as hypertension and arteriosclerosis which cause vascular damage but usually do not obstruct the vessel, and the retinopathies associated with collagenoses and anemia. Hypertension is such a common and important disease that hypertensive retinopathy is dealt with in a separate chapter (see Chapter 13, Hypertensive Retinopathy).

ARTERIAL OBSTRUCTIONS

Arterial obstruction may occur at any point between the precapillary arteriole and the greater arteries that arise from the heart.

OBSTRUCTION OF PRECAPILLARY ARTERIOLES

Obstruction of a precapillary arteriole (Fig. 12-1) produces a white retinal patch, or cotton-wool spot. Such lesions are small retinal infarcts although microscopic examination shows that there is relatively little tissue necrosis within them. The area of capillary bed involved is small and collateral flow from surrounding capillaries (see Chapter 17, under section on Vascular Changes) may be sufficient to preserve most of the cells. Another factor may be the temporary nature of the obstruction in many cases. These white opaque patches produce scotomas in the acute phase, but most clear without leaving a residual field defect. Cotton-wool spots occur in a wide range of diseases including hypertension, diabetes, the collagenoses, severe anemia, leukemia, bacterial endocarditis, following severe hemorrhages, and in Purtscher's retinopathy (Fig. 12-2) (see Chapter 10, under section on Cotton-wool Spots).

Fluorescein angiography usually shows that the capillary bed beneath the cotton-wool spot is incompletely perfused and the feeding arteriole is abnormal.

The natural history of these white patches varies in different diseases. They last only a few days or weeks in treated hypertensive disease but may remain for months in diabetic patients. Their long life in diabetes may be related to a very slow and incomplete restoration of capillary flow.

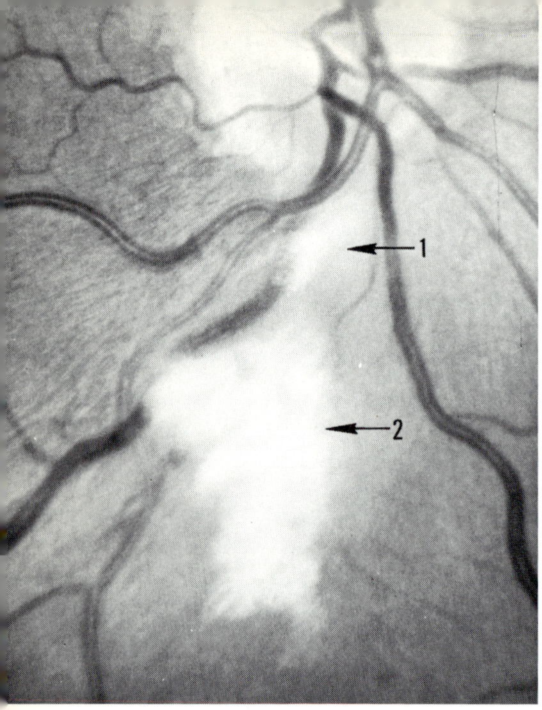

Fig. 12-1. A single (**1**) and an aggregate (**2**) of several cotton-wool spots.

Fig. 12-2. *A*, Purtscher's retinopathy in right eye. The veins are full and dark and there are superficial hemorrhages and multiple fresh, cotton-wool spots at the posterior pole. This developed shortly after an attack of alcoholic delirium and acute pancreatitis. *B*, Left eye of same patient. Corrected vision was 20/50 in each eye.

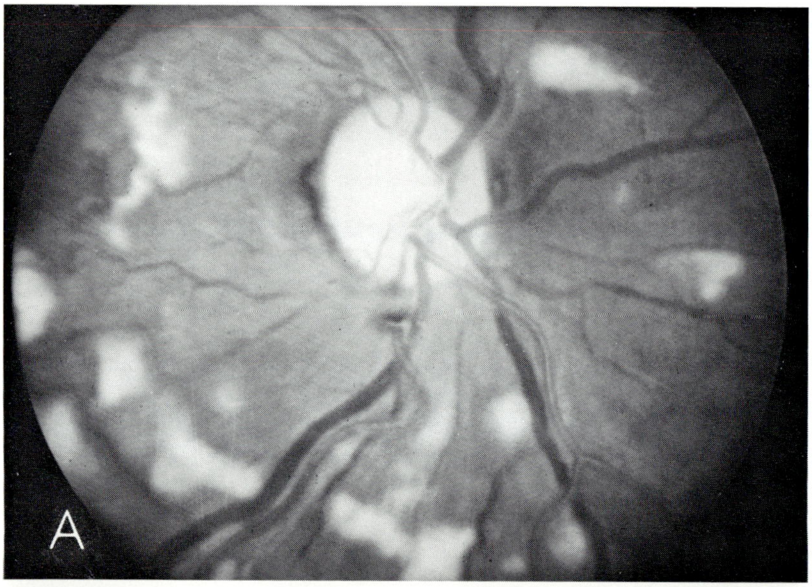

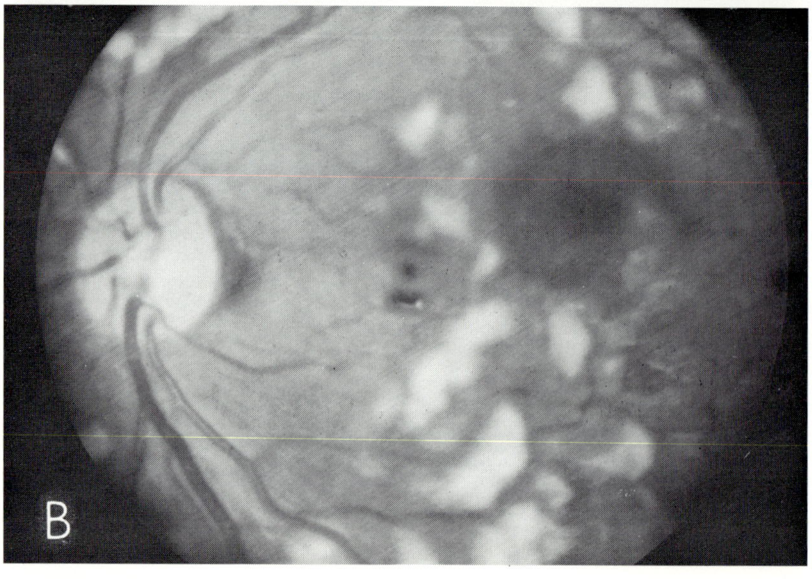

The pathology of the obstructive process in the precapillary arteriole which leads to formation of a cotton-wool spot is incompletely understood. In hypertension, focal arteriolar necrosis such as is seen in other organs is probably responsible. The nature of the obstructive process in diabetes is not known, but blocked arterioles can be demonstrated by fluorescein angiography. It is not known whether anatomic obstruction of a vessel takes place during formation of cotton-wool spots in anemia or following severe gastrointestinal hemorrhage. Conceivably local impairment of flow resulting from a reduced oxygen-carrying capacity of the blood, or low blood pressure can lead to cotton-wool spot formation without complete obstruction.

COLLAGEN DISEASES

Patients with disseminated lupus erythematosus, polyarteritis nodosa, dermatomyositis, and scleroderma may well develop retinopathy. The clinical picture is dominated by the formation of multiple cotton-wool spots and some superficial hemorrhages with superficial retinal edema. Macular stars are occasionally seen. Many of these patients have hypertension and the retinopathy which they develop is indistinguishable from that found in accelerated hypertension. Although retinopathy has rarely been observed in normotensive patients, the relative importance of hypertension and the vascular involvement of the underlying disease has not been determined. Patients with lupus erythematosus or polyarteritis who are hypertensive and have retinopathy lose their cotton-wool spots, hemorrhages, and retinal edema when the blood pressure is reduced. In these patients it seems reasonable to ascribe the retinopathy to the hypertension and not to direct vascular involvement of the disease. Most patients with early lupus erythematosus who are normotensive have no retinopathy. Indeed we have followed for upwards of 8 years more than 50 patients with proven lupus and have found very few examples of so-called "lupus retinopathy."

Ashton and co-workers[3] feel that fibrinoid change in retinal arterioles may be the common pathogenic factor in the very similar vascular retinopathies of collagen disease and malignant hypertension. In their study of two patients with progressive systemic sclerosis (scleroderma) they found lipid in the wall of retinal precapillary arterioles which had fibrinoid changes. In one patient these vascular changes were clearly responsible for the retinal ischemia causing the cotton-wool spots. Foci of acellular capillaries were found in relation to the degenerate precapillary arterioles. Fibrinoid change was also noted in choroidal arteries and fibrinous material was found in the lumen of the choriocapillaris. Fibrinoid change may result from the extravasation of plasma into an altered vessel wall, presumably where the endothelium is damaged.

ANEMIA

Patients with severe anemia may develop retinopathy with typical cotton-wool spots, superficial hemorrhages, superficial retinal edema, and sometimes a macular star. The arteries appear slightly pale and the veins are dilated. Patients with aplastic anemia often show widespread fans of preretinal hemorrhages or Roth's spots. Rarely, bleeding into the vitreous occurs.

The hemoglobin concentration is usually very low before retinopathy develops, often below 2.5 gm per 100 ml.

Retinal hemorrhages are rare in hemophilia, Cooley's anemia, and thrombocytopenia alone. The combination of anemia and thrombocytopenia enhances the incidence of retinal hemorrhages and here, the more severe the thrombocytopenia the more frequent are the retinal hemorrhages.[71]

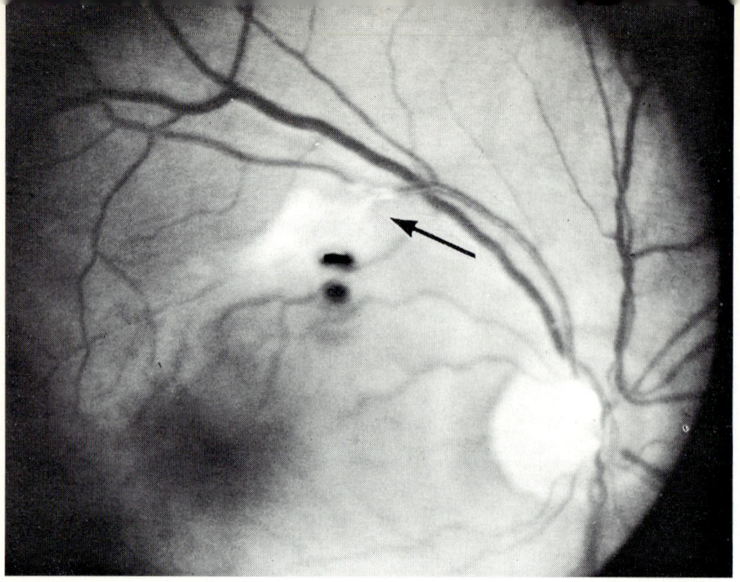

Fig. 12-3. Acute occlusion of a small branch retinal artery. Site of occlusion is indicated by **arrow**.

Merin and Freund [60] found that children under the age of 14 years were especially resistant to anemic retinopathy.

Fluorescein studies in anemic patients show that capillary filling is incomplete beneath cotton-wool spots but arterial obstruction has not been demonstrated (Bulpitt, C., Personal communication). Reversal of anemia by treatment leads to complete regression of all associated retinal abnormalities.

OBSTRUCTIONS OF BRANCH RETINAL ARTERIES

The vast majority of branch retinal artery obstructions are due to embolism and almost all occur at bifurcations (Fig. 12-3). On the other hand not all emboli produce lumen obstruction. Cholesterol crystals commonly do not. It is not unusual to see one or more resting at an arterial bifurcation without producing other signs or symptoms. Often a slight tap on the globe will dislodge them and permit them to move downstream either to disappear into the periphery or relocate at some more distal bifurcation. Arterial lumen narrowing may produce little retinal pathology and present no symptoms until a critical level of flow restriction is reached. It has been shown that two-thirds of the channel may be occluded without retinal infarction, or indeed without evidence of abnormal reaction beyond the obstructive site.[5] On the other hand, fluorescein angiography often shows some degree of lumen patency in classic retinal infarctions.[31] Clinical evidence suggests that infarction is an all-or-none phenomenon. If flow is sufficient to sustain normal function, the retina appears normal; if not an infarct appears. Uncommonly, one may see a case which wavers between these two extremes for a short period. The flow is either promptly reestablished by dislodgement of the embolus (Fig. 12-4) or more commonly the obstructed retinal area eventually becomes infarcted (for stagnation venous obstruction see Chapter 14, under section on Stagnation Thrombosis). Such cases may show a faint haze in the embarrassed retinal region with scattered accentuated white spots suggestive of cotton-wool patches.

Late in severe arteriosclerosis, branch artery obstruction may occur at any site on the arterial tree. In such cases occlusions are not limited to bifurcations. Very rarely, focal necrotic arteriolar lesions with lumen blockage may be seen at any site on larger arterioles in nonhypertensive patients. The latter has been seen in four patients all of whom had similar lesions on arteries and veins leading to obstructions of both vessel systems (Fig. 12-5)

When a major branch arteriole is blocked at the disc, one may sometimes find a hemianopic scotoma suggesting involvement of the adjacent arterial branches. The infarcted retina may be denser white in one quadrant than the other. As time passes, the least involved quadrant may rapidly clear and resume function, while the more involved one remains infarcted. Such an occurrence suggests one of two things: (*1*) either the em-

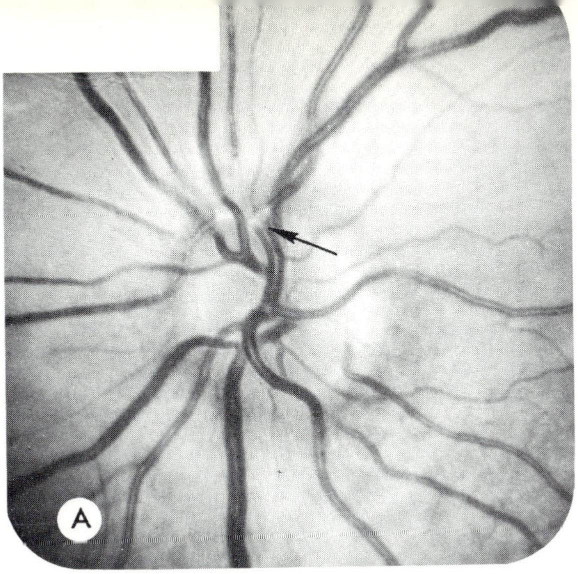

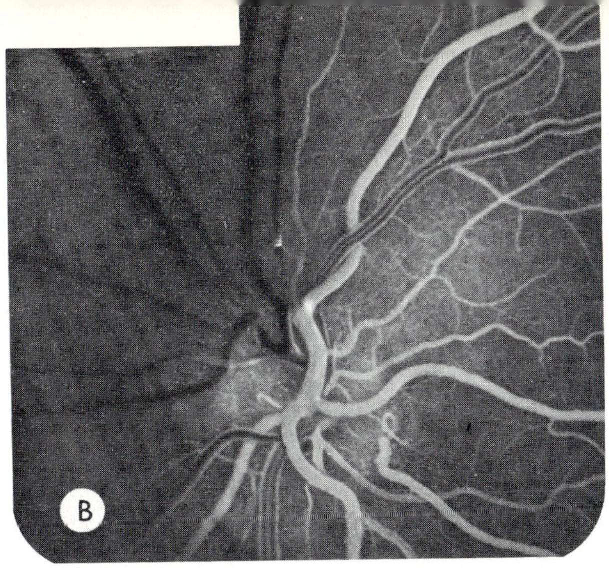

Fig. 12-4. Acute obstruction of the superior retinal artery due to an embolus. Initially, there was a more marked cloudy swelling in the upper nasal quadrant than in the upper temporal area. Following ocular massage, the embolus moved downstream freeing the superior temporal branch. The cloudy swelling in this quadrant cleared.

A, Site **(arrow)** of the embolus after massage.

B, Fluorescein angiogram. Arterial phase shows free flow in the superior temporal artery, and obstruction of the superior nasal artery.

C, Arteriovenous phase shows retrograde flow **(A).** The side of the obstructed branch artery containing the dye is filled from the perfused capillary bed. Another similar site **(B)** in the most obstructed branch, fills from perfused capillaries. Here, flow is in the normal direction.

D, Late phase of the angiogram shows the slow granular flow past the obstruction.

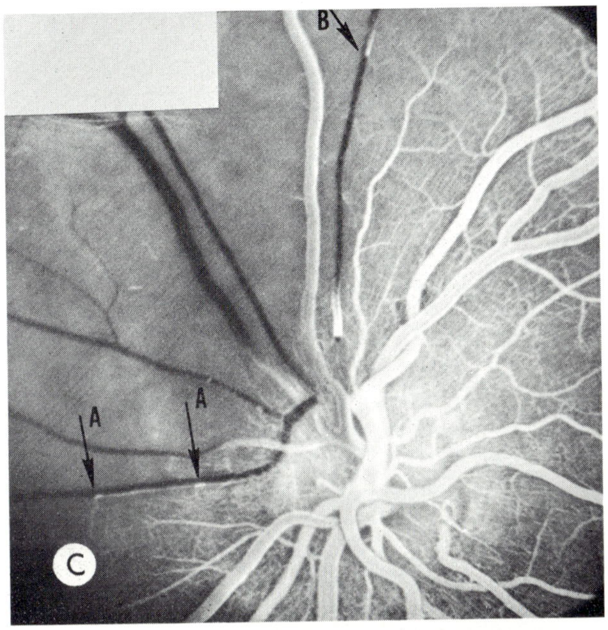

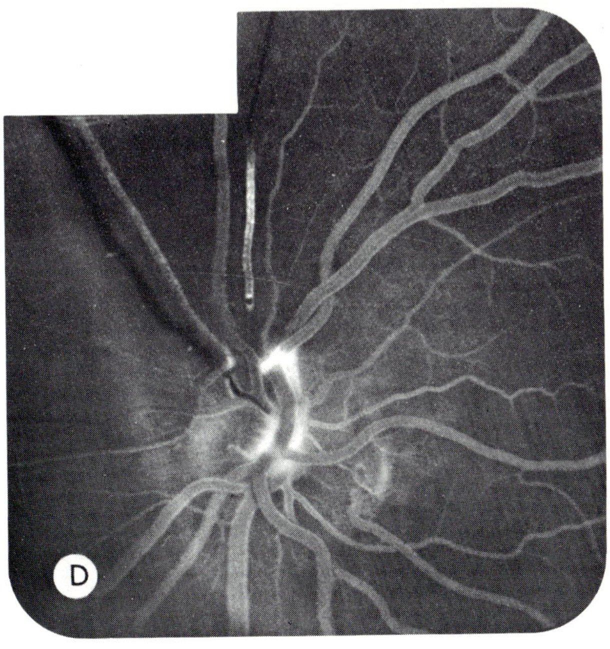

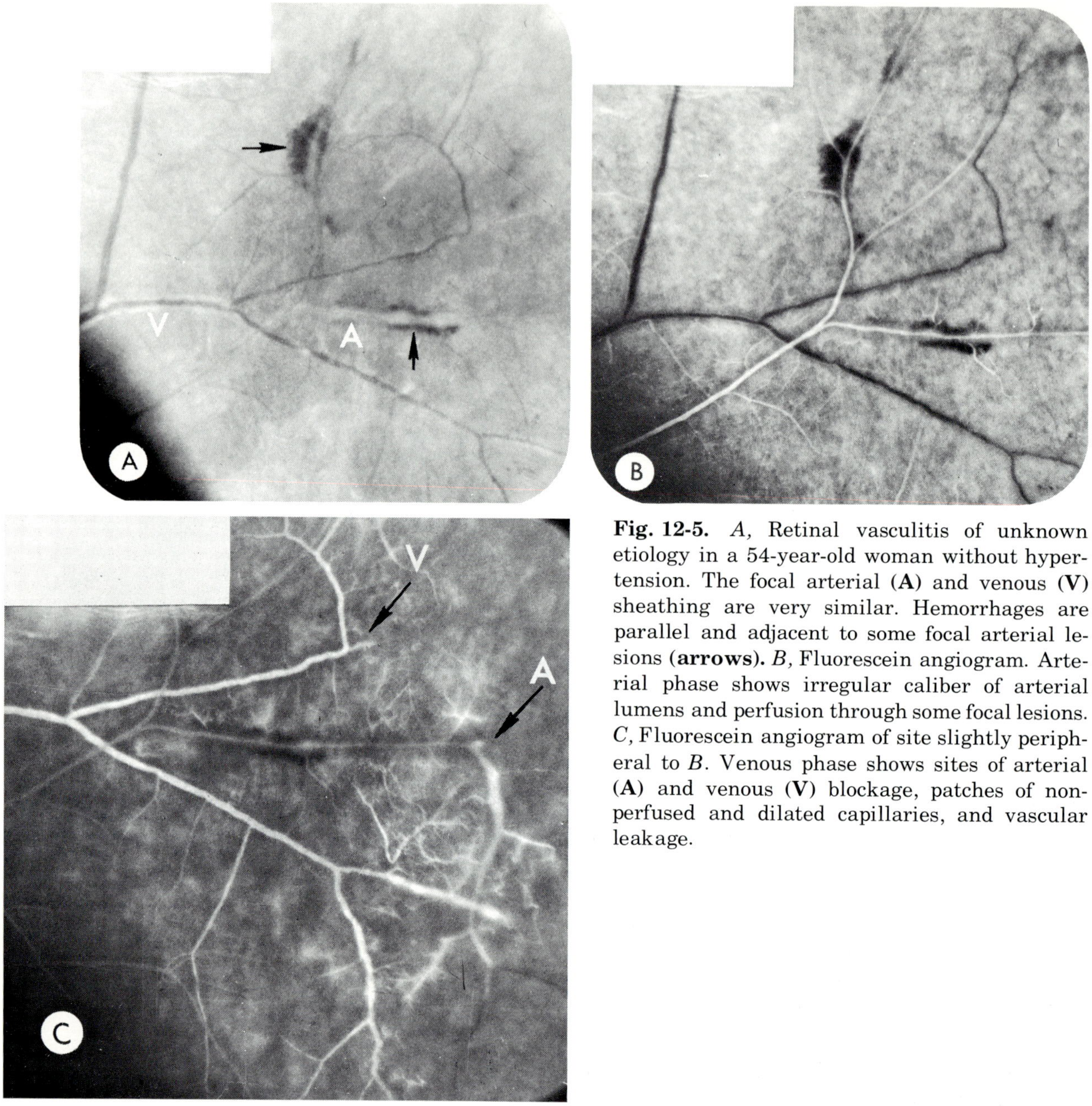

Fig. 12-5. *A,* Retinal vasculitis of unknown etiology in a 54-year-old woman without hypertension. The focal arterial **(A)** and venous **(V)** sheathing are very similar. Hemorrhages are parallel and adjacent to some focal arterial lesions **(arrows).** *B,* Fluorescein angiogram. Arterial phase shows irregular caliber of arterial lumens and perfusion through some focal lesions. *C,* Fluorescein angiogram of site slightly peripheral to *B*. Venous phase shows sites of arterial **(A)** and venous **(V)** blockage, patches of nonperfused and dilated capillaries, and vascular leakage.

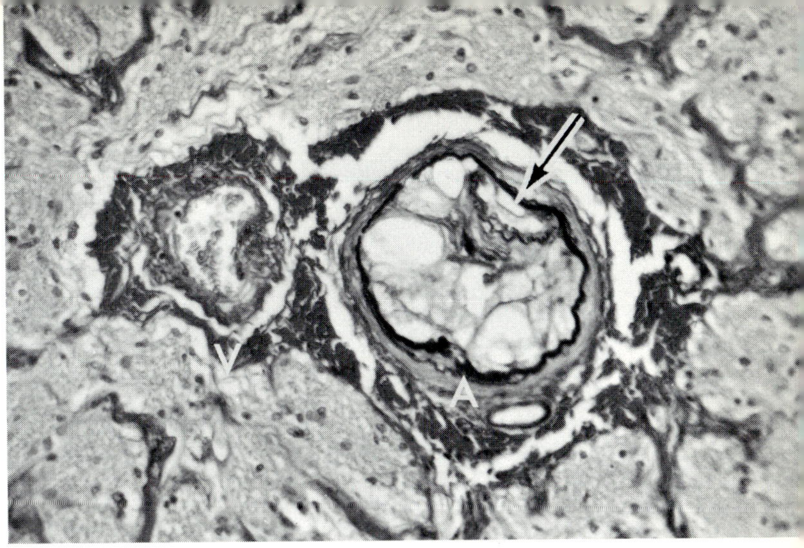

Fig. 12-6. Central retinal artery obstruction at the lamina cribrosa. The atheroma reduces the lumen to a narrow slit **(arrow)**. Artery **(A)**; vein **(V)**. (Courtesy of Dr. G. Kurz.)

bolus partially obstructed an adjacent channel temporarily, or (2) the trauma of embolus impaction produced temporary spasm in the adjacent arteriole.

Obstructions of branch and central retinal arteries have so many common features that they will be discussed together in the next section.

OBSTRUCTIONS OF THE CENTRAL RETINAL ARTERY

Most central retinal artery obstructions are due either to emboli (see Chapter 10, under the section on Retinal Emboli), atheroma or hemorrhage beneath the atheroma [22a] at the level of the lamina cribrosa and they usually occur in patients with hypertension and arteriosclerosis. Rarer causes include cranial arteritis, polyarteritis [6,28] secondary syphilis, orbital granuloma,[33a,17] loa loa microfilaria,[20] and trauma. While a terminal thrombotic episode may complete the lumen closure initiated by an atheroma or some endarteritic pathology, it is unlikely that primary thrombosis occurs in any retinal artery. It is unlikely that arteriolar spasm ever acts as a basic mechanism of retinal artery closure. The usual site of obstruction is at the lamina cribosa; the intraneural segment of the artery or its exit from the nerve may also be involved (Fig. 12-6).

Pressure exerted upon the globe during anesthesia has produced central retinal artery occlusion in previously healthy eyes. While factors incident to anesthesia may play some part, the sustained rise in intraocular pressure is of primary importance.[33]

High, sustained acute rises in intraocular pressure, as in untreated angle closure glaucoma, impair the blood supply to the retina and also to the optic nerve just behind the lamina cribrosa. Even a few days of such pressure levels leads to infarction of this optic nerve segment and subsequently to cavernous optic atrophy.[95]

The patient is usually aware of a retinal arterial obstruction from the time of its occurrence. The positive scotoma of branch obstruction or the total loss of vision with central artery occlusion are both dramatic. Occasionally, transient obscurations of vision immediately precede permanent loss, but persisting loss from onset is much more common.

Once the central retinal artery has become occluded, the involved retina becomes edematous, white, and opaque (Fig. 12-7). The veins darken and commonly show sludged blood while arterioles are narrowed and less frequently show sludging. Severe sudden blockages may even show transient reversal of arterial flow or dark, segmented arterial columns which either move back

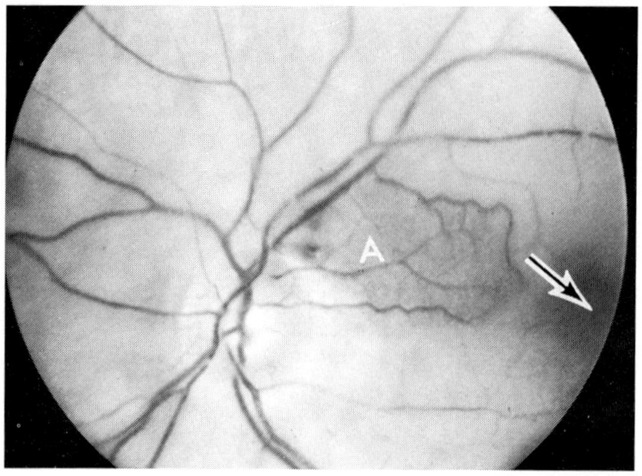

Fig. 12-7. Acute central retinal artery obstruction with a patent cilioretinal artery **(A)**. A part of the cherry red spot at the macula can be seen **(arrow)**.

Fig. 12-8. A cherry red spot at the macula in Tay-Sach's disease.

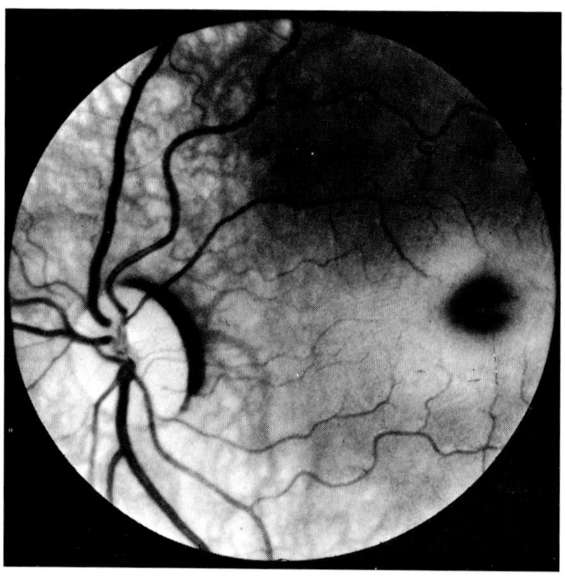

and forth with each pulse wave or remain stationary. The foveal area being uninvolved by the infarction transmits its normal red choroidal color as the "cherry red" spot of central retinal artery obstruction (Fig. 12-7). This cherry red spot differs from those of the lipoidoses where lipid material is deposited predominantly in ganglion cells. In the latter, an opaque white zone surrounds the fovea in the region of densest ganglion cell distribution (Fig. 12-8). It then fades in all directions in direct proportion to the decreasing ganglion cell population. This accentuated white ring about the fovea with fading toward the disc is not seen in central retinal artery obstruction where the opaque whiteness is more uniform posteriorly, or actually increases toward the disc. It is thus evident that ganglion cell death is not solely responsible for the opacity of the latter.

Rarely, a few small retinal hemorrhages, usually superficial and due to capillary wall damage, may be seen.

As all visual function promptly ceases in infarcted retinal areas, total visual failure is an early symptom of all central artery occlusions where a cilioretinal artery is lacking. Preservation of some central visual function in the face of a severely infarcted retina indicates the presence of such a cilioretinal artery. Some patients who have only vague light perception following an occlusive episode may, within a week or two, be able to count fingers as they learn to use a small viable retinal area adjacent to the disc supplied by a cilioretinal artery. Such occurrences have been mistaken for improvement in the central artery obstruction. As the cilioretinal and central retinal arterial systems are independent of each other, involvement of one in no way affects the other.

Microscopically, clumping of the nuclear chromatin and rupture of the cytoplasmic membranes in the inner retinal cells may occur as early as 3.5 hours after total arterial block [51] and after 2 to 3.5 hours irreversible changes take place in the electrical activity of the retina and optic tract.[38] As autolysis proceeds, fluid is imbibed[51] and the inner retinal layers become opaque, vascular endothelium and intramural pericytes degenerate leaving large numbers of cell-free functionless capillaries[50] (Fig. 12-9). The dead material of the inner retina is absorbed or ingested by phagocytes and removed. Gliosis replaces the nerve fiber, ganglion cell, and inner plexiform layers, and some superficial cells of the inner nuclear layer. As these layers under normal conditions, and their replacing gliosis are both clinically invisible, little fundic change except that of the vessels and disc is noted after central retinal artery obstruction. The retinal veins invariably return to their original state without residual sheathing or alteration. The retinal opacity clears within several weeks and the arterial tree may resume its preocclusive appearance (Fig. 12-10). On the other hand, the arteries may be irregularly narrowed, more burnished than normal, show fine white striping, or an irregular and denser white coating, which may hide the blood column in places[54] (Fig. 12-11). More rarely, severe arteriosclerosis with glinting reflections develops in arterial walls. The disc may be clearly outlined and pale, or have a more ragged border with increased disc gliosis. In this instance gliosis may sheath disc vessels, fill the physiologic cup, and produce a dirty gray disc color with indistinct markings.

Collateral vessels are rarely seen following a central retinal artery occlusion. Central and branch artery occlusions often recanalize. If branch arteries remain closed collaterals may form, although these are often of small caliber and not obvious on clinical examination. Fluorescein angiograms can demonstrate them supplying blood from adjacent patent vessels (Fig. 12-12). Collateral inflow is too late to maintain the viability of the retina in the ischemic area. Pigment alterations, retinal microaneurysms, preretinal new vessel formation and fibrosis do not occur following retinal arterial obstructions.

Branch and central retinal artery obstructions produce identical reactions in the retinal areas they supply. In branch occlusion, the retinal zone downstream to the site of the obstruction becomes infarcted and opaque. The unobstructed retinal regions retain their normal appearance and function. The border between the two is irregular and fuzzy (Fig. 12-13) but corresponding field defects have straight edges.

Thus arterial obstructions between the lamina cribrosa and the precapillary arterioles usually cause complete loss of function. The resulting picture of retinal infarction completely overshadows the basic obstructing mechanism and the subsequent course of all such obstructions is the same.

While this is the common course of events there are rare exceptions. Occasionally, blockage of a branch or the central retinal artery will be of such a degree to permit retinal cells to waver back and forth at critical survival and functional levels. In such cases blood sludging is less common and may be visible only with coincident pressure on the globe to further reduce the rate of flow. Very mild retinal haze with scattered, more opaque cotton-wool-like patches may be seen associated with an occasional superficial retinal hemorrhage. The white patches lie at the posterior pole and often near the macula. Veins appear a little dark and arteries are irregularly narrowed. Both vision and fundus appearance may show daily fluctuations and visual fields may vary. This state, however, does not long persist. The critical zone is so narrow that usually in a matter of several days there is either improvement in blood flow and resolution, with varying degrees of residual defect, or the occlusion progresses and retinal infarction ensues.

With early recovery centrocecal or paracentral scotomas may remain with field recovery elsewhere, or more extensive, irregular field defects may persist.

Some cases of this type may suddenly convert to the typical apoplectic picture of central retinal vein obstruction. This is known

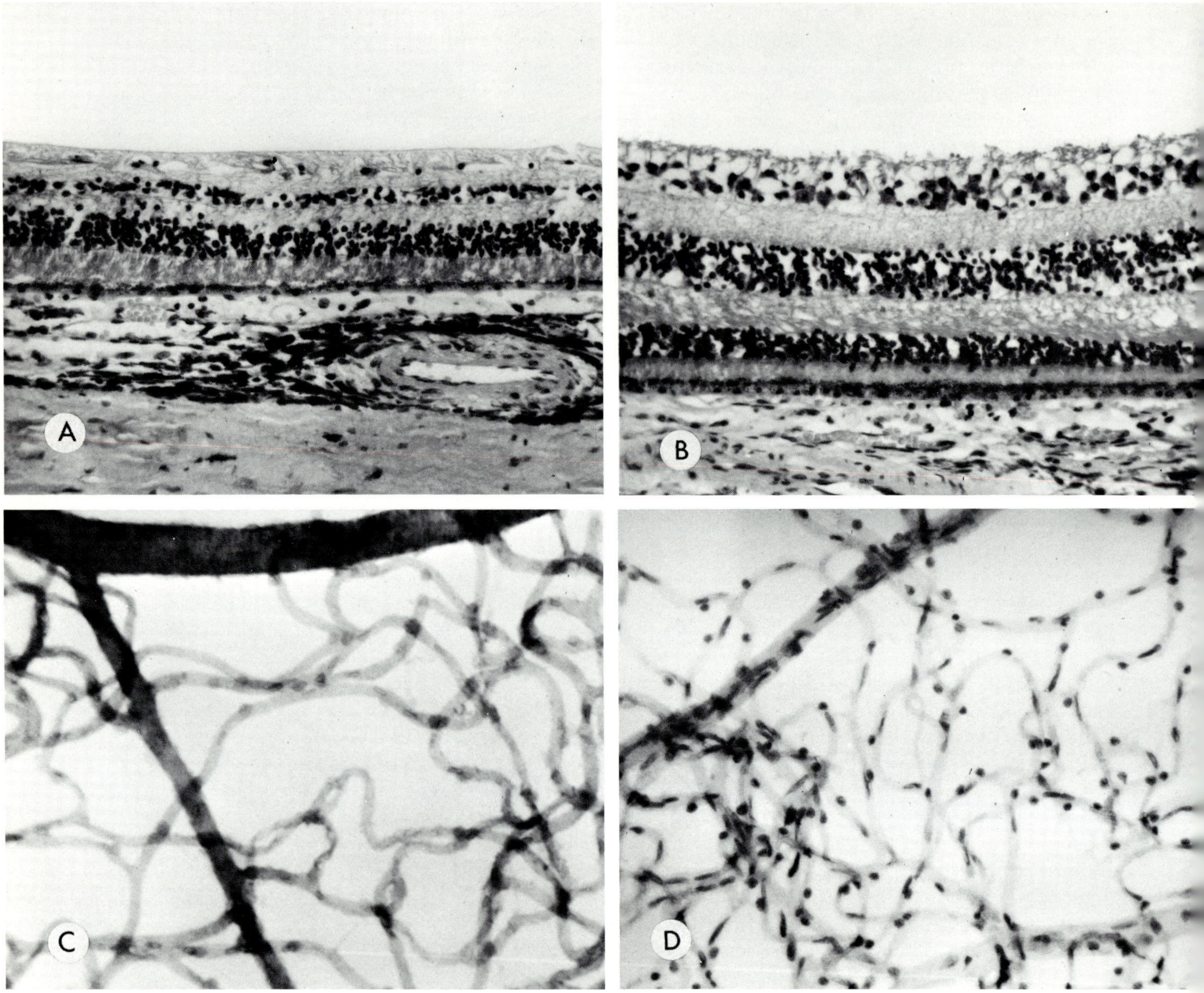

Fig. 12-9. Effect on the retina and its vessels of central retinal artery occlusion shown in Figure 12-6.

A, Histologic appearance shows reduction of ganglion cell-nerve fiber layer and thinning of the inner nuclear layer, with replacement gliosis. The outer retinal layers nourished by the choroid are well preserved (H&E, ×200).

B, Histologic appearance of the normal fellow eye in this patient. The entire retina is well preserved (H&E, ×200).

C, Retinal-digest preparation of the involved eye shows degeneration of the endothelial cells and intramural pericytes in the capillary bed.

D, Retinal-digest preparation of the normal fellow eye showing well-preserved capillary cellularity.

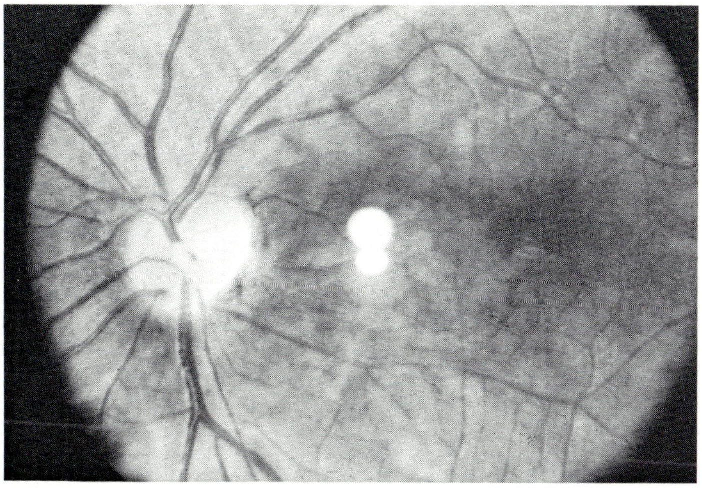

Fig. 12-10. *Above.* The appearance of central retinal artery obstruction some time after the obstructive episode. There is narrowing of the inferior temporal artery but the other arteries appear relatively normal.

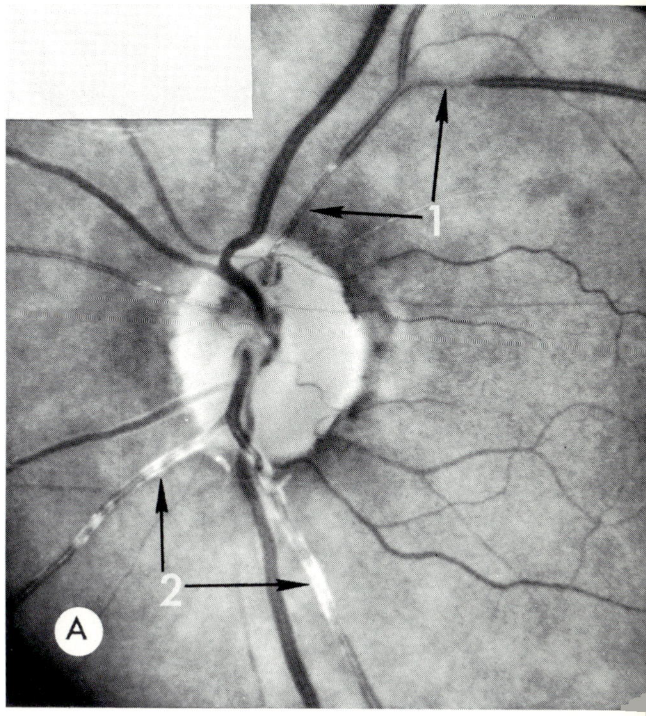

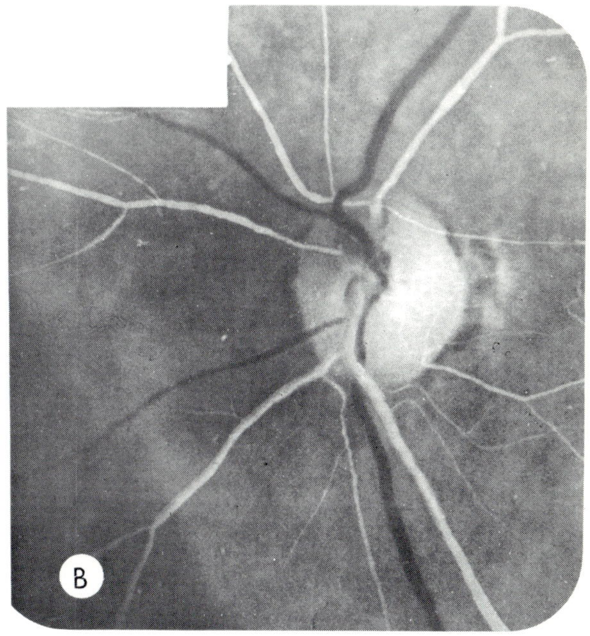

Fig. 12-11. *Right. A,* Nine months after a central retinal artery obstruction. Note marked arterial irregularity (1) and severe arteriosclerosis (2). *B,* Fluorescein angiogram made 9 seconds after dye injection. Arterial phase shows no delay in filling but marked narrowing and irregularity of arterial lumens.

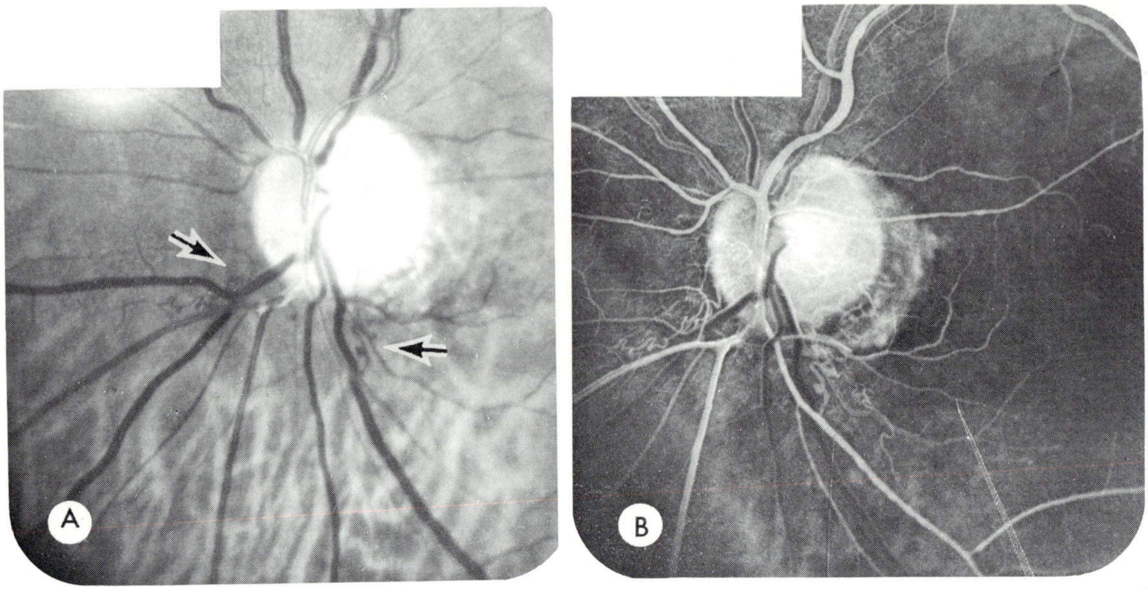

Fig. 12-12. *A*, Left eye, 2 years after an obstruction of the inferior retinal artery at the disc. Arterial collaterals **(arrows)** developed too late to preserve retinal function. *B*, Arterial-phase fluorescein angiogram demonstrates arterial collaterals in *A*.

Fig. 12-13. Obstruction of the inferior retinal artery. Note the irregular junction between the infarcted and normal retina **(black arrows).** A previous branch vein obstruction with collateral circulation **(C)** was an incidental finding.

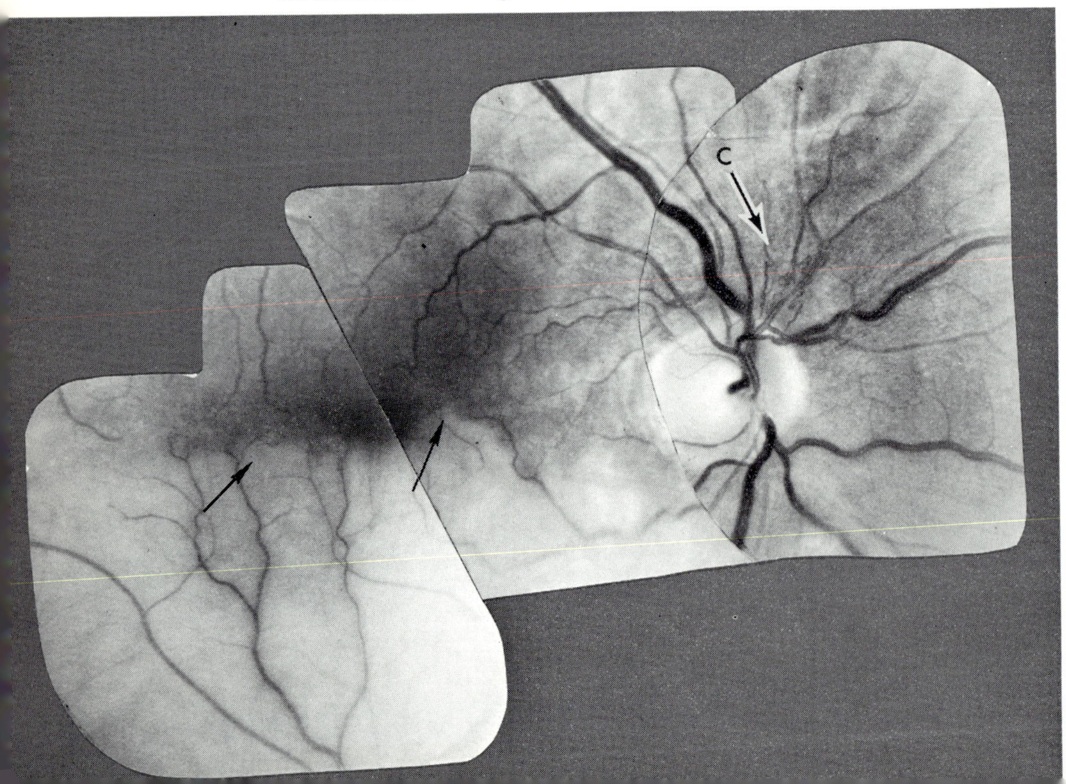

as stagnation thrombosis where the reduced arterial inflow leads to venous underfilling and eventual occlusion. These fundi usually show less venous distention and fewer hemorrhages due to the reduced blood flow to the retina.

Most central artery obstructions which never waver transiently between life and death of retinal cells occur in older individuals. The arteries are often straightened with acute angle bifurcations. These changes with narrowing of the arteries have been attributed by Friedenwald[29] to arteriosclerosis of the intraneural portion of the central retinal artery. He thought that the decreased arterial blood volume and vessel contracture were responsible for this change. This explanation is completely unproved and older individuals often have such arterial configurations without blockage.

There is no known way to prophesy a branch or central retinal artery obstruction. It is fortunately very rare for an individual to have a central retinal artery obstruction in one eye and a second one in the fellow eye, except in cranial arteritis.

Central retinal artery obstruction occurring in systemic diseases such as secondary syphilis, polyarteritis, or sickle cell disease are usually acute in onset and result in complete inner retinal infarction. They seldom occur unless the basic disease is in a severe stage and are therefore usually seen among in-patient hospital populations. Their ocular course is the same as in any other central artery obstruction. If there is retinopathy prior to the obstructive episode, it invariably disappears with the onset of optic atrophy.

ARTERIAL OBSTRUCTIONS BEHIND THE LAMINA CRIBROSA

Diseases affecting the arteries between the lamina cribrosa and the heart commonly cause patchy abnormalities of the arterial wall. Clinical localization of the site of obstruction may be difficult because the arterial lumen may be narrowed or obstructed at more than one point between the aorta and the eye. In the following section each disease entity is discussed under the title of the artery which demonstrates the most severe involvement.

OBSTRUCTIONS OF THE OPHTHALMIC ARTERY

The common diseases attacking the ophthalmic artery are cranial arteritis and arteriosclerosis. Emboli obstructing the ophthalmic artery have not been demonstrated microscopically. They must, however, be considered as a possible source of obstruction, for they are found commonly downstream and larger emboli could reasonably be expected to obstruct an upstream vessel of somewhat larger bore.

Ophthalmic artery obstructions may be divided into three groups: (*1*) those obstructing the artery sufficiently forward to produce the clinical picture of central retinal artery obstruction; (*2*) those obstructing the artery sufficiently near its source to involve posterior ciliary arteries as well; and (*3*) those obstructions producing sudden or slow ischemia of the optic nerve. In a diffuse disease process there may not always be a single obstruction at a specific site, but the various clinical entities produced do suggest that the major interference with flow is in each case at a different location.

Blockage producing the clinical picture of central retinal artery obstruction must exert its major effect in the peripheral portion of the artery beyond the exit of the ciliary vessels. It produces either the typical picture of central retinal artery obstruction or a milder form of this appearance where vision fails suddenly, but the retina shows only a generalized posterior haze accentuated into more opaque cotton-wool-like patches here and there in the posterior fundus. The arteries are usually narrowed and a rare flame-shaped hemorrhage near the disc may be seen. Vascular blood sludging is uncommon but may be produced by pressure upon the globe. The electroretinogram (ERG) in such cases is normal except for a slight reduction in the b-wave.

Blockage proximal to the exit of posterior ciliary vessels also produces the appearance of central retinal artery occlusion either in its typical or milder form. In addition, however, the ERG is extinguished and after a short interval, mild to severe pigment migration and proliferation occurs posteriorly. Any central retinal artery obstruction with an extinguished ERG and later pigment dispersal (Fig. 12-14) therefore indicates infarction of the entire posterior retina due to critical interference with both the retinal and choroidal blood flow.[14]

Those obstructions producing sudden or slow ischemia of the optic nerve suggest that their major interference is with the nutrient vessels of the optic nerve.

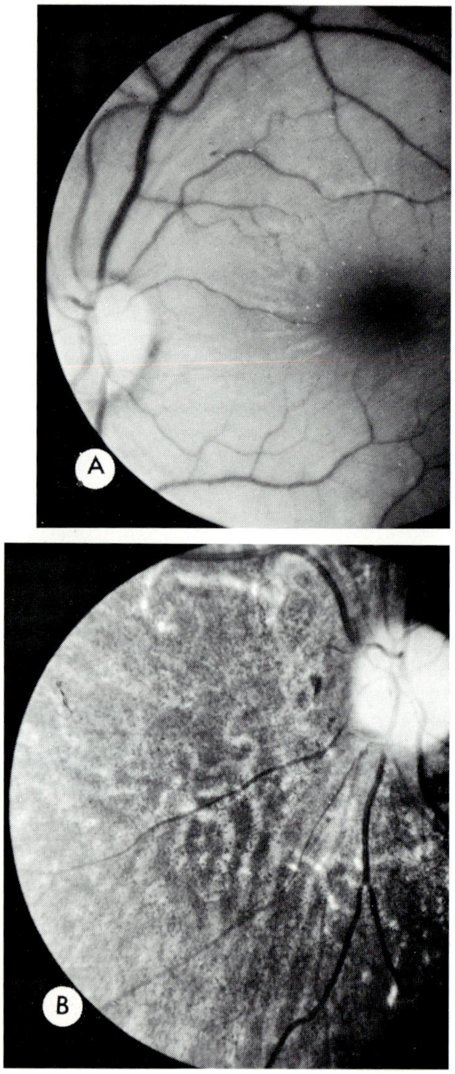

Fig. 12-14. *A,* Acute ophthalmic artery obstruction involving the posterior ciliary arteries in a 27-year-old woman immediately following caesarean section. At the time of this photograph, the ERG was extinguished. *B,* The same eye 2 months later showing optic atrophy, narrowed retinal arterioles, and dispersal, granularity, and clumping of the pigment epithelium. (Courtesy of Dr. R. Carr.)

CRANIAL ARTERITIS (TEMPORAL ARTERITIS; GIANT-CELL ARTERITIS)

Cranial arteritis[21,91,92] occurs about equally in men and women over the age of 55 and the incidence increases with age. While giant-cell arteritis may attack large, medium, and small arteries in many locations throughout the body, ocular involvement is most commonly associated with disease of cranial arteries—the temporal and occipital in this order of frequency. Reports of disease affecting the carotid, chiasmal, ophthalmic, retinal, and posterior ciliary arteries have been recorded in patients showing ocular involvement.[18,85] This disease has not been unequivocally demonstrated in branch retinal or choroidal arteries not having an internal elastic lamina, possibly due to its absence.[15] Disease of the

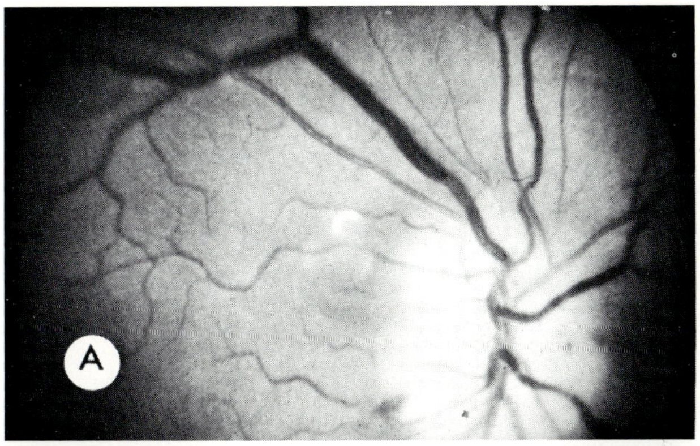

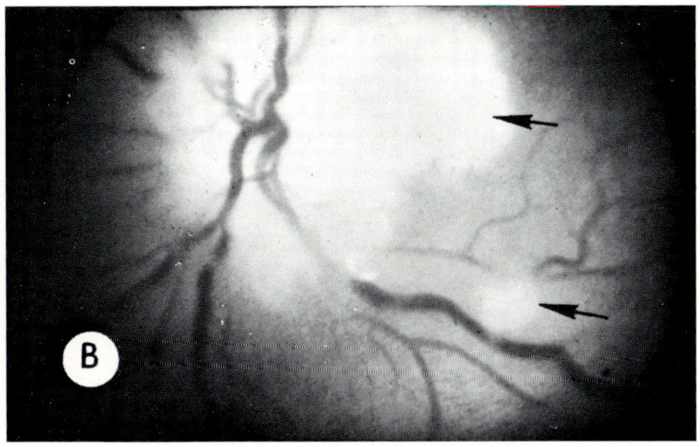

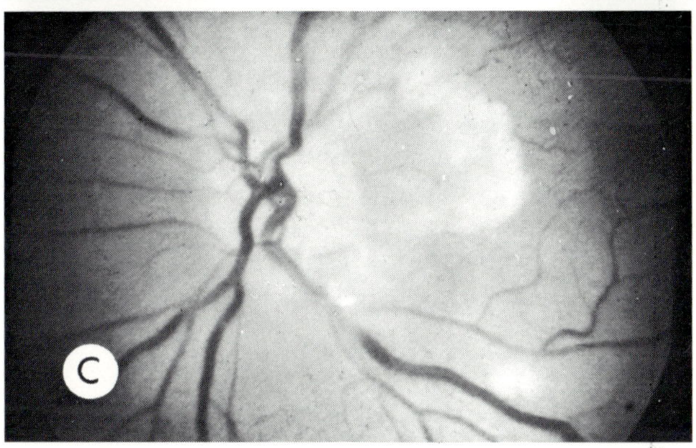

Fig. 12-15. *A*, Cranial arteritis. Ischemic optic neuropathy in right eye. Note the pale, slightly elevated disc with blurred margins and a single superficial hemorrhage on the disc border at eight o'clock. The veins are full and dark and the superior temporal artery is beaded. *B*, Same patient, with ischemic optic neuropathy in left eye. The disc is pale and more elevated than in the right eye and there are several cotton-wool spots **(arrows)** temporal to the disc. *C*, Appearance of left eye several days after *B*. The disc edema is receding and the cotton-wool spots are fading. Patient is blind in both eyes.

ciliary arteries at the circle of Zinn is thought to be necessary for the production of ischemic optic neuropathy—the most common clinical form of ocular involvement in cranial arteritis. Although widespread and variable in distribution, cranial arteritis has been included in this section, for ocular cases most commonly show involvement of the ophthalmic artery and some of its branches. The incidence of the ocular complications is high, but difficult to assess since the introduction of steroid therapy in the earlier stages of the generalized disease. In one series 12 of 72 patients were blind in both eyes;[92] another tally from the literature showed 54 of 250 patients to be bilaterally blind.[7]

Patients often give a history of general malaise, anorexia, weight loss, and headache. Scalp tenderness on combing the hair or resting on a pillow, and pain or fatigue on mastication are common complaints. Some patients present with sudden loss of vision, other symptoms being either absent or so mild as to be brought out only upon close questioning.[79] However, patients with ocular involvement commonly have a 2- to 3-month history of systemic symptoms.

Sudden monocular visual loss is the usual initial ocular complaint. Less commonly amaurosis fugax precedes permanent loss of vision. The latter is often total but may be altitudinal, quadrantic, or rarely, central.

Cases with binocular onset are rare. Involvement of the second eye, if it occurs, usually follows in a few days or weeks. Instances of diplopia and ptosis have been recorded.[92]

Involved cranial arteries show irregular tortuosity, nodular thickening, and poor or absent pulsations. A diseased artery may demonstrate a red overlying skin erythema or, rarely, an ischemic ulcer of the scalp.

The fundus usually shows an ischemic optic neuropathy. The disc is pale, edematous and elevated as much as 2 diopters (D). An occasional flame-shaped hemorrhage may be seen (Fig. 12-15). The arteries are narrowed and often there are cotton-wool spots in the posterior fundus. Blood sludging in veins and arteries is uncommon, but may be brought out by slight pressure on the globe. At times a mild, superficial retinal edema is visible. Less commonly seen, and suggesting a peripheral obstruction, is the classic pattern of retinal infarction with a cherry red spot at the macula. Very rarely, narrowed arterioles and a normal optic nerve head in the absence of light perception suggests severe posterior involvement of the optic nerve.

The erythrocyte sedimentation rate (ESR) is usually raised, often markedly so, but in rare cases normal values have been reported.[92]

The vascular pathology of this disease includes a narrowed, thrombosed or obliterated lumen, marked intimal thickening, fragmentation of the internal elastic lamella with giant cells, and often calcium particles in its vicinity and round cell infiltration of the media and, to a lesser degree, of the adventitia. Epithelioid cells and eosinophils may be present (Fig. 12-16). Spirochetes have been demonstrated in some biopsy specimens of temporal arteritis, suggesting syphilis as an etiologic agent.[80]

In addition to the vascular pathology, ischemic optic neuropathy shows infarction of the optic nerve, or some portion of it just behind the lamina cribrosa (Fig. 12-17).

Once the eye has become involved, and usually irrespective of treatment, the ocular signs evolve in 2 or 3 weeks to the picture of secondary optic atrophy with narrowed retinal arterioles. Stagnation thrombosis of the central retinal vein is a rare complication and late rubeosis iridis with hemorrhagic glaucoma has been reported.[94]

The duration of cranial arteritis is not accurately known, but it probably continues for well over a year. About half of all patients show some ocular involvement. A high index of suspicion is essential for early diagnosis of this disease. Prompt and adequate steroid treatment for as long as necessary – 6 months to several years – usually prevents progression of the visual loss although an initial loss rarely recovers. The institution of treatment should not await the biopsy report, nor should the disease necessarily be excluded by a negative biopsy. Relapses may occur if treatment is stopped too early. While reduction of the sedimentation rate is a good guide to treatment, it may not return to normal and therapy must be gauged by improvement in general symptoms. In occasional patients the disease may progress in spite of vigorous treatment.

Rarely, periarteritis nodosa may mimic this disease.[91]

ARTERIOSCLEROSIS OF THE OPHTHALMIC ARTERY

Some older patients may first be seen with a very similar clinical picture that does not appear to be due to cranial arteritis. Visual loss is usually not so severe, and central scotoma are more often seen. Neither improvement nor progressive loss of vision is usual. Histologic study has revealed an ischemic area located at, or just behind, the lamina cribrosa, a site also involved in temporal arteritis.[16]

Differential diagnosis between this condition and cranial arteritis is difficult. The

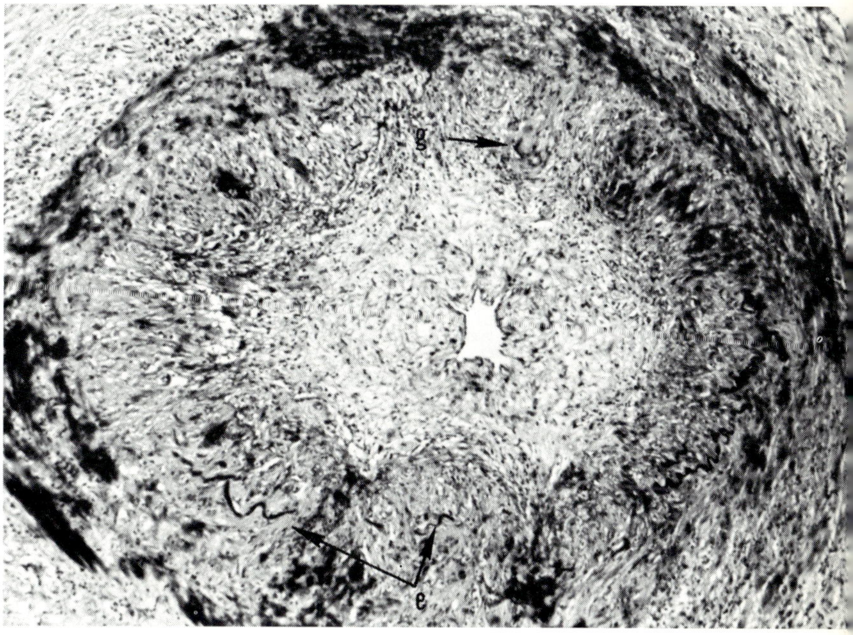

Fig. 12-16. The vascular pathology of cranial arteritis. Note the narrowed lumen, intimal thickening, fragmentation of the internal elastic lamella **(e)** and the giant cells **(g)**.

Fig. 12-17. Cranial arteritis. Histologic appearance of an ischemic optic nerve infarction **(arrows)**. (From Henkind, Charles, and Pearson. *Amer. J. Ophthal. 69:*78, 1970.)

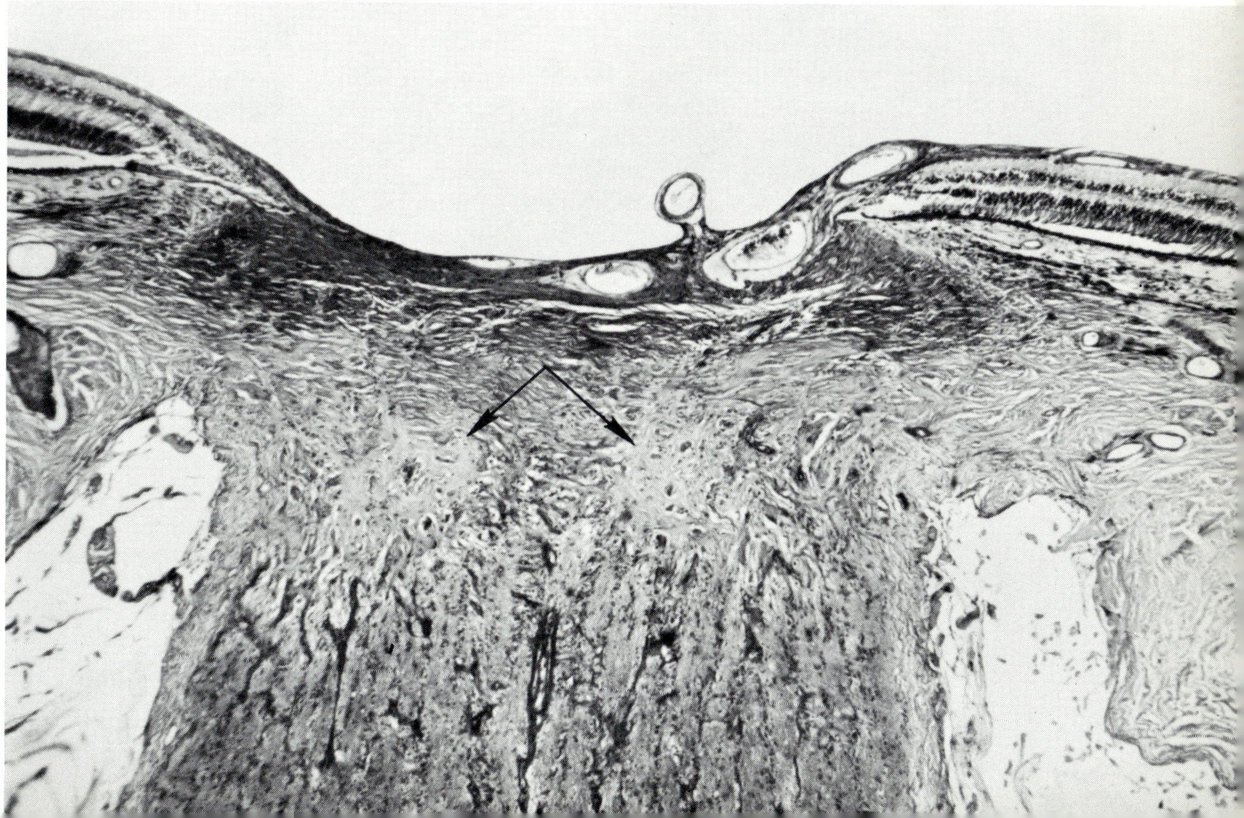

signs and symptoms of cranial arteritis are lacking in arteriosclerosis and the patients are more likely to have hypertension and clinical evidence of arterial disease elsewhere in the body. The cranial arteries are pulsatile and nontender. On biopsy they may show arteriosclerotic changes but no evidence of giant-cell arteritis. The ESR is usually normal, but can be elevated.[21] If doubt remains concerning the diagnosis it may be necessary to initiate treatment with corticosteroids.

ISCHEMIC OPTIC NEUROPATHY

Acute ischemic optic neuropathy more frequently occurs just behind the lamina cribrosa and is thought to result from disease of the posterior ciliary arteries at the circle of Zinn together with some involvement of the ophthalmic artery. Its clinical picture and the fact that it may be due to cranial arteritis or arteriosclerosis have been discussed above. Cases have also been reported in patients with both arteriosclerosis and diabetes[61] but these behave just like the arteriosclerotic group, the diabetes being usually mild with insignificant or no retinopathy. These do not improve, contrary to the course of diabetic involvement of oculomotor nerves. It therefore seems unlikely that these cases represent diabetic microangiopathy of nutrient vessels to the nerve itself. Occasionally an acute ischemic optic neuropathy will occur further back in the optic nerve in which case there will be no disc signs and usually little change in the retinal arteries or any alteration in the fundus. Visual loss and field change will depend on the position and degree of optic nerve infarction. A primary type of optic atrophy develops subsequently, depending in time on the distance of the lesion from the optic disc. These lesions are often indistinguishable from retrobulbar neuritis, especially when milder and selectively involving the papillomacular bundle.

Cases occurring after cataract extraction[68] and in pernicious anemia[26] have a much higher rate of improvement and should not be considered due to infarction until microscopic proof is available.

There is a chronic ischemic optic neuropathy which occurs in older patients. It is rare and in our experience has been seen only in patients over the age of 75 years. The site of vascular obstruction is unknown. This disease produces an appearance identical with glaucomatous disc excavation but without glaucoma (relative, soft, pseudo, or low tension glaucoma). Central scotoma, arcuate, quadrantic, altitudinal, and nasal field defects have all been seen in this condition. The disease may be present in one or both eyes, but in the latter case, one eye is usually much more involved than the other. The fact that it remains stationary or progresses very slowly permits a good visual prognosis. Cases occurring in these older individuals are thought to be due to arteriosclerosis of the nutrient vessels of the optic nerve.[49] Pituitary tumors, luetic cavernous optic atrophy, and congenital coloboma of the optic disc[8] have all given the fundus appearance of this low tension glaucoma. Pressure on the optic nerve from calcified carotid arteries[59] is a rare, verified cause of chronic optic atrophy with cupping which may simulate a slow ischemia of the optic nerve.

RETINAL ISCHEMIA FOLLOWING BLOOD LOSS

Following massive hemorrhage, usually from the gastrointestinal tract, some patients develop visual impairment with retinal hemorrhages, cotton-wool spots, and, in some instances, papilledema. In most cases both eyes are affected but a few monocular examples have been seen.

Usually these patients are so acutely ill from blood loss that the retina is not examined until the patient complains of visual disturbance some days later. At the time of the hypotensive episode the pupils are usually dilated and fixed but the fundus appearance is variable. There may be narrowed arteries and a pale disc. Blood sludging may indicate an extremely low retinal blood flow. Later, scattered flame-shaped hemorrhages, cotton-wool spots, and mild superficial retinal edema may be found. Rarely, the fundus appears normal despite the patient's visual symptoms or the picture of a typical central retinal artery obstruction with a cherry red spot at the macula may be seen. Later, optic atrophy, either partial or complete, and widespread pigment dispersal and proliferation are commonly visible.

The visual outcome in these cases is highly variable and the prognosis given should be guarded. About half the patients have visual improvement and a much smaller group regain normal vision. Some mild cases show no recovery, and others, with severely reduced vision in the beginning, show remarkable improvement.[19] One eye may recover fully while the fellow eye remains blind.

Visual fields are also variable and often unalike in the two eyes. Altitudinal defects and general depression of the field are most frequently found. Central scotoma probably of optic nerve origin and hemianopic defects probably from central involvement have also been seen.

There are few pathologic studies of this condition. One patient seen clinically and examined microscopically[4] showed several cotton-wool patches and flame-shaped hemorrhages in the posterior fundus. Typical cytoid bodies of cotton-wool exudates, retinal edema and splinter hemorrhages were found microscopically. Despite intensive search, no structural changes were found in any retinal arteriole including those in the immediate vicinity of the cotton-wool spots.

The ocular ischemia after blood loss has not been explained. The clinical picture and the few pathology reports suggest that it usually behaves as an insufficiency of the ophthalmic artery and its branches. Rarer cases with central scotoma or hemianopic defects suggest insufficiencies of nutrient vessels to the optic nerve or to the upper visual pathways respectively.

OBSTRUCTION OF THE INTERNAL CAROTID ARTERY

Insufficiency of the internal carotid artery is usually due to narrowing or closure of the vessel due to arteriosclerosis. The cross-sectional lumen must be reduced to about 2 to 4 square mm or less for a significant drop in blood flow above the lesion to occur.[11] This represents a reduction in the lumen of an average internal carotid artery by 80 to 90 per cent. Final closure results from a terminal thrombosis at the site of an ulcerous atheromatous plaque or hemorrhage beneath the plaque.[36] These occlusions are mainly located in the first curved portion of the internal carotid artery just beyond the common carotid bifurcation. The atheromatous disease is by no means limited to this site, but is usually present to some degree in other major arteries to the head or spread along the more involved carotid. The terminal thrombosis may not remain limited, but can extend distally into the brain or into the ophthalmic artery.

Insufficiency or closure of the internal carotid artery is usually unilateral, less than 10 per cent of the cases being bilateral.[42] It generally affects middle-aged or elderly men more often than women, and is often associated with systemic arteriosclerosis and hypertension.

As the ophthalmic artery is the first branch of the internal carotid, closure of the carotid can exert a profound influence on the ocular blood supply. Collaterals between the external carotid artery, which seldom undergoes occlusion, and the ophthalmic artery are common,[76] and have been frequently demonstrated in patients with internal carotid artery obstruction.[44,53,57,72] This could account for some of the misleading ophthalmodynamometry readings[81] particularly in slow obliterations which permit sufficient time for collateral conduits to enlarge. Collateral circulation would also account for those cases in which the ophthalmic artery has been surgically clipped in young individuals without adverse visual effect.[87]

Cases of internal carotid artery occlusion have been divided into several categories:[37,83]

1. An explosive type with sudden stroke and often a fatal outcome
2. A slowly progressive type with transient attacks of neurologic deficits progressing to hemiplegia
3. Those with visual signs and symptoms
4. A completely silent type
5. Those which may mimic a tumor or produce psychiatric disturbances

Those patients with ocular findings can have highly variable signs and symptoms. The most frequent ocular manifestation is a homonymous hemianopic field defect considered to be due to insufficiency of the middle cerebral artery. Amaurosis fugax, central retinal artery or branch retinal artery occlusion, cholesterol or atheromatous emboli in retinal arteries, cotton-wool patches, and lowered ipsilateral central retinal artery pressure are the more common findings. Rarer cases may show signs of ophthalmic artery obstruction, ischemic optic nerve disease, Horner's syndrome, pupillary changes, diplopia, ptosis, late hemorrhagic glaucoma, and congestion of ipsilateral conjunctival vessels.

Amaurosis fugax, a transient partial or complete loss of vision lasting for several minutes or somewhat longer, affects about 40 per cent of patients with carotid insufficiency. When adequately described, the lower field of vision usually blanks out first and returns last when the attack recedes. Hollenhorst[42] examined four patients during their episodes of visual loss and found that two had cholesterol emboli moving in their retinal arteries, one had absent retinal circulation during the attack, and one had normally appearing vessels. All four had fixed pupils during the period of blindness. Platelet emboli have also been observed in retinal arteries during amaurotic attacks (see Chapter 10, under section on Retinal Emboli). Kellogg and Smith[46] have described a patient with transient monocular blindness which occurred when the patient turned his head. This was due to a redundant carotid artery, surgically corrected with complete alleviation of the ocular symptom. There have also been cases of amaurosis fugax in which no carotid artery obstruction was found by angiography.[25]

Sudden, prolonged loss of vision may occur as a result of embolization of the retinal arteries by atheromatous material. In these cases the blockage is usually fixed but vision may rarely improve if the embolus moves down the vascular tree. Hollenhorst,[40] in his series of 86 patients with intermittent carotid insufficiency, has noted eight with ipsilateral central or branch artery occlusions. Six of 38 patients with complete occlusion of the carotid artery were similarly affected.

The uniocular presence of scattered cotton-wool patches and dilated retinal vessels with dark veins should suggest insufficiency of the ipsilateral carotid artery. Such findings were present in about 12 per cent of patients with internal carotid occlusion.[40] A similar finding of unilateral cotton-wool spots and associated venous dilatation has been observed after carotid artery ligation in the treatment of carotid-cavernous fistula.[75,85]

Ophthalmodynamometry may reveal a lower arterial pressure in the affected eye, but for reasons already given, this test is not always reliable. A difference of 20 per cent in the two eyes is usually considered significant.[82]

Hollenhorst[41,42] was the first to point out that patients with hypertensive retinopathy and carotid artery disease had an asymmetric fundic appearance. He found less hypertensive retinopathy, including less arterial narrowing, on the side of the occluded carotid artery. This finding is not invariable, however, and the retinopathy can be more pronounced on the involved side.[62] Ligation of the carotid artery may cause a similar asymmetric retinopathy in hypertensive individuals.[47]

A lowered central retinal artery pressure or carotid artery occlusion has also been noted on the side of least retinopathy in cases of asymmetric diabetic retinopathy.[31a]

Miller[62] has suggested that ipsilateral retinopathy, unequal retinopathies, central retinal artery occlusions, carotid or ocular bruit, and a decreased ipsilateral central retinal artery pressure should alert one to the possibility of internal carotid artery occlusion. Amaurosis fugax and atheromatous or cholesterin crystal emboli are also suggestive of carotid arteriosclerosis. It must be remembered that eyes with prior optic atrophy show neither papilledema nor any vascular retinopathy.

VENOUS STASIS RETINOPATHY

Kearns and Hollenhorst[45] have found a very different type of retinopathy in 5 per cent of their patients with internal carotid artery occlusion. They described widened arteries and markedly dilated veins with blot hemorrhages about small venous tributaries in the mid- and peripheral retina. Sludging of venous blood, retinal microaneurysms, and retinal neovascularization were also occasionally seen. They called this condition "venous stasis retinopathy." A comparable retinopathy has been described by Madsen[56] in two patients with ophthalmic artery insufficiency, and by Quint[67] in three patients with carotid artery thrombosis. Sanders and Hoyt[73] have described a hypoxic retinopathy in cases of carotid-cavernous fistulae. Their patients showed dilated and tortuous retinal veins, retinal microaneurysms, blot hemorrhages adjacent to the venous tree, retinal edema and an occasional cotton-wool patch. Fluorescein angiography revealed vascular leakage as in vein obstruction. The possible influence of the raised venous pressure (impedance to venous outflow) in the production of this picture was not considered. It is our opinion that what is called stasis retinopathy is actually stagnation venous occlusion, the underfilling of the retinal artery eventually leading to collapse and partial occlusion of the central retinal vein. The reduced arterial inflow would mitigate to some extent the venous congestion and produce a picture of an incomplete venous occlusion rather than that of the typical apoplectic retina. The prodromal signs of central retinal vein obstruction usually include small blot hemorrhages about peripheral venous tributaries; and small blot hemorrhages in this same distribution can also be seen in the late recovery stages of central vein obstruction, when some venous insufficiency persists. Finally, were this picture produced by prolonged retinal hypotension, one should find a retinopathy similar to that of pulseless disease (see below). Until there is microscopic confirmation of stagnation venous occlusion, however, venous stasis retinopathy cannot be excluded as an entity.

PULSELESS DISEASE (AORTIC ARCH SYNDROME; TAKAYASU'S DISEASE)

Pulseless disease is produced by a slowly progressive obliteration of the major vessels arising from the aortic arch. Every vessel is not involved in each case but generally there is sufficient obliteration to produce a slowly decreasing flow of blood to the head and upper extremities. Vinijchaikul has reviewed the subject and presented a clinicopathologic study of eight patients.[90] The disease is now recognized as being primarily of the aorta, often extending down the descending aorta, involving the renal arteries, and producing hypertension. In its typical form it occurs primarily in young women and children. The aorta shows a panarteritis with intimal thickening, fibrosis, and vascularization of the media, fragmentation of elastic fibers, and mild lymphocytic infiltration with thickening of the walls of the vasa vasorum in the adventitia. Aneurysmal dilatations also appear and a superimposed thrombosis may eventually occur. The etiology is still obscure.

The pulseless syndrome is actually due to slow closure of some or all of the major vessels from the aortic arch. Takayasu's arteritis is only one of the diseases responsible for this syndrome. Other cases have been due to syphilis, and arteriosclerosis, and giant cell arteritis also has been suggested. Some of these cases occur in older individuals. One report[70] cited a case secondary to excessive radiation in childhood. Cases due to arteriosclerosis more often involve men with widespread vascular disease, and the left subclavian, innominate, and left carotid arteries are more often involved.[89] These cases usually occur in older individuals.

The ocular findings in this syndrome constitute some of the early signs of the condition. Pinkham[66] reviewed the ocular manifestations in all reported cases up to 1954 and Ostler[65] has more recently listed these. The condition is rare and no single observer has carefully recorded the retinal reaction in the different disease stages. In fact, detailed descriptions of retinal findings are sparse. The major ocular signs and symptoms derived from reported cases will therefore be indicated in their probable order of occurrence as the disease progresses, and the retinal reaction described in one early proved case personally observed. For a more detailed list of ocular findings, see Ostler's listing in Reference 65.

The ocular, upper extremity, and head manifestations are the result of a chronic, slowly progressive decrease in the arterial flow to these regions. Recurrent blurring of vision (bilateral amaurosis fugax), lasting only 1 or 2 minutes is the most common and probably the earliest ocular symptom of the syndrome. It may also be associated with lightheadedness or dizziness and is aggravated by raising the head; becoming increasingly severe upon standing or walking. The central retinal artery pressures are markedly reduced at this stage. Light flashes may be seen from time to time. The fundi are pale and the retinal vessels are dilated. The pupils are also dilated, especially so with attacks of amaurosis fugax. Peripheral retinal arteries are obliterated and both large and small retinal hemorrhages appear, the latter occurring especially toward the periphery. Cotton-wool patches sometimes appear in the posterior fundus and at any stage the central retinal artery may become occluded with secondary disc atrophy. Because of the optic atrophy such an eye would not show further significant retinal reaction.

Later in the disease visual field defects appear and commonly show a progressive peripheral loss. The eye becomes hypotonus and the iris begins to show a patchy atrophy. Most cases show a mild enophthalmos probably due to atrophy of the orbital content.

Late in the disease there is retinitis proliferans, vitreous hemorrhage, and the retinal vessels form a rosary of arteriovenous anastomoses around the disc.[12] Ashton[2] has noted the similarity between this and the late stages of vaso-obliteration in his experimental retrolental fibroplasia. Peripheral to the arteriovenous communications, retinal vessels are very narrowed, obliterated, or not visible. Rubeosis iridis, cataract, and late detachment of the retina may occur. The sedimentation rate can be markedly elevated in some patients.

Tarkkanen et al.[88] have reported 14 patients with the aortic arch syndrome in which the eye findings were correlated with proved blockage of various major arteries. Three had innominate artery obstructions. Two of these had had attacks of transient blurrings of vision and showed asymmetric ophthalmodynamometry readings. The third had had no visual symptoms and had symmetric pressure readings. None of the three showed any other ocular findings. One of the first two patients was described, and at angiography, backflow from the right vertebral artery entered the right subclavian and carotid vessels. Normal flow resumed following surgical removal of the obstruction, ophthalmodynamometry readings became symmetric, and no further visual blurrings occurred.

One patient had an obstruction of the left common carotid artery and stenosis of the left subclavian artery. Her only ocular finding was a reduced central retinal artery pressure in the left eye—diastolic readings of 75 in the right eye and 45 in the left eye.

Ten patients had obstruction of the left subclavian artery proximal to the left vertebral artery. Three had had occasional visual symptoms but all had normal ophthalmodynamometry readings and normal ocular findings.

These cases demonstrate that the eye findings may be completely normal in the early phases of the disease.

One case of the aortic arch syndrome with early retinal pathology has been personally observed. A 30-year-old woman had 20/20 vision and ocular tensions of 8 mmHg in each eye. Ophthalmodynamometry revealed central retinal artery pressures of 20/10 right eye and 10/0 left eye. In the posterior fundi both arteries and veins were full and the arteries were slightly burnished with mild beading in places suggesting the changes seen posteriorly in angiomatosis retinae or Leber's disease (see Chapter 11, under section on Anomalous Vascular Formations). There were good foveal reflexes and a few fine yellow dots at both maculae. These were either drusen or small fatty exudates. The major findings were in the retinal periphery, especially temporally, and both eyes were alike. The peripheral capillary bed was greatly dilated and readily visible. These channels were most numerous about small venous tributaries; small arterial branches had a relatively free capillary zone about them. The mesh of the network suggested that many capillary channels were obliterated, while the remaining patent ones were dilated. Multiple microaneurysms were visible in the area, and numerous dilated capillary arteriovenous anastomoses were present. Peripheral to these loops the retina appeared avascular with a light gliotic sheen. The vitreous was detached posteriorly in each eye. No retinal hemorrhages nor retinitis proliferans were seen. The peripheral retinal areas were very similar to the abnormal vascular area of Leber's disease shown in Figure 11-9*A*.

Fluorescein study of pulseless disease[77] revealed a decreased rate of flow in the retinal circulation, dilatation of capillaries in the temporal periphery and at the macula, beading of the veins, retinal microaneurysms, and leakage of dye through capillary and venous walls. Surgical correction of the arterial blockage and normalization of the retinal arterial pressures at this stage, in one case, resulted in the disappearance of retinal abnormalities and a normalized fluorescein angiogram.

Later in the disease, peripheral arteriovenous communications with nonperfusion of more peripheral vessels and leaking neovascular tufts, especially from the disc, were demonstrated.

The retinal reaction in the later stages of the aortic arch syndrome, by having certain features of both, bridges the gap between the types of retinal response seen in arterial and venous blockage.

TREATMENT

Cotton-wool spots require no treatment themselves. They are secondary manifestations and successful treatment of the local or systemic disease responsible for them is usually coincident with their disappearance.

Obstruction of a branch or central retinal artery should be handled as an ocular emergency. Some fresh emboli may be moved downstream by tapping on the eye or by initially exerting firm pressure on the globe with the sudden release of the fingers. Vasodilators should be tried although they are usually unsuccessful. We have observed the dislodgement of one embolus in a branch artery after the inhalation of amyl nitrite in a patient who had severe rheumatic heart disease which was the probable source of the embolus. Prompt paracentesis of the anterior chamber should be attempted. The technique for this differs from the usual procedure. The incision should be made if possible, without loss of aqueous. Then, by depressing the posterior lip of the wound, the aqueous is suddenly and rapidly evacuated in order to produce maximum vasodilatation. The paracentesis can be periodically reopened. We have had no success with retrobulbar Priscoline.

Once in the hospital, anticoagulation with heparin is in order and inhalation of 5% carbon dioxide and 95% oxygen can be started. These are usually given for 5 or 10 minutes every hour. They must be given by nasal catheter or a tight-fitting mask to be effective. 5% carbon dioxide exerts a sufficiently strong vasodilating effect on retinal arteries to overcome any oxygen vasoconstriction. Signs of carbon dioxide intoxication, such as a rising blood pressure, should be avoided. Breathing into a paper bag is a useless procedure.

As arterial obstructions are not always complete, every patient should receive maximal therapy promptly for several days. If, in 4 or 5 days, no improvement occurs, treatment can be stopped.

Thrombolytic agents may be toxic and have had insufficient trial as yet for their evaluation.

Obstructions of the central retinal artery, or ischemic optic neuritis in patients over 55 years of age should always suggest temporal arteritis. A search for other signs of the disease and careful questioning for suggestive early symptoms is mandatory. An immediate sedimentation rate should be obtained. If there is any question regarding the diagnosis, prompt steroid therapy should be instituted. This should not await a positive biopsy, nor should a negative biopsy in the presence of other suggestive evidence warrant stopping the administration of steroids. In established cases of cranial arteritis, large doses of steroids are given initially and the dosage is tapered with a decrease in the sedimentation rate. In some patients the sedimentation rate will remain high with the improvement in general symptoms and signs. In these patients the latter can be used as a guide in dosage. In reduced dosage, steroids must be continued for several months and in some cases for several years. In a personally observed case, a shock position in bed, steroids and anticoagulants saved the vision of a second eye. At the onset of therapy, this eye was blanking out whenever the patient sat up in bed. This was unusual, for once the second eye becomes involved some visual loss can be expected. Steroids are also indicated in cases of orbital closure due to orbital granuloma.[33a]

Arterial obstructions due to arteriosclerosis are not often responsive to treatment. Medical evaluation and direction are indicated. In some patients anticoagulation may be helpful and over the longer term some form of regular exercise, a low fat diet, and the avoidance of heavy meals may be advised. An elevated cholesterol should be lowered and the hematocrit kept below 45.

Arterial blockage following blood loss and that due to mask pressure at anesthesia should be avoided, for treatment of both is usually unsuccessful.

Acute attacks of glaucoma with high intraocular pressures should be promptly controlled. A sustained pressure of this degree for even a day or two is likely to produce permanent damage to the retina or optic nerve, secondary to vascular ischemia.

In older patients with hypertension, sudden lowering of blood pressure with antihypertensive drugs may produce ocular arterial insufficiency. These should be treated by promptly stopping the drug, shock position of the patient in bed, paracentesis of the anterior chamber, etc. Carbonic anhydrase inhibitors to reduce intraocular pressure may be helpful.

Carotid artery insufficiency and the aortic arch syndrome lie in the province of the vascular surgeon. Early cases may be amenable to surgical correction. Others may be treated by anticoagulation. It is the duty of the ophthalmologist to be aware of the early ocular signs and symptoms of these diseases and to offer the patient prompt referral.

OBSTRUCTION OF CHOROIDAL VESSELS

Because of their large lumens and free anastomoses, embolic obstructions producing signs of choriocapillary blockage are rare. In fact, several anterior and probably posterior ciliary arteries as well, can be severed without apparent consequences. It is only when three or more recti muscles are severed from their globe insertions that any adverse effect of anterior ciliary artery circulation is likely. The ability of an area of choroid to receive its blood supply from any one of several ciliary arteries, probably explains why choroidal involvement occurs primarily in diffuse disease processes.

For descriptive purposes choroidal arterial insufficiency can be divided into obstructions of the choriocapillary vessels and small arteries, obstructive disease of several or all large ciliary arteries, and choroidal sclerosis. Since sufficient obstruction of anterior ciliary arteries to cause an adverse effect produces disease of the anterior segment, it is not pertinent to this discussion.

OBSTRUCTION OF CHORIOCAPILLARY VESSELS AND SMALL CHOROIDAL ARTERIES

The effect of severe accelerated or malignant hypertension upon the retinal vessels has been considered in Chapter 13, Hypertensive Retinopathy. In its acute phases the retinal pathology overlies and may obscure changes produced in the choroid. In rare instances the choroidal vessels may be preferentially involved,[32] and choroidal disease can be more readily appreciated.

In the severe phase of hypertension, leakage of fluid from the choriocapillaris through overlying and defective pigment epithelium may produce retinal detachment. Klien[48] has shown such leakage histologically and it has been shown to occur from multiple choroidal sites by fluorescein angiography.[32]

If the hypertension is brought under sufficient control for some recovery to ensue, the subretinal fluid absorbs, the retina returns to its normal position, and the residual effects of the choroidal vascular damage become apparent. These changes are dependent upon the hypertension itself and have been reported in such diverse diseases as toxemia of pregnancy, malignant hypertension, glomerulonephritis, and collagen disease.[32,48,63]

Microscopically, severe arteriosclerosis with narrowed lumen is found in larger choroidal arteries and patchy thrombosis, with fibrinoid necrosis and obliteration of small choroidal arteries and choriocapillaries occurring. As a result of the small vessel damage, the overlying pigment epithelium is severely altered with areas of pigment loss and pigment proliferation.

Clinically such areas appear in different forms and may be seen anywhere in the fundus although they are more common posteriorly. They appear as small, bright yellow zones with central knots of proliferated pigment epithelium, about three or four times the width of a retinal artery, overlying "thrombosed" choroidal vessels as originally described by Elschnig in severe nephritis.[27] These are commonly called Elschnig's spots. Klien[48] described similar lesions about the papilla, with central clumps of pigment surrounded by yellowish halos no more than 1/3 dd in size. Other forms may appear as larger, ragged, yellowish white lesions with intermingled and border pigment clumps (Fig. 12-18).

These spots heretofore[23] have been considered to be of grave prognostic import. With improved control of serious hypertension, they may be seen more frequently and offer a less ominous prognosis.

Siegrist[78] has described two cases show-

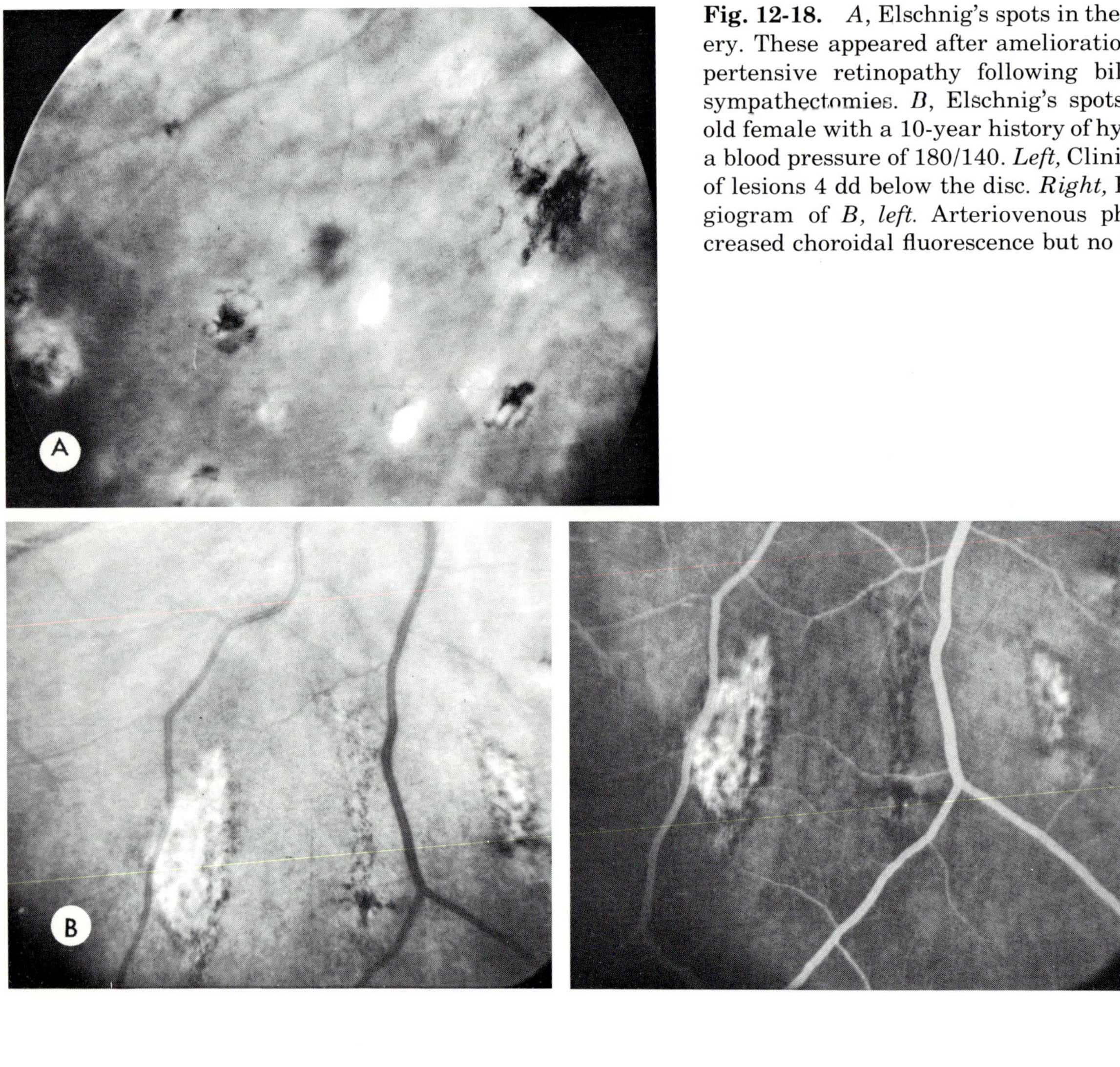

Fig. 12-18. *A,* Elschnig's spots in the retinal periphery. These appeared after amelioration of severe hypertensive retinopathy following bilateral lumbar sympathectomies. *B,* Elschnig's spots in a 60-year-old female with a 10-year history of hypertension and a blood pressure of 180/140. *Left,* Clinical appearance of lesions 4 dd below the disc. *Right,* Fluorescein angiogram of *B, left.* Arteriovenous phase shows increased choroidal fluorescence but no leakage.

ing rosary chains of clumped pigment with yellowish zones about them, overlying pink choroidal vessels. Sclerosed choroidal vessels did not have such superimposed lesions. One case studied histologically showed the pigment clumps overlying a larger, relatively normal choroidal vessel. The choriocapillaris beneath the clumps was absent. In this case some cerebral arteries showed very narrowed lumens and wall pathology with giant cells suggesting cranial arteritis. Both Siegrist's and Elschnig's spots probably represent slight clinical modifications of obliterated choriocapillary channels from different causes and should not, therefore, be considered as different entities.

Sickle cell disease in its severe ocular form may produce choroidal infarcts. These are most frequent in the periphery of the fundus and may produce scars 2 or 3 dd in size depending upon the area of choroidal vascular blockage by sickled cells. Healing takes place, leaving irregular white chorioretinal scars with proliferated pigment at the borders.

The tendency for giant-cell arteritis (cranial arteritis) to attack the small ciliary arteries at the circle of Zinn and produce ischemic optic neuropathy has been discussed (see under section on Cranial Arteritis). This disease has not as yet been reported to produce choroidal infarction although ciliary artery involvement has been demonstrated histologically.[55]

Polyarteritis has also been repeatedly demonstrated in choroidal arteries[9,30,34,35,39] and grayish white foci with blurred outlines have been seen clinically in the periphery of the fundus.[10] These later changed into clearly outlined, yellowish white scars containing some proliferated pigment epithelium. Typical changes of the disease in choroidal arteries and areas of obliterated capillaries with dispersal of the overlying pigment epithelium were found histologically. The discrepancy between the rare report of clinically observed choroidal infarcts and the relatively frequent histological finding of diseased choroidal vessels is probably explained by the presence of anterior segment pathology or the accompanying hypertensive retinopathy.[92] Some patients at this stage of the disease are so ill that careful ocular examination cannot be made.

PRIMARY CHOROIDAL SCLEROSIS

Primary choroidal sclerosis occurs in three different forms; around the disc, in the macular area without peripheral involvement, and as a diffuse disease usually sparing the macular area. The genetic characteristics may differ in these various forms. The mode of inheritance is autosomal, either dominant or recessive in the peripapillary and macular variety and usually autosomal dominant in the diffuse type.[13,24,43] In many patients no related family history can be obtained.[43] This is often true in all forms of the disease and some of these cases may not be genetically determined.

In older patients it is not unusual to see choroidal sclerosis temporally and adjacent to the disc. It often appears as a crescent hugging the disc border. Some pigment epithelium is missing, sclerosed choroidal vessels can be seen and there may or may not be a fringe of proliferated pigment at the border. It is of no significance, but because it produces an enlarged blind spot on field testing, it should be taken into consideration when other disease is suspected. Rarely, a uniform white ring with no pigment at its border and no visible sclerosed choroidal vessels may surround the disc. The edge of the ring has been mistaken for the disc border, the true disc border suggesting the edge of a glaucomatous cup. As this occurs in patients of glaucoma age, often with some lens opacity, it may be difficult to interpret with the ophthalmoscope. The true diagnosis is readily made upon contact lens and slit-lamp examination. Both of these types are limited to the immediate disc area, are not genetically determined, and are considered one of the senile changes of the eye.

The inherited variety of peripapillary choroidal sclerosis starts around the disc and extends away from it in an irregular fashion, with diffuse borders. This type can progress to involve the macular area as well. Peripheral vision is retained, the ERG is essentially normal and, unless the macula is involved, the patient is unaware of its presence.

The macular type[74] is better known as central areolar choroidal sclerosis or dystrophy (Fig. 12-19). It apparently starts as a diffuse macular granularity, similar in the two eyes with retention of good foveal reflexes and otherwise normal fundi.[13] At this stage visual acuity may be in the 20/60 to 20/70 range. It may also develop with a fairly rapid loss of central vision over the course of several months. A case of this type revealed bilateral, oval, somewhat depigmented macula-centered lesions with diffuse foveal reflexes. The oval areas were surrounded by a granular change in the pigment epithelium, the whole region being about 1 dd in size. The involved region had a golden sheen when viewed at an angle, and the visual acuity was reduced to 20/100 and 20/400 in the two eyes. The remainder of the fundus was normal.[13] The mother of these two patients had fully developed macular lesions. They were oval, about twice the size of the disc, and had sharp borders with mild pigment proliferation in places. Just beyond the sharp margin temporally in each eye there were deep, discrete white dots and the retina in this area gave a silvery sheen. In the center of the lesions nonsclerotic, large and small choroidal vessels were visible. The vision in the two eyes was 20/400 and 20/300. Both fundi were otherwise normal. In this patient the ERG was reduced in all photopic and scotopic responses bilaterally.[13]

Other cases of the fully developed maculopathy show round or oval, sharply punched-out central areas, similar in the two eyes and having a yellowish white background with various degrees of readily visible choroidal sclerosis. Pigment proliferation at the border of the lesions is usually minimal or absent and pigment migration into the overlying or surrounding retina is not seen. The remainder of both fundi is normal in appearance.

Diffuse choriodal sclerosis (Fig. 12-20) usually starts in the midretinal zones or posteriorly around the disc. It progresses slowly in a very irregular manner, often leaving the macula and a very peripheral area uninvolved. During its course involved areas show varying degrees of the disease and uninvolved islands may appear transiently as the disease proceeds.

In some patients it never becomes very severe, either because of the patient's age at onset or because of the slowness of the process. In some of these individuals the disease does not appear to be familial and no family history is obtained. They have no sense of night blindness, and if the macula is not involved, no loss of visual acuity. The inherited form is usually much more extensive and in its late stages, may be confused with other diseases.

The earliest sign of any type of choroidal sclerosis is a change in the pigment epithelium. First the pigment in these cells becomes rarified and the area appears granular, lighter in color, and it may show a metallic sheen. It is best appreciated by retroillumination. Very shortly the pigment is so depleted that the choroidal vessels are easily seen. At first the tessellated choroidal vessels appear almost normal being only slightly paler than their normal pink color. This stage can be confused with a normal tessellated fundus, especially if the tessellation is limited to the vertical meridian below the disc, as can be seen in cases of very mild coloboma of the choroid. When it appears in other sectors as well, early choroidal scle-

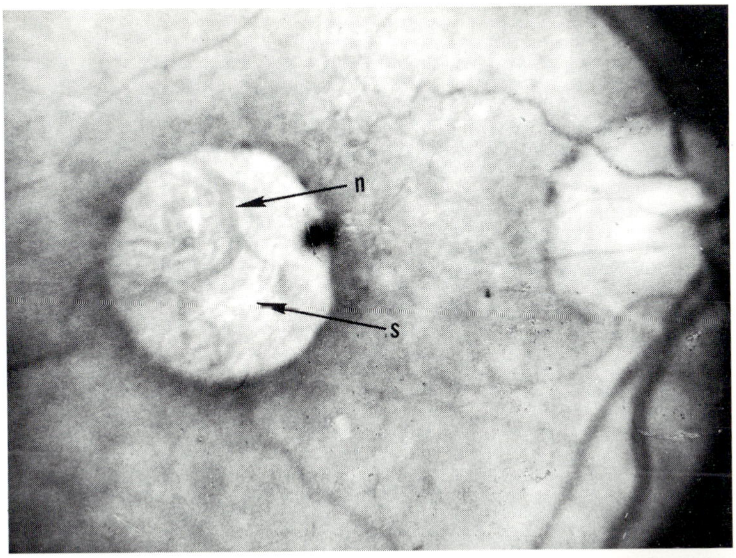

Fig. 12-19. Central areolar choroidal sclerosis. There is an oval area of absent pigment epithelium at the macula with minimal border pigmentation. Some larger choroidal vessels appear normal (**n**); others are sclerotic (**s**).

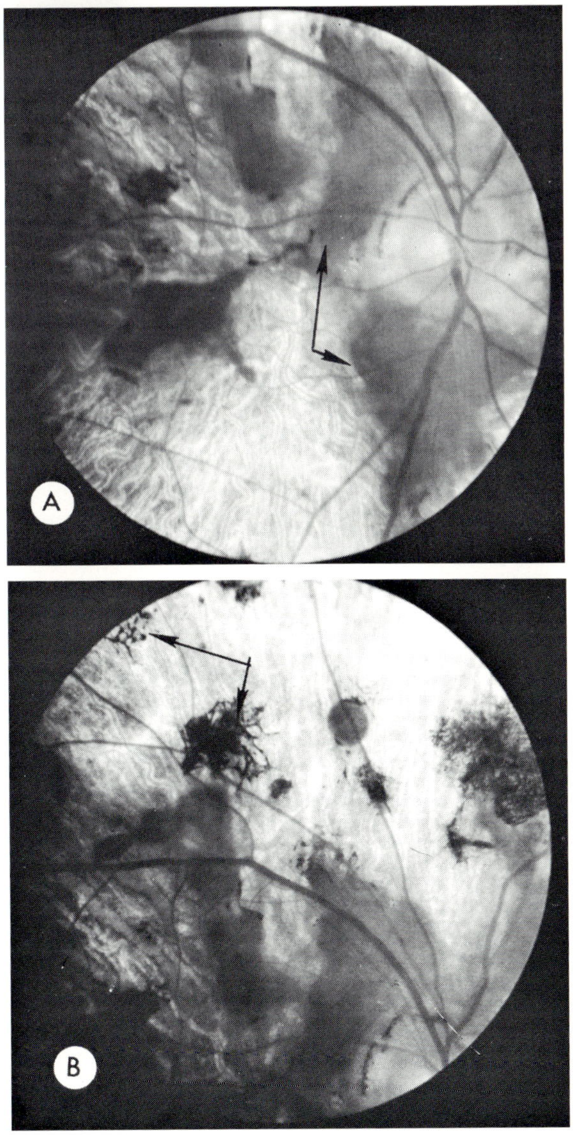

Fig. 12-20. *A*, Diffuse choroidal sclerosis. Disc and macular area of right eye. Islands of normal pigment epithelium are indicated by **arrows.** *B*, Appearance of same eye above the disc. Note proliferated pigment epithelium (**arrows**) which has migrated into the overlying retina above areas of choroidal sclerosis.

rosis should be suspected. As the pigment epithelium loses its pigment early in the disease, the choroidal vessels are readily seen and the degree of sclerosis is dependent upon the changes visible in them. They are first a pale pink, then orange, and finally take on increasing whiteness as the sclerosis increases. The blood column, at first of normal uniform width between any two vascular connections, becomes increasingly narrowed and irregular until finally it is hidden from view. At this severe stage the vessels appear as white irregular cords containing no visible blood. Larger vessels may course through such an area and show varying but usually lesser degrees of these same changes. Sometimes the larger vessels in such an area show no discernible sclerosis. In extreme degrees, patches of vascular channels may become matted together in a yellow white amalgam and all definition of individual channels disappears. Except in central areolar choroidal sclerosis, pigment may migrate into the overlying retina, or form clumps of proliferation at its original level. The migrating pigment may form clumps unrelated to overlying retinal vessels or may sheath veins. Some patients show peripheral spicules simulating retinitis pigmentosa. The peripapillary and the diffuse disease both proceed in a very patchy manner. Areas of severe sclerosis with absent overlying pigment appear adjacent to uninvolved areas with normal overlying pigment. The transition between two such regions is often quite abrupt, producing a smooth curvilinear line of demarcation.

Microscopically the choriocapillaris was obliterated and Bruch's membrane was either little affected [1] or irregularly thinned and thickened, basophilic, fibrillated, and fragmented.[43] Larger vessels were present and patent and did not show arteriosclerosis. The pigment epithelium overlying the obliterated choriocapillaries was completely absent—no sign of it being visible. Where some choriocapillary blood supply remained, plaques of proliferated pigment epithelium were seen. Overlying the more diseased areas, rods and cones with their nuclei were absent, and nuclei of the inner nuclear layers and external limiting membrane lay against patches of pigment proliferation or remnants of Bruch's membrane without any replacement of connective tissue. Both of these pathology reports were in cases of central areolar choroidal sclerosis [84] but comparable findings could be expected in all types of choroidal sclerosis. One eye of Ashton's patient was injected with intravascular neoprene. The choriocapillaris and some larger vessels in the involved area failed to fill demonstrating their complete occlusion. In the other eye, examination of the posterior ciliary arteries revealed no pathology.

In its late stages, the inherited form of diffuse choroidal sclerosis may be confused with late retinitis pigmentosa, choroidremia, or extensive luetic chorioretinitis. The latter is mentioned in the older literature but is almost nonexistent today and therefore offers no problem. The patches of white sclera with total absence of choroidal vessels as seen in choroidremia do not occur in choroidal sclerosis. Although axial posterior subcapsular cataracts have been reported in diffuse choroidal sclerosis,[58] they are so rare in our experience as to be an aid in differentiating diffuse choroidal sclerosis from retinitis pigmentosa. This form of choroidal sclerosis does have an extinguished ERG and patients are usually night blind with it. In fact some authors have included it with the tapetoretinal degenerations.

Fluorescein angiography in the late stages of the diffuse disease showed filling of larger choroidal vessels but only patchy filling of a few remaining patent choriocapillaries.[22]

Although the pathology has not demonstrated choroidal arteriosclerosis, the term "choroidal sclerosis" is so broadly accepted that no attempt should be made at present to change the name.

Secondary choroidal sclerosis, as is seen in regions of healed chorioretinitis, is an incidental finding; the choroidal vessels show the same clinical appearances described above, and this subject needs no elaboration.

TREATMENT

Treatment of choroidal artery obstruction usually involves general medical treatment of the primary disease responsible. There is no treatment for choroidal sclerosis. Often, if a reasonably good visual prognosis can be given, the patient is satisfied.

REFERENCES

1. Ashton, N.: Central areolar choroidal sclerosis. *Brit. J. Ophthal. 37:*140, 1953.
2. Ashton, N.: Pulseless disease and oxygen studies (letter). *Amer. J. Ophthal. 38:*418, 1954.
3. Ashton, N., Coomes, E. N., Garner, A., and Oliver, D. O.: Retinopathy due to progressive systemic sclerosis. *J. Path. Bact. 96:* 259, 1968.
4. Ashton, N., Pears, M. A., and Pickering, G. W.: Neuroretinopathy following hemorrhage with a discussion on the nature of cytoid bodies. *Brit. J. Ophthal. 45:*385, 1961.
5. Ball, C. J.: Atheromatous embolism to the brain, retina and choroid. *Arch. Ophthal. 76:* 690, 1966.
6. Bernstein, A.: Periarteritis nodosa without peripheral nodules diagnosed antemortem. *Amer. J. Med. Sci. 190:*317, 1935.
7. Birkhead, N. C., Wagener, H. P., and Shick, R. M.: Treatment of temporal arteritis with adrenal corticosteroids. *JAMA 163:*821, 1957.
8. Blazar, H. A., and Scheie, H. G.: Pseudoglaucoma. *Arch. Ophthal. 44:*499, 1950.
9. Böck, J.: Ein Beitrag zur Periarteritis nodosa am Auge. *Z. Augenheilk. 78:*28, 1932.
10. Boeck, J.: Ocular changes in periarteritis nodosa. *Amer. J. Ophthal. 42:*567, 1956.
11. Brice, J. G., Dowsett, D. J., and Lowe, R. D.: The effect of constriction on carotid bloodflow and pressure gradient. *Lancet 1:*84, 1964.
12. Caccamise, W. C., and Okuda, K.: Takayasu's or pulseless disease. *Amer. J. Ophthal. 37:*784, 1954.
13. Carr, R. E.: Central areolar choroidal dystrophy. *Arch. Ophthal. 73:*32, 1965.
14. Carr, R. E., and Siegel, I. M.: Electrophysiologic aspects of several retinal diseases. *Amer. J. Ophthal. 58:*95, 1964.
15. Cogan, D. G.: *Neurology of the Visual System.* Springfield, Ill., Thomas. 1966, p. 168.
16. Cogan, D. G.: *Neurology of the Visual System.* Springfield, Ill., Thomas. 1966, p. 186.
17. Conrad, W. C., and Penner, R.: Sickle-cell trait and central retinal artery occlusion. *Amer. J. Ophthal. 63:*465, 1967.
18. Cooke, W. T., Cloake, P. C. P., Govan, A. D. T., and Colbeck, J. C.: Temporal arteritis; a generalized vascular disease. *Quart. J. Med. 15:*47, 1946.
19. Cordes, F. C.: Retinal ischemia with visual loss. *Amer. J. Ophthal. 45:*79, 1958 (April, part II).
20. Corrigan, M. J., and Hill, D. W.: Retinal artery occlusion in loiasis. *Brit. J. Ophthal. 52:*477, 1968.
21. Cullen, J. F.: Ischemic optic neuropathy. *Trans. Ophthal. Soc. U.K. 87:*759, 1967.
22. Curry, H. F., and Schonberg, S. S.: Fluorescein photography in choroidal sclerosis. *Arch. Ophthal. 81:*177, 1969.

22a. Dahrling, B. E.: The histopathology of early central retinal artery occlusion. *Arch. Ophthal. 73:*506, 1965.

23. Duke-Elder, S.: *System of Ophthalmology. Diseases of the Uveal Tract.* London, Kimpton, 1966, vol. IX, p. 629.
24. Duke-Elder, S.: *System of Ophthalmology. Diseases of the Uveal Tract.* London, Kimpton, 1966, vol. IX, p. 702.
25. Eadie, M. J., Sutherland, J. M., and Tyrer, J. H.: Recurrent monocular blindness of uncertain cause. *Lancet 1:*319, 1968.
26. Ellis, P. P., and Hamilton, H.: Retrobulbar neuritis in pernicious anemia. *Amer. J. Ophthal. 48:*95, 1959.
27. Elschnig, A.: Die diagnostische und prognostische Bedeitung der Netzhauterkrankungen

bei Nephritis. *Wien. Med. Wschr. 54:*494, 1904.

28. Evans, H.: Periarteritis nodosa with marked eosinophilia. *Proc. Roy. Soc. Med. 37:*40, 1943.
29. Friedenwald, H.: The Doyne Memorial Lecture: Pathological changes in the retinal blood vessels in arteriosclerosis and hypertension. *Trans. Ophthal. Soc. U.K. 50:*452, 1930.
30. Friedenwald, J. S., and Rones, B.: Ocular lesions in septicemia. *Arch. Ophthal. 5:*175, 1931.
31. Gass, J. D.: A fluorescein angiographic study of macular disfunction secondary to retinal vascular disease I. Embolic retinal artery obstruction. *Arch. Ophthal. 80:*535, 1968.

31a. Gay, A. J., and Rosenbaum, A. L.: Retinal artery pressure in asymmetric diabetic retinopathy. *Arch. Ophthal. 75:*758, 1966.

32. Gitter, K. A., Houser, B. P., Sarin, L. K., and Justice, J., Jr.: Toxemia of pregnancy. An angiographic interpretation of fundus changes. *Arch. Ophthal. 80:*449, 1968.
33. Givner, I., and Jaffee, N.: Occlusion of the central retinal artery following anesthesia. *Arch. Ophthal. 43:*197, 1950.

33a. Godfrey, R. C.: Occlusion of the retinal artery in two cases of orbital granuloma. *Brit. J. Ophthal. 53:*703, 1969.

34. Goldsmith, J.: Periarteritis nodosa with involvement of the choroidal and retinal arteries. *Amer. J. Ophthal. 29:*435, 1946.
35. Goldstein, I., and Wexler, D.: Ocular pathology of periarteritis nodosa. *Arch. Ophthal. 2:*288, 1929.
36. Gordon, N.: Ocular manifestations of internal carotid artery occlusion. *Brit. J. Ophthal. 43:*257, 1959.
37. Graham, M. V.: Carotid artery disease. *Trans. Ophthal. Soc. U.K. 88:*5, 1968.
38. Hamasaki, D. I., and Kroll, A. J.: Experimental central retinal artery occlusion. *Arch. Ophthal. 80:*243, 1968.

38a. Henkind, P., Charles, N. C., and Pearson, J.: Histopathology of ischemic optic neuropathy. *Amer. J. Ophthal. 69:*78, 1970.

39. Herson, R. N., and Sampson, R.: Ocular manifestations of polyarteritis nodosa. *Quart. J. Med. 18:*123, 1949.
40. Hollenhorst, R. W.: Ocular manifestations of insufficiency or thrombosis of the internal carotid artery. *Trans. Amer. Ophthal. Soc. 56:*474, 1958.
41. Hollenhorst, R. W.: The ocular manifestations of internal carotid thrombosis. *Med. Clin. N. Amer. 44:*897, 1960.
42. Hollenhorst, R. W.: "The Neuro-Ophthalmology of Strokes," in *Neuro-Ophthalmology,* ed. by Smith, J. L., St. Louis, Mo., Mosby, 1965, vol. 2, p. 109.
43. Howard, G. M., and Wolf, E.: Central choroidal sclerosis: a clinical and pathologic study. *Trans. Amer. Acad. Ophthal. Otolaryng, 68:*647, 1964.
44. Huber, A.: Arteriography and phlebography in the diagnosis of orbital affections. *Bull. N. Y. Acad. Med. 44:*409, 1968.
45. Kearns, T. P., and Hollenhorst, R. W.: Venous stasis retinopathy of occlusive disease of the carotid artery. *Mayo Clinic Proc. 38:* 304, 1963.
46. Kellog, D. R., and Smith, L. L.: Recurrent monocular blindness due to a redundant carotid artery. *Arch. Surg. 95:*908, 1967.
47. Kirby, T. J., and Hollenhorst, R. W.: Asymmetric hypertensive retinal changes after ligation of the internal carotid artery. *XVII Concilium Ophthalmologicum, Acta 1954 1:* 335, 1955.
48. Klien, B. A.: Ischemic infarcts of the choroid (Elschnig spots). *Amer. J. Ophthal. 66:*1069, 1968.
49. Knapp, A.: Course in certain cases of atrophy of the optic nerve with cupping and low tension. *Arch. Ophthal. 23:*41, 1940.
50. Kornzweig, A. L., Eliasoph, I., and Feldstein, M.: Occlusive disease of retinal vasculature. *Arch. Ophthal. 71:*542, 1964.
51. Kroll, A. J.: Experimental central retinal artery occlusion. *Arch. Ophthal. 79:*453, 1968.
52. Lauber, H.: Treatment of atrophy of the optic nerve. *Arch. Ophthal. 16:*555, 1936.
53. Lorentzen, S. E.: Occlusion of the central retinal artery: a follow-up. *Acta Ophthal. 47:* 690, 1969.
54. Lin, P. M., and Scott, M.: Collateral circulation of the external carotid artery and the internal carotid artery through the ophthalmic artery in cases of internal carotid artery thrombosis. *Radiology 65:*755, 1955.
55. MacFaul, P. A.: Ciliary artery involvement in giant cell arteritis. *Brit. J. Ophthal. 51:* 505, 1967.

56. Madsen, P. H.: Venous stasis retinopathy in insufficiency of the ophthalmic artery. *Acta Ophthal. 44:*940, 1966.
57. Marx, F.: An arteriographic demonstration of collaterals between internal and external carotid arteries. *Acta Radiol. 31:*155, 1949.
58. McKay, R. A., and Spivey, B. E.: Generalized choroidal angiosclerosis. *Arch. Ophthal. 67:*727, 1962.
59. McLean, J. M., and Ray, B. S.: Soft glaucoma and calcification of internal carotid arteries. *Arch. Ophthal. 38:*154, 1947.
60. Merin, S., and Freund, M.: Retinopathy in severe anemia. *Amer. J. Ophthal. 66:*1102, 1968.
61. Miller, G. R., and Smith, J. L.: Ischemic optic neuropathy. *Amer. J. Ophthal. 62:*103, 1966.
62. Miller, S. J. H.: Carotid insufficiency. *Trans. Ophthal. Soc. U.K. 80:*287, 1960.
63. Morse, P. H.: Elschnig's spots and hypertensive choroidopathy. *Amer. J. Ophthal. 66:* 844, 1968.
64. Naunton, W. J., and Forester, R. M.: Severe vitreous hemorrhage in a premature infant. *Brit. J. Ophthal. 39:*563, 1955.
65. Ostler, H. B.: Pulseless disease (Takayasu's disease). *Amer. J. Ophthal. 43:*583, 1957.
66. Pinkham, R. A.: The ocular manifestations of the pulseless syndrome. *Acta XVII Concilium Ophthalmologicum 1954 1:*348, 1955.
67. Quint, K. R.: Fundusveränderungen bei Karotisthrombose. *Klin. Mbl. Augheilk. 142:*559, 1963.
68. Reese, A. B., and Carroll, F. D.: Optic neuritis following cataract extraction. *Amer. J. Ophthal. 45:*659, 1958.
69. Reese, A. B., and McGavic, J. S.: Relation of field contraction to blood pressure in chronic primary glaucoma. *Arch. Ophthal. 27:*845, 1942.
70. Rotman, M., Seidenberg, B., Rubin, I., Botstein, C., and Basniak, M.: Aortic arch syndrome secondary to radiation in childhood. *Arch. Intern. Med. 124:*87, 1969.
71. Rubenstein, R. A., Yanoff, M., and Albert, D. M.: Thrombocytopenia, anemia and retinal hemorrhage. *Amer. J. Ophthal. 65:*435, 1968.
72. Sachs, E. Jr.: Arteriographic demonstration of collateral circulation through ophthalmic artery in internal carotid artery thrombosis. *J. Neurosurg. 11:*405, 1954.
73. Sanders, M. D., and Hoyt, W. F.: Hypoxic ocular sequelae of carotid-cavernous fistulae. *Brit. J. Ophthal. 53:*82, 1969.
74. Sandvig, K.: Central areolar choroidal atrophy. *Acta Ophthal. 37:*325, 1959.
75. Schenk, H.: Ueber das Auftreten einer Retinopathia traumatica Purtscher nach Unterbindung der Arteria carotis communis. *Klin. Mbl. Augenheilk. 127:*669, 1955.
76. Shea, M.: Carotid-ophthalmic anastomoses. Frequency of external carotid and ophthalmic artery anastomoses. *Brit. J. Ophthal. 40:* 497, 1956.
77. Shikano, S., and Shimizu, K.: *Atlas of Fluorescence Fundus Angiography.* Philadelphia, Saunders, 1968, p. 87.
78. Siegrist, A.: *IX Congrès Periodique International d'Ophtalmologie. Utrecht 14–18 Août, 1899.* Amsterdam, Van Mossen, 1900, p. 131.
79. Simmons, R. J., and Cogan, D. G.: Occult temporal arteritis. *Arch. Ophthal. 68:*8, 1962.
80. Smith, J. L., Israel, C. W., and Harner, R. E.: Syphilitic temporal arteritis. *Arch. Ophthal. 78:*284, 1967.
81. Smith, M. C., and Hoyt, W. F.: Chronic occlusive disease of the carotid arteries with non-diagnostic or misleading pressures on the retinal arteries. *Amer. J. Surg. 102:*661, 1961.
82. Smith, V. H.: Carotid insufficiency. *Trans. Ophthal. Soc. U.K. 80:*253, 1960.
83. Smith, V. H.: Pressure changes in the ophthalmic artery after carotid occlusion: an experimental study in the rabbit. *Brit. J. Ophthal. 45:*1, 1961.
84. Sorsby, A., and Crick, R. P.: Central areolar choroidal sclerosis. *Brit. J. Ophthal. 37:*129, 1953.
85. Spencer, W. H., and Hoyt, W. F.: A fatal case of giant cell arteritis (temporal or cranial arteritis) with ocular involvement. *Arch. Ophthal. 64:*862, 1960.
86. Swan, K. C., and Raaf, J.: Changes in the eye and orbit following carotid ligation. *Trans. Amer. Ophthal. Soc. 49:*435, 1951.
87. Tamler, E., and Takahashi, E.: Collateral circulation to the eye. *Amer. J. Ophthal. 52:* 381, 1961.
88. Tarkkanen, A., Tala, P., Karjalainen, K., and Virkkula, L.: Ocular manifestations of the aortic arch syndrome. *Ann. Chir. Gynaec. Fenn. 56:*141, 1967.

89. Thompson, B. W., Read, R. C., and Campbell, G. S.: Aortic arch syndrome. *Arch. Surg. 98:* 607, 1969.

90. Vinijchaikul, K.: Primary arteritis of the aorta and its main branches (Takayasu's arteriopathy). *Amer. J. Med. 43:*15, 1967.

91. Wagener, H. P., and Hollenhorst, R. W.: The ocular lesions of temporal arteritis. *Amer. J. Ophthal. 45:*617, 1958.

92. Whitfield, A. G. W., Batemen, M., and Cooke, W. Trevor: Temporal arteritis. *Brit. J. Ophthal. 47:*555, 1963.

93. Wise, G. N.: Ocular periarteritis nodosa. *Arch. Ophthal. 48:*1, 1952.

94. Wolter, J. R.: Secondary glaucoma in cranial arteritis. *Amer. J. Ophthal. 59:*625, 1965.

95. Zimmerman, L. E., DeVenecia, G., and Hamasaki, D. I.: Pathology of the optic nerve in experimental acute glaucoma. *Invest. Ophthal. 6:*109, 1967.

chapter 13

Hypertensive Retinopathy

Severe retinopathy in patients with Bright's disease was recognized long before the blood pressure was measured in man, and the connection with hypertension was established. In 1859, Liebreich [30] described the main retinal features of accelerated hypertension. He noted radial streaks of blood among the nerve fibers, small white points, and larger oval or round milk-white spots, a reddish papilla, engorged veins, and abnormal arterioles in Bright's disease.

The arterial abnormalities of benign hypertension were described in 1898 by Marcus Gunn.[16] He described arterial narrowing and irregularity, tortuosity, a bright arterial light reflex, loss of transparency of the arterial wall, and venous nipping. Gunn wrote that the patients had often suffered from migraine and had a family history of arterial disease. His description was enlarged in 1916 by Foster Moore [36] who noted that arteriolar irregularity developed over a few months in a patient with trench nephritis. Moore noted that the line of a vein was often displaced at the crossing but banking was less common. He found it difficult to say when vessels were narrowed because of the wide variation seen in normal eyes. Bull, in 1886,[9] pointed out that patients with Bright's disease and neuroretinitis had a very poor prognosis. He followed up 86 such patients until death and found that 57 died within a year of neuroretinitis being diagnosed.

Volhard and Fahr in 1929 [44] firmly established the connection between renal disease, hypertension, and retinopathy and ascribed the pathology in both organs to "angiospasm." They believed that the rise in blood pressure was also caused by vascular spasm. Volhard and Fahr assumed that patients who had proteinuria could not have essential hypertension. Although this is no longer thought to be correct the mistake is understandable because most patients with accelerated hypertension and retinopathy do develop proteinuria.

The work of Keith, Wagener, and Barker [23] is a landmark in the scientific clinical study of hypertensive retinopathy. These workers were able to associate different grades of hypertensive retinopathy with differences in the prognosis. A patient with severe arteriolar changes but no hemorrhages or exudates had a life expectancy of about 5 years while patients with accelerated hypertension and papilledema lived, on the average, only 6 months. Since the publication of their paper the grading system of Keith and his colleagues has been widely used to compare the severity of hypertension in different series of treated patients.

CLINICAL FEATURES

ARTERIAL CHANGES

The most common disease of large arteries is atherosclerosis and this term is often used to describe arterial disease in general. Such usage is incorrect. Atherosclerosis is a patchy, nodular, fatty infiltration of the intima often associated with fibrosis and is found in arteries down to about 300 μ in size, roughly the diameter of the ophthalmic artery. The arterial changes in smaller vessels found in hypertension and presumably in aging are a diffuse fibrosis and hyalinization most correctly called arteriosclerosis. As the smaller retinal vessels are arterioles the changes in them should be termed "arteriolarsclerosis."

In hypertension interpretation is complicated by two other types of vascular change.

The first is smooth muscle hypertrophy which takes place in normally reactive arterioles as a result of pressure elevation. The hypertrophied artery may itself become the victim of arteriosclerosis with replacement of smooth muscle by fibrous tissue.

The second is focal arteriolar necrosis. Such damage to small arteries of 20 μ in diameter or less is common in accelerated hypertension and resembles the fibrinoid necrosis seen in other organs. Focal damage to the wall of such small vessels is hard to detect clinically unless it causes the formation of a cotton-wool spot but such areas are readily seen on fluorescein angiograms.

The diagnosis of early hypertensive vascular changes in the retinal arterioles is complicated by the close similarity of many of the features to those seen in the eyes of normotensive elderly men and women. The retinal arteries in aged people may run a straighter course than in young people and be slightly narrowed and pale in color. Such vessels have a wall in which the smooth muscle has been partly replaced by collagen.[29]

In the young patient with severe hypertension the arteries are usually considerably narrowed. Earlier writers have spoken of a ratio of arterial to venous caliber of 1:4 but this is almost certainly an exaggeration. In our experience the most severely narrowed vessels among hypertensive patients (Fig. 13-1) are about half the expected normal diameter. It is easy to overestimate the degree of narrowing and if the veins are engorged the arteries appear narrowed in comparison (Fig. 13-2). Retinal edema may obscure the retinal arteries and also lead to a misjudgement of the extent of the narrow-

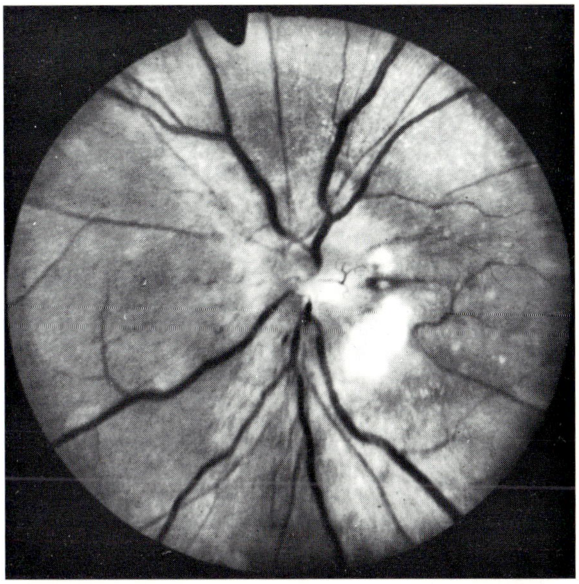

Fig. 13-1. Malignant hypertension in a 19-year-old male. The arteries are conspicuously narrowed but measurement showed that they average about half the normal caliber.

Fig. 13-2. Superior temporal quadrant of a patient with malignant hypertension. The veins are dilated and the arteries inconspicuous amid cotton-wool spots and retinal edema. Although the arteries appear thread-like, measurement showed that they were about half normal caliber. (From Hodge and Dollery. *Quarterly Journal of Medicine 33:* 1964.)

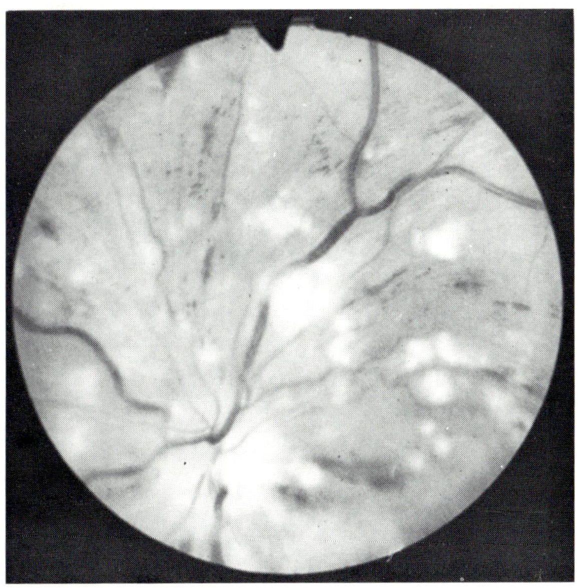

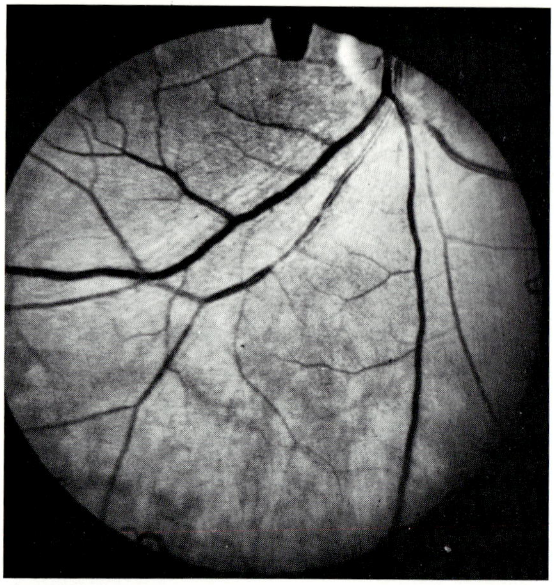

A

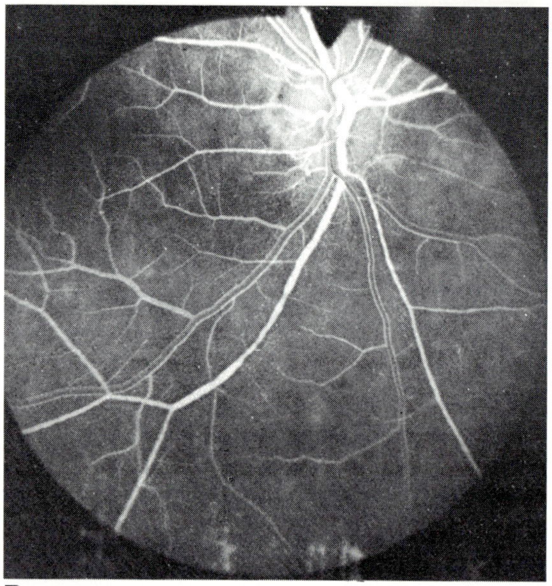

B

Fig. 13-3. *A*, From a color transparency showing focal narrowing of a retinal artery in a hypertensive patient. *B*, Fluorescein angiogram of the vessel shown in *A*. The internal caliber of the vessel is very irregular.

ing. Arteries may also appear narrowed at the disc edge as they dip over into the retina. It is unwise to judge vessel narrowing within 1 dd.

If the pressure elevation is maintained structural changes in the vessel wall become manifest in only a few weeks or months. The wall becomes thicker and in consequence the light reflex increases. At a later stage the reflection may take on a burnished coppery color and in some cases become silvery white. The dark column of venous blood normally seen dimly through the arterial blood column at arteriovenous crossings become invisible. Parallel zones of concealment appear on either side of the artery at vein crossings and in a small proportion of cases venous obstruction leads to banking of the blood column upstream from this point. The outline of the arterial wall becomes irregular and focal narrowing may appear.

Older patients with a slow rise of pressure or with hypertensive changes occurring after the sclerosis of aging show a somewhat different pattern. Severe general narrowing of the arteries is less common but irregularity of the vessel caliber is prominent (Fig. 13-3). Leishman[29] has suggested that the narrowed areas were those which contained contractile elements while the wider ones were fibrosed sections blown out by the high pressure. This explanation of the pathogenesis of focal narrowing may be partially correct but as some of these narrowed areas show severe structural changes[17] it may not be the whole story. The main arteries are often wide, tortuous, and irregular, but the smaller branches seem narrow and inconspicuous. Severe crossing changes are common and thrombosis of branch retinal veins may occur as a complication.

Fluorescein studies of the retinal arteries in hypertensive patients often show minor irregularities of the lumen. Occasionally, side branches are considerably narrowed at their origin from the main artery, probably

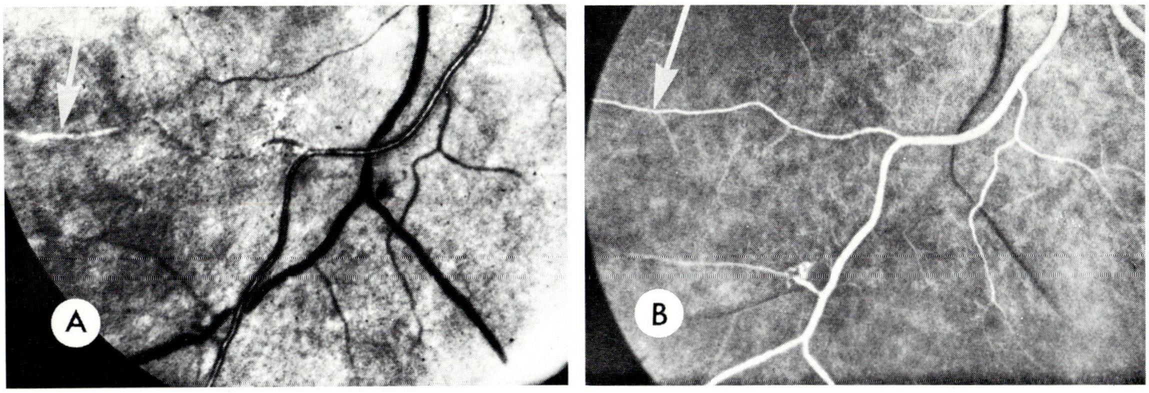

Fig. 13-4. *A*, From a color transparency of a hypertensive patient with a retinal artery which shows arteriosclerosis. In places the lumen of the vessel is completely obscured **(arrow).** *B*, Fluorescein angiogram of the same area as in *A*. Flow passes through the sclerosed section of the artery **(arrow).**

as a result of thickening of the wall. Complete occlusion of the arteries is rare, even when a vessel has pipe-stem sheathing without a visible lumen (Fig. 13-4). Fluorescein flows through although the lumen may be very irregular at this point.

To make use of the clinical features in the evaluation of an individual patient it is important to know how well they correlate with other aspects of hypertensive cardiovascular disease.

QUANTITATIVE ASPECTS

There are two main problems in interpreting hypertensive retinal vascular changes. The first is the frequency with which these changes occur in hypertension and the second is the extent to which they may be confused with the features of aging.

Bechgaard, Kopp, and Nielsen,[5] who examined the eyes of 500 hypertensive patients with pressures higher than 160/100 mmHg, threw some valuable light on the first point. The diameter of the retinal arteries of two-thirds of these patients was judged to be normal, 24 per cent were narrow, and 10 per cent very narrow. Minor irregularities of caliber were seen in 20 per cent and major ones in 7 per cent of patients. There were abnormal arteriovenous crossings in 37 per cent and an increased light reflex in 46 per cent. Bechgaard's data are a valuable corrective to the widely held view that almost all hypertensive patients have abnormal retinal arteries. They illustrate particularly the unreliability of change in caliber as a clinical sign of hypertension. Stokoe and Turner[42] pointed out how difficult it is to derive a meaningful ratio of arterial to venous caliber because of the variations in the normal branching pattern. They could find arteries and veins whose relative caliber could be assessed in only 153 out of 320 retinal quadrants which they examined.

The study of van Buchem, Heuvel-Aghina, and Heuvel[8] is a useful clinical comparison of the effects of hypertensive and aging changes. These workers used four grades of vascular change; diffuse narrowing alone; a widened light reflex; crossing changes; and copper wiring. Among men with a blood pressure less than 141/91 mmHg, 6.2 per cent had narrowed vessels while one-third with a blood pressure above 160/110 mmHg had narrowing. A widened light reflex was present in about a third of the group with a blood pressure less than 141/91 mmHg and a fifth of those with a pressure exceeding 160/110 mmHg.

Crossing changes were present in a quarter of men with a blood pressure less than 151/91 mmHg and a third of men whose blood pressure exceeded this level. Copper-wire arteries were present in 3 per cent of men with a pressure below 151/91 mmHg and 16 per cent of men with a higher pressure.

Both a widened light reflex and crossing changes in the normotensive men were related to their age. Only 13 per cent of men in the 40 to 44-year age group had crossing changes but this proportion had risen to 43 per cent in the age range of 55 to 60 years. The only important drawback of this study was that it included few men with severe hypertension.

Because clinical studies are subject to uncontrolled observer variation and bias, Kagan, Aurell and Tibblin[22] have tried to derive quantitative indices related to hypertensive vascular changes. They examined retinal photographs from 630 men aged 50 years, and measured the width of arteries and veins by projecting the pictures of a disc area so that the disc filled a circle 10 cm in diameter. The vessels were measured where they crossed a circle 20 cm in diameter. The number of vessels crossing the circle (N), the mean width of the arteries (W) and veins (V) and the sum of the length of all the vessels from the disc edge to the 20-cm circle (L) were measured (Fig. 13-5). The mean values of N, L, and W were greater in the normals than in the hypertensives but the differences in L were not significant. Thus, the value of the clinical sign of straightening of the arteries did not find much support in these measurements. Even though the changes in N and W were significant there was a wide overlap between the normals and the hypertensives. Mean values of W ranged from 16.7 for a diastolic blood pressure < 79 mmHg to 13.8 for one of > 120 mmHg. Values of N over the same range of pressures were 18.9 to 16.7.

The wide range greatly reduces the usefulness of these measurements. For example, in 34 subjects with systolic blood pressure < 120 mmHg the range of N was 14 to 22 and that of W was 11 to 20, while for 25 subjects with a systolic blood pressure exceeding 180 mmHg the range of N was 14 to 22 and that of W was 8 to 18.

These studies show that clinical signs such as straightening of the arteries, arterial narrowing, crossing changes, and widening of the light reflex are unreliable indices of hypertensive vascular disease because of their variability and because they are relatively common in older normotensive individuals. They are still useful signs of retinal vascular disease but not necessarily of hypertension.

CLINICAL FEATURES OF RETINOPATHY IN ACCELERATED HYPERTENSION

The incidence of hypertension increases with age but malignant hypertension is most common in middle age and rare after the age 65 years.[23,26,38] The reason for the relative immunity of older people to accelerated hypertension may be related to two factors. Malignant hypertension is a common late complication in patients with chronic renal disease such as glomerulonephritis and most of these patients die in the third to fifth decade. However, even essential malignant hypertension is rare in old age. Leishman has suggested that the arteries and arterioles of elderly people are protected from the acute damaging effect of a high blood pressure as a result of fibrous replacement of smooth muscle in the vessels. He called this "defence by sclerosis."[29]

The earliest feature of accelerated hypertension is the appearance of small linear hemorrhages in the nerve fiber layer and cotton-wool spots which usually lie, in the area of the radial peripapillary capillaries, along the main vessel routes at the posterior pole of the eye (Fig. 13-6). Linear or flame-shaped hemorrhages vary in size from tiny streaks near the limit of visibility to substantial hemorrhages up to 100 μ wide and ten times as long. Cotton-wool spots begin as a greyish white discoloration of the retina and grow rapidly in size and optical density. When fully developed at 24 to 48 hours after they first appear, they are shiny white with faintly frayed edges and usually measure between 100 μ and 1 mm in diameter. Large cotton-wool spots may deflect an adjacent vein which then curves round the edge of the spot. As they clear, cotton-wool spots lose their fluffy whiteness and develop a granular appearance (Fig. 13-7). If the patient is not treated for several weeks or months, hemorrhages and cotton-wool spots of different ages may be seen in the same eye.

In the early stages of accelerated hypertension it is unusual to see hard, fatty exudates but these form after a few weeks have passed. They begin as discrete white flecks usually on the disc side of the macula. As they become denser they form a radial spoke-like pattern which may spread to form a complete star figure radiating from the macula (Fig. 13-8). Such exudates may also form above and below the temporal vessels and on the nasal side of the disc, but they are often densest in the macular region.

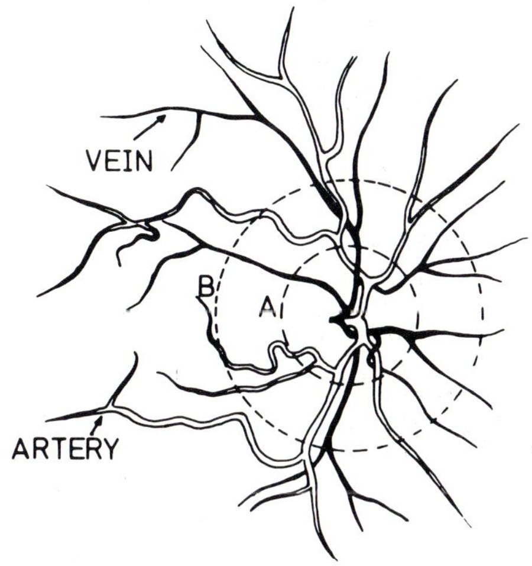

Fig. 13-5. Diagram of the method used by Kagan, Aurell, and Tibblin[22] to quantitate vessel narrowing and straightening in hypertension. The first circle **(A)** fits the edge of the disc (disc ring radius = 10 cm) and the second **(B)** has twice the diameter of **A.**

Fig. 13-6. Map of the location of hemorrhages **(black areas)** and cotton-wool spots **(shaded areas)** in the right retina of a patient with malignant hypertension. Both are found predominantly along the main vessel groups.

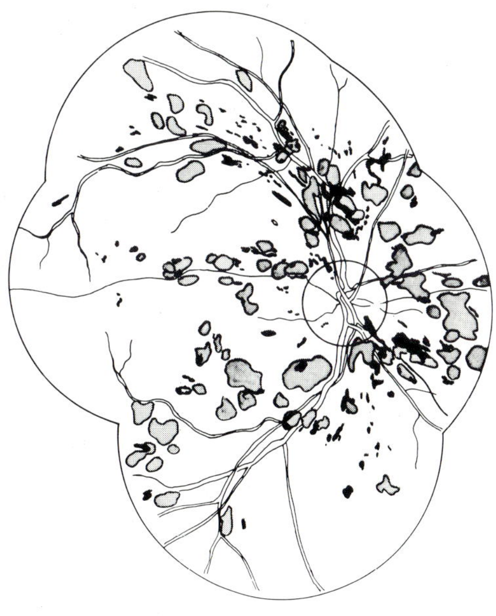

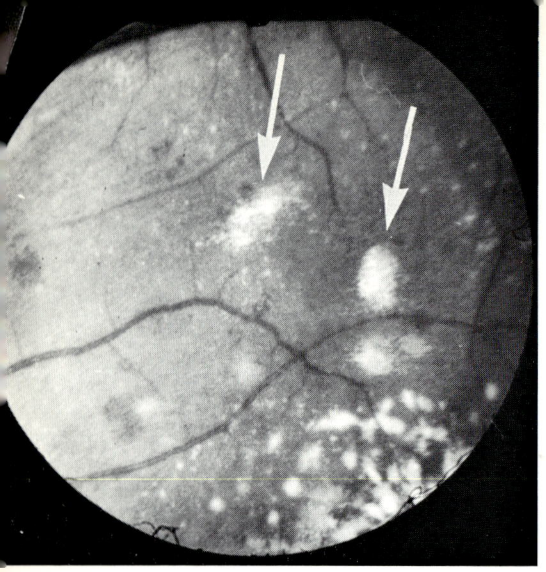

Fig. 13-7. Enlargement of a retinal area in a patient with accelerated hypertension who had received treatment for 2 weeks. Cotton-wool spots **(arrows)** show a granular appearance. (×2)

Fig. 13-8. *A*, Retina of a patient with accelerated untreated hypertension. There are many cotton-wool spots but no fatty exudates. *B*, Same patient after 1 week of treatment. Several fresh cotton-wool spots have formed while some of those present initially are fading. Fine lines of fatty exudate are forming around the macula. *C*, Same patient 2 weeks after *A*. Cotton-wool spots are clearing but the fatty exudate around the macula is increasing. *D*, Three months after *A*. All the cotton-wool spots have disappeared and the amount of fatty exudate is reduced.

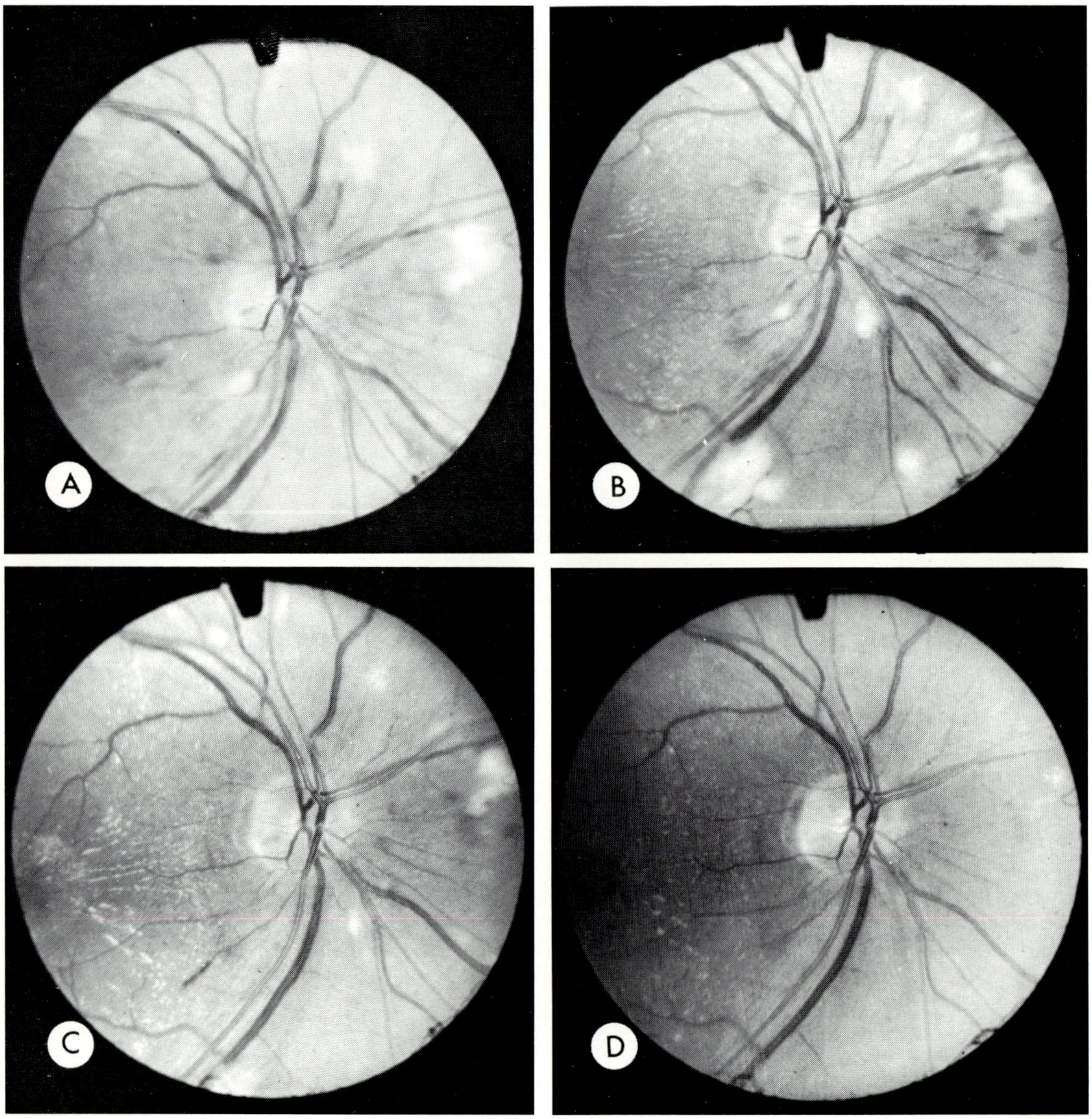

The first change in the optic disc is a pinkish discoloration. Later the nerve head may become orange or brick red in color and the margins become indistinct. It is now unusual to find severe papilledema in hypertensive patients because they are treated before this occurs. However, if for some reason the patient is not treated, severe papilledema may develop with the disc swelling to twice its normal diameter and bulging forward several diopters.

Retinal edema and engorgement of the retinal veins commonly precede papilledema in hypertension. Retinal edema usually begins as a grayish haze on the temporal side of the disc but may spread over the whole of the posterior pole. The swollen veins become dark in color and the narrowed arteries buried in retinal edema may appear thread-like in comparison.

Fluorescein photography has been most helpful in analyzing the microvascular changes which occur in accelerated hypertension. Hodge and Dollery[19] have found that 84 per cent of 464 cotton-wool spots which they examined had associated vascu-

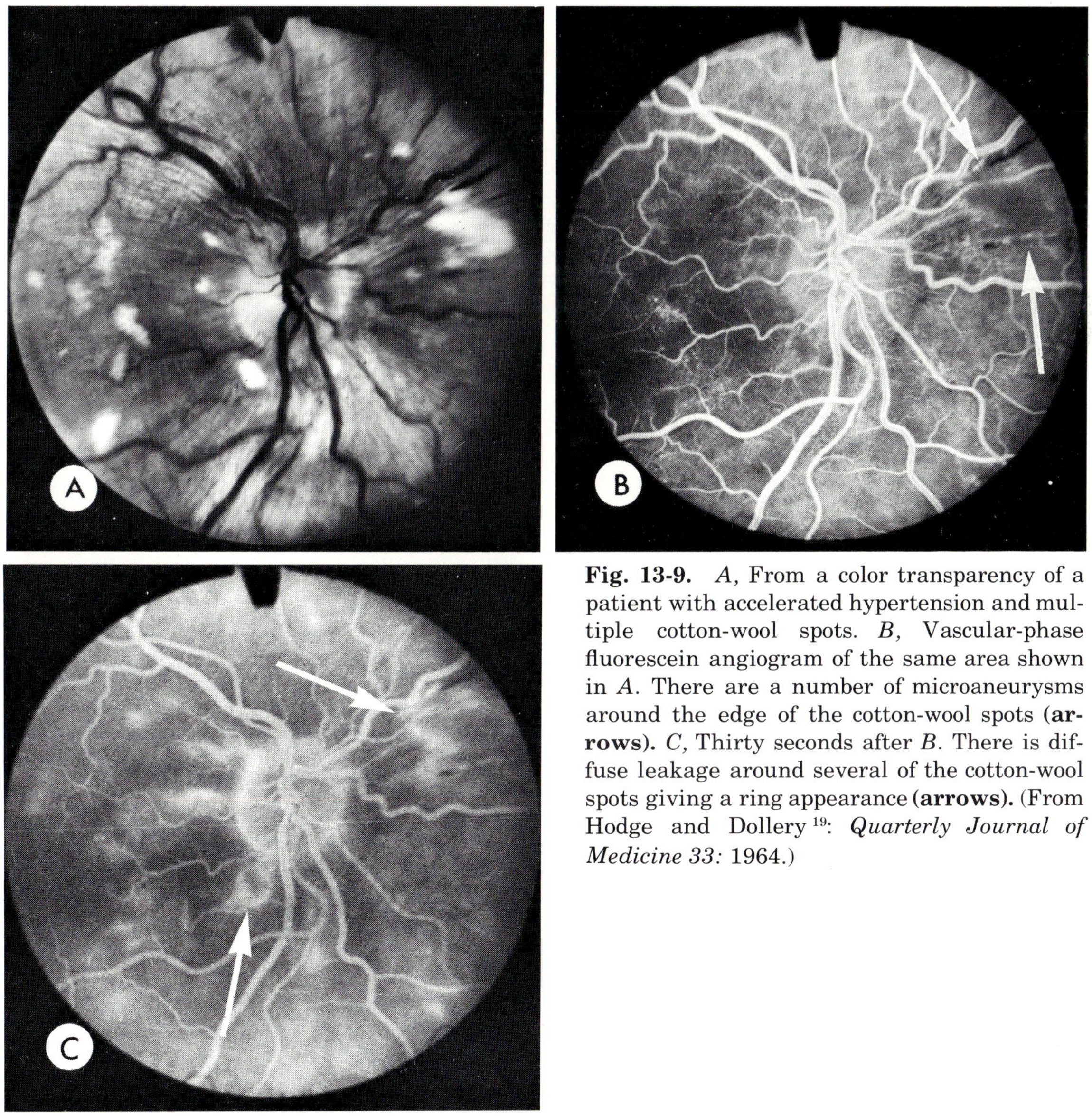

Fig. 13-9. *A,* From a color transparency of a patient with accelerated hypertension and multiple cotton-wool spots. *B,* Vascular-phase fluorescein angiogram of the same area shown in *A.* There are a number of microaneurysms around the edge of the cotton-wool spots **(arrows).** *C,* Thirty seconds after *B.* There is diffuse leakage around several of the cotton-wool spots giving a ring appearance **(arrows).** (From Hodge and Dollery[19]: *Quarterly Journal of Medicine 33:* 1964.)

lar lesions. Aneurysmal dilatation of capillaries was the most common abnormality and there were sometimes many aneurysms in relation to a single cotton-wool spot (Fig. 13-9). Some were arranged like strings of beads along the course of tiny venules, others were connected to veins through minute channels, but the vascular connections of many could not be discerned. Some filled early with the arteries while others were clearly on the venous side of the circulation. Microaneurysms varied greatly in size and some were as much as 100 μ in diameter. Vascular abnormalities were found both within exudates and outside their border, but the greatest number appeared near the edge of the visible cotton-wool spot.[19,35] Of the exudates studied by Hodge and Dollery, 20 per cent showed a ring pattern of microaneurysms around the cotton-wool spot (Fig. 13-9), similar to that demonstrated in pathologic material by Ashton.[1,2] Serial studies showed that microaneurysms changed their appearance only slowly. The larger ones persisted for several weeks, often getting smaller before they finally disappeared. This is different from the life history of diabetic microaneurysms which persist for months or years.

Defects in the capillary bed appeared in fluorescein angiograms as dark areas in the capillary phase and many cotton-wool spots showed such dark areas where the capillaries did not fill. Capillary perfusion usually returned as the cotton-wool spots faded and it was rare to find complete destruction of the capillary bed.

Leakage of fluorescein from microaneurysms surrounding cotton-wool spots was rapid. Cotton-wool spots surrounded by microaneurysms showed a ring pattern of fluorescence which gradually filled in towards the center of the lesion. Increased background fluorescence was observed on at least one occasion in 420 of 464 exudates studied. The tendency to fluoresce often outlasted the visible lesion. Exudates which showed persistent fluorescence were most often those with residual vascular abnormalities.

Of more interest in the pathogenesis of cotton-wool spots are the changes observed which preceded visible retinal damage. Of 18 areas of cotton-wool spots which were studied before the spot appeared 15 showed excessive fluorescein leakage on the occasion of the first study.[19] However, the ring pattern of microaneurysms was seen only after the cotton-wool spot had formed. The most common lesion preceding the formation of a cotton-wool spot was rapid leakage from discrete points on small arteries feeding the area in which the spot was to occur. Such leaking spots on small arteries were prominent in patients with untreated malignant hypertension (Fig. 13-10). These point lesions were quite distinct from microaneurysms as they had an indistinct margin and the initial rate of spread of dye from them was more rapid than from leaking aneurysms. The arteries which leaked fluorescein had a patent lumen at the time they were studied.

Because of the close topographic relationship between arterial leaking points and cotton-wool spots it seems probable that they are related. The pathology of the leaking points appears to be localized necrosis of the wall of small arteries with fatty change.[17] Flow through the damaged artery may not be obstructed and in this case it is probable that a cotton-wool spot will not appear. Obstruction of the artery at the point of leakage, perhaps only for a few hours by swelling of the wall or adherence of platelets, leads to ischemic damage to the tissue downstream and the formation of a cotton-wool spot. The microaneurysms and capillary changes that form at the periphery of a cotton-wool spot must represent a vascular response to this tissue damage. They are not causally related to the formation of the cotton-wool spot itself.

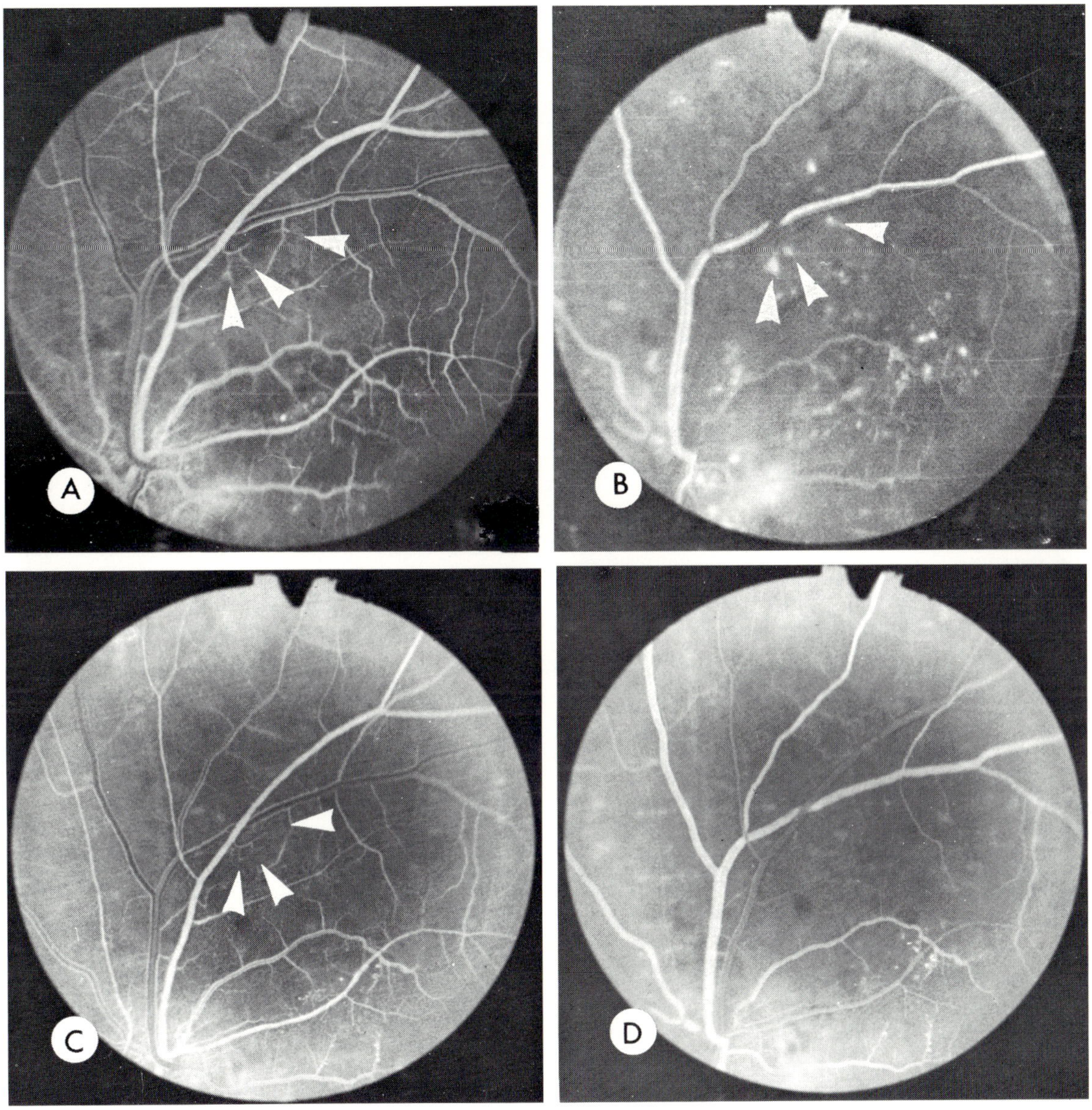

Fig. 13-10. *A*, Arterial-phase fluorescein angiogram of a patient with untreated malignant hypertension. **Arrowheads** indicate small arterial branches supplying areas which contained cotton-wool spots.

B, Venous phase of the same study as *A*. Dye (**arrowheads**) is leaking from the small arteries.

C, Arterial-phase examination taken 4 weeks after *A*. The same branch arteries are identified (**arrowheads**).

D, Venous phase of *C*. There is no leakage of dye from the arteries.

(From Hodge and Dollery[19]: *Quarterly Journal of Medicine 33:* 1954.)

These observations show that leakage and exudation is not an essential part of the life cycle of a cotton-wool spot although leakage from arteries and surrounding capillaries is very common. Thus, it seems preferable to refer to them as cotton-wool spots rather than as soft exudates.

Cotton-wool spots, retinal hemorrhages, and papilledema may be found in a number of other conditions besides accelerated hypertension. Thus, they may appear after severe gastrointestinal hemorrhage and in severe anemia, while hemorrhages and cotton-wool spots may be found in normotensive diabetics. The accompanying clinical features, found on a general medical examination, usually suffice to make the differential diagnosis. It is important not to confuse the retinopathy of accelerated hypertension with a local condition such as central vein obstruction. The presence of papilledema in a hypertensive patient without hemorrhage or cotton-wool spots should lead to suspicion of an alternative explanation such as a rise in intracranial pressure. More than one series of patients with "malignant hypertension" has contained a patient who had a silent meningioma.

PROGNOSTIC SIGNIFICANCE OF HYPERTENSIVE RETINOPATHY

Bull [9] in 1886 appears to have been the first to recognize the poor prognosis associated with neuroretinitis.

In 1939, Keith, Wagener, and Barker [23] proposed a classification of hypertensive retinopathy which is still widely used. There is no doubt that this work was a substantial contribution to the understanding and identification of hypertensive vascular disease but it has also given rise to many difficulties. Their classification was as follows:

Stage I: Slight narrowing or sclerosis of the retinal arteries. Most patients were free of symptoms.

Stage II: More marked arteriolarsclerosis with a widened arterial light reflex, compression of veins at arterial crossing, general and focal arterial narrowing. The blood pressure was usually higher than in patients with Stage I changes and the prognosis was worse.

Stage III: Retinal edema, exudates and hemorrhages with diffusely and focally narrowed arteries. High levels of blood pressure were usual and the patients often had symptoms of headache, breathlessness, and nocturia. The urine often contains protein. The mean survival time was 15 months.

Stage IV: Papilledema with the other features of Stage III. Renal failure was an early feature. The mean survival time was only $4\frac{1}{2}$ months and 70 per cent of patients were dead within 1 year.

Difficulties in the interpretation of vascular narrowing and arteriolarsclerosis have led many workers to abandon the first two stages of the Keith-Wagener classification. The link between the retinal changes and prognosis is not sufficiently decisive. Other "risk factors" such as the level of the blood pressure, the serum lipids, smoking habits, and physical activity have proved more reliable for assessing prognosis. Most internists and ophthalmologists now make a note of the retinal vascular changes which they have observed under specific headings and if possible make a photographic record. Classification under a particular Keith-Wagener staging conveys less information than a full clinical description of the fundus.

There is much wider acceptance of the continued usefulness of Stages III and IV because untreated patients in these categories have a very poor prognosis. Pickering,[38] who has criticized Stage III as being too heterogeneous, believes a distinction should be made between the patient who has cotton-wool spots and flame-shaped hemorrhages and the patient with fatty exudates and blot hemorrhages. The patient with cotton-wool spots and flame-shaped hemorrhages may rapidly progress into malignant hypertension, while the outlook for the patient with fatty exudates and blot hemorrhages is much better. This view has much to commend it, but treatment of patients with Stage III has greatly improved prognosis and among those treated there is no difference in prognosis according to whether they have many exudates or few, hard or soft. The mean survival time of these patients is now about 10 years or about eight times longer than those in Keith and Wagener's series dating from an era before treatment was possible (Fig. 13-11).[7,20,21]

Stage IV retinopathy has been used by many investigators as a means of identifying a group with a particularly poor prognosis. Different series throughout the world have all shown that between 80 and 90 per cent of untreated patients die within 1 year. There is a good correlation between Stage IV retinopathy and the presence of fibrinoid necrosis and onionskin proliferation in renal arterioles.[26]

The prognosis of Stage IV hypertension has also improved greatly with treatment. The mean survival time of 4½ months in Keith and Wagener's series has stretched to 3 to 4 years and is chiefly determined by the deterioration of glomerular filtration rate prior to the initiation of therapy (Fig. 13-12).

The time may come when it would be helpful to abandon the Keith-Wagener classification. Stages I and II are confusing and indistinct. Stages III and IV identify a type of hypertension that has entered an accelerated phase but the term malignant no longer seems appropriate because of the improved prognosis brought about by treatment. The term "accelerated hypertension" qualified by a description of the individual features present is a reasonable alternative.

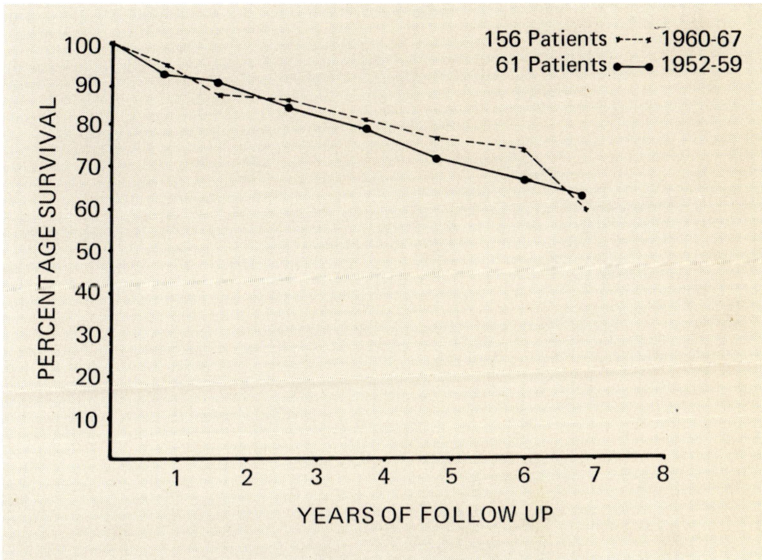

Fig. 13-11. Plot of survival against years of follow-up in treated patients who had Keith-Wagener Stage III retinopathy before treatment began. Mean survival before the availability of treatment averaged about 15 months.

Fig. 13-12. Plot of survival against years of follow-up in treated patients who had Keith-Wagener Stage IV retinopathy before treatment began. Prior to the availability of treatment mean survival in this group was about 4½ months.

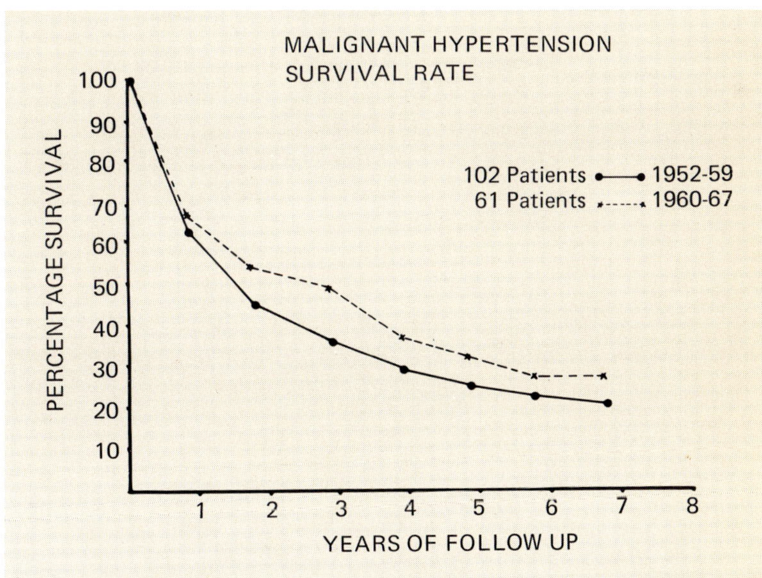

COMPLICATIONS OF HYPERTENSIVE RETINOPATHY

As hypertension is one of the most common causes of retinal vascular disease it is not surprising that it is a frequent precipitating factor in occlusion of both arteries and veins.

In the series of 45 patients with retinal vein occlusion studied by Kohner in 1965,[27] 25 had hypertension.

RESPONSE OF RETINAL VESSELS TO BLOOD PRESSURE REDUCTION

Among treated hypertensive patients there is still a substantial mortality from vascular disease, particularly involving the coronary vessels. If the changes in the retinal vessels were reversible they might give a useful clue to changes taking place elsewhere.

One of the most interesting studies on this subject was undertaken by Lockhart and his colleagues[31] who used four grades of severity to assess caliber changes and arteriolarsclerosis. Among 39 patients who survived during a period of observation lasting several months the most striking changes were the regression of hemorrhages, exudates and papilledema. There was no change in the constriction grading and a slight but nonsignificant reduction in the sclerosis grading.

Lockhart and his colleagues' results were disappointing as they suggest that the changes in larger arteries were not reversible. More recent work using vessel caliber measurements has confirmed their findings but shown some interesting differences between large and small retinal arteries. Hill and Dollery[18] studied groups of patients whose blood pressure had been brought under good control either by renal surgery or use of antihypertensive drugs. Eight of 21 patients showed a pattern of change in which the larger retinal arteries narrowed slightly when blood pressure was lowered while the smaller vessels became significantly wider. Recently these results have been extended.[39]

Patients were selected because their blood pressure had been brought under control by a number of different means. Three young hypertensive patients with a short history of hypertension showed a general dilatation of their retinal arteries when the blood pressure was reduced, but the increase in size was less marked in the larger vessels (Fig. 13-13). A similar pattern was seen in six patients treated with intravenous doses of the vasodilator drug, hydralazine. The blood pressure was reduced to nearly normal levels but here again there was only a slight increase in diameter of the larger arteries and a much greater increase in the smaller ones.

A different pattern was seen among six patients studied upright and recumbent while on sympathetic blocking drugs. There was a reduction in mean blood pressure from 145 to 115 mmHg. The larger arteries became narrower while the smaller ones dilated. The same pattern occurred in seven patients who had successful renal surgery which permanently reduced their blood pressure to normal (Fig. 13-14).

The retinal arteries of hypertensive patients are often narrowed and effective treatment might be expected to return them to normal by bringing about a general increase in diameter. Such a permanent change was seen in only the three young patients with a short history of hypertension. Although hydralazine also caused this type of change the effect was temporary, lasting only during the period of drug action.

The main arteries of the patients treated with hydralazine were judged to be still narrowed even at the peak of the drug effect.

One difficulty in this investigation was the problem of deriving a meaningful index of arterial narrowing.

The patients treated by surgery or with sympathetic blocking drugs present an interesting problem. Small arteries dilated in each case but larger ones became narrower. It is noteworthy that the small arteries dilated in every case when the blood pressure was reduced even though the methods used for lowering pressure were varied. As the retinal vessels have no sympathetic adrenergic vasomotor nerves[32] it seems probable that small vessel dilatation is a local autoregulatory response to the fall in blood pressure. Possibly these small vessels retain their reactivity because, being further down the arterial tree, they are not exposed to such a high pressure.

Why do the larger arteries narrow? These vessels are less reactive to oxygen than normal vessels and in many patients clinical examination shows that they are sclerosed.[39,40,41] Presumably replacement of smooth muscle by collagen has rendered these vessels unresponsive to autoregulatory stimuli, instead they react like inert tubes and become narrower when the pressure falls. This theory does not entirely explain why these vessels can still dilate to a limited extent with hydralazine or constrict with a small amount of oxygen. It must be assumed that fibrous replacement of smooth muscle is incomplete.

In this investigation many areas of caliber irregularity, some amounting to severe focal narrowing, were studied before and after the blood pressure was reduced. The great majority were unchanged by pressure reduction. This finding is supported by Pickering[38] who states that he has never seen a narrowed area dilate. In experimental hypertension reversible focal narrowing often occurs but it is uncommon in man.

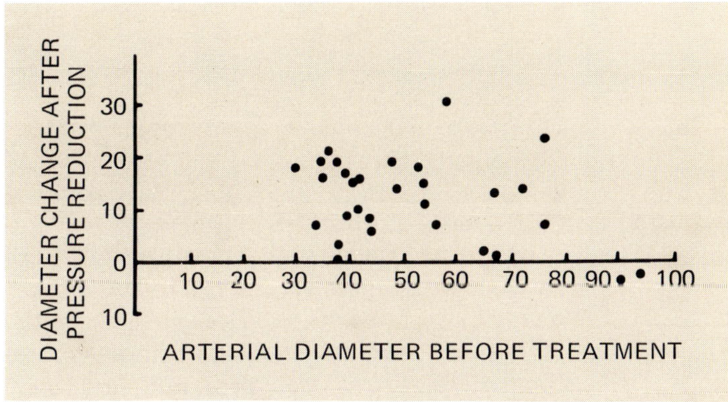

Fig. 13-13. Plot of changes in retinal artery caliber versus initial caliber prior to treatment in three young hypertensive patients. Mean blood pressure was reduced from 138 to 98 mmHg. (From Ramalho and Dollery. Hypertensive retinopathy: Calibre changes in retinal blood vessels following blood-pressure reduction and inhalation of oxygen. *Circulation 37*:580, 1968. By permission of the American Heart Association, Inc.)

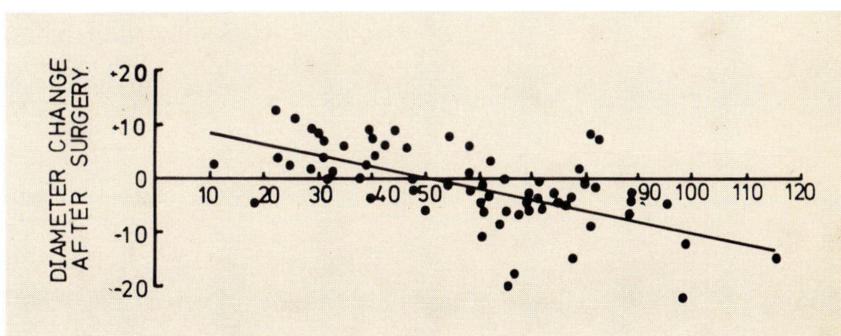

Fig. 13-14. Plot of changes in retinal artery caliber versus initial caliber in seven hypertensive patients treated by renal surgery which reduced the mean blood pressure from 155 to 101 mmHg. The abcissa indicates the caliber of vessels in micra. (From Ramalho and Dollery. Hypertensive retinopathy: Calibre changes in retinal blood vessels following blood pressure reduction and inhalation of oxygen. *Circulation 37*:580, 1968. By permission of the American Heart Association, Inc.)

RESPONSE OF EXUDATIVE HYPERTENSIVE RETINOPATHY TO TREATMENT

Lowering the blood pressure does not produce an immediate change in the hemorrhages, exudates, or papilledema seen in the retinae of patients with malignant hypertension. Even if the pressure has been brought down to a level which is nearly normal, cotton-wool spots continue to form for a day or two. After 2 or 3 days have passed, the formation of cotton-wool spots ceases.[11,33] Formation of fresh cotton-wool spots after these early days strongly suggests poor control of blood pressure and should be considered as a danger signal.

The cotton-wool spots begin to pass through their characteristic life cycle. They lose their fluffy appearance and become gray white and finely granular. The exudate often breaks up into a number of small islands before it finally disappears. During this stage the resolving cotton-wool spot has been confused with deep fatty exudates but the material it contains is more finely divided and it is not difficult to distinguish them clinically.

The rapidity of resolution varies with the initial size of the cotton-wool spot. Small ones may disappear in 2 weeks but larger ones may take 8 weeks or more. The speed of clearing has been measured by plotting the area of the white spot against time (Fig. 13-15). It takes about 4 weeks for the initial area to be reduced by half.

After a cotton-wool spot has cleared the retina in that area usually looks normal. Red spots within, or at the margin, of cotton-wool spots usually correspond with the microaneurysms demonstrated on fluorescein photographs. Most microaneurysms become obliterated during the period in which the cotton-wool spot resolves but occasionally one or two may remain. Neame[37] and Fishberg[13] have stated that soft exudates which are not absorbed leave behind white dots indistinguishable from fatty exudates. Such spots were seen in only three of over 200 cotton-wool spots investigated.[19] In this case it seemed that the spots were hard exudate occupying the position of the cotton-wool spot purely by chance. Leishman[29] has stated that a white thread, signifying a thrombosed arteriole could often be seen in the bed of a cotton-wool spot. In our experience such white threads are rare. None of 200 cotton-wool spots investigated by Hodge and Dollery[19] showed this appearance.

Hemorrhages often lie in close proximity to cotton-wool spots and fresh hemorrhages may appear within the border of a cotton-wool spot as it clears. However, fresh hemorrhages are as uncommon as fresh cotton-wool spots in hypertensive patients once the blood pressure has been brought under control.

Fluorescein studies of cotton-wool spots show that they commonly have a leaking point on the feeding arteriole before treatment is initiated. The cotton-wool spot itself is surrounded by a ring of microaneurysms and these, too, leak fluorescein. The point sources of leakage resolve quickly when the

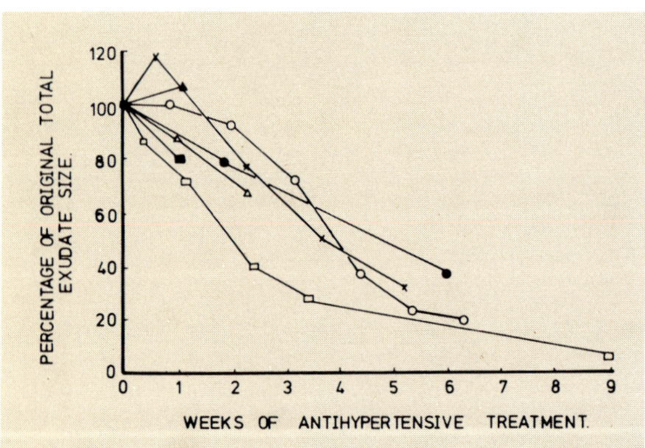

Fig. 13-15. A plot of the total area covered by cotton-wool spots, as a percentage of the pretreatment value in seven patients followed-up for 9 weeks after antihypertensive treatment began. (From Hodge and Dollery. *Quarterly Journal of Medicine 33:* 1954.)

blood pressure is reduced. They disappeared within 4 to 7 days in three out of four patients studied. The disappearance may have been even more rapid as the patients were not restudied earlier. The circulation returns to the dark, nonperfused area in the center of the cotton-wool spot as the lesion clears. The capillary bed which reopens in the base of the cotton-wool spot may be somewhat coarse and contain a few microaneurysms but after a few weeks it usually appears normal (Fig. 13-16).

Patients with the acute onset of malignant hypertension often have no fatty exudates in their fundus at the time, but these appear and increase over the next few days and weeks (see Fig. 13-8). This is the normal evolution of the retinal reaction and does not indicate that the disease process is escaping from control. Fatty exudates often appear in parts of the retina that have previously been normal. They are not related to the position of previous hemorrhages or cotton-wool spots.[33] The fatty exudates are usually arranged in radial spokes around the macula, but almost invariably these spare the fovea and so have little or no adverse effect on vision.

Fatty exudates evolve much more slowly than cotton-wool spots. It may take a year or more for a dense, macular star figure to resolve but it always does so if the blood pressure is kept under good control (Fig. 13-17).[24,33]

Papilledema that is present at the time treatment is begun may progress for several days after the blood pressure is returned to normal and give rise to alarm that the disease is uncontrolled or some other cause of disc swelling is present. A normal disc, or one of doubtful appearance, may develop papilledema during this period. However, once blood pressure has been under control for a few days the papilledema begins to regress. The speed with which it does so depends chiefly upon the degree of the disc swelling. Slight disc swelling may return to normal within 2 or 3 weeks but more severe cases may take several months. If the disc swelling has been very severe and prolonged the disc appearance may never return to normal. Consecutive optic atrophy with a white opaque and fuzzy disc outline may occur. Papilledema of long duration and sufficient severity to cause optic atrophy is now very uncommon because most patients with hypertension are treated long before they get into such a state.

Patients who complain of blurred vision at the onset of malignant hypertension usually lose this symptom within about 2 to 3 months of the institution of hypotensive therapy.[14]

EXPERIMENTAL HYPERTENSIVE RETINOPATHY

In 1937 Keyes and Goldblatt[25] reported the retinal changes which they had observed in eight dogs and one monkey whose blood pressure had been raised by the method of renal artery constriction developed by Goldblatt and his colleagues in 1934.[15] The retinal appearances in one of the dogs was followed for a period of 2 years. The first pathologic change was bilateral superficial retinal hemorrhage. Some of the small arteries had a keen light reflex and were very wavy in their course. Edema formed and ultimately the retina detached. The optic disc of one eye became swollen and remained edematous for 9 months.

There were conspicuous changes in the retinal vessels of this animal. The main arteries showed a greatly thickened intima and hyperplasia of the muscle with some degree of hyaline replacement. Some arteries were locally occluded but the lumen on either side was patent.

In the one monkey studied there were

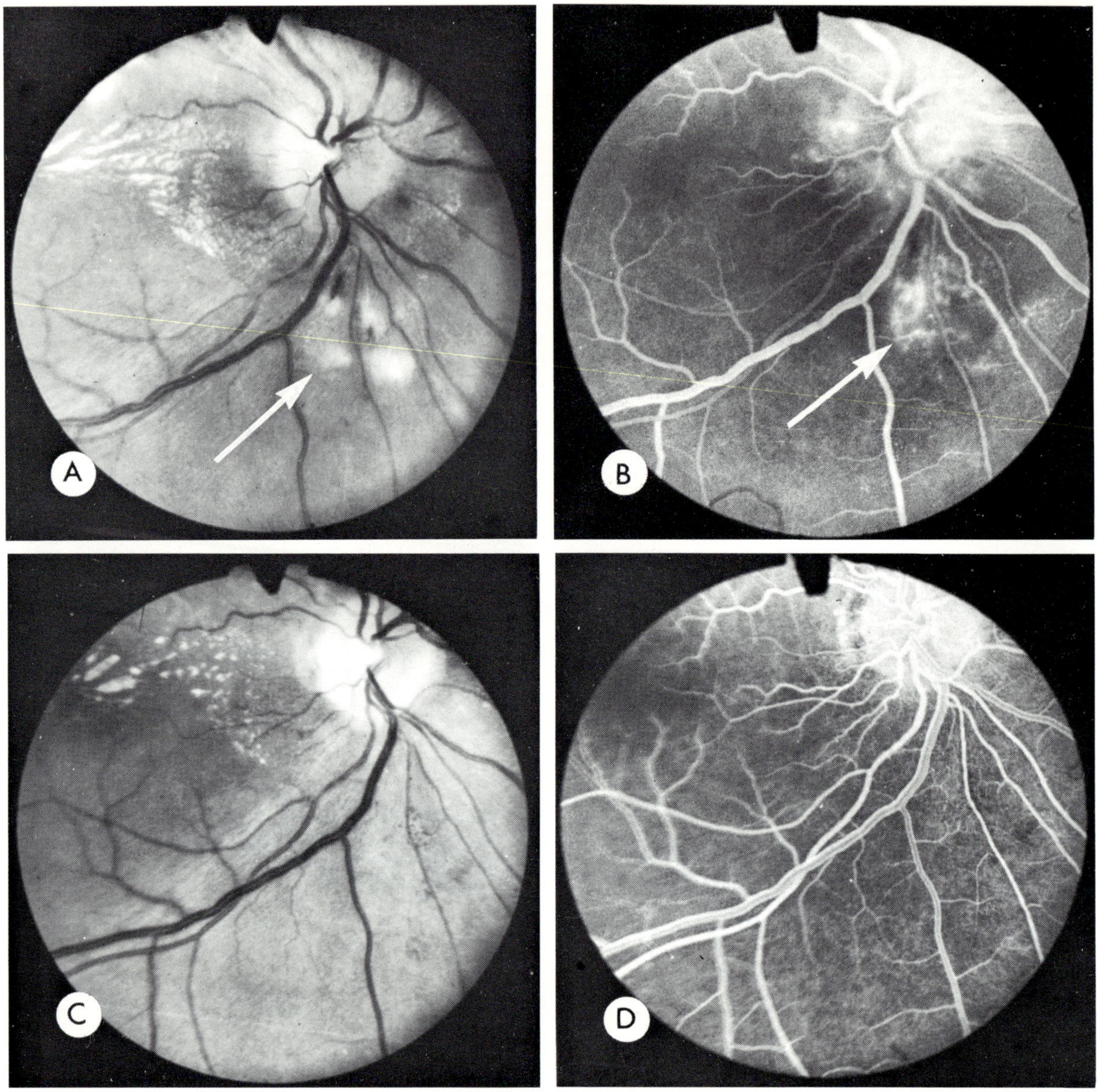

Fig. 13-16. *A*, From a color transparency of the retina of a patient with untreated accelerated hypertension. There are a group of cotton-wool spots beneath the disc **(arrow).**

B, Venous-phase fluorescein study of the same area as *A*. Fluorescein leakage has occurred in the vicinity of the cotton-wool spots **(arrow).**

C, From a color transparency of the same area as *A* but after 5 weeks of treatment. The cotton-wool spots have cleared.

D, Fluorescein angiogram taken on the same date as *C*. There are a few minute dilated capillaries in the area previously occupied by the cotton-wool spots but no dye leakage.

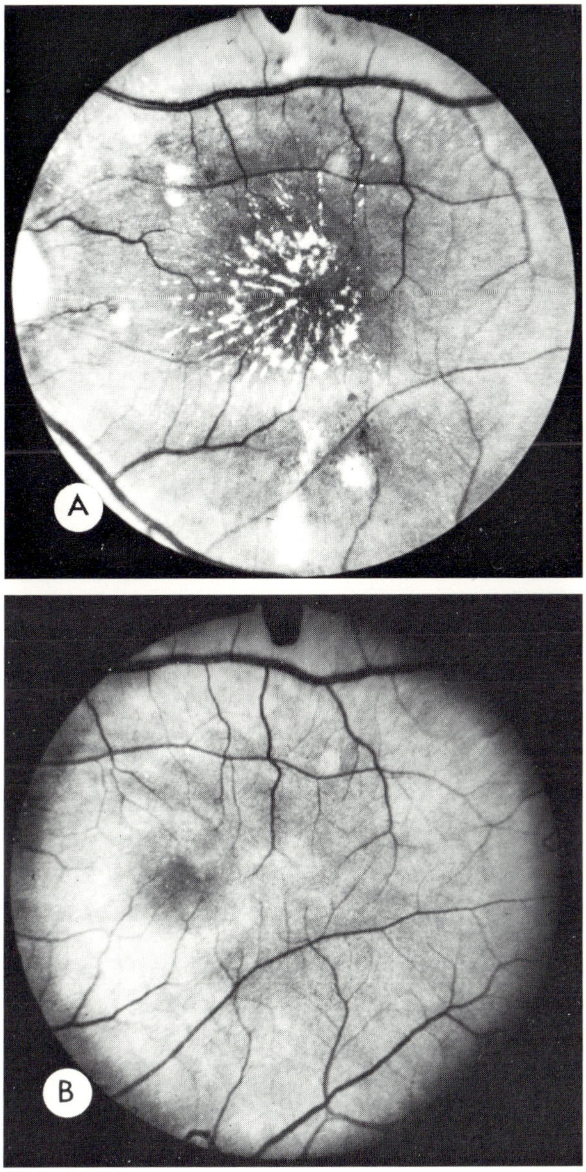

Fig. 13-17. *A*, From a color transparency showing a macular star figure in a patient with accelerated hypertension shortly after initiating treatment. *B*, The same area as *A* taken 1 year later. The fatty exudate forming the star figure has completely cleared.

hemorrhages, edema, and a copper-wire appearance of the arteries. This animal had a blood pressure of 300/220 mmHg.

Laughlin, Thomas, and Friedenwald,[28] in 1940, reported the retinal changes in a dog with severe hypertensive retinopathy. The animal had bilateral Goldblatt clamps and the blood pressure was 250/140 mmHg or higher. The retinal arteries showed variations of caliber like a string of sausages. Near the disc there were hemorrhages and two cotton-wool spots. In the left eye the retina was partly detached and there was an old hemorrhage in the vitreous.

Histologic examination of the retinal vessels showed the appearance of arteriolarsclerosis with medial hypertrophy and hyalinization. Correlation of the irregular narrow vessels with histologic examination showed three types of change: (*1*) clinical narrowing without histologic change; (*2*) organic changes without clinical narrowing; and (*3*) organic changes and narrowing corresponding with the clinical findings. Fibrous thickening of the media without narrowing was the most common change in vessels with a normal caliber. Narrowed vessels showed slight to moderate medial hypertrophy. These workers concluded that some of the localized areas of narrowing without structural change must present a true functional constriction of the smooth muscle in the wall.

Byrom[10] and more recently Uyama[43] have induced chronic hypertension in male rats by excising one kidney and constricting the artery of the other. Byrom found occasional hemorrhages, edema, and retinal detachment but the most common changes were in the vessels. In mild or moderate hypertension (systolic blood pressure up to 170 mmHg) there was very slight diffuse narrowing of the arteries. At higher levels of blood pressure (up to 220 mmHg) diffuse narrowing was also common but there was often focal arterial narrowing as well. In these animals deepening of the level of ether anesthesia reversed the focal narrowing and also reduced the blood pressure by about 35 mmHg. If ether was discontinued the narrowing returned in the same places. When the high blood pressure was of some weeks' duration it became increasingly difficult to abolish the narrowing with ether. When the hypertension was cured by removing the renal artery clip, with a single exception, vasoconstriction disappeared within a few hours. The animals had been hypertensive for 2 to 18 months.

Serial sections were examined in 36 eyes. Focal arteriolar necrosis was found in several vessels of one eye and in one vessel in seven other eyes. In one animal with chronic hypertension a large retinal artery was focally narrowed by proliferative endarteritis and fibrinoid necrosis. However, in the great majority no microscopic changes were observed to account for the changes in caliber.

Engerman, Meyer, and Buesseler [12] have caused hypertension in rats by administering corticosteroids and salt. They reported that fibrinoid arteriolar necrosis was common in the eye of these animals. Other features included exudates and retinal detachment. Bellhorn [6] has studied the effect of age on the focal and general narrowing of retinal arteries in hypertensive rats and found that the changes were more prominent in younger animals than in older ones with comparable degrees of pressure elevation. The older rats may be comparable with older humans who have arteries that show less narrowing with pressure elevation and oxygen breathing than younger people.[39]

Ashton, Peltier, and Garner [4] have reported hypertensive retinal changes in macaque monkeys with renal artery clip or encapsulation. The features included cotton-wool spots, hemorrhages, fatty exudates, and vascular changes. Retinopathy closely resembled that observed in accelerated hypertension in man. Fluorescein studies of these animals showed that many arteries leaked fluorescein. Some of the leaking points were on arteries related to cotton-wool spots but many were not. Some arteries of about 20 μ in diameter were completely occluded and the distal vascular bed filled either through capillary or larger-diameter collaterals (Fig. 13-18).

The capillary bed underlying some cotton-wool spots did not fill either directly or through collaterals, a feature which suggested that the capillaries were closed. Some areas with occluded arteries did not have cotton-wool spots and others with cotton-wool spots had patent ones. As the life cycle of the cotton-wool spot in the monkey is short, it may be that occluded arteries without cotton-wool spots had this feature earlier but that it had been resolved. Similarly, areas with patent vessels and cotton-wool spots may have had a temporary arterial obstruction which later cleared. During a previous investigation with glass microspheres in pigs it was found that obstruction of only a few hours' duration was necessary to ensure the formation of a cotton-wool spot.[3] Electron microscopic studies of these eyes showed that fibrin had leaked through the wall of vessels and some smooth muscle cells were necrotic.

INTERPRETATION

It is instructive to compare the features of experimental hypertensive retinopathy with studies of the cerebral circulation using transparent skull windows. Byrom [10] reported general and focal narrowing of the cerebral arteries in hypertensive rats. When the hypertension was mild there was a diffuse general narrowing of the arteries but in animals with encephalopathy the brain was pale and the small arteries were much narrower. Not infrequently the vessels had a beaded appearance with alternating dilated and constricted segments. When the renal artery clip was removed the vessels returned to normal.

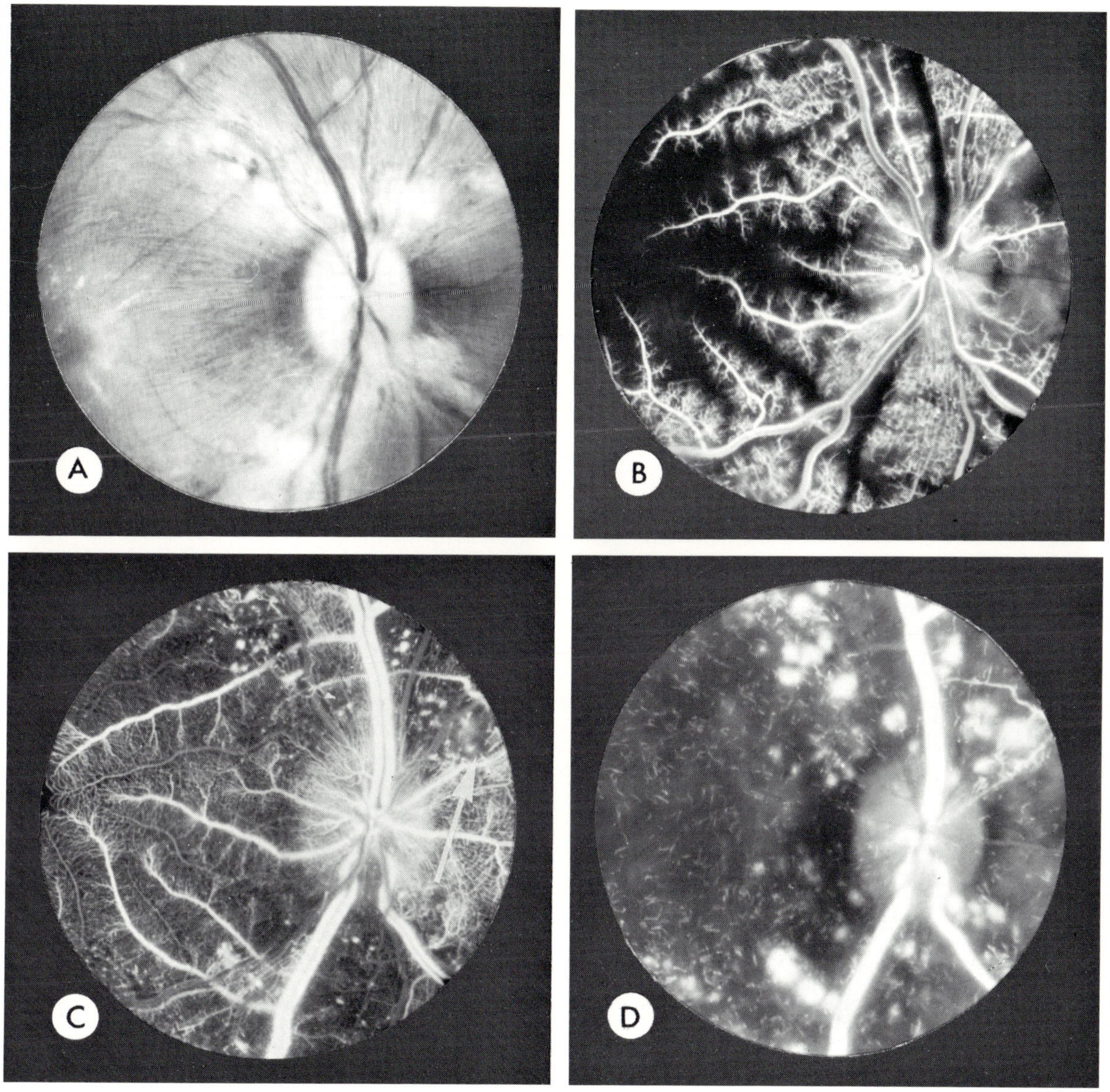

Fig. 13-18. *A*, From a color transparency of a rhesus monkey with accelerated hypertension. A number of cotton-wool spots are present. *B*, Arterial phase fluorescein angiogram of the same area as *A*. *C*, Capillary filling is complete except for small areas beneath some cotton-wool spots (**arrow**). *D*, There are many points of dye leakage. Some, but not all, of which are related to cotton-wool spots.

Meyer, Waltz, and Gotoh[34] have studied the cerebral vessels in 12 monkeys and five cats through a transparent window. The animals were made hypertensive and the cerebral vessels constricted. In cats there was often focal as well as diffuse narrowing but in the monkey the narrowing was always generalized without focal narrowing and the same is true of the retinal arteries in the monkey.[4]

It is interesting that all features of hypertensive retinopathy in man have been reproduced in animals. Evidence concerning the pathogenesis of vascular change is of particular importance. There is no doubt that reversible narrowing can occur in rats, cats, dogs, and monkeys. It is noteworthy that focal arterial narrowing has not been demonstrated conclusively in the monkey. Both focal and general narrowing must represent an increase in arterial tone. Later it appears that structural changes take place which make the narrowing irreversible. In the rats studied by Byrom arterial narrowing was not permanent even after 2 years of hypertension. However, in the dog observed by Laughlin, Thomas, and Friedenwald there appeared to be narrowed areas associated with structural change as well as others in which the histologic structure was normal. If the animal is older the vessels seem to be less reactive and show less marked changes as the pressure rises.

Thus the results in animals are in good agreement with the findings of Ramalho and Dollery in hypertensive man.[39] As blood pressure rises normal retinal arteries constrict. If the elevation of pressure is severe focal necrosis of the vessel wall leads to leakage and to ischemia of the tissue downstream. Smooth muscle in the wall of retinal arteries is damaged by persistent pressure elevation and the vessel becomes less reactive as muscle is replaced by fibrous and hyaline tissue. If the arterial wall is already sclerotic as a result of aging or other pathology its ability to constrict is reduced and features of hypertensive retinopathy are less prominent.

REFERENCES

1. Ashton, N.: Retinal microaneurysms in the non-diabetic subject. *Brit. J. Ophthal. 35:* 189, 1951.
2. Ashton, N.: Diabetic retinopathy. A new approach. *Lancet 2:*625, 1959.
3. Ashton, N., Dollery, C. T., Henkind, P., Hill, D. W., Paterson, J. W., Ramalho, P. S., and Shakib, M.: Focal retinal ischemia: Ophthalmoscopic, circulatory and ultrastructural changes. *Brit. J. Ophthal. 50:*281, 1966.
4. Ashton, N., Peltier, S., and Garner, A.: Experimental hypertensive retinopathy in the monkey. *Trans. Ophthal. Soc. U.K. 88:* 167, 1968.
5. Bechgaard, P., Kopp, H., and Nielsen, J. H.: 1,000 hypertensive patients followed from 16–22 years. *Acta Med. Scand. 154 (Suppl. 312):*175, 1956.
6. Bellhorn, R.: "Experimental Hypertensive Retinopathy in Rats." (M.Sc. Thesis, New York University School of Medicine, 1966.)
7. Breckenridge, A., and Dollery, C. T.: Prognosis of treated hypertension. *Quart. J. Med. 39:*411, 1970.
8. van Buchem, F. S. P., Th. v.d. Heuvel-Aghina, J. W. M., and v.d. Heuvel, J. E. A.: Hypertension and changes of the fundus oculi. *Acta Med. Scand. 176:*539, 1964.
9. Bull, C. S.: Analysis of 103 cases of exudative neuroretinitis, associated with chronic Bright's disease. *Trans. Amer. Ophthal. Soc. 4:*184, 1886.
10. Byrom, F. B.: The nature of malignancy in hypertensive disease. Evidence from the retina of the rat. *Lancet 1:*516, 1963.
11. Dollery, C. T., Ramalho, P. S., and Paterson, J. W.: "Retinal Vascular Alterations in Hypertension," in *Hypertensive Therapy.* Ed. by Gross, F. Berlin, Springer, 1966, p. 152.
12. Engerman, R. L., Meyer, R. K., and Bues-

seler, J. A.: Effects of alloxan diabetes and steroid hypertension on retinal vasculature. *Amer. J. Ophthal. 58:*965, 1964.

13. Fishberg, A. M.: *Hypertension and Nephritis.* Philadelphia, Lea & Febiger, 1954, p. 371.
14. Gass, J. D. M.: A fluorescein angiographic study of macular dysfunction secondary to retinal vascular disease. III. Hypertensive retinopathy. *Arch. Ophthal. 80:*569, 1968.
15. Goldblatt, H., Lynch, J., Hanzal, R. F., and Summerville, W. W.: Studies on experimental hypertension. I. The production of persistent elevation of systolic blood pressure by means of renal ischemia. *J. Exp. Med. 59:*347, 1934.
16. Gunn, M.: On ophthalmoscopic evidence of general arterial disease. *Trans. Ophthal. Soc. U.K. 18:*356, 1898.
17. Harry, J., and Ashton, N.: The pathology of hypertensive retinopathy. *Trans. Ophthal. Soc. U.K. 83:*71, 1963.
18. Hill, D. W., and Dollery, C. T.: Caliber changes in retinal arterioles. *Trans. Ophthal. Soc. U.K. 83:*61, 1963.
19. Hodge, J. V., and Dollery, C. T.: Retinal soft exudates. A clinical study by color and fluorescence photography. *Quart. J. Med. 33:*117, 1964.
20. Hodge, J. V., and Smirk, F. H.: The effect of drug treatment of hypertension on the distribution of deaths from various causes. *Amer. Heart J. 73:*441, 1967.
21. Hood, M., Aurell, M., Falkheden, T., and Bjork, S.: "Analysis of Mortality and Survival in Actively Treated Hypertensive Disease," in *Antihypertensive Therapy.* Berlin, Springer, 1966, p. 370.
22. Kagan, A., Aurell, E., and Tibblin, G.: Signs in the fundus oculi and arterial hypertension. *Bull. WHO 36:*231, 1967.
23. Keith, N. M., Wagener, H. P., and Barker, N. W.: Some different types of essential hypertension: Their cause and prognosis. *Amer. J. Med. Sci. 197:*332, 1939.
24. Kempner, W.: Radical dietary treatment of hypertensive and arteriosclerotic vascular disease, heart and kidney disease and vascular retinopathy. *GP 9:*71, 1954.
25. Keyes, J. E. L., and Goldblatt, H.: Experimental hypertension. IV. Clinical and pathologic studies of the eyes. *Arch. Ophthal. 17:*1040, 1937.
26. Kincaid-Smith, P., McMichael, J., and Murray, E. A.: The clinical course and pathology of hypertension with papilledema (malignant hypertension). *Quart. J. Med. 27:*117, 1958.
27. Kohner, E. M.: Retinal vein occlusion. *Proc. Roy. Soc. Med. 57:*816, 1964.
28. Laughlin, R. C., Thomas, C. B., and Friedenwald, J. S.: The retinal arterioles in experimental renal hypertension: the significance of localized caliber constriction. *Bull. Johns Hopkins Hosp. 67:*79, 1940.
29. Leishman, R.: The eye in general vascular disease, hypertension and arteriosclerosis. *Brit. J. Ophthal. 41:*641, 1957.
30. Liebreich, R.: Ophthalmoskopischer Befund bei Morbus Brightii. *Graefe Arch. Ophthal. 5:*265, 1859.
31. Lockhart, G., von Noorden, G., Dustan, H. P., Corcoran, A. C., and Page, I. H.: The course of retinopathy in treated malignant hypertension. *Arch. Intern. Med. 106:*205, 1960.
32. Malmfors, T.: The adrenergic innervation of the eye as demonstrated by fluorescence microscopy. *Acta Physiol. Scand. 65:*1, 1965.
33. McMichael, J., and Dollery, C. T.: Hypertensive retinopathy. *Trans. Ophthal. Soc. U.K. 83:*51, 1963.
34. Meyer, J. S., Waltz, A. G., and Gotoh, F.: Pathogenesis of cerebral vasospasm in hypertensive encephalopathy. II. The nature of increased irritability of smooth muscle of arterioles in renal hypertension. *Neurology 10:*859, 1960.
35. Mizobe, A., Murai, S., and Mizushima, N.: Fluorescein studies of hypertensive retinopathy. *Jap. Circ. J. 31:*789, 1967.
36. Moore, R. F.: Retinitis of arteriosclerosis and its relation to renal retinitis and to cerebral vascular disease. *Quart. J. Med. 10:*29, 1916.
37. Neame, H.: In: *The Eye and its Diseases.* Ed. by Berens, C. Philadelphia, Saunders, 1950, pp. 610–626.
38. Pickering, G. W.: *High Blood Pressure.* London, Churchill, 1955, p. 273.
39. Ramalho, P. S., and Dollery, C. T.: Hypertensive retinopathy. Caliber changes in retinal blood vessels following blood-pressure reduction and inhalation of oxygen. *Circulation 37:*580, 1968.
40. Sieker, H. O., and Hickam, J. B.: Normal and impaired retinal vascular reactivity. *Circulation 7:*79, 1953.
41. Sieker, H. O., Hickam, J. B., and Gibson,

J. F.: The relationship between impaired retinal vascular reactivity and renal function in patients with degenerative vascular disease. *Circulation 12:*64, 1958.

42. Stokoe, W. L., and Turner, R. W.: Normal retinal vascular pattern. Arteriovenous ratio as a measure of arterial caliber. *Brit. J. Ophthal. 50:*21, 1966.

43. Uyama, M.: A clinical observation of the rat eye with experimental hypertension. *Acta Soc. Ophthal. Jap. 70:*1321, 1966.

44. Volhard, F., and Fahr, K. T.: *Die Brightische Nierenkrankheit. Klinik, Pathologie und Atlas.* Berlin, Springer, 1914.

chapter 14

Diseases of Capillary and Venous Insufficiency

All superficial retinal capillaries, both the radial peripapillary straight channels and the main superficial bed lying at the base of the nerve fiber layer, are supplied directly by the retinal arterioles and are more prone to attack in arterial diseases. The deep retinal capillaries represent a denser network with a finer mesh lying at the outer side of the inner nuclear layer. This bed receives blood via connections from the superficial capillary bed. It has been thought that the deep capillaries also received blood directly from retinal arterioles which bypassed the superficial network.[157] On repeated search, Shakib[202] has been unable to demonstrate electron microscopically a retinal arteriolar channel at the level of the deep capillary bed. Not only has he failed to demonstrate a direct arteriolar connection with the deep bed, but the change from capillary to postcapillary venule, readily visible at this level, is only one of lumen size. Electron microscopically, retinal capillary and postcapillary venular walls are identical. There is increasing evidence that small venules are not simply inert collecting channels. The work of Cunha–Vaz[47] demonstrates the increased permeability of these vessels in experimentally induced disease states. The absence of arterioles and the numerous venous drainage channels at the level of the deep capillary bed suggests a closer relationship of the deep capillaries to the venous rather than to the arterial circulation. This makes the preponderant involvement of the deep network in retinal venous disease more understandable.

Diseases primarily attacking retinal veins and capillaries are much more common and have a much more varied etiology than those primarily attacking retinal arterioles. In obstruction of either veins or capillaries, circulatory alterations are marked but the retinal tissue mainly survives. Irrespective of the etiology of the obstruction, and once the latter occurs, all capillary and venous obstructive diseases undergo a similar course of events. It is this feature which makes much of their advanced clinical pathology so similar.

The key to understanding retinal capillary and venous diseases is to acquire a thorough knowledge of the slowly altering course of events ensuing between the obstructive episode and the final retinal readjustment and stabilization. The key to their etiologic diagnosis is recognition of the obstructive mechanism. The former is most clearly demonstrated by tracing the course of events after vein obstruction secondary to arteriosclerosis. Here the arterial disease can be mild enough to produce no retinal pathology other than the vein obstruction. In such cases the retinal reaction to uncomplicated vein obstruction can be clearly identified. Once this knowledge is gained, the retinal pathology sequential to the obstructive mechanism and that due to the obstruction itself can be separated in the more complicated venous obstructive diseases. The latter key, the obstructive mechanism itself, will be considered in each disease category.

Capillary obstructive diseases may also involve veins and those first obstructing veins commonly show subsequent capillary obliterations as well. This overlap prevents any clear-cut division of the two. Following a list of the known mechanisms by which veins or capillaries may be obstructed, vein obstruction secondary to arteriosclerosis will be described. The course of events following simple vein obstruction can then be applied to the remaining disease categories.

Mechanisms of Obstruction

1. Arteriosclerosis – spread of arterial wall disease to the veins at juxtapositions, arteriovenous crossings, or at the lamina cribrosa
2. Primary venous thrombosis
3. Vein closure by proliferating endothelial cells
4. Stagnation thrombosis – underfilling of the central retinal artery with secondary closure of the vein
5. Senile capillary obliterations in the periphery and at the macula
6. Diabetic retinopathy – extension of capillary disease to the veins
7. Retrolental fibroplasia – oxygen obliteration of immature capillaries
8. Pressure on the vein from without as in tumor or glaucoma
9. Inflammatory obstructions:
   - (a) Peri- or endophlebitis as in Eales's disease
   - (b) Nonspecific uveitis
   - (c) Toxoplasmosis
   - (d) Peripheral chorioretinitis or pars planitis
   - (e) Sarcoidosis
   - (f) Behçet's disease
   - (g) Periphlebitis as a rare occurrence in other diseases
   - (h) Septic thrombosis
10. Coats's disease
11. Changes in the blood constituents:
    - (a) Sickle cell disease
    - (b) Malaria
    - (c) The hyperviscosity syndrome:
      1. Dysproteinemias
      2. Polycythemia
      3. Leukemia
      4. Cystic fibrosis of the pancreas
12. Parasitic obstructions
13. Rickettsial retinopathy
14. Phlebosclerosis
15. Trauma

VEIN OBSTRUCTION SECONDARY TO ARTERIOSCLEROSIS

Vein obstruction due to this mechanism always occurs at arteriovenous crossings, where artery and vein are adjacent, or at the lamina cribrosa. At all such sites the artery and vein share a common adventitial sheath. Most branch obstructions occur temporally where arteriovenous crossings are much more numerous.[110] Most also occur at points where the artery overlies the vein. This too is purely dependent upon the statistical frequency of this type of crossing. Although blockage can occur where the vein overlies the artery or where the two vessels are adjacent but do not cross, this is less frequent.

This type of obstruction is most common in patients with hypertension but can be seen in individuals who do not have, nor, have they ever had, hypertension. These obstructions are more frequent with increasing age and are rare below the age of 40. Those occurring in hypertensive patients are related to the reactive sclerosis of the arterial wall. Thus, hypertension of short duration, even when severe is not as apt to lead to retinal vein obstruction as when the hypertension is of longer duration, even though mild.

As the course of events in branch and central retinal vein obstructions has many different features, they can best be described separately. For descriptive purposes all vein obstructions can be divided into acute and chronic.

BRANCH VEIN OBSTRUCTIONS

Acute branch obstructions have a fairly rapid onset but not as immediate a one as in branch artery blockage. The vein peripheral to the obstruction dilates, darkens, and becomes more tortuous. There is both deep and superficial retinal edema in its drainage area. This is due to fluid leakage through dilated capillary walls and in places, usually near the point of obstruction, through the venous walls as well. Dot-and-blot deep retinal hemorrhages predominate and are readily visible in the periphery about small obstructed venous radicles (Fig. 14-1). Obstructions near the disc commonly show superficial flame-shaped hemorrhages and these often have a predilection for the distribution of the superficial radial peripapillary capillaries. Cotton-wool patches, when present, are more frequent in this same distribution. Here, they are rarely profuse, but commonly multiple. They never occur in the more peripheral branch vein obstructions. Here also, superficial hemorrhages are usually absent. If the tributary obstruction involves the disc, the involved sector becomes elevated, edematous, and has indistinct margins. Not only are major obstructed veins serpentine in the retinal plane, but they dip up and down in the edematous retina and may reach either the internal or external limiting membrane. If macular venous drainage is unaffected, visual acuity is unchanged, and patients may be unaware of the obstructive episode.

Collateral circulation via the deep capillary bed to adjacent patent venules begins promptly although this is clinically invisible. Sometimes the collateral load on these small adjacent capillaries and venules will be so great that both fluid and red blood cells will seep through their dilated walls. This is most common and most important in the case of small patent veins draining the macula, for they inevitably recover their integrity, and retinal function in their distribution is preserved. Thus, in a major temporal branch vein obstruction where a patent venule lies between the obstructed branch and the fovea, an excellent prognosis can be given. This is true even though there may be edema and hemorrhages in the distribution of the overloaded venous collateral, with foveal involvement, and a temporary reduction in visual acuity. The latter is seldom below 20/200 in such cases and visual recovery without treatment often occurs within several weeks. In cases where the intervening patent venule only drains a part of the foveal area, some protection is afforded, but some degree of macular damage is likely, and the visual prognosis must be guarded.

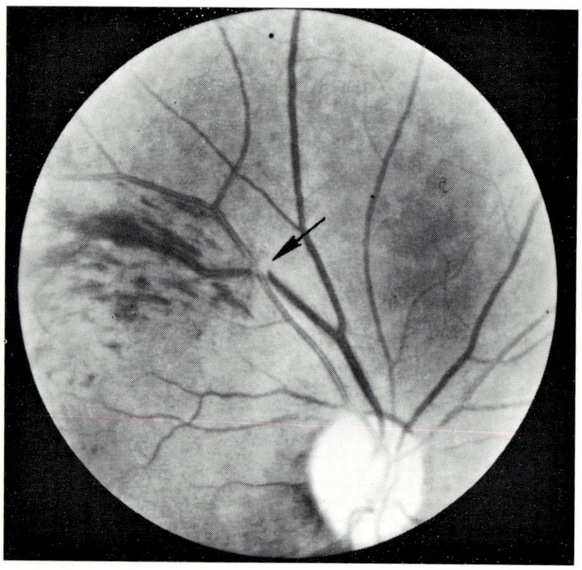

Fig. 14-1. Acute superior temporal branch vein obstruction due to arteriosclerosis in a 61-year-old woman. The vein overlies the artery at the point of obstruction **(arrow).**

If the macular area is unprotected, and its drainage is involved by the obstructive episode, the retinal edema in that sector of the fovea will be exaggerated. This progresses fairly rapidly to a microcystic edema of the macular wedge. In a major temporal vein obstruction, the horizontal division between involved and uninvolved macula can be dramatic.

From this acute phase on to full circulatory adjustment and retinal stabilization, the course of events and their time sequence is extremely variable. In our present state of knowledge, only generalizations are permissible. These changes are best considered individually.

Fatty exudates may appear at any time after 2 months following the obstructive episode. They first appear in the external plexiform layer but when large may extend to other layers. Two distribution patterns occur. The earliest is usually a scattering of exudates within the area of obstructed drainage or at its border in unobstructed retinal zones. There is no uniformity of distribution; they often occur in broad arc-like swathes. Very occasionally, a few will line up in Henle's layer, if its drainage is affected, but a well-developed macular wing does not occur. The other pattern, usually appearing later, is that of a well-developed arc or ring of exudates surrounding a number of large microaneurysms. This form develops around patches of obliterated capillaries within the area of obstructed venous drainage. Fatty exudates may persist for months and have been observed to last as long as 4 years. Probably, there is a continual slow formation and absorption rather than a true persistence of the individual exudates. Exudates fade with the improvement in retinal circulation and are usually absent in the presence of good collateral formation.

Cotton-wool patches disappear early and are seldom present in older obstructions.

In the early acute phases the obstructed vein wall has a hazy, veiled appearance probably due to serum leakage. Later, the wall develops an increasingly prominent halo sheathing. Although this may become well developed and then decrease as circulation improves, mild degrees of it are often permanent. For this reason it represents a most important sign of prior impedance of venous flow. Very rarely, and only when collateral circulation is excellent or good recanalization has occurred, it may be clinically absent. Ghost veins, or ghost segments of veins with obliterated lumens are late features. Sometimes a venous segment will disappear clinically. The venous segment usually undergoing the most marked change is that portion between the obstruction and the next *peripheral* major branch. When this segment becomes a ghost vessel or when its lumen is very narrowed, an identical change takes place between the obstruction and the next patent venous branch toward the disc. This does not represent a migration of a thrombus for the latter does not occur in retinal vein obstructions. It results from the alteration inflow pattern incident to collateral formation.

When examining a retina long after a branch vein obstruction has occurred, a missing vein segment can make the site of the original obstruction difficult to pinpoint. If one bisects the acute angle made by the still visible vein trunk and its main branch taking part in the collateral circulation, the arrow so formed will invariably point to the arteriovenous crossing at the site of original obstruction (Fig. 14-2).

Late in vein obstruction, the halo-sheathed vein may have a narrowed uniform lumen, or alternately may show dilated and narrowed segments. Marked degrees of this may give it a beaded appearance.

Retinal edema and retinal hemorrhages arise through seepage from dilated capillary and small vein walls. They are therefore prominent from the beginning of the occlusive episode. As collateral circulation improves, first the hemorrhages and later the edema recede. Flame-shaped hemorrhages are the first to disappear. Blot hem-

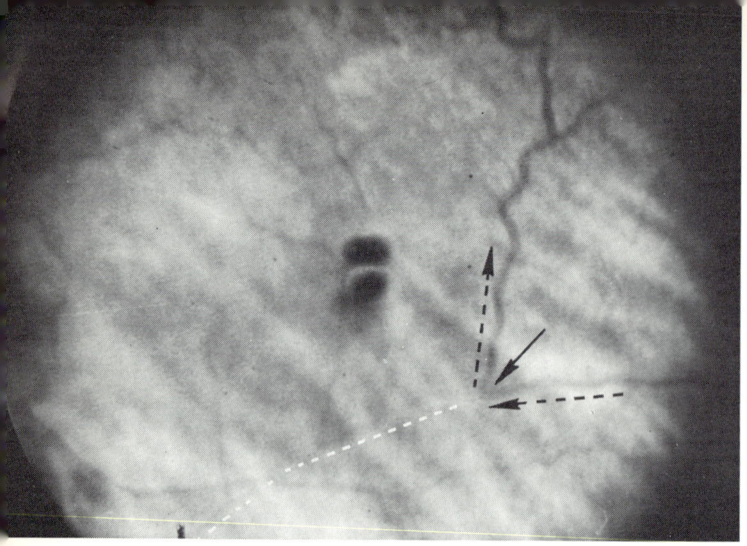

Fig. 14-2. Old inferior temporal retinal vein obstruction in left eye of a 62-year-old man with hypertension. The direction of blood flow **(dotted arrows)** is from the periphery through a macular collateral to the superior temporal vein. The **solid arrow** bisecting the sharp angle made by these vessels points to the ghost vein **(dotted white line)** and site of original obstruction.

orrhages are much more persistent and may come and go for a number of years. They are often the last to disappear in the far periphery around small venous tributaries of the obstructed vein. After all retinal hemorrhage has gone a persistent deep retinal edema remains, and, in mild degrees, this may be permanent when venous compensation is incomplete. In the stage of persistent retinal edema, it is often possible to visualize small, irregular, knobbed capillaries in places between larger vessels where ordinarily they would not be seen. For reasons presently unknown, patches of capillaries in the obstructed region will close permanently. These are the loci of the large aneurysms and circinate exudates forming the ring figures mentioned above.

In this type of retinal vein obstruction the limiting membranes of the retina are uninvolved and demonstrate their marked degree of natural strength.[34,223] Intraretinal hemorrhage and edema can thicken the retina to four times its normal width without either membrane giving way.[33] Rarely, a massive hemorrhage at the onset of vein obstruction will break through into the vitreous.

Venous collaterals begin to form just after the onset of an acute branch vein obstruction. At first they are simply dilated capillaries hidden by other retinal pathology, and they remain clinically invisible. When they are seen, they appear as a brush of vessels anywhere between branches of the obstructed vein and adjacent patent venules. They tend to occur in two places: about the point of blockage connecting the peripheral obstructed venous segment with its patent proximal segment, or at either side of the macula connecting the superior and inferior temporal veins if either of the latter is obstructed. They can, however, occur anywhere, sometimes connecting adjacent veins near the ora serrata. The course of blood flow within the obstructed channels becomes variable after the obstructive episode. Depending upon the position of the collaterals, flow in some segments may be normal and discward, and in others reversed toward the more peripheral collaterals. Indeed, a segment of an accompanying arteriole has been observed serving as a venous conduit in collateral formation.[241] Ordinarily, brush-like early collaterals slowly decrease in number ultimately forming one or more well-developed definitive channels. Collateral formation also accounts for the venous loops and parallel channels sometimes seen in the very late stages of branch vein obstruction.

Retinal venous collaterals enlarge slowly. Rudimentary ones may be clinically visible at 3 months and fairly definite ones by 6 months. They continue to develop over the months and may not become stabilized for 4 to 5 years (Fig. 14-3).

Capillary microaneurysms invariably form after branch vein obstruction and are always limited to the drainage area of the

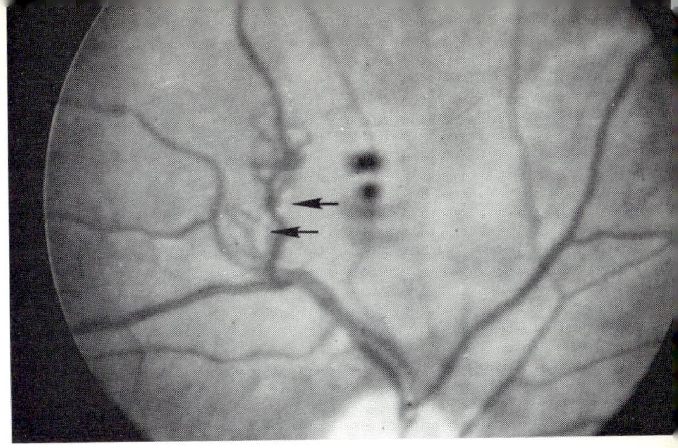

Fig. 14-3. Venous collateral formation 5 years after a branch retinal vein obstruction in a hypertensive woman 60+ years of age. Note the gray ghost segment of the original vein passing under the artery at the original site of obstruction **(arrows).** The main collaterals now overlie the artery.

obstructed vein. Just when they form is not known, but they can be visible clinically 3 months after the obstructive period. As hemorrhages and exudates recede aneurysms become more prominent. They vary in size, the largest usually occurring within the ring exudate formations. They hyalinize and eventually disappear as has been described (see Chapter 11, under section on Retinal Microaneurysms). Some microaneurysms seem very persistent. As with hemorrhages, it is not known whether individual aneurysms persist for years or whether there is a slow turnover in their formation. Aneurysms and fine, dilated, knobbed capillaries are most likely to persist near the macula, if a macular draining vein has been obstructed. At times, their position here may represent one of the few persisting clinical signs of a previous well-recovered temporal branch vein obstruction.[239]

It is very common for the artery accompanying the obstructed vein to show an increasing arteriosclerosis as time passes. This change is subtle, the arterial wall becoming slowly paler with a brighter reflex which is often intensified at bifurcations and bends in the arteriole. Within about 6 months a denser, yellowish material can be seen in the arterial wall and segments of its blood column may be hidden from view. This change has been previously described in detail (see Chapter 10, under section on Arteriosclerosis after Vein Obstruction). Increased arteriosclerosis is associated with poor collateral formation and persisting venous decompensation in its milieu. When collateral formation is good arteriosclerosis may not develop at all. Once definitely present, it may persist for years, either slightly decreasing over months or progressing to arteriolar closure and retinal infarction.[110]

The macular changes seen after obstruction of a macular draining vein are generally milder, the smaller the obstructed vein. These are discussed under Central Vein Obstructions.

Unless a branch vein obstruction occurs at or adjacent to the disc, the latter remains unchanged throughout the course of this disease. If involved, the hemorrhages and edema of that disc quadrant slowly absorb. Collaterals between the obstructed vein and the patent central vein or the choroidal circulation may develop on the disc surface or deeper in its substance. Because of these, or because of a persisting capillary dilatation, this quadrant of the disc usually remains hyperemic in appearance. Disc atrophy following an uncomplicated branch vein obstruction has not been observed.

Only branch vein obstructions at or adjacent to the disc are followed by retinitis proliferans from the disc itself. The disc is, however, the most frequent site of retinitis proliferans in such cases. It most often has a moderate fibrous component from the beginning and fibrosis may predominate. Such proliferans grows from the center of the disc, where there is no restricting internal limiting membrane, and extends toward the obstructed retinal quadrant. Its time of onset has not been documented but it is more frequently reported as a delayed development.

Low-grade preretinal fibrosis, whose contracture produces retinal folds and vascular distortion has only been seen as a late manifestation in cases of persistent venous decompensation. This type of proliferans may occur elsewhere in the zone of obstructed venous drainage but is most common within the temporal vessel arcade in cases of temporal vein blockage. Finally, tufts of reté proliferans may develop preretinally anywhere in the zone of impeded circulation. These have not been observed earlier than 3 months following vein obstruction. They may remain for long periods with little increasing fibrosis. Their fragility predisposes them to rupture with resulting preretinal or vitreous hemorrhage. New reté tufts may form from time to time in spite of repeated obliteration by photocoagulation. Sometimes they are adjacent to the burn area and sometimes quite a distance from it. Far peripheral tufts may be a source of bleeding and should not be overlooked. In cases of rapidly developing and adequate collaterals, retinitis proliferans may never develop at all.

Blockage of a nonmacular venous tributary of the second or third order produces an insignificant field defect. Obstruction of a major nasal vein produces a mild depression of the corresponding temporal field. Interference with a major temporal vein produces a mild depression of the corresponding nasal field and a central or paracentral scotoma. Some patients recover without discernible field defect. Rare patients will show a centrocoecal arcuate defect.

Obstruction of any vein not draining the macula has no permanent effect on visual acuity. If macular drainage is involved a final visual acuity anywhere from normal to 20/200 is usual although in rare cases it may be less than 10/200.

Rubeosis iridis and hemorrhagic glaucoma have rarely been reported following a branch vein obstruction.[110]

Total occlusion had always been considered necessary to produce the clinical picture of an acute branch vein obstruction. Seitz[201] and Rabinowicz, Litman, and Michaelson,[179] have shown that complete blockage does not always occur in such cases and fluorescein studies have supported this contention (Fig. 14-4). It must, therefore, be assumed that the clinical picture of an acute branch vein obstruction is due to an impedance of flow not necessarily associated with complete obstruction of the venous lumen.

The blockage in chronic branch vein obstruction occurs at the same sites as in the acute variety but the impedance of venous flow develops much more slowly. It may take place over years, may be intermittently progressive or may reach a certain point and become stabilized. A sudden and sufficient increase in obstruction can convert a clinically chronic picture into an acute one.

As arteriovenous crossing defects increase, they produce the phenomenon of banking (see Chapter 10, under section on Arteriovenous Crossing Changes). Mild degrees of banking may produce no discernible effect on fluorescein flow but eventually turbulence appears and the normal laminated venous fluorescein flow pattern is converted into solid lumenal filling at the point of crossing. Bonnet[22] has described a slightly more advanced change at such a point as the prethrombosis sign (Fig. 14-5). All of his eight patients ultimately developed the clinical picture of branch vein obstructions at these same sites. Of these, one obstructed within a month, and another 14 years later. The crossing region showed a few hemorrhages with or without exudates, a white halo about the vein or a white line beside the artery, and localized transudate.

It is clinically impossible to determine when or even whether a moderately banked vein will progress to clinical obstruction. One such patient observed personally for 17 years has not yet shown such obstruction.

In estimating the future course of events at a particularly suggestive crossing, one

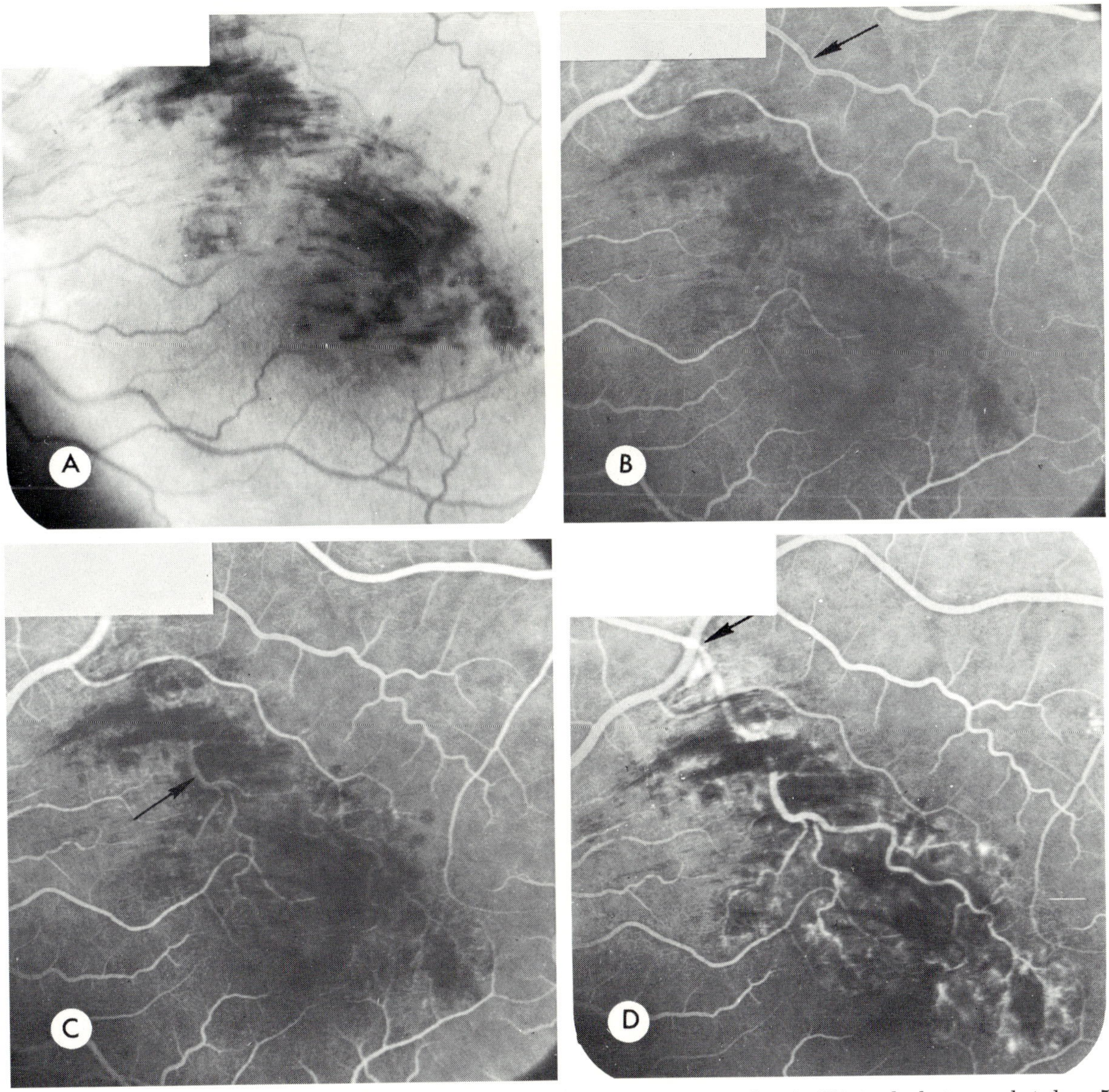

Fig. 14-4. Branch vein obstruction in left eye of a 67-year-old female. *A,* Clinical photograph taken 5 days after obstructive episode. *B,* Fluorescein angiogram of *A.* Note absence of dye in obstructed vein and its presence in an adjacent patent vein **(arrow).** *C,* Fluorescein angiogram of a later phase. Obstructed vein has begun to show dye **(arrow).** *D,* Fluorescein angiogram taken still later, showing passage of dye through the narrowed site of obstruction **(arrow).**

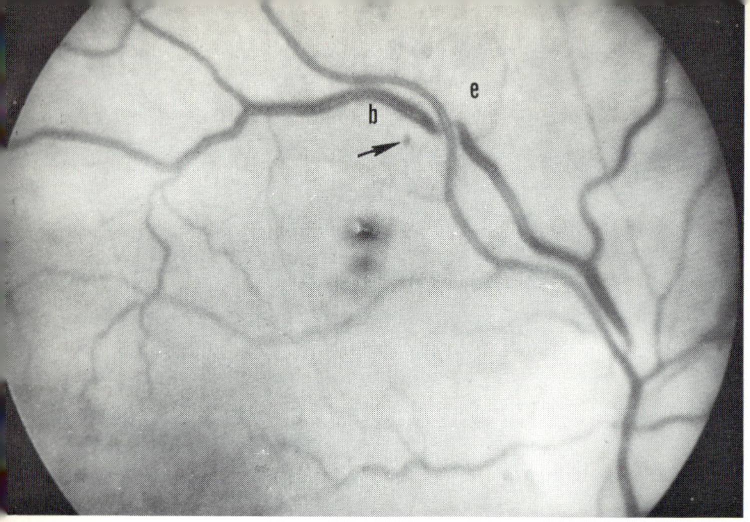

Fig. 14-5. Bonnet's prethrombosis sign of the left, superior temporal vein in a 74-year-old woman with hypertension. Note the arteriovenous crossing defect, the venous banking **(b)**, the microaneurysm **(arrow)**, and the retinal edema **(e)**.

must search for increasing signs of venous insufficiency. These not only occur in the region of the crossing but may be seen anywhere in the zone of venous drainage beyond the crossing. In addition to those signs described by Bonnet, a darkening and increased tortuosity of the vein, an occasional aneurysm, and a dilatation of capillaries to the point of clinical visibility, all just peripheral to the crossing, may occur. In addition, small, blot hemorrhages about the very peripheral venous twigs near the ora are a valuable early sign. Deep retinal edema may occur anywhere peripherally to the crossing defect but is most commonly seen just beyond it, in the far periphery or if macular drainage is involved, somewhere in this latter area.

When these chronic obstructions are slowly progressive and have no acute complications, they proceed over months or years to develop collaterals as in the later stages of acute obstructions. They differ from the latter in never showing an acute apoplectic phase. Edema tends to be limited to the deep retina, blot hemorrhages are sparse and scattered and both flame-shaped hemorrhages and cotton-wool patches are rare except at the point of crossing. Fatty exudation is thinly spread as deep droplets imparting a yellowish fundus reflex in the area of venous drainage. Aneurysms, while always present, may not be as profuse clinically and vascular proliferans is rarer. Chronic venous insufficiency involving the macula often produces in this region an exaggerated deep retinal edema, microcystic macula, and mild preretinal fibrosis, which draws the retina into folds and distorts the vascular pattern.

Chronic branch vein obstructions are easily overlooked in the presence of hypertensive retinopathy where they are common but somewhat obscured by the coincidental and more superficial pathology due to hypertensive disease.

The visual prognosis is usually much better in chronic than in acute branch vein obstructions involving macular drainage.

CENTRAL VEIN OBSTRUCTIONS

Acute central vein obstructions show exactly the same retinal phenomena as acute branch occlusions except that the entire retina is involved. The macular area is especially sensitive and in early stages shows an exaggerated deep retinal edema and microcystic change with loss of the foveal reflex. On two occasions widespread retinal edema and hemorrhages with dark, dilated, tortuous veins have been observed in which the macular areas were singularly free of pathologic signs, retaining their foveal reflexes and good visual acuity (Fig. 14-6). A cilioretinal vein draining the macula could have produced this picture but was not identified in either case. No explanation for this very rare phenomenon was apparent.

Macular changes, varying only in degree, are the same in branch vein obstruction involving macular drainage and central vein obstruction. In spite of the degree of microcystic edema at the macula, so long as the central cyst does not rupture, the condition is entirely reversible (Fig. 14-7). The prognosis for full visual recovery is good so long as the central cyst is intact, and so long as there is neither pigment alteration nor preretinal macular fibrosis. The pigment epithelium beneath the macula may disperse, proliferate, or show both features, producing a mottled appearance. Preretinal fibrosis can vary greatly in degree. A circinate lesion, i.e., a ring of fatty exudates surrounding large microaneurysms, may rarely, and as a late phenomenon, involve the macula and reduce vision permanently. When recovery is incomplete and venous decompensation persists, low degrees of edema, recurrent small hemorrhages, microaneurysms, and dilated capillary channels may persist in the macular region causing vision in such cases to be impaired. A persistent decompensation such as this is apt to be associated with some degree of preretinal macular fibrosis.

In central retinal vein obstruction all collaterals must develop at the disc. These are commonly found between the retinal and ciliary circulations. Collaterals between obstructed retinal branch veins and the patent central retinal vein behind the obstruction have not been identified. In both of these features central vein obstructions differ from branch obstructions. Also, some degree of recanalization of the obstructed central vein is commonly seen in microscopic specimens of eyes which have been removed following an obstructive episode. Retinociliary collaterals on the disc or within its substance are the *sine qua non* of a prior vein obstruc-

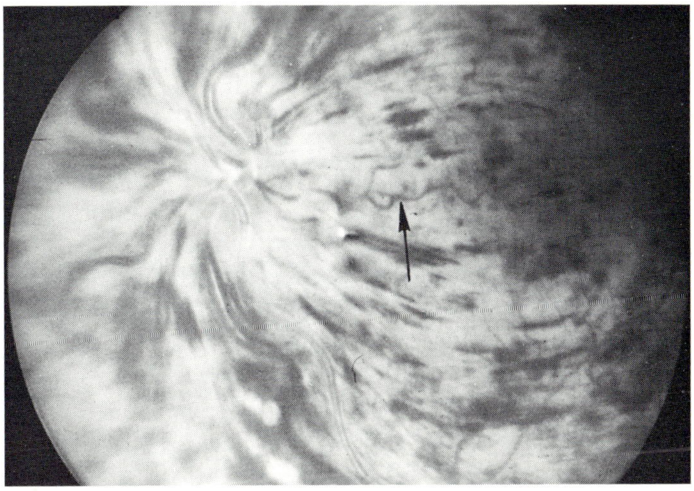

Fig. 14-6. Acute obstruction of the central retinal vein in the left eye of a 66-year-old woman with hypertension. Her vision is 20/30 and the macula is almost free of edema. Note the clearly visible small vein draining the macular area **(arrow).**

Fig. 14-7. Incomplete central retinal vein obstruction in left eye of a 38-year-old nonhypertensive man. Vision is 20/30. Note the potentially reversible macular cyst **(arrow).**

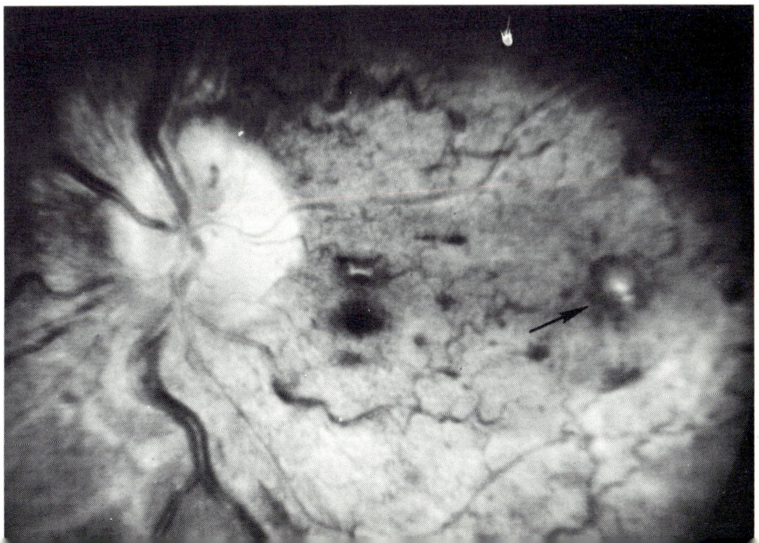

tion at this point. They can be easily overlooked (see Chapter 10, under section on Venous Collaterals).

Retinitis proliferans, especially at the disc, is more apt to occur and more likely to be extensive following central rather than branch vein obstructions. As in branch vein obstruction, it may occur in either the reté or the fibrotic form. Reté tufts of new vessels are usually seen first and fibrosis later, but fibrosis can predominate from the start.

Optic atrophy, which has not been seen following branch vein obstruction, is a rare late occurrence after central vein occlusion. The usual late appearance of the disc is one of hyperemia. The patients observed personally with late optic atrophy have given the clinical appearance of an associated or subsequent arterial insufficiency in addition to the vein blockage.

Although hemorrhagic glaucoma was reported in almost one-half of his cases of central retinal vein obstruction, Braendstrup[24] thought his cases were too selective, and suggested that a 10 per cent incidence would be more accurate. Duke-Elder[62] placed the incidence at about 20 per cent. This complication is most common in older patients 3 to 4 months after the obstructive episode. It has been reported as late as 4 years after the occurrence.[24] Early and adequate collateral circulation appears to deter its development.

In all other respects, the changes in the vein wall, hemorrhages, microaneurysms, cotton-wool patches, fatty exudates, increased arteriosclerosis, and retinal edema, the course following acute central retinal vein obstruction is similar to that following acute branch vein obstruction. They differ mainly in the extent of the retinal area involved.

Fluorescein angiography, performed after an acute central retinal vein obstruction, shows irregular leakage of dye through large vein walls. Patchy capillary leakage occurs as well. It is most clearly identified at the macula where, in the late stages of the delayed venous phase, fluorescein begins to leak from perifoveal capillaries about 0.5 dd from the fovea. Over a period of about 15 minutes the dye spreads into the spaces of the microcystic macula forming a characteristic macular fluorescein star identical to that seen in microcystic macular edema after cataract extraction (see Fig. 10-17).

The terms chronic and prethrombosis are seldom used in connection with occlusions of the central retinal vein. Here, the comparable clinical condition is spoken of as an impending or partial central vein obstruction.

Klien[122] has drawn attention to prodromal transient obscurations of vision as one of the earliest symptoms of impending central retinal vein obstruction (Fig. 14-8). This symptom is due to the varying deep retinal edema, exaggerated at the macula, which appears early in the state of venous insufficiency. The fundic background, especially at the posterior pole, takes on a yellowish hue due to sheet-like, widely dispersed, deep, retinal fatty droplets.[128] These can be clinically identified as individual deposits by using the slit lamp and sufficient magnification. The deep retinal edema over this yellowish hue lightens its color and is partially responsible for the apparent darkening of venous color. In addition to the apparent darkening due to the lighter background against which the veins are seen, the slowed venous blood flow due to its impeded drainage, is less saturated with oxygen and is therefore actually darker than normal. Such veins are also dilated and more tortuous as compared either with their normal state or to those of the normal fellow eye. The retinal capillaries become dilated and clinically visible in areas where normally they cannot be seen. This is often seen best in retinal areas near the disc or within the temporal vessel arcades. These capillaries are often irregular and knobbed and actual microaneurysms may be seen among them in any or all of the four quadrants. An occasional blot hemorrhage may

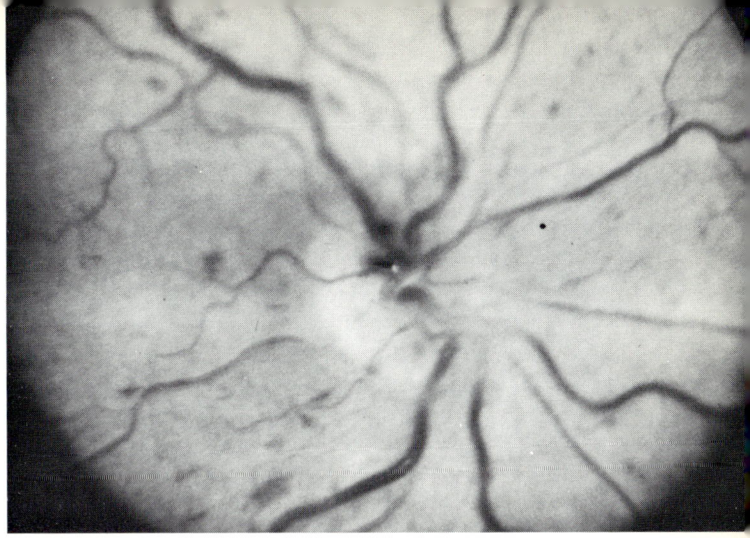

Fig. 14-8. Impending central retinal vein obstruction in right eye of a 61-year-old woman with hypertension for the previous 17 years. There was transient blurring of vision in this eye several days prior to the photograph. Vision is 20/30. Note the dilated, slightly tortuous veins and the scattered deep retinal hemorrhages and edema.

be seen near the disc or further out in the retina, but they are especially prone to occur early about the very peripheral venous twigs where they are most easily seen with the slit lamp and Goldmann mirror. Here, their appearance in all four quadrants indicates an attack upon the central retinal vein and their absence in one or more quadrants indicates early branch vein obstruction. This is a most helpful early diagnostic sign.

The retina may have some of these early features and remain this way for months. Progression is indicated by the onset of retinal hemorrhages and increasing deep retinal edema. From this point on, progression may be slow and steady or the retinal picture suddenly may be converted to one of acute central retinal vein obstruction. Slowly progressive obstructions are less apt to show flame-shaped hemorrhages and cotton-wool patches as early features and less apt to have retinitis proliferans as a later complication. With the added time element, collaterals at the disc are more likely to provide some degree of retinal protection. All of the features enumerated in the later stage of chronic branch vein obstruction, except for the intraretinal collaterals, may, however, occur. As in branch obstructions, these slowly developing central retinal vein occlusions in the presence of hypertensive retinopathy are easily overlooked, being somewhat hidden by the more obvious and superficial pathology due to the hypertensive disease.

The clinical diagnosis of an acute or chronic branch vein obstruction due to arteriosclerosis, in the absence of other retinal pathology, is relatively simple. It occurs only at arteriovenous crossings or rarely where the artery and vein are adjacent to one another, other crossing defects of variable degree are always present and the retinal signs enumerated above are readily seen. An acute vein obstruction in the presence of other retinal pathology has such an overriding and typical appearance that its diagnosis is easily made. On the other hand, chronic branch vein obstructions in the presence of other retinal pathology, particularly in the presence of well-developed hypertensive retinopathy, are easily overlooked and must be diligently sought out. There is an increasingly high incidence of these branch vein obstructions in long-standing hypertensive retinopathy, and they often account for the otherwise unexplained visual loss. In the absence of arterial occlusion, significant visual loss due purely to hypertensive retinopathy is extremely rare.

The diagnosis of acute and partial central retinal vein obstructions due to arteriosclerosis is much more difficult. In acute obstructions, the apoplectic retina masks the arteriosclerotic pathology. By the time the retina has cleared sufficiently for adequate visualization, so much secondary change has occurred, especially the increased arteriosclerosis incident to the venous obstruction itself, that evaluation is most difficult. Under these conditions, increased patient age, established hypertensive retinopathy, arteriosclerosis, crossing defects, impending central retinal vein occlusion, and prethrombosis signs or actual branch vein obstructions due to arteriosclerosis, all in the fellow eye, would strongly suggest this diagnosis.

Impending or partial central retinal vein obstruction due to arteriosclerosis must also be diagnosed by inference since the site of obstruction is at or behind the lamina cribrosa and not clinically visible. In the absence of other retinal pathology, retinal arteriosclerosis with crossing defects, prethrombosis signs or actual prior branch vein obstructions due to arteriosclerosis are strongly suggestive signs. As in branch vein obstructions, signs in the fellow eye, increased patient age, and established hypertensive retinopathy are also suggestive. In the presence of well-developed hypertensive retinopathy, the signs of central retinal vein obstruction due to arteriosclerosis may be considerably obscured by the overlying hypertensive pathology. The increasing incidence of central vein obstruction with the increasing duration of hypertension and its associated arteriosclerosis should make one constantly alert to this possibility. Meticulous study will usually permit the separation of the retinal pathology incident in each. A complicating central retinal vein obstruction can often account for an otherwise unexplained loss of vision in hypertensive retinopathy. It is well to remember that retinopathies are generally much milder in appearance with high myopia, glaucoma, and old chorioretinitis and are absent in optic nerve atrophy. Except in the latter case when retinal signs are absent, evidence in this group may be sparse, and diagnosis of vein obstruction may be more difficult.

The actual pathology of either a branch or central vein obstruction due to arteriosclerosis is not known. Thickening, fibrosis, and hyalinization of the arterial wall exerts an influence on the veins only at points of their common adventitial sheath. As arteriosclerotic crossing pathology progresses, a point is reached when the normal laminated fluorescein pattern in the vein becomes turbulent at the crossing site. This effect, readily visible in the retina, undoubtedly occurs also at the lamina cribrosa prior to central vein obstruction. The sequence of events from the onset of turbulence, through partial to complete occlusion is unknown. The arterial wall change, which appears rather uniform at retinal arteriovenous crossings is not necessarily so uniform at the lamina cribrosa. Klien[121,123] has demonstrated a disproportionate thickening of the central connective tissue strand between artery and vein as etiologically important in some central vein occlusions.

PRIMARY VENOUS THROMBOSIS AND VEIN CLOSURE BY PROLIFERATING ENDOTHELIAL CELLS

Von Michel,[229] who first described the clinical entity of central retinal vein obstruction, divided his cases into three groups: (*1*) complete, due to thrombosis; (*2*) partial, due to proliferation of the endothelium; and (*3*) minimal, in the periphery, due to both thrombosis and endothelial proliferation, or to either. He then proceeded to describe what has subsequently been named "stagnation thrombosis" (see following section), in which the actual thrombosis was a terminal secondary event dependent upon other preceding factors.

Coats[33,34,38] favored true thrombosis as the most frequent mechanism of central vein obstruction. Verhoeff[223,224,226,227] disagreed, and stated that thrombosis may occur in septic obstructions, but that all others were due to proliferation and blocking by venous endothelium. Their varied opinions probably resulted from a lack of fresh pathologic material. The descriptions of their specimens were often quite alike, but the interpretations differed. Ennema and Zeeman[69] confirmed the findings of both Coats and Verhoeff, but suggested the term "venous obstruction" rather than the more specific diagnosis of venous thrombosis.

Klien[120,121,123,127,128] believes that primary thrombosis in circulatory stagnation is probably not rare although very difficult to prove microscopically. She also believes that vein obstructions basically due to other causes may have a terminal thrombotic phase.

The crux of the argument between true thrombosis and endothelial proliferation as mechanisms of retinal vein obstruction lies in the lack of microscopic material from prodromal and early stages of such blockages. The marked stimulus to endothelial proliferation of both hypoxia and vascular ligation (especially in veins)[3] would ensure endothelial cell multiplication coincident with the early stages of retinal vein obstruction. Therefore, the primary or secondary nature of such findings at a somewhat later stage of examination would necessarily be in doubt.

Seitz[201] has studied microscopically three cases which had been observed clinically; two showed arteriovenous crossings in a stage of prethrombosis and one was considered to represent an actual fresh clinical branch retinal vein obstruction. In all he found evidence of endothelial cell swelling and proliferation and degenerative venous wall changes. In none did he find any evidence of early primary thrombosis. The case of clinical branch vein obstruction showed microscopically a still patent though narrowed venous lumen. Rabinowicz, Litman, and Michaelson[179] also described two cases of branch retinal vein obstruction each of which showed microscopically a narrowed, but still patent, venous lumen. A narrowed, but still patent venous lumen, can also be demonstrated by fluorescein angiography in some cases of fresh clinical branch vein obstruction. The failure of complete lumen closure suggests endothelial proliferation rather than primary thrombosis.

There are other findings which, at least in branch retinal vein occlusions, argue against primary thrombosis as the closure mechanism. No migration of a retinal vein "thrombosis" has been reported nor has one ever been observed personally by the authors. Second, and even third retinal vein obstructions have been seen in a single eye, but they bore no progressive relation to one another and each appeared as an independent episode. On the other hand, migration of thrombi in systemic primary venous thrombosis is common. Multiple primary thromboses in systemic veins are not unusual in some collagen diseases and in carcinomatosis, while retinal vein obstructions bear no relation to either of these conditions.

Although no firm conclusion can yet be drawn, the weight of evidence is against primary thrombosis as a common mechanism of either branch or central retinal vein obstruction. A terminal thrombotic episode following other basic alterations cannot, however, be ruled out and is, indeed, rather likely.

STAGNATION THROMBOSIS

In the first clinical report of central retinal vein obstruction, von Michel[229] has described the mechanism of stagnation thrombosis. This type of vein closure is probably more common in central vein occlusions[200] but has been observed in branch vein obstructions.[130,239] Typically, the patient is symptomless until the decreasing arterial inflow is eventually incapable of sustaining normal retinal function. Vision fails dramatically, and at this stage the fundic picture is that of a central retinal artery obstruction. Overnight, or as long as 10 days later in a case reported by Klien,[120] the fundus converts to a picture of central retinal vein obstruction and some degree of visual improvement occurs. All of the findings described in central retinal vein obstruction are present but mild. The mildness of the retinal signs is in part attributable to the decreased arterial inflow producing lessened intraluminal venous and capillary pressures. These cases either proceed through the normal course of central retinal vein obstruction or, at some later time, the central retinal artery also closes. Following closure of both vessels, the disc becomes atrophic with ragged edges and the retinopathy disappears. The veins show residual halo sheathing and the arteries are very narrowed and sclerosed. Some macular pigment mottling or fibrotic scarring can usually be seen.

In stagnation thrombosis the decreasing arterial inflow produces an underfilling of the veins and eventual collapse of the central retinal vein. The intraocular pressure, the venous pulse, and the structural bends in the vein at the disc, especially in cases of cupping, make the vessel more vulnerable to this type of closure. A terminal thrombotic episode is thought to occur.

Microscopic examinations of patients clinically diagnosed as having central retinal vein obstruction have demonstrated a considerable pathology of the accompanying central retinal artery.[34,227,237] Hayreh[99] has been able to produce the clinical picture of experimental central retinal vein obstruction in the rhesus monkey only by occluding both central retinal artery and vein. These findings, together with the prevalence of this type of occlusion in older patients more likely having some arterial pathology, suggest that the incidence of stagnation thrombosis may be higher than was previously thought.

SENILE CAPILLARY OBLITERATION IN THE PERIPHERY AND AT THE MACULA

Kuwabara, Carroll, and Cogan,[136] in a retinal-digest study, have found widespread loss of cellularity in the peripheral capillaries of old people. Endothelial cell loss was followed by the loss of intramural pericytes. The vessel walls sometimes remained intact and otherwise appeared normal. In other places the wall was described as ragged with an irregular contour. It was their opinion that such capillaries were not functional.

Generally, this change was found in persons over the age of 50. Although there was considerable variation from case to case, the peripheral capillary pathology increased directly with increasing age and appeared directly correlated with the degree of peripheral cystic retinal degeneration.

Wolter[247] has described hyalinization, obliteration and atrophy of peripheral retinal vessels in a 70-year-old man. There was an associated proliferation of the perivascular glia and peripheral cystic degeneration of the retina.

These findings lend support to the hypothesis that peripheral cystic retinal degeneration is, at least in part, dependent upon a peripheral vascular insufficiency.

Kornzweig, Eliasoph, and Feldstein[132] have made a study of retinal digest preparations from patients mostly 70 years of age or older. They counted the number of acellular capillary strands (non-functional capillaries) in the perifoveal macular region. These strands were greatly increased in myopia and diabetes and moderately increased in glaucoma. Those eyes with early senile macular degeneration did not show a significant increase in strands, but, with more advanced macular degeneration, the ischemic perifoveal capillaries were definitely increased in number. It was the authors' opinion that these findings suggested a relationship between defective perifoveal retinal circulation and senile macular degeneration.

CAPILLARY AND VEIN OCCLUSIONS IN DIABETIC RETINOPATHY

Capillary and vein occlusions in diabetic retinopathy are discussed in Chapter 15, Diabetic Retinopathy.

CAPILLARY AND VEIN OCCLUSIONS IN RETROLENTAL FIBROPLASIA

HISTORICAL BACKGROUND

Terry[216] first reported retrolental fibroplasia in premature infants in 1942. Owens and Owens[165] have described the disease clinically, showed it to be a retinopathy, and determined that it developed postnatally. Unsworth,[219] independently, also has noted the postnatal development of retrolental fibroplasia. Heath,[100,101] Tyner and Frayer,[218] Friedenwald, Owens, and Owens,[82] Reese, Blodi, and Locke,[183] Manshot,[149] and Friedenwald[81] clearly have outlined the pathologic course of the disease. The etiology was very speculative at first, but Campbell in Australia,[29] and Evans in England[70] were the first to definitely incriminate the role of oxygen in published reports. Crosse and Evans,[44] Locke,[146] and Kinsey and Hemphill[117] have substantiated this association of early oxygen administration and retrolental fibroplasia and the latter stated that the first 10 days of oxygen exposure were critical.

Gyllensten and Hellström[94] were the first to demonstrate retinal damage from oxygen exposure in newborn animals. However, Ashton, Ward, and Serpell[15] and Patz et al.[174] independently were the first to produce unequivocal retrolental fibroplasia in the experimental animal.

Thus, in a span of 12 years, an iatrogenic, blinding disease of rapidly increasing incidence was first recognized, its cause discovered, and its almost total prevention accomplished. As devastating as this story is, it should not be told without noting the tremendous advances in the basic knowledge of retinal pathophysiology derived from its study. The recent surge of interest in retinal disease can be dated from these investigations.

CLINICAL COURSE

This bilateral disease occurs in otherwise normal premature infants of low birth weight who have been subjected in their early postnatal period to an oxygen concentration of over 40 per cent. Most cases occur when the birth weight is below 1500 gm but rare instances have occurred in full term infants of normal birth weights, and in an occasional child not exposed to oxygen.[173] As the oxygen vasoconstricting effect could only produce the disease if retinal vessels were immature, its rare appearance in full-term infants was not explained until Cogan[39] demonstrated with retinal digests from full-term infants that the normal temporal periphery was incompletely vascularized at birth.

In the susceptible child exposed to excessive oxygen, severe retinal vasoconstriction can be seen. This is the first indication that the disease may later develop. Then after a variable period, under normal atmospheric conditions, retinal vasodilatation and tortuosity becomes apparent, most markedly in the veins. This is followed by retinal hemorrhages, superficial retinal edema, and preretinal neovascular formations. If localized, these findings are usually in the temporal periphery. As the proliferative phase develops, the retinal edema and hemorrhages become more widespread, new vessels may develop from the disc area, and retinal detachment appears, usually starting also in the temporal periphery. With rupture of the new vessels, vitreous hemorrhage occurs. From this point on, there is progressive retinal detachment and the highly vascular proliferation of the early stages becomes progressively more fibrotic. This cicatricial phase proceeds until the detached and disorganized retina is bound down in a sparsely vascular, highly fibrotic, retrolental mass.

For purposes of classification the disease has been divided into five active stages and five cicatricial stages.[185] Spontaneous regression is most apt to occur in the first two active stages of the disease. With the onset of retinal detachment in Stage III spontaneous regression is unlikely.

If spontaneous regression begins early, the final vision may be normal and mild scarring in the temporal periphery may be the only abnormal retinal finding. If peripheral scarring is more severe, the retina may be displaced toward the scar and an ectopic macula produced. As the macula does not fully mature until 6 months postnatally, such maculae, although displaced, may be otherwise normal in appearance with good foveal reflexes and function. Still more severe temporal scarring may produce retinal traction lines from the disc temporally. These cases usually show a deformed, slightly tilted disc with a pale nasal side and an arc of proliferated pigment epithelium at the nasal border. The retinal vessels are drawn across the disc temporally as a brush, some of which passes through the macular zone. At some point the nasal vessels turn back in a more normal direction. In spite of this distortion such eyes may have unexpectedly good vision (20/30 to 20/50). More severe scarring than this materially reduces vision. A small area of poorly vascularized nasal retina may remain undetached and allow light perception. With total detachment and scarring behind the lens no light perception will result.

Children with these milder degrees of cicatricial retrolental fibroplasia may hold their head in an abnormal position for best visual acuity, and their near vision may be much better than would be anticipated from their corrected distance acuity.

Myopia is common, even in the mild degrees of cicatricial retrolental fibroplasia and appears proportional to the severity of the disease.[252]

In cases of Stage V cicatricial retrolental fibroplasia, corneal scarring, iris atrophy, posterior synechia, shallow anterior chambers, pupillary membrane, and cataract may be seen. If such cases do not develop glaucoma and buphthalmos, the globe may be small and enophthalmic.

Duke-Elder[63] estimates that about 25 per cent of the infants developing retrolental fibroplasia progress to a moderately severe or severe cicatricial stage.

Although the disease may become completely quiescent and remain so for some years, retinal detachments in late childhood or during the teens are not uncommon.[72]

PATHOPHYSIOLOGY

The work of Ashton and his group[6–8,11,12,15,16] and the corroborative studies of Gyllensten and Hellström,[95,96] and of Patz and his collaborators[171–175] have been fundamental in explaining the pathogenesis of this disease.

With sufficient exposure to high oxygen concentrations, immature retinal arteries, followed by capillaries and then veins, narrow and become obliterated first in the periphery and then back to the disc. Mature retinal vessels narrow but cannot be obliterated; nor has this occlusive effect been produced in vessels elsewhere in the body.

When retinal vaso-obliteration is incomplete, arteriovenous anastamoses develop at the posterior edge of the zone of vascular closure. In extreme cases these can develop near the disc and, here, have suggested the similar formations seen in advanced pulseless retinopathy (see Chapter 12, under section on Pulseless Disease).

With prolonged oxygen exposure, all retinal vasculature back to the disc can be obliterated,[63] and fluorescein angiograms of such retinae show normal choroidal filling but no retinal circulation.[173] In spite of the complete cessation of retinal circulation, Patz[173] found insignificant changes in retinal neural elements examined electron microscopically. This substantiated the earlier light microscopic finding of normal ganglion cells in early retrolental fibroplasia. In normal atmospheric conditions, ganglion cells show chromatin clumping and irreversible change within 3.5 hours following interruption of their retinal vascular blood supply.

In the experimental animal, if the oxygen vaso-obliterative effect is of short duration, retinal vessels become engorged and retinal hemorrhages and edema appear upon return to air breathing, but vaso-proliferation does not occur. If the oxygen exposure is sufficiently prolonged to ensure permanent occlusion of numerous capillaries, then upon return to air breathing retinal vaso-proliferation invariably follows.

Although both Patz[171] and Ashton[12] had suggested earlier that the choroidal circulation might be responsible for the retinal vaso-obliteration in experimental retrolental fibroplasia, no fully satisfactory explanation of the mechanism of closure was given.

In 1961[243] it was proposed that the rise in oxygen tension in the older choroidal circulation permitted its nourishment of the entire retina rather than just the outer retinal layers as in normal atmospheric conditions. In such a state, the retinal vessels were no longer necessary and underwent obliteration.

The following year Ashton and Pedler[14] showed that immature retinal capillaries, exposed to sufficient oxygen, closed with vacuolization and degeneration of endothelial cells. These degenerating cells then retracted into patent vessels, leaving only a thin strand of tissue behind representing the remnant of the obliterated capillary. They noted the similarity of this to the normal retraction seen in capillary beds of developing vascular systems. Similar vascular changes elsewhere in the body tissues of their experimental animals were not found.

After sufficient oxygen exposure and return to normal atmospheric conditions, the oxygen level in the choroid returns to its normal value and is no longer able to support the inner retinal layers. The larger retinal arteries and veins reopen, but widespread blockage of retinal capillaries impedes the reestablishment of normal retinal circulation. This results in an inner retinal hypoxia. The preservation of normal ganglion cells at this stage proves that the hypoxia is of an insufficient degree to produce death of neural elements. It is, however, sufficient to evoke vaso-proliferation. Patz,[173] by fluorescein angiogram has demonstrated this widespread capillary blockage and leakage of dye. Thus, hypoxia would explain the early retinal vasodilatation, and capillary leakage of early retinal edema—these two findings representing the first clinical evidence of the onset of retrolental fibroplasia. The early vasoproliferation from the superficial retinal capillaries has been shown in histologic section,[243] in inked specimens,[15] and by fluorescein angiogram.[173] These vessels first leave the retina in the periphery where the internal limiting membrane is poorly developed or at the disc, in the center of which this membrane is absent.

With increasing vaso-proliferation and the pull of contracting associated fibrous elements, the retina becomes detached. Outer retinal layers, now removed from their choroidal blood supply and dependent on diffusion from an embarrassed retinal circulation, become sufficiently hypoxic to stimulate vasoproliferation downward beneath the retina.[12,243] The fibrovascular proliferation, at first highly vascular and later predominantly fibrotic now involves the entire retina. With the ensuing contracture, the retina is pulled into a scarred mass behind the lens.

Ashton [16] showed that the oxygen vaso-obliterative effect was inversely proportional to the degree of maturity of the retinal vessels. In newborn kittens the vaso-obliteration was complete, back to the disc, but in somewhat older animals (1 or 2 weeks postnatally) vaso-obliteration occurred only in the retinal periphery. These older animals upon reexposure to air showed vasoproliferation only in the retinal periphery where the vascular closure had taken place. In a discussion of retinal neovascularization, Wise [239] has noted the similarities in the position of new vessel formation in these older animals and in human branch vein obstruction. In both, the vaso-proliferation occurred only in areas of prior vascular closure.

It is probable that the maturity of the retinal vessels and the duration of the oxygen vaso-obliterative phase are both factors in those milder cases of retrolental fibroplasia with earlier healing and less terminal defect.

Dollery (see Chapter 6, under section on Calculation of Retinal Oxygen Diffusion) has suggested that choroidal oxygen levels under the circumstances productive of retrolental fibroplasia are such that the entire retina can be adequately supplied with oxygen from the choriocapillaris. It is presumed that the oxygen acts on the retinal circulation by producing severe arteriolar constriction and that capillary collapse and retraction is a secondary phenomenon. What is not yet known is why immature retinal vessels react with complete occlusion and mature retinal vessels only with narrowing.

DIFFERENTIAL DIAGNOSIS

In the differential diagnosis of cicatricial retrolental fibroplasia, the milder cases must be separated from the severe ones producing a white pupil. The two lesions which might be confused with mild cicatricial retrolental fibroplasia are discussed first. Then the differential diagnosis of diseases producing leukokoria, in their approximate order of frequency, will be given.

Juvenile Retinoschisis

This disease is usually bilateral and starts in early infancy. It is thought to have a sex-linked recessive inheritance.[210] The past medical history is normal, the size of the globes are normal, and the anterior segments are negative. Posteriorly, there is a thin diaphanous veil most commonly present in the lower retinal periphery. The veil contains retinal blood vessels between which are small and large oval dehiscenses. Large holes and sparse tissue about the vessels may give the appearance of a strand of tissue through the vitreous. There are pigmentary changes in the area of schisis and demarcation lines at its border. The macula is often cystic and may show mild puckering with radiating traction lines. In spite of this the vision is often good at first. The disease may be stationary for periods but is usually progressive over the years. Some patients have an associated night blindness. Retinal detachment may complicate the problem, and, if the detachment is well forward, it may produce a pale white pupillary reflex. Microscopically the schisis differs from senile retinoschisis in that the retinal splitting occurs in the nerve fiber layer.[251]

Falciform Retinal Folds

These are large congenital folds in otherwise normal eyes, extending from the disc to the ciliary region, and involving persistent hyaloid vessels.[150] They are usually symmetric, if bilateral, and most commonly appear in the lower temporal quadrant. Rarer cases occupy the line of the fetal fissure or occur along other retinal meridians. The hyaloid vessels can be seen along the crest of the fold with a slight tented detachment of the retina to either side. The disc is usually normal in appearance and there is no distortion of the remaining retinal vasculature nor displacement of the fovea as in retrolental fibroplasia. Although pigmentation is not necessarily present, there may be some along the line of the fold. Some cases appear to have an autosomal, probably recessive hereditary character.

More severe cases may show proliferation of the hyaloid tissue as a plaque on the posterior lens surface. Rarely, retinal detachment or pseudoglioma has been reported in the fellow eye.[232] Such cases would show a white pupillary reflex.

Microscopically[61] the fold consists of a dysplasic overproliferation of the inner layer of the optic cup. The outer layer of the optic cup is not involved in the fold. The retina is tented and slightly detached on either side of the fold. Hyaloid vessels and connective tissue can usually be seen on the crest. Retinal rosettes and dysplasic cells are prominent.

It is thought that the anomaly originates before the 13-mm stage of fetal development due to an attachment of primary vitreous and persistent hyaloid vessels to some portion of the inner layer of the optic cup.[150]

Leukokoria

A number of different diseases can have as their presenting sign a white pupillary reflex. This condition, formerly called "amaurotic cat's eye" or "pseudoglioma," has been given the name of leukokoria by Reese.[186] The differential diagnosis of diseases producing leukokoria can be very difficult. When retinoblastoma cannot be excluded with certainty, enucleation and histologic examination is in order.

Cicatricial Stage V Retrolental Fibroplasia. Retrolental fibroplasia in this state[181] is almost always bilateral although it may be of a different severity in the two eyes. The usual history is that of prematurity and oxygen exposure. The white tissue behind the lens is sparsely vascular or avascular, smoothly concave, and contains no calcium. Connective tissue traction on the ciliary processes produces the large serrations known as dentate processes. These can be seen by looking under the pupillary edge of the iris. The lens is usually clear, but if cataractous, the capsule is not ruptured and the opacity is usually equatorial and mild. Some patients develop glaucoma and buphthalmos while others show corneal scarring, iris atrophy, posterior and peripheral anterior synechiae, shallow anterior chambers, and pupillary membranes. When glaucoma is not present the globes may be atrophic, small, and enophthalmic producing a dark recess in the upper lid. Strabismus and uncoordinated wandering nystagmus are common. Mental retardation may be present, especially in these severe cases.

Retinoblastoma. Retinoblastomas are progressive malignant tumors, often bilateral, but usually in such cases much more advanced in one eye. They occur sporadically or show an autosomal dominant inheritance. The tumor is usually detected between the ages of 1 and 3 although cases have been reported which developed later (at 16 [154] and 48 years of age [225]). Bilateral disease during the first year of life is very rare. The globe is white and of normal size with a normal anterior segment, anterior chamber depth, and intraocular pressure. The latter only rises late in the disease. The interior of the eye shows a creamy white, nodular mass containing chalky deposits of calcium. In most cases these can be seen clinically as well as demonstrated by x-ray. Large vessels may be seen on the surface of the mass or small vessels near the surface sometimes give a pinkish color to the area in which they lie. The tumor mass is convex behind the lens unless it presses against the posterior capsule of the lens. Dentate processes are not seen. Rarely, seedling tumors on the anterior surface of the iris or posterior cornea may suggest mutton-fat keratitic precipitates. The less involved eye may have one or more tumors scattered anywhere in the fundus.

While yellow retinal exudates suggesting Coats's disease are quite rare, they have been observed with retinoblastoma.

Some cases undergo tumor necrosis with hemorrhage, and inflammatory signs may then mask the tumor's presence. Spread of the tumor outside of the globe, or extension up to the optic nerve enlarging the optic foramen are late occurrences.

This lesion is never seen in microphthalmic eyes and the infants harboring the tumor are full-term and otherwise normal.

Iridocyclitic Membranes. Fetal toxoplasmosis or infections, or postnatal diseases such as septicemia, scarlet fever, meningitis, or gastrointestinal infections may produce severe iridocyclitis with the later development of an iridocyclitic membrane behind the lens. Irrespective of etiology, this condition has been called "metastatic ophthalmia."

Iridocyclitic membranes are usually monocular although bilateral cases do occur. Often one eye is much more involved than the other and clues as to the etiology can be gained from a careful study of the less involved eye.

Postnatal infections occur in normal-sized globes while microphthalmos may be present with fetal disease.

All of the usual signs of iridocyclitis such as keratitic precipitates, anterior chamber flare, anterior peripheral and posterior synechiae, iris atrophy, ectropion uveae, and secondary cataract may be present. Those patients developing secondary glaucoma may show corneal scarring and buphthalmos, while other globes undergo atrophy. If the pupil can be dilated and the gray white iridocyclitic membrane seen, dentate ciliary processes may be visible under the pupillary border. The membrane itself may contain a few vessels, but composed as it is of detached retina and connective tissue, no view of the interior is possible.

Persistent Hyperplastic Primary Vitreous. Persistent hyperplastic primary vitreous (persistent tunica vasculosa lentis; persistent posterior fetal fibrovascular sheath of the lens) has been most clearly described by Reese.[181] The condition is usually unilateral in otherwise normal full-term infants. If the second eye is involved, the lesion is usually minimal and nonprogressive. The abnormal eye is noted at birth or shortly thereafter. Some patients have nystagmus and strabismus.

The retrolental tissue is densest at the pupillary center and thins toward the periphery. It is pinkish white and always contains blood vessels which often radiate from the center. The tissue varies from a small, white, central plaque to a thick membrane over the posterior lens surface. Contracting retrolental tissue produces large dentate ciliary processes as in retrolental fibroplasia.

The lens, clear at first, is smaller than normal and its equatorial margin is often visible when the pupil is dilated. The latter at times dilates poorly. Some time during the first month after birth there is wrinkling of the posterior lens capsule followed by its rupture and the onset of cataract. As the cataract develops the lens may swell and bulge forward touching the cornea. Corneal opacity, peripheral anterior synechia, and glaucoma may follow this development. Other lenses undergo absorption and contracture without producing corneal touch or glaucoma. These end as small globular masses often containing calcium.

Hemorrhage usually occurs about the fourth month postnatally. It is most frequent retrolentally, and bleeding into the lens itself can occur. Once the lens capsule is ruptured, some cases develop inflammatory signs due to the reaction to lens material.

The iris usually shows abnormally large blood vessels and iris processes are prominent in the angle. The latter may have fetal features but is not congenitally blocked. Ectropion uveae, iris atrophy, and iris vessels entering the retrolental mass may be seen late in the disease. Remnants of the pupillary membrane are usually absent.

The globes usually end with iris bombé, glaucoma, and buphthalmos, or atrophy with band keratopathy.

The retina is ordinarily not detached. In rare cases a band of tissue extends back to the disc area and detached retinal folds above and below the disc can be seen. The retrolental membrane in these cases is mild enough to permit some view of the interior.

Retinal Dysplasia. Retinal dysplasia (congenital encephalo-ophthalmic dysplasia)[133,186] is a bilateral congenital anomaly occurring in full-term infants. The ocular findings are associated with other systemic manifestations often sufficiently severe to cause an early death. The cause of retinal dysplasia, which may actually represent more than one entity, is thought to be some noxious influence acting on the fetus during the early stages of rapid retinal development.

Microphthalmos is usually present and may be mild or severe. The anterior chamber is shallow and both pupillary membrane remnants and posterior synechiae may occur. The lens is somewhat cataractous but often clear enough for some view of the interior. There is a white retrolental mass of vascularized tissue and traction of this tissue on the ciliary processes produces visible dentate processes in some cases.

When the interior can be visualized, persistent primary vitreous or a congenital retinal fold can be seen. These folds are like the falciform folds previously described.

Somewhat later, glaucoma develops due either to intraocular hemorrhage or to an embryonal filtration angle. The cornea becomes steamy with an acute rise in pressure, or a more chronic rise results in a buphthalmic eye.

The more common systemic manifestations include hydrocephalus, mental retardation, cardiovascular defects, polydactylism, cleft lip and palate, umbilical hernia, and malrotation of the intestines. In Reese and Straatsma's series, there was a 70 per cent mortality rate during the first year of life.[186]

Microscopically there is an anomalous infolding of the inner layers of the optic cup forming tubes composed of rods and cones, external nuclear layer, and external limiting membrane. In cross section these produce the typical rosettes of this disease. These are larger, have more cells and cell layers, and show branching tubular configurations, all of which differentiate them from retinoblastoma rosettes. All patients show some persistence of the primary vitreous. Some specimens show colobomas of the iris, choroid, or disc. The other findings have been described clinically. (For further discussion of this see section on 13–15 Trisomy.)

Coats's Disease. Coats's disease (see Chapter 11, under the section on Coats's Disease) when seen in infants is almost invariably unilateral. It occurs postnatally in normal, otherwise healthy children and is not genetically transmitted. Either strabismus or an abnormal pupillary reflex is usually the stimulus for the initial examination.

The globe is of normal size, the anterior segment is normal, the anterior chamber is of normal depth, and the lens is clear. The vitreous is usually clear and great sheets of yellow retinal and subretinal exudation mixed with hemorrhage produce mounds of retinal detachment. Dilated retinal vessels, large microaneurysms and vascular malformations can usually be seen in one or more areas. As the exudative phase progresses the retina comes forward and the depth of the anterior chamber lessens. Within a period of several years the retinal mounds either flatten with scarring and absorption of exudate, or intraocular hemorrhage, rubeosis iridis, and hemorrhagic glaucoma lead to loss or atrophy of the globe. Dentate processes are not seen and calcium is not present.

Angiomatosis Retinae. Retinal angioma (see Chapter 11, under section on Angiomatosis Retinae) is an hereditary disease with autosomal dominant transmission, incomplete penetrance, and varying expressivity. It is usually monocular but if binocular, it is more advanced in one eye. The lesion develops postnatally in apparently normal, full-term infants. The globes are of normal size and the anterior segments are negative. The fundus is similar to that in Coats's disease except for the presence of the retinal angioma with its enlarged feeding and draining vessels. If allowed to progress the clinical picture becomes indistinguishable from Coats's disease and the later ocular complications are the same in each.

Congenital Cataract. Congenital cataracts, when occurring without other ocular defects, usually offer no problem in the differential diagnosis of leukokoria.

Congenital Rubella Syndrome. Zimmerman[256] has most clearly defined the ocular defects in congenital rubella. One or both eyes may be involved. The globe is only mildly microphthalmic with a corneal diameter varying between 8 and 10 mm. If congenital glaucoma is present, the cornea may be cloudy due to rupture in Descemet's membrane. There is active iridocyclitis or evidence of its sequellae. The iris shows a patchy atrophy and the pupil is difficult to dilate due to hypoplasia or absence of the dilator muscle. The chamber angle is immature. The cataract is densest centrally with a relatively clear peripheral cortex, or has a less dense but uniform opacity. The infant is underweight and poorly developed and usually has some of the other congenital defects of rubella such as hydrocephalus, mental retardation, cryptorchidism, and anomalies of the large vessels or heart.

Microscopically the lens has a normal capsule and lens epithelium which serves to differentiate it from Lowe's, Miller's and Down's syndromes. The persistence of cell outlines and nuclei in the center of the opaque lens tissue appears to be a specific feature of the rubella cataract. Colobomata, persistent hyperplastic primary vitreous, and retinal dysplasia are not seen.

The Oculocerebrorenal Syndrome of Lowe. This is a genetic disease of males transmitted by heterozygos females. Curtin, Joyce and Ballin[48] have reviewed the ocular findings in this rare and only recently recognized syndrome of abnormal amino acid metabolism.

Affected infants show retarded growth and development, cryptorchidism, a renal dysfunction which is mainly tubular, hyporeflexia, decreased muscle tone, and ocular defects.

The primary ocular defect is thought to be in the lens and to begin at the fifth week of fetal life. The cataract involves the capsule, cortex, and nucleus with imperfectly formed nucleated fibers in a distorted pattern throughout the lens. The posterior polar region is degenerated with vitreous adherent to the capsule. The lack of lens growth is thought to account for the maldevelopment of the ciliary body, peripheral retina and the angle. It is the latter which produces the congenital glaucoma of this disease.

Norrie's Disease. Norrie's disease[232] is an extremely rare affliction affecting the retinal sensory cells, the first and second neurones of the visual path, the cerebral cortex and mesencephalon and presumably the auditory nerves. It has a sex-linked recessive inheritance with complete penetrance and varying expressivity.

Clinically, the disease appears bilaterally and is equally severe in the two eyes, occurs in males only, and is usually discovered in the first few months of life. Infants are born blind or develop blindness soon after birth. Early, the cornea and lens are clear, and a gray or grayish yellow retrolental mass containing a few vessels on its surface can be seen. The posterior retinal detachment, vitreous opacities, and intraocular hemorrhages can rarely be seen. In the beginning the eyes are of normal size and show a wandering nystagmus.

Later in the course of the disease there are mild inflammatory signs, aqueous flare, peripheral anterior and posterior synechiae, ectropion uveae, cataracts, shallow anterior chambers, and elongated dentate ciliary processes as in retrolental fibroplasia may be seen. With cornea-lens contact, the cornea becomes hazy and scarred, angle closure glaucoma and buphthalmos develop or the globe may become atrophic and shrunken. These changes become stationary as a rule by the eighth or tenth year.

One-third of the patients show severe and one-third show moderate mental retardation and one-third have normal mentality. One-fourth to one-third have mild or severe hearing defects but this is a late development.

Microscopic examination shows all of the anterior segment pathology described clinically. The vitreous cavity is full of vascularized scar tissue with prominent collagenous fibers and excessive proliferated pigment epithelium. Ganglion cells and retinal sensory cells are absent. Persistent hyperplastic primary vitreous and evidence of old hemorrhage are both present. The cellular components consist of foreign body giant cells, lymphocytes, and plasma cells. There is aplasia of the myelin sheaths and axones in the optic nerve.

Incontinentia Pigmenti. Incontinentia pigmenti[41,144,232] is another rare disease probably of either genetic or viral transmission. The name is derived from the fact that the basal cells of the skin lose their pigment to the corium, thus, seemingly being incontinent of pigment. The disease occurs in full-term infants, and, of the cases reported, eight have appeared in males and 170 in females.[232]

Shortly after birth an erythematous, vesicular, and bullous skin eruption appears on the extremities and trunk in a splotchy, linear distribution. These are followed by a papular or verrucoid reaction which subsequently disappears leaving the characteristic pigmentation. Lesions of all ages may be seen at any one time.

The skin lesions are associated with other anomalies of ectodermal and mesodermal tissues. Alopecia, nail and dental defects, and abnormalities of musculoskeletal, cerebrospinal, and ocular tissues have been reported. Any combination of these defects may appear. It has been estimated that perhaps one-third of the patients show eye defects.

The ocular lesions may be monocular or binocular and apparently start posteriorly, with normal anterior segments and globe size in the beginning. Ill-defined, gray white, edematous, vascularized fundic lesions with a few scattered retinal hemorrhages progress to gray, elevated retinal masses with increasing disc pallor. These masses can progressively enlarge until the retina is detached in a funnel-shaped, fibrovascular, retrolental membrane with visible dentate processes.

The late changes occurring in the anterior segment are no different from those described in other inflammatory retrolental membranes.

The microscopic examinations have thus far shown no specific lesion. There is a detached disorganized retina ensnarled in a mildly inflammatory, retrolental, fibrovascular membrane with the usual anterior segment pathology.

13–15 Trisomy. 13–15 Trisomy[40,159,250] (Bartholin–Patau's syndrome) occurs in infants having an extra chromosome in the 13–15 group. A high proportion of the patients reported have shown ocular defects.

The infants are born at full-term and the defects are present at birth. There may be no eye abnormalities, the defects may be relatively mild in one eye and severe in the other,[105,250] or, more commonly, the ocular defects are severe in both eyes. The ocular anomalies include microphthalmia, shallow anterior chambers, infantile angles, peripheral anterior and posterior synechiae, remnants of the pupillary membrane, iris coloboma, cataract, and vascularized white retrolental membranes. These clinical findings, the microscopic features which have been reported and the systemic defects, make this syndrome indistinguishable from the previously discussed category of retinal dysplasias. The presence of intraocular cartilage in some cases[40,159] may be specific for the syndrome or may be related to the severity of the microphthalmia.

Hunter and Zimmerman[105] have reported 14 well-documented cases of unilateral retinal dysplasia with normal fellow eyes (one patient had myopia), and one bilateral case in a patient with a sex-linked recessive inheritance. None of these patients had other congenital anomalies. They believe that most cases showing dysplasic changes in the retina will be familial, will not have a chromosome anomaly, and will have no systemic defects. Most will be associated with some unilateral, congenital, eye anomaly of unknown etiology.

These authors also point out that within the 13–15 trisomy group, accurate chromosomal typing is not yet able to distinguish which of the three chromosomes is in triplicate; nor can partial trisomy or mosaicism yet be identified. This failure could account for the variety of ocular lesions seen from patient to patient. In spite of this fact, all cases diagnosed as retinal dysplasia should have chromosmal typing.

Microphthalmia. Microphthalmos[61] is a term used to cover a number of different conditions in which the small eye is one of the outstanding ocular features. It is seen with coloboma, colobomatous cyst, or as microphthalmos in one eye and coloboma in the other. It is also associated with a huge number of other ocular or systemic defects. Some of these have been separated from the general group as syndromes. Abnormalities of fingers and toes, polydactyly, harelip, cleft palate, and dental, skeletal, cardiovascular, genitourinary, and central nervous system abnormalities have all been seen with microphthalmos.

Microscopic study of enucleated eyes have shown, in addition to the above, corneal opacities, staphyloma, cataract, aniridia, persistent pupillary membrane or hyperplastic primary vitreous, bone formation in the choroid, retinal gliosis, and dysplasia.

Such a diverse group includes some hereditary cases in which dominant, recessive, and sex-linked transmission have all been recorded.

The very small eyes of microphthalmia at birth and the associated pathology usually make the diagnosis relatively easy if the infants are seen at this time. If seen later, after secondary atrophy or phthisis has developed subsequent to other primary pathology, and particularly if the history is inadequate, differential diagnosis may be more difficult. Sex-linked microphthalmia is apparently exceedingly rare and only this category might be confused with cases showing the late changes of Norrie's disease.[232]

When a patient is seen late in any of the conditions producing leukokoria and, especially when the history is inadequate, the differential diagnosis is much more difficult to make. In trying to reconstruct the course of events in an individual patient, when one is faced from the beginning with a shrunken globe and badly scarred cornea, then old trauma, corneal ulcers, ophthalmia neonatorum, keratomalacia, or xerophthalmia may cause confusion. In cases with normal-sized or buphthalmic globes and corneal pathology, Hurler's disease or congenital glaucoma may have to be considered.

PRESSURE FROM WITHOUT AS IN TUMOR OR GLAUCOMA

Pressure upon the central retinal vein, exerted by an enlarging malignant melanoma, has led to occlusion of the vein.[5] Retinal vein occlusions may also occur in cases of tumor necrosis with secondary endophthalmic inflammation. In these cases the veins are probably closed by the secondary inflammation rather than by a direct effect from the tumor. There has been no microscopic study of the vein closure in these cases, so the mechanism must remain unknown.

Papilledema has been reported in cases of acute angle closure glaucoma.[255] The mechanism of this development is unknown, but the profound pressure exerted on the relatively weak lamina cribrosa might in some way interfere with the capillary circulation of the disc, especially its venous drainage, and thereby produce the disc congestion.

Central retinal vein obstruction occurring at the onset of chronic open-angle glaucoma usually has the characteristic fundus picture of an acute apoplectic retina (see section on Central Vein Obstructions). Especially, if the eye shortly develops rubeosis iridis and hemorrhagic glaucoma, the question arises as to which preceded which. Has a slowly rising intraocular pressure produced central retinal vein obstruction subsequently complicated by hemorrhagic glaucoma? Or, has the central retinal vein become obstructed primarily and glaucoma developed only after the rubeosis iridis? In these patients, careful observation of the second eye, which often subsequently develops chronic open-angle glaucoma without central vein obstruction, suggests that chronic glaucoma was primary in the first eye.[221]

The effect of a raised intraocular pressure in early glaucoma on the peripapillary radial capillaries and its part in the production of the arcuate scotoma is discussed elsewhere (see Chapter 2, under section on Radial Peripapillary Capillaries). For the effects of a raised intraocular pressure on the dynamics of retinal circulation (see Chapter 17, under section on Effect of Altered Intraocular Pressure on Retinal Circulation); and, on the retinal capillaries with the production of arteriovenous shunts (see Chapter 15, under section on Capillary Closure).

The usual type of vein obstruction due to glaucoma is occlusion of the central retinal vein late in any kind of chronic glaucoma. This obstruction is much more common than the literature would indicate and usually develops insidiously in cases with moderate to marked cupping of the disc. Verhoeff[224] has examined microscopically the central retinal vessels in 39 patients with secondary glaucoma due to anterior segment pathology. In every patient one or both vessels were affected by an endovasculitis in the region of the lamina cribrosa. While the central vein was more often affected than the artery, the reverse also occurred, and in six patients both vessels were equally affected. In 13 patients the central vein was completely or almost completely obstructed. In eight others it was only mildly involved in spite of deep cupping and advanced glaucoma. Verhoeff found that the obstructive mechanism was the same as he had found in other central vein occlusions, namely, subendothelial proliferation of connective tissue and final blockage by endothelial cell proliferation.

Salzmann[190] studied 100 glaucomatous eyes and found 19 with prepapillary proliferation of connective tissue. He found obliterative and proliferative changes in the blood vessels of the retina and optic nerve and mentioned especially occlusion of the central retinal vein. Fine, new-formed vessels were described within the prepapillary connective tissue and their connections with small retinal vessels were noted.

Clinically, these central retinal vein obstructions develop slowly, often with minimal or absent retinal hemorrhages. The veins simply darken, may show slight dilatation and increased tortuosity and slowly develop halo sheathing. Retinal edema is often not clinically apparent and microaneurysms are not often clinically visible although injected retinal vascular specimens and retinal digests show them in profusion in late glaucoma. Cotton-wool exudates are not seen nor have late fatty exudates been noted. The disc never becomes edematous, but the slow formation and enlargement of disc venous collaterals attests to central retinal vein occlusion. Some patients develop a small tuft of preretinal fibrous tissue which may contain microscopic new vessels often not clinically apparent. Late macular pigment mottling, a ruptured macular cyst, or mild preretinal macular fibrosis is sometimes seen and may account for the final loss of central vision in late cases. Proliferative retinopathy elsewhere in the retina must be quite uncommon, for we have not observed it.

The raised intraocular pressure and the increased number and sharpened bends in the vein due to the disc cupping are both thought to be contributing factors in these vein occlusions. The accompanying pathology of the central retinal artery is also a likely factor[54] and decreased inflow may in part account for the mildness of the retinal picture. The atrophy of many retinal cells in late glaucoma would also make such a retina less reactive.

INFLAMMATORY OBSTRUCTIONS

Inflammatory involvement of retinal blood vessels has in the past been loosely termed retinal vasculitis or perivasculitis and has been divided into primary and secondary types. A retinal vasculitis affecting both arteries and veins has been exceedingly rare in our experience (see Chapter 12, under section on Obstructions of Branch Retinal Arteries). With careful clinical examination during the early stages of this group of diseases, it is possible to separate the primary attack upon the veins from the subsequent, secondary arterial lesions. Part of this problem results from inexact clinical observation and part from the lack of fresh material for microscopic examination. The vast majority of early pathology reports contain abundant evidence of venular and perivenular cellular infiltration and little or no evidence of a similar reaction about arteries. The arterial changes are predominantly of an arteriosclerotic nature. Microscopic examinations long after the disease has been in progress cannot be relied upon, for late, nonspecific, inflammatory infiltrates in vascular walls and around vessels have been observed in such noninflammatory retinopathies as hypertension and Coats's disease.[246]

A number of diverse conditions either start as a retinal periphlebitis or endophlebitis (see section on Eales's Disease), or very shortly develop a secondary periphlebitis. Some lesions may subside without vein obstruction, others partially obstruct veins, and still others lead to clinical vein obstruction.

EALES'S DISEASE

Although not the first to report the condition [56] Eales [66] in 1880, described five cases of recurring hemorrhages into the retina and vitreous in young men. There was a predilection for the left eye and epistaxis, constipation, and headache were usually associated findings. The vessels of the retina, especially the veins were engorged and tortuous in all cases.

Between this report and the present time there have been many articles on this subject. Among the more recent reviews are those of Jefferson and Cloake,[109] Elliot,[67,68] Kimura, Carricker and Hogan,[115] Wise,[239] Donders,[56] and Ashton.[9] As the clinical descriptions increased, the diagnosis was more frequently made and a number of diverse conditions presenting a periphlebitis and intraocular bleeding were included under its title. When other conditions producing periphlebitis became separated from the general category of Eales's disease, fewer cases meeting all of the present criterion for its diagnosis were seen. There does remain, however, a group of cases where all known causes of retinal periphlebitis can be excluded, and this group, especially if complicated by vitreous bleeding, still should be called Eales's disease until a more definitive diagnosis can be made.

Clinical Picture

Eales's disease occurs predominantly in young, male, otherwise healthy individuals. It occurs rarely above the age of 40 and we have not observed it in patients over 45. The disease does appear to start more frequently in the left eye but may begin in either. Usually, the periphlebitis first appears in the retinal periphery but cases initially involving the central retinal vein at the level of the lamina cribrosa have occurred.[67] These patients are first seen as having an acute central retinal vein obstruction and are usually diagnosed as such. The proper diagnosis is reached only when the periphlebitis involves peripheral venous tributaries and can be seen. Sometimes such peripheral lesions are first seen in the second eye.

The first change to be seen is darkening and irregularity of a venous branch. The vein is generally dilated with narrowed sites along its course. At this stage no change in the vein wall or perivascular region is apparent but mild deep retinal edema in the area of venous drainage can be seen. Within several days white periphlebitic foci (cuffing) appear scattered along the venous segment. They have no predilection for arteriovenous crossings or venous branches and

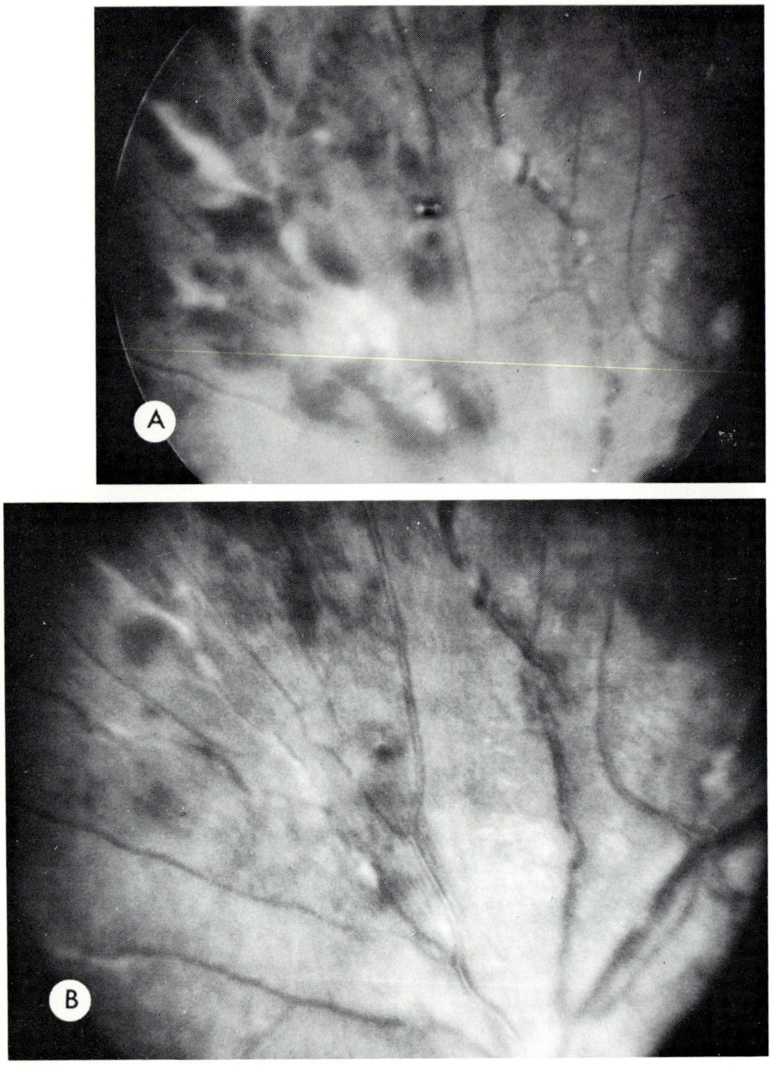

Fig. 14-9. Eales's disease in a 21-year-old male. Sudden blurring of vision in left eye occurred 2 weeks prior to time picture was taken. There is blood in the vitreous below. *A*, Above the disc shows mild and severe periphlebitis which partially obstructs the vein to the left. The arteries are free of inflammatory cuffing. *B*, Same eye shows spontaneous regression 3 weeks later.

have a completely random distribution. By this time a few retinal blot hemorrhages appear in the area of venous drainage and a slight haze can often be seen along both sides of the venous blood column between the more obvious white cuffs. These periphlebitic foci may be so mild that the venous blood column can still be recognized through their substance or so dense and fuzzy white as to completely obscure the blood column. They are often more marked on one side of the vein than the other and extend into the perivascular retina well beyond the vein wall. Nearby arteries are not involved and even cuffs on a vein at an arteriovenous crossing extend only a minimal distance along the artery to either side. Donders [56] also saw no arteritis in any of his 100 patients.

The periphlebitis may get no worse than this with only signs of mild impedance to venous flow before subsiding. Remarkable improvement in an involved venous segment can occur as quickly as within 2 or 3 weeks (Fig. 14-9). The periphlebitic foci may absorb, the vein resume its normal caliber, regularity and color and all hemorrhages and edema resolve within 3 months. Often only a faint halo-vein sheathing is all that remains.

On the other hand, the periphlebitis of the vein segment may be progressive and extend along the vein in an irregular fashion hiding extensive lengths of the vessel from view. The vein then becomes clinically obstructed at one or more sites and the retinal hemorrhages and edema increase peripherally in the pie-shaped sector of venous drainage (Fig. 14-10). If venous segments in the posterior fundus are attacked, cotton-wool patches may appear peripherally to an obstruction site. Obstructed peripheral veins produce no cotton-wool spots.

At any time a nearby or distal vein may become similarly involved. In the absence of serious vitreous bleeding, when the smouldering periphlebitis can be visualized, all stages of activity and resolution can be seen in the fundus at one time.

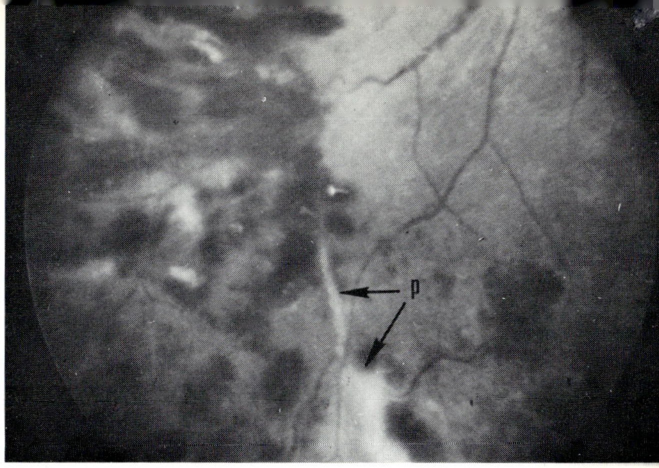

Fig. 14-10. Eales's disease in a young male. This photograph was taken prior to vitreous bleeding. Note the periphlebitis **(p)** and the vein obstruction. The arteries are free of inflammation.

Bleeding into the vitreous can occur at any stage and vitreous hemorrhage may be the cause of the initial complaint. Once serious vitreous bleeding has occurred the course of the retinal disease is obscured.

A similar process may occur in the second eye from the beginning, shortly after the disease starts in the first eye, several years later or the second eye may never become involved.

Sometimes, when intermittent vitreous hemorrhages are mild, the course of events can be periodically visualized. Later, all of the sequellae following vein obstruction begin to appear. New vessel formations proliferate in the areas of venous blockage or, if blockage is extensive, neovascular formations may develop from the disc zone. These are usually first of the reté type and later more fibrotic. Where their connections with retinal vessels can be seen, they are usually venous. Older obstructed veins begin to show halo sheathing and microaneurysms become visible. From this point on, the delicate new vessels are usually the source of fresh bleeding episodes. At this stage and when visible, the retinal veins show beading, loops and coils, parallel intraretinal channels, and the usual collateral formations. Arteries show an increasing arteriosclerosis. When retinal veins draining the macular area become involved, microcystic macular edema, macular cyst or rupture of the cyst may be seen.

During the later stages of the disease the contracture of the fibrous tissue tents and then detaches the retina. Rubeosis iridis appears and progressive disease leads to hemorrhagic glaucoma, cataract, and loss of the eye.

At no time in the earlier stages of Eales's disease is there evidence of any chorioretinitis or uveitis. Until there is bleeding into the vitreous, it is quite clear except perhaps in cases of early posterior detachment of the vitreous, where vitreous opacities may be seen.

In the more severe cases of Eales's disease neovascular formations are early and profuse. They develop much more rapidly than in diabetic retinopathy and they are more profuse than in vein obstruction secondary to arteriosclerosis. If, during the early course of the disease, a spontaneous remission occurs, early neovascular formations and small amounts of preretinal fibrous tissue can absorb and completely disappear.[67,80,169] Heavy fibrous bands may "shrink" somewhat during a long quiescent period or after the disease is no longer active, but they do not disappear.

In those cases that run their course and become quiet without developing rubeosis or sufficient cataract to prevent a view of the fundus, all of the late changes described after vein obstruction due to arteriosclerosis may be seen. Fatty exudates occur but are not as prominent a feature as they are in vein obstruction due to arteriosclerosis. This could be due to the fact that bleeding prevents their being seen at the time of their most likely occurrence.

Fluorescein Angiography

Fluorescein angiograms taken during active Eales's disease are very similar to those seen in retinal vein obstruction. There is spotty leakage of dye from retinal veins and capillaries, and profuse leakage from new vessel formations. In the presence of microcystic edema of the macula, there is late leakage from perifoveal capillaries and delayed formation of the star pattern seen in central retinal vein obstruction.

Pathology

No early case of Eales's disease has been available for study. Sections at a later stage have shown an inflammatory reaction of the vein wall, perivenous space, and even involvement of the adjacent retina. Nonspecific lymphocytic cuffing of retinal veins has been a common finding.[56,116] Other cases have shown perivenous plasma, epithelioid, and even giant cells. Eosinophils have not been seen. Some cuffs are signet ring in configuration which would correspond to the clinical observation of more marked periphlebitis to one side of the vein than the other. Hyalinization and thinning of the vein wall, narrowing and obstruction of the lumen, endothelial cell proliferation, thrombosis, necrosis, and rupture of the vein have all been reported.[9,116,147] Hemorrhages into the retina and vitreous, and retinitis proliferans from the veins or disc were usual. Granulomatous nodules have been demonstrated in a single case in the arachnoid and below the pia behind the globe.[147] Tubercle formation about the veins has occasionally been seen[80,228] and rarely tuberculosis bacilli have been demonstrated in periphlebitic foci.[89] Ashton[9] has cited three other instances of this finding in the literature. Arterial pathology has hardly been mentioned in the reports, although rare periarterial round cell accumulations have been seen.[17] The finding is usually one of arteriosclerosis, a secondary change, as can be readily observed clinically. Cases of Eales's disease have also shown no signs of uveitis.[9,116]

Venous collaterals, microaneurysms, retinal detachment, cataract, glaucoma and rubeosis iridis are all late secondary manifestations of the disease.

One feature of this disease may in part account for the early vitreous hemorrhages and the ease with which new vessels grow into the vitreous. In many cases the internal limiting membrane is involved in the perivenous inflammatory reaction and therefore cannot act as a barrier to the spread of retinal hemorrhage into the vitreous, as it does in ordinary central or branch vein obstructions.[33,227]

Etiology

The etiology of Eales's disease is still obscure. The theoretical concept that the periphlebitis represents an allergic reaction of a previously sensitized tissue to tuberculoprotein, when again exposed to this antigen, has most support. The often nonspecific nature of the perivenular reaction, the rapidity with which it waxes and wanes, the high incidence of tuberculin skin sensitivity, the occasional focal reaction to tuberculin skin testing and the rare finding of tuberculosis bacilli in the retinal lesions, all support this concept.

Schmid[195,196] and Hager[97] vigorously denied Marchesani's contention that thromboangiitis obliterans might be a cause of Eales's disease and Ashton[9] concluded that this idea should be dismissed from consideration until some supporting evidence becomes available.

Sifverskiöld[206] has described three patients with Eales's disease having paraplegia and pleocytosis in the spinal fluid. Veirs[222] has mentioned the intracranial manifestations of the disease, and central nervous system signs or symptoms in association with Eales's disease have frequently appeared in the literature. Ballantyne and Michaelson[17] have found symptoms suggesting central nervous system involvement in about 17 per cent of the reported cases.

While this association with Eales's disease undoubtedly does occur, care must be taken that the retinal periphlebitis in cases of multiple sclerosis are not mistakenly called Eales's disease. The periphlebitic cuffing in the active states and the halo sheathing in quiescent intervals, which occur in multiple sclerosis, can be extensive and quite similar to that seen in Eales's disease, but this is rare. An occasional retinal hemorrhage beyond a venous cuff and one case of vein obstruction with later collateral formation have both been reported (see Chapter 10, in section on Venous Sheathing in Multiple Sclerosis). However, clinically visualized microaneurysms, retinitis proliferans, vitreous bleeding and none of the late sequellae of Eales's disease have been seen in multiple sclerosis. The periphlebitis of multiple sclerosis has usually been mild, has only been present in a small proportion of the cases, and its course is usually a smouldering one, very different clinically from Eales's disease. In a single patient personally observed, the perivenous cuffing was extensive and changed in appearance and distribution quite rapidly, often within the week. The veins were very irregular with dilatations and narrowings. There were, however, none of the other features of Eales's disease and the late manifestations of multiple sclerosis made the diagnosis obvious.

Ashton[9] has written that the similarity of the perivenular cuffing in these two diseases suggested that their development might result from similar allergic mechanisms to different antigens. He has cited as evidence for this, the increasing emphasis being placed on the possible role of allergic factors in producing a complex autoimmune reaction in demyelinating diseases. This concept could be applied as well to the different diseases producing similar periphlebitic retinal reactions.

Prognosis

Elliot[67] and Donders[56] have shown that the eventual prognosis in cases of Eales's disease is not nearly so bad as was formerly thought. With an average follow-up of 6 years, Elliot has reported 54 per cent (25 of 46 eyes) had a final vision of 20/50 or better, while only 26 per cent (12 of 26 eyes) had a final vision of less than 20/200. His patients showed periodic exacerbations and remissions for a period varying from 6 months to 14 years (average 2.9 years) before the disease became finally quiescent. The degree of retinal recovery following severe episodes of activity can be surprising.

PERIPHLEBITIS IN NONSPECIFIC UVEITIS

Clinical Picture

Sufficiently severe uveitis, whether anterior or posterior, produces a secondary retinal vascular reaction. The vascular reaction is variable, some cases of relatively mild uveitis producing a fairly marked reaction while other more severe inflammations have less effect. These are exceptions, however, for generally, the more severe is the uveitis, the worse is the vascular reaction.

The optic disc becomes hyperemic and may show edema, the veins are congested and darkened and show some increased tortuosity. The retina develops deep retinal edema exaggerated into a microcystic macula and an occasional deep retinal hemorrhage may be seen. A hazy whiteness appears along the venous walls with indiscriminately scattered periphlebitic cuffing throughout the fundus. Veins near a posterior focus of chorioretinitis show these changes more prominently, but they are also seen to a lesser degree about more distant veins. Retinal arteries are singularly free of this reaction.

Early in uveitis of this degree, posterior vitreous detachment is common. White, fuzzy fluffs can be seen adhering to the posterior surface of the receding vitreous and lying scattered upon the retinal surface. These details can best be seen with intense illumination, contact lens and slit-lamp examination. It is the fluffs lying on the retinal surface and overlying retinal arteries which have caused the erroneous interpretation of a periarterial cuffing in such cases.[242]

Retinal arteries become brighter and more burnished with thickened walls. This reaction is often exaggerated at arterial bifurcations and bends in the artery. It is this arterial reaction as well as the venous congestion which produces the arteriovenous crossing defects.

In cases of severe uveitis, acute retinal vein obstructions, both reté and fibrotic retinitis proliferans, increasingly severe arteriosclerosis, and vitreous hemorrhage may be seen.

If the uveitis is brought under control before destruction of the eye, and eventually becomes quiescent, the retinal vascular reaction also subsides. The vitreous clears, the fluffs on the posterior vitreous face and retinal surface, and the periphlebitic haze and focal cuffing all disappear and transient halo sheathing of veins can be seen. The halo sheathing is also reversible and may disappear completely although in many cases mild degrees of it may be permanent. The severe arteriosclerosis is also reversible but some degree of mild arteriosclerosis and arteriovenous crossing defects always persist. Retinal hemorrhages and edema disappear and a microcystic macula can return to a normal appearance with reappearance of its foveal reflex. In severer cases pigment mottling at the macula or a ruptured macular cyst may be sequellae. When the inflammation is over, the retinal veins resume their normal appearance except for the residual halo sheathing and except in those cases in which vein obstruction has occurred. In these, venous collaterals, narrowed, halo-sheathed venous segments, ghost veins, and sometimes venous retinochoroidal anastomoses in an area of healed chorioretinitis may be seen. It is rare, clinically, to see retinal microaneurysms during the course of the uveitis or when all active reaction has subsided.

Pietruschka[176] was the first to point out the signs indicating obstruction to venous outflow in uveitis. He concluded that the retinal changes seen in uveitis were more likely secondary to this venous outflow impedance than to any direct effect of the inflammation. Wise[242] has confirmed these observations and called attention to the similarity of the retinal reaction in uveitis, excepting the inflammatory features, and that seen in a recovering central retinal vein obstruction. Fluorescein angiograms in uveitis also show similarities to those in central vein obstruction. There is leakage of dye from some veins and capillaries in the acute phase and a typical late macular star formation in the presence of microcystic macular edema.[84]

Pathology

Fuchs[83] has drawn attention to the retinal perivenular accumulation of lymphocytes in uveitis. He believed toxins from the uveitis acting through the vitreous upon the retina caused venous dilatation and transmural migration of these cells.

Samuels[191] in a microscopic study of 59 cases of iritis serosa following surgery or trauma found round cells distributed along retinal capillaries and, especially, clustered lymphocytes about veins. These findings were particularly prominent at the posterior pole but were present well out toward the ora. The distribution along veins was irregular, forming heavy signet rings in some places.

Zeeman[254] found similar changes about retinal veins in uveitis and noted in some cases marked round cell accumulation about the central retinal vein, even extending behind the lamina cribrosa. He has concluded that these changes indicate some interference with retinal circulation.

Klien[125] also has found aggregates of lymphocytes and monocytes about retinal capillaries and veins in uveitis. She described extensive perivenular cuffing of round cells with narrowing of the venous lumen. There were also extensive cellular infiltrations along superficial retinal capillaries and those connecting the two major retinal capillary beds.

None of these authors have demonstrated periarterial cellular collections as a feature of this pathology. This is in keeping with our own clinical observations and those of Knapp[129] who has stated unequivocally that the perivenous lymphocytic cuffing seen in uveitis does not occur about arterioles except where arterioles pass through an area of perivenous pathology.

Although retinal microaneurysms are rarely seen clinically during the course of uveitis or even after it has subsided, Ashton[5] has demonstrated their profusion in this disease. These, more likely, result from the venous embarrassment, rather than from the inflammation.

TOXOPLASMOSIS

Toxoplasmic retinochoroiditis shows all of the features described in nonspecific uveitis. In some of these cases the vitreous remains sufficiently clear to follow the retinal vascular reaction throughout the course of the disease until it becomes quiescent. The periphlebitis of this disease is usually prominent and vein obstructions are common. These often occur silently in that they do not show the widespread hemorrhages and other features seen in acute vein obstructions. They are more likely to occur in the region of active inflammation. Sometimes microaneurysms can be transiently seen near the retinochoroidal lesion. Severe arteriosclerosis in a segmental distribution, most marked at the height of the inflammation, is not uncommonly seen. These patchy wall changes may be seen on any artery regardless of the position of the retinochoroiditis. They disappear as the inflammation subsides, but mild arteriosclerosis and arteriovenous crossing defects remain permanently. When all inflammation has subsided, venous collaterals, halo-sheathed narrowed veins, occasional ghost veins, and, sometimes, retinochoroidal anastomoses within the toxoplasmic scar may be seen. These connections have also been observed in old congenital toxoplasmic scars.

PERIPHERAL CHORIORETINITIS (CHRONIC CYCLITIS; PARS PLANITIS; PERIPHERAL UVEITIS)

Peripheral chorioretinitis[25,26,102,116,235] is a chronic disease, common in children and young adults and rare over the age of 50 years. It may be unilateral but is usually bilateral and unilateral cases may become bilateral after an interval of several years. The etiology of this disease has not been determined. Some authors feel that the affliction is strictly a cyclitis[102,115] while others believe the peripheral choroid is also involved.[25,26] Our own observations suggest frequent choroidal involvement.

The disease is of varying severity, some cases smouldering along for years, worse or better from time to time, and others, having a much more severe course with angle closure glaucoma, retinal detachment, optic atrophy, or the formation of a retrolental cyclitic membrane.

The anterior segment is usually quiet, the eye white and painless, but fine keratitic precipitates and a slight flare are common. Peripheral anterior and posterior synchiae develop in the more severe cases. Milder disease usually shows neither of these.

Early posterior cataract, fine anterior vitreous floaters, or macular edema may lead to the initial examination.

The peripheral inflammation produces fine debris, or larger stringy opacities with vitreous and preretinal snowball-like clumps in the anterior vitreous. Exudate tends to collect dependently overlying the pars plana and extending both anteriorly and posteriorly in severe cases. Small areas of active and pigmented, healed, foci of chorioretinitis, although often absent, are by no means rare.

Retinal Vascular Reaction

The early retinal vascular reaction is a characteristic feature in many cases and may in some actually suggest the disease's presence. The optic disc is hyperemic, the retinal veins are dilated and dark, and there is a generalized deep retinal edema best seen posteriorly where it is exaggerated at the macula, forming a microcystic hillock. The most peripheral retinal veins, especially those lying inferiorly, show typical periphlebitic reactions. Such reactions may be mild, as an irregular perivenular haze or more severe with intermittent cuffing. Peripheral arteries do not show this reaction. Retinal hemorrhages are rare and microaneurysms if present are hidden by the reaction and not clinically visible.

In severe cases the periphlebitic reaction can extend back to the disc and perivascular round-cell infiltration in an edematous disc has been demonstrated microscopically.[115] The central retinal vein can become obstructed, for venous disc collaterals to the choroid have been personally observed. In such cases the occlusion is a slow one, and the picture of acute occlusion of the central retinal vein is not seen. While fatty exudates are rarely seen, cases with central vein obstruction do have a somewhat yellowish fundic reflex suggesting their fine distribution in the deep retina.

Peripheral veins frequently become occluded and converted into white cords (ghost vessels). As the inflammation quiets, the perivenular reaction may subside and peripheral halo sheathing of veins may be visible. Arteries show at first mild and, later, more severe arteriosclerosis. Cases of complete obliteration of arteries and veins with optic atrophy have been reported.[25]

Eyes showing severe occlusive peripheral periphlebitis may develop retinitis proliferans while vitreous bleeding has been observed in several instances.[25]

The posterior retinal edema is usually an early feature and can be present with the mildest of peripheral inflammatory reaction. This edema is not always proportional to the severity of the peripheral chorioretinitis. Some severer cases may show less macular edema than other milder ones.

Fluorescein angiography shows typical leakage from edematous disc capillaries and a delayed macular star in cases of microcystic macular edema. This star is similar to that seen in Eales's disease, central retinal vein obstruction, or the macular edema following cataract extraction.

While vitreous shrinkage and traction on the macula has been suggested as the cause of the macular edema and elevation in some cases,[235] we have not observed this. Like others,[26,102] we believe that involvement of the disc, posterior retina, and macula occur as a result of the perivenular inflammatory reaction.

SARCOIDOSIS

Gould and Kaufman[93] have reviewed the reported cases of sarcoid involving the fundus and have added a case of their own.[92]

According to their review, the fundic lesions occurred equally in the sexes and had a wide age distribution. There were systemic manifestations of sarcoidosis in 80 per cent of the patients and 13 per cent had an associated uveoparotid fever. The true incidence of fundic lesions is hard to evaluate, for most patients have serious anterior uveal involvement and cloudy media, preventing an adequate view of the interior. Only one-third of the reported cases have had no apparent anterior uveitis.

Crick[42] has examined the eyes of 103 patients with systemic sarcoidosis, 63 of whom had their diagnoses confirmed by biopsy. There were 21 patients with ocular involvement. Seventeen of these had anterior uveitis and 13 showed chorioretinal lesions.

The fundic lesions of sarcoid were first reported by Walsh[231] and later described as candlewax drippings by Franceschetti and Babel.[79] They are of two main types, one primarily in the choroid with secondary retinal involvement[42,79,142] and the other a retinal periphlebitis.[43,74,79,92,142,148] Both show discrete, fuzzy white, waxy, opaque lesions scattered in the fundus or as periphlebitic foci around retinal veins. Heavy strands, discrete snowballs, or chains of grayish white, opaque, spherical bodies, varying from small dots to 1/3 dd in size, are sometimes seen in the preretinal vitreous.[139] They move with eye movements, cast shadows on the retina, and are most common in the dependent peripheral vitreous or, at times, lie on the retinal surface. Both types of lesions are more frequent in the periphery, but also occur posteriorly and sometimes involve the disc as large sarcoidal masses.[90] They often persist unchanged for long periods if no treatment is instituted.

The choroidal lesions are made up of epithelioid cells and lymphocytes some of which break through Bruch's membrane into the retina.[42,142] Giant cells are seen in some lesions and caseation is absent, as with all sarcoid lesions. Nonspecific chorioretinal lesions are also present in about 40 per cent of the patients.[93] The same types of cellular accumulation, which produce the choroidal nodule, occur about retinal veins as periphlebitis. The vein walls may be severely involved and the venous lumens occluded.

If the periphlebitis is severe, venous narrowing at the point of cuffing, banking, tortuosity, darkening of the blood column, beading and retinal hemorrhages may be seen. With frank vein obstruction, reduplication of the channel or collaterals to patent veins, retinitis proliferans, vitreous bleeding, retinal detachment, and all the sequellae of vein obstruction may follow.

Fine and Flocks[75] reported a case of bilateral neuroretinitis due to sarcoidosis. Although rare, this lesion is of interest because apparently there is an increased incidence of central nervous system involvement associated with the presence of fundal sarcoidosis.[93]

BEHCET'S DISEASE

The literature on Behçet's disease has been well reviewed by Mavioğlu.[153] It is an illness that is most prevalent in the Near East and in Japan[204] usually affecting men between the ages of 15 and 40.[198] Although it has been considered by some to be basically vascular or allergic in origin, the recovery of a virus from several patients[160,198,199] has given support to this etiologic concept originally held by Behçet himself. The virus is thought to lie dormant in the epithelium of the skin and neuroepithelium of the iris, ciliary body, and retina. Trauma to the skin or some other factor is believed to activate the virus and to allow both the viremia and secondary vascular reaction to proceed.[160]

The disease is characterized by recurrent attacks, as often as once or twice a month, which continue with slow diminution over a period of 15 or 20 years ultimately leading to blindness in most cases. The few lethal cases are those in which the central nervous system is involved. Aphthous ulcers of the oral mucous membrane, ulcers of the genital organs, and hypopion iridocyclitis were the original lesions in the syndrome described by Behçet. Since then erythema nodosum, thrombophlebitis, skin infections, joint pains and swellings, orchitis, and fever have been added.

Because of the acute attacks of iridocyclitis with hypopion and cloudy vitreous, the early vascular reaction within the eye is not always seen clinically. Reports of patients where the interior of the eye could be examined have been conflicting. Some authors believe retinal arteries are first involved, some believe retinal veins are first attacked, some find early pathology of both, and still others believe the initial reaction is in the choroid.[108,151,160,198,199] Vitreous opacities, retinal hemorrhages, edema, and exudation have been seen by many observers while others have seen new vessel formations and vitreous bleeding.[108,253]

The available histopathologic findings[73,203] have suggested a diffuse uveal involvement with early loss of the retinal visual elements and an attack upon the retinal blood vessels, primarily the veins. Vascular occlusions due to perivasculitis, vasculitis, and thrombosis lead to hemorrhagic infarction of the retina with its almost total destruction. Obstructions of both central retinal vessels have been seen. The cellular infiltration consists of lymphocytes and plasma cells predominantly, but histocytes, neutrophils, and eosinophils have been observed. A primary attack upon the retinal veins would more likely explain the numerous retinal hemorrhages, the pre- and subretinal neovascular and fibrotic membranes, and the rubeosis iridis commonly found in these reports. The optic nerve is usually atrophic. Systemic lesions show an early attack upon collagen fibers of skin and vessels with subsequent profuse repair.[203]

Shikano and Shimizu[204] have described the early retinal reaction of a patient undergoing an acute attack of Behçet's disease. The optic disc was edematous, the retinal veins showed stagnation, and the posterior fundus was yellowish white with exudation. There was one heavily ensheathed retinal vein, and many retinal hemorrhages. The fluorescein angiogram revealed a normal arterial phase, dilated capillaries, and leakage from both disc capillaries and retinal veins. In another patient, during a quiet interval after several attacks, the fluorescein angiogram revealed dye leakage from disc and retinal capillaries and small retinal veins, but no abnormality during the arterial phase. None of the fluorescein angiograms, even those taken later in the course of the disease, showed leakage from the choroid as might be expected with diffuse choroidal involvement.

The weight of evidence in this disease therefore tends to support the concept of inflammatory attack upon the retinal veins and capillaries with subsequent thrombotic or inflammatory occlusions.

PERIPHLEBITIS AS A RARE OCCURRENCE IN OTHER DISEASES

Brucellosis

There are a few reports[33] of retinal venous involvement as a rare complication of brucellosis. None of these very clearly describes the retinal lesion. Solanes et al.[207] have mentioned one case of periphlebitis among 87 cases of brucellosis. It was not further described. Foggitt has reported[78] retinal periphlebitis in a patient with brucellosis. The fundic appearance suggested partial obstruction of the involved vein. White[238] has noted retinal vasculitis in a single patient with brucellosis. The fact that this patient subsequently developed retinitis proliferans suggests that the vascular involvement was venular.

Cryptococcus Neoformans

Beck, Hutchings, and Makay[18] have reported retinal perivascular choroidal "tubercles" in a case of cryptococcus neoformans occurring in a 32-year-old male. Although they called this Eales's disease, it is not clear whether this was primarily a choroidal lesion with involvement of a vein overlying the lesion by chance, or whether true retinal periphlebitis was present.

Infectious Mononucleosis

Jones[111] has described a patient having the appearance of a central retinal vein obstruction during the course of infectious mononucleosis. Three gray white perivascular cuffs were described on inferior retinal veins and a similar lesion was assumed to have occurred about the central vein. The author spoke of this case as being similar to the central retinal vein obstructions occurring in influenza.

Leprosy

Landau[138] has described a case of retinal periphlebitis which he has attributed to leprosy. The exudate was present around an engorged retinal vein and was situated near the disc. The posterior position of the lesion, the presence of a strongly positive Mantoux test, and the fact that the patient had been bacteriologically negative for 15 years, cast considerable doubt on a leprous etiology of this periphlebitis.

We have observed fundic lesions in two patients with active leprosy which was proved by nasal smears. Both patients had the corneal and iridic lesions of the disease. There were indolent, small, white spots, scattered in the far peripheral retina. They had a dim luster, and their edges were not fuzzy as is usual in periphlebitis. Their distribution suggested that perivascular involvement was purely a chance phenomenon.

Syphilis

Duke-Elder[64] has noted the rarity of periphlebitis due to syphilis. Most reports were of individual cases occurring in young patients probably having the congenital disease. Uveal inflammation was regularly present in these cases.

We have observed a case of secondary syphilis having a central retinal artery obstruction in one eye and a central vein obstruction in the other. No periphlebitic lesions were seen. In this patient the disease was probably primarily arterial with purely happenstance closure of the adjacent vein in the second eye.

SEPTIC THROMBOSIS

In the older literature[34,37,223,226,227] there are reports of central retinal vein obstruction occurring as a result of systemic sepsis such as influenza, thrombophlebitis, and pneumonia. These obstructions were more common in the young, had a good prognosis and were generally considered as being due to true thrombosis.

In our experience, obstructions such as these are seldom seen today. Unusual cases of central vein obstruction in apparently healthy patients in their twenties and thirties are still seen in which no cause for the obstruction can be found. These, too, usually have an excellent prognosis. There are also reports of such cases in the literature.[141,166,167,213]

Rare cases of central vein obstruction due to orbital sepsis, which is often secondary to sinus infection, are still occasionally seen.

It may well be that the era of antibiotics and improved medical care has reduced the incidence of this group of retinal vein obstructions.

COATS'S DISEASE

Coats[35,36] originally described occasional arterial obstructions in his microscopic studies of this disease, but the predominant obstructions were venous. These included mechanical obstructions such as lumen narrowing and kinks in the vessels, blockage by periphlebitis, and endothelial proliferation, and finally the filling of the venous lumen by a homogenous coagulum.

Reese[182] has reported a PAS-positive, thick, homogenous material at the level of the basement membrane which increased in thickness until in places it occluded the vascular lumen.

Wise and Horava[246] have found the earliest vascular lesion in this disease to be a swelling of the deep capillary bed endothelium. This was followed by a patchy obliteration and necrosis of these capillaries. PAS-positive material was found at a slightly later stage within vascular lumens, trapped in their walls and outside of the vessels, streaming down through and beneath the retina.

It seems probable that the lumen narrowings and kinks in the vessels seen by Coats were late secondary phenomena or part of the vascular malformations of this disease. The periphlebitis he has described is undoubtedly a late secondary manifestation, for this disease is noninflammatory and neither this change nor blockage by endothelial cell proliferation was observed in the early pathologic studies.[246] The blockage by a homogenous coagulum, as described by Coats, is probably the same PAS-positive material noted above by these later observers. This is the same type of material that makes up the massive exudation of this disease.

The initial vascular lesion in Coats's disease therefore seems to be a patchy and widespread dilatation of the deep capillary bed leading, in severe cases, to destruction of large areas of the bed. For an hypothesis to explain this reaction of the deep capillary bed as secondary to the anomalous vascular formations (see Chapter 11, under the section on The Interrelationships of Anomalous Vascular Formations).

CHANGES IN BLOOD CONSTITUENTS

Certain changes in the blood constituents often produce vascular retinopathies. Such changes could, therefore, be expected to produce retinal signs of arterial, capillary, and venous pathology with an attack upon both of the major capillary beds. While this is theoretically true, clinical and microscopic studies have revealed that the major attack is made upon the capillary and venous side of the circulation. Therefore, these diseases have been included in this chapter where they most clearly simulate diseases of capillary and venous obstruction.

SICKLE CELL DISEASE

For purposes of identification normal hemoglobin has been designated by the letter A, sickle hemoglobin by S, and other abnormal hemoglobins by the letters C, D, E, Thal (thalassemia), etc. Normal hemoglobin is composed of two alpha-peptide chains and two beta-peptide chains. The alpha-chains contain 141 amino acids and the beta-chains contain 146. The alpha-chains are the same in A, S, and C hemoglobin. These hemoglobins vary because of the varying single amino acid in the 6 position of the beta-peptide chain. Glutamic acid occupies this position in normal hemoglobin, valine in S hemoglobin, and lysine in C hemoglobin. It is this biochemical variability which accounts for the different electrophoretic patterns of these hemoglobins and makes their laboratory identification relatively easy.[234]

The S hemoglobin is found predominantly in the Negro race and is most prevalent in Central and West Africa. This is an area of high malarial incidence and, for unknown reasons, sickle cell disease and malaria tend to be mutually exclusive. Hemoglobin C is more commonly found along the Gold Coast in Ghana, and thalassemia in southern Mediterranean regions. Among American Negroes, abnormal hemoglobins occur in about 10 per cent of the population, 8.5 per cent of which have sickle cell trait (A S), 0.4 per cent sickle cell anemia (S S), 0.1 per cent sickle cell hemoglobin C disease (S C), and 2.2 per cent C trait disease (A C).[163] Hook and Cooper [103] gave somewhat different figures. They estimated that among patients having sickle cell disease, 8 to 11 per cent are A S, 2 to 3 per cent are A C, 1 in 600 is S S, 1 in 1500 is S C, and 1 in 6000 is C C. These figures may vary in different studies due to the locality in which census is taken.

Patients with sickle cell anemia and sickle cell hemoglobin C disease are most likely to have retinopathies. Rarer instances of positive retinal findings have been reported in patients with A S, A C, and S Thal hemoglobinopathies and possibly in S D disease.[91] The retinal and choroidal vessels are unaffected in patients with the C C and S F varieties of hemoglobin.[234] Rudd, Evans, and Peeny's patient did not have an electrophoretic study and may well have been one with S C disease rather than S F [189] and it is not clear that thalassemia played any part in the retinopathy reported by Kahán et al.[112]

The varying clinical retinopathies seen in these different hemoglobinopathies are not as yet fully known, but an attempt at this separation is being made.[162,234] As the vascular retinopathy is dependent upon the sickling phenomenon and its production of vascular occlusions, and as sickling is present in varying degree in all hemoglobinopathies with retinopathy, a dependable, clinical differentiation may not become possible.

In the presence of an abnormal hemoglobin and a lowered oxygen tension, red blood cells become sickled and rigid. They become unable to alter their shape and pass through small vascular channels. Thus, they tend to pile upon one another and block capillaries and small veins. Obstruction of small arteries also occurs, but the process probably begins in the capillaries and small veins where the oxygen tension is normally the lowest. Once blockage begins, further depletion of oxygen and increasing acidosis tend to aggravate the sickling phenomenon. The raised blood viscosity in the presence of sickled cells may also be a factor in the retinopathy (see Hyperviscosity Diseases).[171]

Clinical Picture

Following a general discussion of the fundic changes seen in sickle cell disease, some of the clinical appearances suggestive of the individual hemoglobinopathies will be noted. This section has been based extensively upon the study of Lieb, Geeraets, and Guerry.[143] For the systemic manifestations of this disease, the reader is referred to this work.

Sickle cell retinopathy has been classified into four grades of increasing severity. Each grade may contain features described in less severe grades.

Grade 1. The retinal veins show increased dilatation and tortuosity and may appear darker than normal. The arteries either show no change or are slightly burnished and may nick the veins at crossings. The disc is often hyperemic and in the far periphery, especially temporally, an occasional retinal hemorrhage may be seen. Patients showing Grade 1 changes have either no systemic manifestations of the disease or very mild ones present for no more than 2 years. There has usually been no sickle cell crisis.

Grade 2. The most marked changes are in the temporal periphery. The small veins show constrictions and dilatations with halo sheathing in places. Some appear very dark and thrombosed, while others suggest a static circulation which later begins to move. Both intraretinal collateral venous formations and dilated capillary channels, which cannot always be distinguished from one another, begin to appear. Reté new vessel formations on the retinal surface can be seen and some of these may show early fibrosis. Microaneurysms are seen in areas of vascular insufficiency and sclerosis and obstruction of small arterial tributaries develop. These patients have had systemic manifestations of the disease for up to 10 years and many have had a sickle cell crisis.

Grade 3. The most marked changes extend around the full retinal periphery. Venous thromboses and arterial obstructions increase with increasing intraretinal, preretinal, and subretinal hemorrhages. Some of the superficial of these are salmon pink in color and can resemble peripheral retinal holes. Cholesterin deposits appear in the region of vein obstructions or at their borders. Atrophic retinal zones with subsiding retinopathy are seen in regions of arterial closure. The choroid becomes involved and patches of choroidal infarction with hyperpigmented borders are seen. These look like scars of old chorioretinitis. Cholesterin crystals may appear in the vitreous. In this grade, the systemic manifestations are more severe, some patients having shown them for more than 10 years. Others have required hospitalization for sickle cell crises.

Grade 4. This group shows extensive fibrotic and vascular retinitis proliferans, recurring vitreous hemorrhages, retinal detachment, and occlusion of either the central retinal vein or artery may develop. Generally this group shows the most severe systemic manifestations of the longest duration.

Other rarer findings reported by Lieb, Geeraets, and Guerry[143] were papilledema in two patients and angioid streaks in 6 per cent of their patients. One of these also had pseudoxanthoma elasticum. Geeraets and Guerry[86,87] have extended their studies on the angioid streaks and found them in both S S and S C hemoglobinopathy. The pathology of the angioid streaks, that in one long ciliary artery and in systemic arteries of two other patients were strikingly similar to those seen in pseudoxanthoma elasticum. Paton[168] independently, has described angioid streaks in two cases of S S disease in which both Paget's disease and pseudoxanthoma elasticum were excluded.

Goodman, von Sallmann, and Holland[91] have reported chalk white arteries, veins and capillaries in the peripheral retina of a patient with S C disease, and Boniuk and Burton[21] have confirmed this observation. This change is thought to be due to hemolysis of trapped intravascular, sickled, red blood cells.

Hemorrhagic glaucoma with rubeosis iridis may complicate the end stages of sickle cell retinopathy.[87]

While this classification is useful, not all cases fall neatly into this grouping. Patients having S C disease may be seen with well-advanced retinopathy before a diagnosis of the hemoglobin disease has been made. With in-patient populations, the "routine" medical consultant, unless properly appraised, may find so few signs or symptoms of the disease as to deem intensive study unnecessary. In several of our patients, it has only been at the insistence of the ophthalmologist, that the proper diagnosis has been reached. Patches of fibrotic retinitis proliferans may appear early and bleeding into the vitreous from new vessel formations may be an early phenomenon. Retinal edema often extends well posterior to the area of most intensive retinopathy and we have observed both macular edema and rarely a macular cyst.

Welch and Goldberg[234] have described vascular "sea fans" in S C disease and have not observed them in the other hemoglobinopathies. These are fed by a retinal artery, drained by a vein, and spread out preretinally over an atrophic, nonvascular, peripheral retinal area. They fill with fluorescein in the arterial phase and leak dye profusely as any other neovascular proliferans. These authors have also described a sunburst type of peripheral pigmentation "fed by a retinal artery" as being seen in S S disease. A similar pigmentation not "fed by a retinal artery" was noted in some of the S C cases. It was implied that the obliterated feeding retinal artery was in some way related to the pigment sunburst in the S S cases. Our interpretation of this lesion is somewhat different. Retinal artery obstructions, in our experience, are never associated with pigment alteration. The artery lying in the nerve fiber layer may close, but the resulting inner retinal infarction in no way affects the pigment epithelium nourished by the choriocapillaris. We believe these sunbursts are the result of sickle cell interference with choriocapillary circulation and bear no relation to retinal vasculature.

Arteriovenous anastomoses in the periphery have been reported by a number of observers[162,234] and it is not clearly stated where these occur. We have observed them only at the posterior border of infarcted avascular, peripheral zones. In this position their appearance is similar to the arteriovenous anastomoses seen peripherally in pulseless disease. "Sea fans," although fed by an artery and drained by a vein, should not be considered true arteriovenous anastomoses.

Malaria

In the postmortem examination of a soldier who died of malignant malaria, Dudgeon[58] was able to demonstrate sections showing many brain vessels thrombosed with malarial parasites and many parasites in retinal vessels. Although there has been no actual microscopic demonstration of a retinal vascular occlusion due to malarial parasites, this finding in cerebral vessels and the clinical observation of occluded retinal vessels strongly suggests a similar mechanism in the retina.

Positive retinal findings are usually present only in severe cases of malaria. Blatt[20] has noted that retinal hemorrhages were the most frequent ocular complication of malaria, and occurred in tertian malaria at the period of greatest toxicity, i.e., when the parasites entered the red blood cells. He thought that the stickiness of the intima and slowing of the blood stream resulted in thrombosis and closure of the vessel, and that the eye changes were secondary to vascular closure, rather than being primarily due to malaria per se. Davis[51] also believed that the large peripapillary and macular hemorrhages in malaria were due to vascular blockage by parasites.

Kiep,[114] Fisher,[77] and Friedenwald[80] have reported retinal vein occlusions with subsequent retinitis proliferans and venous collateral formation in malaria, and Kiep has stressed the preponderance of venous rather than arterial obstructions.

Other retinal findings in malaria include tortuous arteries and veins, cotton-wool spots, infarcts of the retina and choroid[51,161] and retinal detachment.[20]

HYPERVISCOSITY DISEASES

General Considerations in the Hyperviscosity Syndrome

Viscosity is the property of a fluid to resist flow. The science concerned with these properties is called rheology (i.e., the study of the deformation and flow of matter). A fluid's viscosity is defined as the ratio of its sheer stress—the force imposed per unit area of fluid plane in dynes per square centimeter (dyn/em^2)—to sheer rate, the velocity gradient between the adjacent planes of layers of fluid during flow.[236]

In ideal (Newtonian) fluids such as water, the rate of flow is proportional to the pressure or sheer stress propelling it, and the Law of Poiseuille applies. Biologic fluids, such as blood, are non-Newtonian, much more complicated, and do not obey Poiseuille's law. Their viscosities are variable and depend on many factors, among which the flow rate is predominant. These other factors include the size of the blood vessel, the hematocrit, the degree of red cell aggregation, the internal viscosity of the red and white blood cells, and the viscosity of the plasma.[208] Various means have been used to measure the viscosity of biologic fluids but none is completely satisfactory. These viscosity measurements are complicated and different methods give different values. There is not as yet any standard procedure acceptable to all. Measurements in comparison to water with an Ostwald viscosimeter at 37° C is a method frequently used.

Capillary tube viscosity studies have shown a nearly linear viscosity-hematocrit relation for hematocrit levels up to 50 per cent. Higher hematocrit values lead to an exponential increase in viscosity. Dintenfass[53] has also shown that the blood viscosity is elevated in patients with leukemia. The apparently higher internal viscosity of white rather than red blood cells may be a factor in these cases.

Clinically, plasma and serum viscosity values are more frequently determined than that of whole blood. The fact that the plasma viscosity is the rheologically critical fluid in the microcirculation[236] probably explains why the most marked examples of hyperviscosity retinopathy are seen in the dysproteinemias, for the viscosity of the nonred cell fraction of blood is primarily dependent upon the protein constituents. The protein concentration, its molecular character, and degree of hydration (salvation) are all important factors. Of the blood proteins, the globulins have a more marked effect on viscosity than do the albumins.

The tendency to blood sludging in the hyperviscous state is readily visible in the conjunctival vessels of such patients. This sludging and reduced rate of flow, together with the hypoxia produced by the inefficient delivery of oxygen to the tissues[131] is responsible for the similarities of the retinopathies seen in various hyperviscous states. Mild degrees of hyperviscosity have little effect on the fundic appearance, but in severer cases, the retinal changes may be profound. Dintenfass[53] has stated that the presence of high viscosity plasma in vivo would be expected to endanger the circulation in a manner analogous to, but not identical with that encountered in polycythemia or in acidosis. He believes that an increased blood viscosity from whatever cause, decreases the velocity of blood flow, and that all other complicating features, such as vascular leakage and obstruction result from this feature.

Behrman[19] has stated that the high "flow resistance" of the retinal circulation at the lamina cribrosa results in a limited ability of the retinal venous circulation to accommodate to an increasing blood viscosity as compared to that in other systemic vessels. He believes that this accounts for the early appearance in the retina of the characteristic features of hyperviscosity. It is our feeling that the high oxygen demand of retinal tissues is also important. Clinically, signs do appear early in the fundus, and the retinal picture in some cases is marked and seemingly out of proportion to the general state of the patient.

Dysproteinemic Retinopathy

The blood viscosity produced by abnormal serum proteins is dependent upon the concentration and type of abnormal protein. The highest viscosities are produced by the IgM macroglobulins whose molecular weight is about 1,000,000. The gamma globulins associated with multiple myeloma (IgG) have a molecular weight of 160,000 and do not ordinarily produce the extreme elevations of serum viscosity seen in Waldenström's macroglobulinemia. Thus, high concentrations of myeloma proteins are required to increase the blood viscosity to symptomatic levels.[131] After an initial slight ascent, the viscosity curve rises steeply with increasing concentrations of IgM globulin while the serum viscosity rises linearly and more gently with increasing concentrations of myeloma IgG globulins. In addition, most IgM proteins remain within the vascular compartment, while only 40 per cent of the IgG protein and albumin are within the vessels.[71] All of these factors tend to produce the most dramatic examples of the hyperviscosity syndrome in the cases of Waldenström's macroglobulinemia, while milder examples are more common in cases of multiple myeloma.

The most common features of the hyperviscosity syndrome produced by abnormal proteins are bleeding from the mucous membranes, retinopathy, neurologic disorders, congestive heart failure, and a high sedimentation rate. A purpuric skin rash may be present and Raynaud's phenomenon may occur especially when cryoglobulins are present. Symptoms are not present with blood viscosities below 4 and may be absent with viscosity levels of 8 to 10.[71]

The retinopathy starts with dilatation and tortuosity of the veins. It has not been determined at exactly what blood viscosity level this occurs, but conjunctival sludging has been reported at a viscosity of 4.6[76,197] and minimal retinal venous dilatation with several small hemorrhages has been observed at this same level.[197] Venous dilatation and tortuosity together with hemorrhages and exudates have been seen at blood viscosities of 6.5.[30] Blood sludging in retinal veins is not seen early in the retinopathy, but it can often be induced by pressure on the globe. The disc shows an early hyperemia.

Progressive retinopathy reveals increasing dilatation, tortuosity, and darkening of the veins, increasing nicking of the veins by the arteries at crossings, hemorrhages, and exudates. The hemorrhages are both superficial and deep and extend to the far periphery. The exudates are in the posterior fundus and consist of superficial cotton-wool patches and gray white, ill-defined lesions of about this same size, but occurring most prominently in the deeper retina. These are probably collections of abnormal protein-containing serum which has leaked through the damaged vascular walls. Some are PAS-positive like the serum within vascular lumens; others fail to take this stain.[30] The fundic picture can closely resemble that of a central retinal vein obstruction although the vein be proven patent at microscopic examination.[1]

Retinal microaneurysms have been observed in the retinal periphery[52,85] but they are not as commonly seen, nor are they seen in the numbers that one might expect.

In the late stages of macroglobulinemic retinopathy tremendous sausage-like veins develop. Beading and sometimes sludged venous blood may be seen. The arteries become more burnished and greatly indent the veins at crossings. The retina has a glistening reflex and may show no clinical signs of edema in spite of the most marked vascular dilatation (Fig. 14-11). Other cases of milder

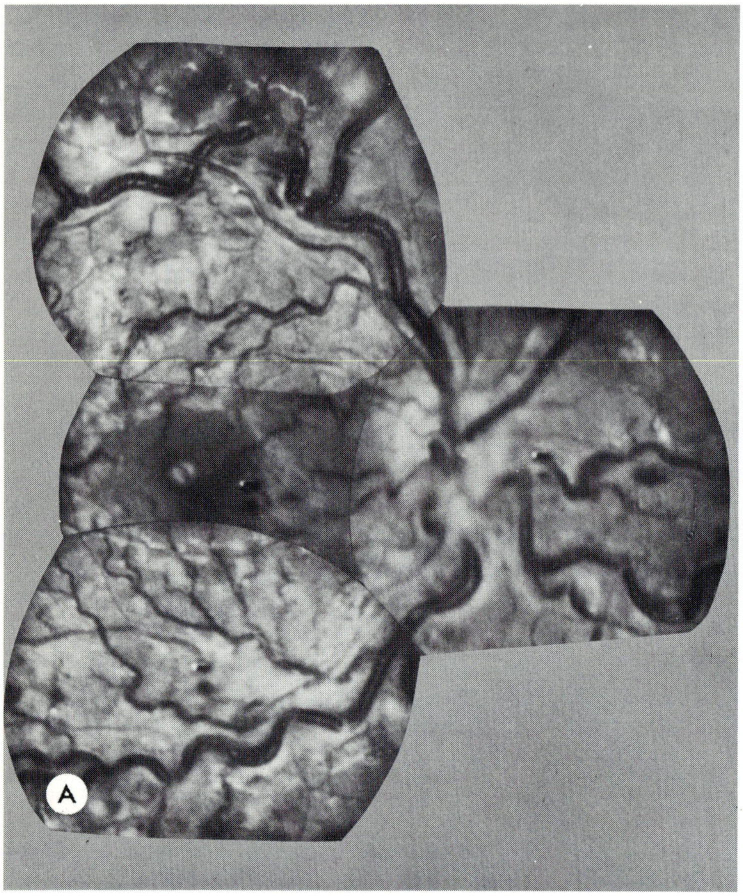

retinopathy, as in multiple myeloma, often do show clinical edema of the retina. This suggests that leaking highly viscous serum is less apt to produce the clinical appearance of retinal edema than is a serum of lower viscosity. These cases may show a white fuzziness about the venous blood columns (Fig. 14-12). An increased density of this haze, especially when present at a narrowed venous segment, looks clinically like mild cuffing as is seen in periphlebitis.

Peripheral, branch, and central venous thromboses may occur (Fig. 14-12)[211] as well as vitreous hemorrhage and rubeosis iridis with glaucoma.[57] Neovascularization around the papilla progressing to fibrotic retinitis proliferans has also been observed.[4]

In a case of multiple myeloma, Delaney and Liaricos[52] have reported peripheral chorioretinal destruction due to invading myeloma cells. The retinal vessels stopped abruptly at the edge of the pigmented scar between the equator and ora serrata.

Fluorescein angiography in a patient with Waldenström's macroglobulinemia revealed dilated capillaries around the papilla, mi-

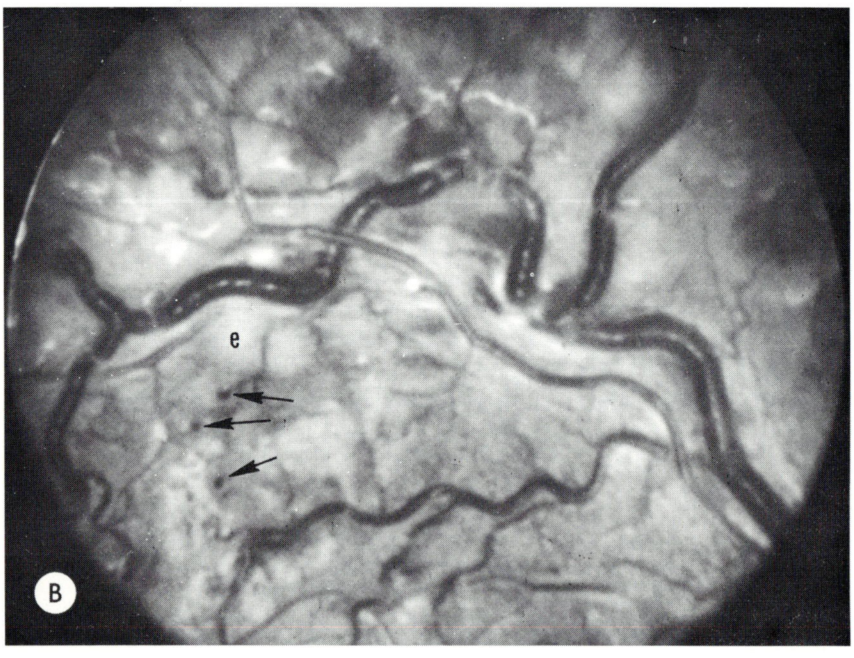

Fig. 14-11. *A*, The right fundus of a 23-year-old woman with cryomacroglobulinemia. Blood serum viscosity 24 minutes, control 1 minute. Note the engorged tortuous veins and the cotton-wool patch at the lower border of the disc. (From Carr and Henkind. *Amer. J. Ophthal.* *56:*23, 1963.)

B, Enlarged detail of *A* showing venous beading, microaneurysms **(arrows)**, and dysproteinemic exudate **(e).**

croaneurysms, no leakage from retinal vessels, and a much delayed fluorescein transit time.[188]

The dysproteinemic retinopathy can be reversed by lowering the blood viscosity (Fig. 14-13).[131,197] This is usually accomplished by plasmapheresis. Clearing of the retinopathy occurs as the serum viscosity decreases, but return to a normal appearance does not occur until sometime after the serum viscosity has approached normal levels.

The first microscopic study of dysproteinemic retinopathy was that of Spalter.[211] In addition, his report contains a very clear exposition of the fundamentals of this syndrome. This article and others[10,13,30,193] have defined the major features of the retinal pathology.

The retina is edematous in both reticular layers. The veins and some capillaries, especially those of the deeper bed, are dilated and contain the homogenous PAS-positive abnormal serum proteins. Some of this same material is pocketed extravascularly in both reticular layers, and probably accounts for the grayish white exudates seen clinically. Retinal hemorrhages are seen in all layers and cotton-wool patches containing cytoid bodies appear in the nerve fiber layer. Retinal microaneurysms are very profuse in the peripheral retina, less frequent in the equatorial retina, and, posteriorly occur only around the macula. Capillary ghosts without endothelium or intramural pericytes are present peripherally and there is a zone showing endothelial cell proliferation just posterior to this. Some endothelial cell pro-

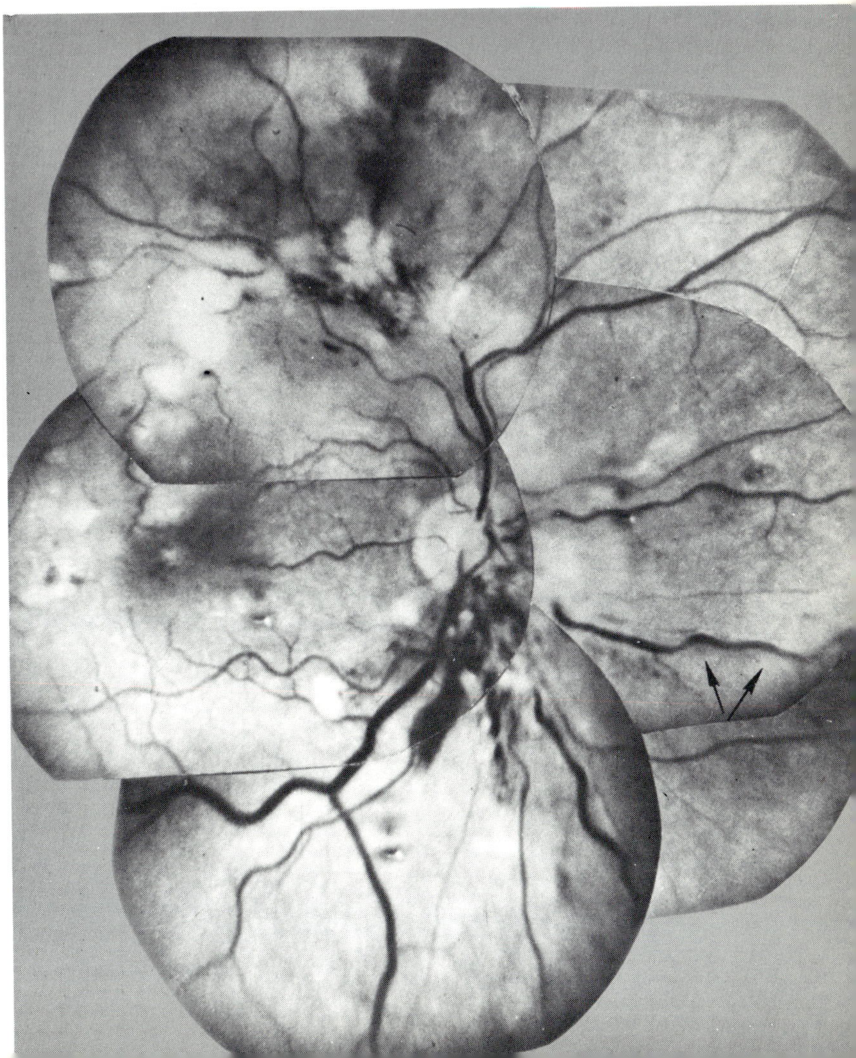

Fig. 14-12. Fundus photograph of a 44-year-old man with dysproteinemia. Prior to the establishment of the diagnosis, his Raynaud's phenomenon had been unsuccessfully treated by sympathectomy. The fundus shows dilated, tortuous, dark veins, crossing defects and a gray white haze (**arrows**) about the veins accentuated in places simulating a periphlebitic cuff. There are cotton-wool patches, deeper gray white exudates, retinal edema, and both superficial and deep hemorrhages in all quadrants. The inferior temporal vein has developed an obstruction at the first arteriovenous crossing. Collaterals subsequently have formed.

liferation in capillaries may also be seen in the posterior fundus. Rudimentary new vessel formation may occur in areas of most marked endothelial proliferation. In the peripheral zone of ghost capillaries, the basement membrane shows severe degeneration and both lamination and sacculation. Some arterioles demonstrate fibrinoid degeneration.

The major retinal effect of the abnormal serum proteins is produced by the increased blood viscosity, slowing of the circulation, and inefficient delivery of oxygen and nutrients to the tissues. Other effects such as increasing the rouleau formation of red blood cells[187] and coating the platelets seem to be of less importance.

Polycythemia

Primary polycythemia, because of its higher red blood cell count and hyperviscosity, is more apt to produce a retinopathy than is secondary polycythemia which is due to such causes as emphysema and congenital heart disease. Mild degrees of secondary polycythemia usually produce no discernible retinal change.

The retinopathy of both primary and sec-

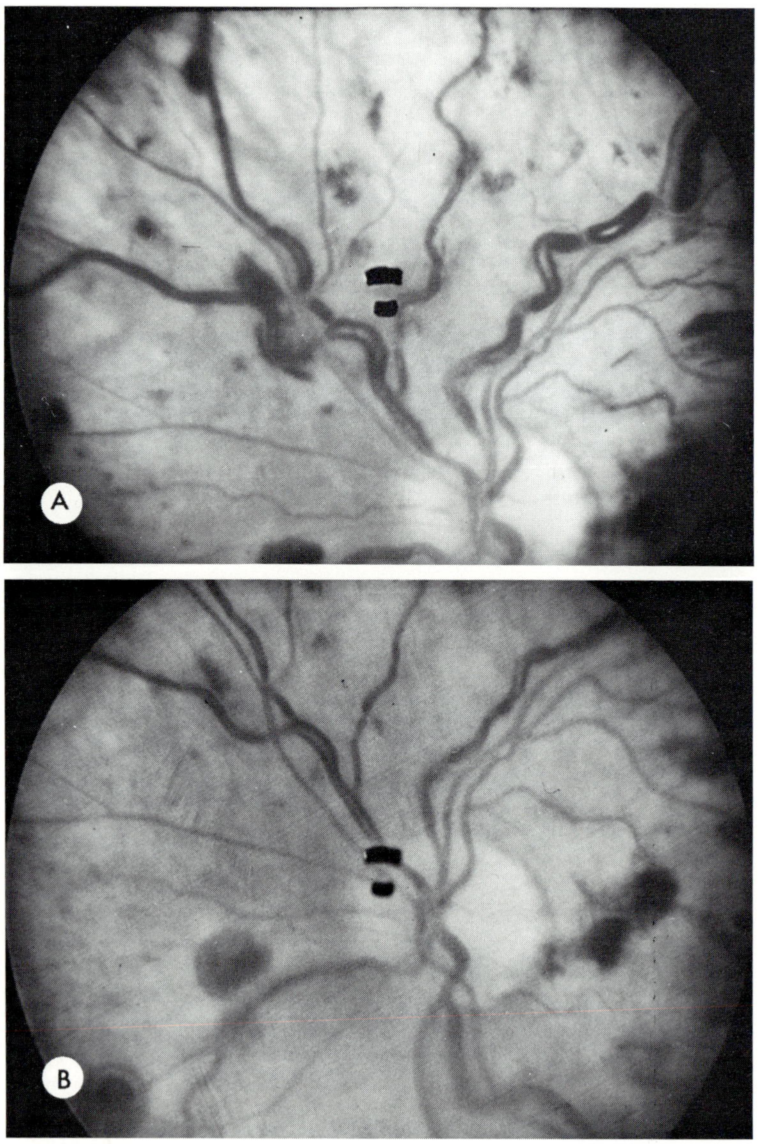

Fig. 14-13. Macroglobulinemia in a 55-year-old woman. *A*, Photograph has been taken above the right disc. Blood serum viscosity 1 minute 17 seconds, control 20 seconds. *B*, Shows same retinal area 2 weeks later after plasmapheresis. Blood serum viscosity is now 22 seconds, control 20 seconds.

ondary polycythemia varies only in degree and is the same in each case. The first change is darkening, dilatation, and increased tortuosity of the retinal veins. The disc is hyperemic and both it and the fundic background may assume a violaceous color. When there is sufficient venous dilatation and tortuosity, arteries may nick the veins at crossings and produce the effect of linked sausages. With the appearance of retinal hemorrhages, which are usually scattered and not numerous, the picture can suggest that of impending central retinal vein obstruction. Deep retinal hemorrhages are more common but superficial ones, especially about the disc, can also occur.

In more severe cases, retinal edema may be seen at the posterior pole, venous ectasis may occur,[49,164] and dilated retinal capillaries may become clinically visible. A small number of severe cases show papilledema.[113,230] Hemangiomatous tumors in the posterior cerebral fossa may produce a secondary polycythemia. Kearns[113] has cited such a case showing increased intracranial pressure and papilledema whose proper diagnosis was not established at first.

The most serious retinal complications of polycythemia are vascular occlusions.[65] In our experience these are rare in patients with polycythemia vera who do not have other retinal vascular disease. Secondary polycythemia with its elevated hematocrit may be an important factor in retinal vascular occlusions, especially those of veins, when it co-exists with other retinal vascular pathology (see section on Treatment).

Leukemia

With minor exceptions, the fundic pictures produced by the leukemias are so similar that they cannot be differentiated on this basis. It has long been recognized that the associated anemia and thrombocytopenia[113,230] may play a part in the retinopathy. Only recently has the influence of hyperviscosity been recognized.

The improved methods of treating leukemias have led to an extended life expectancy and, in consequence, late neurologic complications are more frequently seen. Mild leukemic infiltration of the optic nerve is often mentioned in the older literature. Today, one occasionally encounters severe leukemic infiltration of the optic disc producing a pale elevated disc and leading to optic atrophy if untreated.

The hemorrhagic and exudative features of the retinopathy are more commonly seen in the acute leukemias and the marked vascular and color changes are more often apparent in the later stages of chronic leukemia. Myelogenous leukemia is more apt to have an associated retinopathy than lymphatic leukemia.[23,46] Culler[46] has concluded that decreased platelets do account for some retinal hemorrhages and that anemia is important in the production of hemorrhages and cotton-wool patches when the red blood cell count was below 1.5 million[46] or the hemoglobin was below 40 per cent.[23]

The earliest change seen is dilatation and tortuosity of the retinal veins. Retinal hemorrhages, both superficial and deep, are next to appear. The superficial ones are often of the large thumb-blot variety and, if dense enough in the center, will give a small central light reflex when viewed with the ophthalmoscope. These can be misinterpreted as Roth's spots (see Chapter 10, under section on Roth's spots). True, white-centered hemorrhages (Roth's spots) and cotton-wool patches also appear. The Roth's spots may represent hemorrhage around a cotton-wool patch or the center may be made up of leukemic cells.[2,46] These two different microscopic types cannot always be differentiated clinically. The cotton-wool patches may represent a part of the anemic retinopathy or may be due to plugging of precapillary arterioles by clumps of leukemic cells. Gray white patches of leukemic cells, $1/6$ to $3/4$ of a disc diameter in size, without surrounding hemorrhage, may be confused with cotton-wool spots.[23] They are often in the deeper retina, a location which serves to distinguish them. Their presence has been thought to bear more of a relation to the immaturity and invasiveness of the leukocytes than to their number within the blood stream.[23] Rarely, these nodules are huge and show proliferating leukemic cells.[135] In cases of secondary anemia, mild superficial retinal edema, and a pale, mildly edematous disc may be seen.

As the retinopathy progresses, the veins become more dilated and tortuous and take on the appearance of linked sausages due to nicking by the crossing and often slightly tortuous arteries (Fig. 14-14). In these cases deep yellowish, fatty exudates are sometimes seen. In chronic myelogenous leukemia, fuzzy white striping may develop around the veins, especially in the periphery. This has been attributed to leukemic cell infiltration of the vein wall and perivenous spaces.[23,46] Leukemic cells have been demonstrated microscopically around the veins, but Allen and Straatsma[2] did not find them in sufficient numbers to explain this clinical appearance. In our experience the white striping suggests that at least some component of it is due to halo sheathing. Its position on peripheral veins and its occurrence with other signs of impeded venous flow is compatible with this concept.

Duke, Wilkinson, and Sigelman[59] have studied the retinal digests of 40 patients dying of leukemia, all of whom had no other disease known to produce retinal microaneurysms. No patient dying of acute leukemia had microaneurysms, but significant numbers were found, mainly in the retinal periphery, among those who died of the chronic leukemias. More were found in chronic myeloid leukemia than in lymphocytic disease. They seemed to bear a relation to the height of the white cell count and therefore to the degree of increased blood viscosity. Chronic myelogenous leukemia is also more apt to show exaggerated signs of venous stasis in the periphery than is chronic lymphocytic leukemia.

The choroid shows more leukemic cell infiltration than the retina especially in its posterior aspects. Choroidal infiltration tends to be diffuse whereas that in the retina is more nodular.[2]

The color changes in the leukemic fundus are related to several factors. The anemia and increased white cell count probably produce the lightening of the normal red color seen in retinal vessels. It is thought that leukemic infiltration of the choroid is responsible for the altered fundic background color. This change can be modified by the degree of pigment in the pigment epithelium. Colors such as greenish and orange have been described,[209] but these colors have not been seen by others,[23] nor have we observed them. A gray white color retaining some red value is, however, sometimes seen.

The hemorrhages in leukemic retinopathy are derived from both the superficial and deep capillary beds. Superficial ones will sometimes be large and sheet-like and they may break through into the vitreous. The larger deep ones at times break through beneath the retina.[2] Allen and Straatsma[2] have cited one patient with a massive subretinal hemorrhage which detached the retina and showed new vessels growing subretinally as in Coats's disease. This is in conformity with the concept of neovascular formation presented in Chapter 11.

Mild to frank disc edema has been frequently noted.[2,113,230] Some patients have increased intracranial pressure[230] and others do not.[207,230] Wagener and Rucker[230] have reported a patient with raised intracranial and jugular venous pressures and papilledema. They have incriminated increased blood viscosity as a possible factor, for when blood was withdrawn, the disc edema receded.

According to Borgeson and Wagener[23] leukemic retinopathy may be absent in cases with very high white cell counts (532,000)

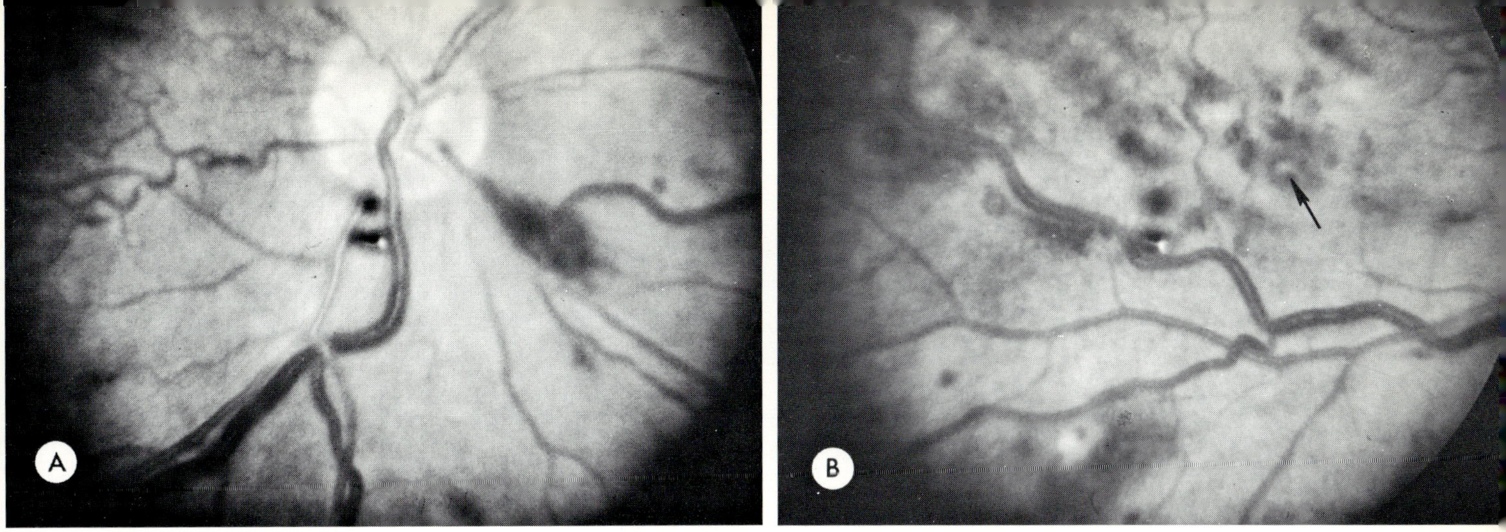

Fig. 14-14. Chronic lymphocytic leukemia in a 68-year-old male with associated hepatosplenomegaly and a white blood cell count of over 1 million. *A*, Left eye shows sausage-like veins and both superficial and deep hemorrhages. *B*, Same eye shows a Roth's spot (**arrow**) and leukemic infiltrates.

or present with very low counts (4300). It may also develop as early as 3 weeks after the onset of systemic symptoms or be absent after 10 years of the disease.

Pancreatic Cystic Fibrosis

The retinopathy occurring in cystic fibrosis of the pancreas was first described by Bruce, Denning, and Spalter.[27] In a subsequent report, Spalter and Bruce[212] have demonstrated a similar retinopathy in adults with other diseases producing chronic pulmonary insufficiency with carbon dioxide retention.

Chronic cystic fibrosis of the pancreas is an hereditary disease with recessive genetic expression, occurring in children and young adults. In its more severe stages there is chronic lung disease, pancreatic insufficiency, and loss of sodium and chloride in the sweat.

The retinopathy starts with dilatation and tortuosity of retinal veins. Papilledema and a few superficial or deep retinal hemorrhages occur usually near the disc. A few patients will also show microcystic edema of the macula or a ruptured central macular cyst. The retinopathy is only present in those patients with chronic and severe pulmonary insufficiency, and, in general, it is proportional to the duration and severity of the pulmonary defect.

In the patients which these authors have studied, chronic pulmonary insufficiency and carbon dioxide retention appear to be most closely related to development of the retinopathy. Secondary polycythemia, chronically elevated venous pressure, and raised intracranial pressure have been excluded as causes. The authors felt that increased cerebral blood flow secondary to the carbon dioxide retention could be the major factor in its production. Although the gamma globulins were usually elevated in those patients having retinopathy, and hyperviscosity was mentioned as a possible contributing etiologic factor, serum viscosity levels were not measured.

This retinopathy may very well *not* be an example of the hyperviscosity syndrome. Because the retinopathy clinically suggests hyperviscosity, it has been placed in this category until its etiology has been proved or until serum viscosity measurements have been shown to be normal.

PARASITIC OBSTRUCTIONS

Toussaint and Danis[217] have reported the case of a 38-year-old male patient with generalized *Loa loa* filariasis and reduced vision in each eye. The patient was too ill for an exact determination of his visual acuity. Both fundi revealed large preretinal hemorrhages scattered from the disc to the equator, intermingled or covering yellow exudation, and several white lines interpreted as obstructed arterioles.

The patient died after 7 days. The postmortem examination revealed intravascular microfilariae, vascular thromboses, and venous stasis in systemic organs and tissues. Nodules containing extravascular parasites, giant cells, and mononuclear histiocytes were noted, as well as numerous microinfarcts.

Microscopically the eyes revealed extensive retinal hemorrhages both superficial and deep, sometimes thickening the retina five times. There was widespread retinal edema and serous exudation especially in the outer plexiform layer and to a milder degree posteriorly beneath the retina. Some extravascular microfilaria were seen within this fluid, but most were intravascular, especially within capillaries and veins. There was perivenous lymphocytic infiltration and superficially, the ganglion cells were absent in the serohemorrhagic areas. The choroid showed almost no involvement.

A retinal digest preparation revealed intravascular microfilaria and microaneurysms, some filled with parasites, and most in the periphery. Some capillary segments contained no intramural pericytes and others showed zones of endothelial cell proliferation.

RICKETTSIAL RETINOPATHY

The rickettsial infections produce similar retinopathies and may, therefore, be considered as a group.

Following the initial infection and an incubation period, the rickettsial organisms enter the endothelial cells of capillaries, small veins and arteries. Harrell,[98] in Rocky Mountain spotted fever, has demonstrated that the rickettsia prefer the nuclei although they are also found in the cytoplasm of these cells. Here they multiply and destroy the cells, first in the capillaries, then in the arterioles and to a lesser extent in the venules. In arterioles they may also destroy the smooth muscle cells. With cell death, thromboses and hemorrhages occur. The thrombi are hyaline with proliferation of the endothelium leading to microinfarcts. Systemically, perivascular accumulations of monocytes are also seen. It is this pathology, which produces the skin rash and central nervous system lesions.

The fundic findings[31,177,178,194] suggest a similar pathogenesis of retinal and choroidal lesions. The first to appear, and the most common retinal finding, is venous engorgement. This appears in the second or third week of the disease and in severe instances progresses to markedly dilated and tortuous vessels of irregular caliber. Slightly pale arterioles nick the veins at crossings and produce the picture of linked sausages. Disc edema and retinal edema, especially in the posterior fundus, are the next most common findings. When the edema is marked the retinal veins may have a hazy white outline or be partly hidden at crossings. This, and the occasional occurrence of a small hemorrhage within the venous wall, both suggest leakage from the retinal veins. The edematous disc is seldom elevated more than 2.5 D and often occurs with a normal spinal fluid pressure, suggesting a local vascular etiology. It was always bilateral in Scheie's cases.[194] Retinal hemorrhages, superficial more often than deep, are few in number and occasional cotton-wool exudates occur. Both arterial and venous occlusions are rare but have been reported.[177,178,194]

Anterior and posterior uveitis are both seen and most of Scheie's cases examined microscopically showed diffuse choroidal infiltration with mononuclear cells. Retinal perivascular cellular infiltration was not seen, nor were intraretinal rickettsial organisms identified. In spite of this, other evidence of vasculitis, perivasculitis, and endothelial cell proliferation in retinal capillaries suggested that the retinal pathology was no different from that described in the central nervous system and systemically.

The retinopathy persists well into the convalescent period. Residual findings consist of enlarged blind spots, occasional peripheral field depression, and rarely, a pigment disturbance adjacent to the macula.

PHLEBOSCLEROSIS

Gibson and Smith[88] have divided venous sclerosis into three clinical types. The first type has been described as intimal, and occurs after venous thrombosis when the circulation is not fully restored. Peripheral to the thrombosis the vein becomes white and fibrous with a smooth contour. The second has been called intramural and it occurs when the sclerosis is sufficiently severe to cause indentations in the lumen and changes in the contour of the vein. This alternate constriction and dilatation of the vein, or beading, occurs prior to thrombosis. Following thrombosis the vein becomes fibrotic. The third type has been called adventitial and it develops after the subsidence of perivenous inflammation or edema. Thereafter, connective tissue ensheathes the vein.

Klien[122] believed that primary phlebosclerosis as an endo- or mesophlebitis was important in the pathogenesis of central retinal vein obstruction. She thought this occurred in senescence but was much more important accompanying such systemic disorders as hypertension and diabetes.

With increased knowledge of these changes, the term phlebosclerosis has dropped from popular usage. The term is a broadly descriptive one used to describe many of the secondary venous changes resulting from other primary causes. These have been singled out and described elsewhere in this text. Primary phlebosclerosis does not occur and therefore cannot be a primary cause of retinal vein obstruction.

TRAUMA

The choroid is more fragile than the retina, and direct, ocular trauma, therefore, more frequently produces choroidal rupture in a healthy eye. More severe injuries of this type may not only rupture the choroid but also damage the retina. Retinal capillaries are most likely broken, and veins more commonly torn than arteries. Relatively mild traumas, heretofore considered important in the production of retinal detachment, are now considered irrelevant or only a possible precipitating incident, where the basic retinal disease bears primary responsibility. Even in these retinal tears, a retinal break across a vein is more common than one involving an artery.

Traumatic ruptures of the choroid and retina may produce severe intraocular bleeding. When the blood is absorbed, and the interior can again be seen, healing with traumatic chorioretinitis proliferans is usually present. In such cases the fibrovascular connective tissue is for the most part derived from the choroid and some pigment proliferation is usually present. Such cases have been commonly reported in war injuries.[45,55,137,170,205]

Michaelson [156] and Michaelson and Kraus [158] have reported this same lesion in penetrating double injuries of the eyeball. In some cases of this type, the proliferative chorioretinitis extends through the vitreous between the wounds of entrance and exit.

Iron is the most important of the retained intraocular foreign bodies. A delayed siderosis may develop and the iron, which collects in the perivascular tissues and produces fibrosis, can indirectly lead to occlusion of retinal capillaries and small veins.[32] This probably accounts for those instances of retinitis proliferans seen in some of these eyes.

Some injuries, particularly bullet wounds, which penetrate the orbit without directly striking the globe, may produce concussion injuries of both retina and choroid. This same type of injury also produces an avulsion of the optic nerve with coincident damage to the major retinal vessels.

A direct, nonpenetrating blow to the eye usually produces a contrecoup effect upon the retina. As the eye is often looking in the direction of the blow when it is struck, the posterior effect is exerted upon the macula. The macular lesion, known as Berlin's edema or commotio retinae, consists of a fuzzy, white, raised edema of the macula with loss of its foveal reflex. This edema appears quickly and is associated with a decrease in central visual acuity. It subsides within a week or 10 days either returning to complete normality, with reappearance of the foveal reflex, or, leaving varying permanent defects. These consist of a fragmented or absent foveal reflex, a macular cyst which often ruptures, and varying degrees of pigment disturbance. Pigment alterations, both mottling and proliferation, are usually slower to develop and increasing pigmentation can occur for some weeks after the injury.

It is thought that the immediate effect is one of vascular constriction followed very shortly by capillary dilatation and leakage. A fluorescein angiogram in one of our patients, taken 4 days after injury but while macular edema was still present, failed to show such leakage, but this may have been too late for its demonstration.

The prognosis can often be approximated shortly after the injury. A mild reduction in vision and a relative central scotoma suggest a good prognosis, while poor visual acuity and a deep scotoma usually mean permanent damage.

Associated with the remote contrecoup effect of these injuries, there is often a direct effect exerted anteriorly, where contact is made. Probably because of Bell's phenomenon (the rolling up of the eye on lid closure), the anterior traumatic chorioretinitis is usually present in the periphery below. Scattered retinal hemorrhages and edema are seen at first. With healing, a permanent mottling of pigment epithelium remains.

While the macula is most frequently involved in commotio retinae, other posterior retinal areas have been involved. These usually offer an excellent visual prognosis.

Sun eclipse burns of the macula are almost invariably bilateral. The lens focuses infrared rays on the macula, and their absorption by the pigment epithelium with the coincident heat production, produces the outer retinal burn. Macular capillaries dilate and leak producing a hazy central edema. The scotoma appears promptly, and unless it disappears very shortly, some permanent visual defect can be expected. The choroid appears to be little involved, probably due to the speed of its circulation and the heat dissipating effect this produces. Residual scars often show a red depigmented center with a fringe of pigment around them. In fortunate cases they are sometimes centered parafoveally and produce less permanent visual reduction than would be expected from their appearance.

Arc-welding or "flash" burns do not affect the macula. The emanation is predominantly in the ultraviolet spectrum and these rays are almost entirely absorbed by the cornea.

The remote effects upon the retinal circulation produced by strangulation or difficult deliveries have been discussed in Chapter 10, under the section on Hemorrhages.

Carotid-cavernous fistulas are usually of traumatic origin but spontaneous cases do occur. Their diagnosis is made from the history and clinical findings other than those seen in the retina. In a series of 25 patients with untreated carotid-cavernous fistula, Sanders and Hoyt[192] have reported mildly dilated retinal veins in 19 eyes. Although not mentioned by the authors, in our experience, the arteries are often darker than normal. Of their 25 patients, only three showed more severe vasculopathy than the venous dilatation. These had marked venous dilatation and tortuosity, scattered deep retinal hemorrhages, and two developed microaneurysms. In one of the three, the retinal pathology developed 3 months after onset of the fistula and this patient showed swelling of the disc as well.

A fluorescein angiogram in another of the three patients showed a very slow development of the arterial phase with some caliber irregularity. The capillary phase demonstrated microaneurysms and both it and the venous phase were prolonged, with leakage of dye from capillaries and large venous trunks.

Hope-Robertson[104] has reported two cases of obstruction of the central retinal vein following nonocular injuries. The first was a man 36 years of age who developed the vascular occlusion 7 days after striking his maxilla on a door handle. The second was that of a 29-year-old male who developed a central retinal vein obstruction 4 days after an automobile accident. There were no evident general injuries in this case. These two unusual cases have not been explained.

PRERETINAL MACULAR FIBROSIS

Preretinal macular fibrosis is placed in the category of venous and capillary obstructive diseases because advanced stages of it are so similar to the retinal reaction seen after obstruction of a macular draining vein. In its development it behaves as though there were first some localized derangement of the deep capillary bed in the macular or paramacular region, followed by obstruction of these capillaries or postcapillary venules. This course of events is by no means proved and the actual etiology is still obscure.

The disease occurs equally in male and female patients and one or both eyes may be involved. Although cases are seen in patients with hypertension and glaucoma, they are by no means limited to this group. Most lesions occur in healthy individuals over 60 years of age without other significant ocular pathology. The earliest one which we have observed was first seen in a patient 46 years of age.

Some paramacular lesions are discovered during the course of periodic ocular examinations before there is macular involvement, and before the patients are aware of any trouble. The first sign is a localized, deep retinal edema with ill-defined borders located almost invariably somewhere within the vascular arcade around the macula (Fig. 14-15). Of 36 patients recently reviewed, we

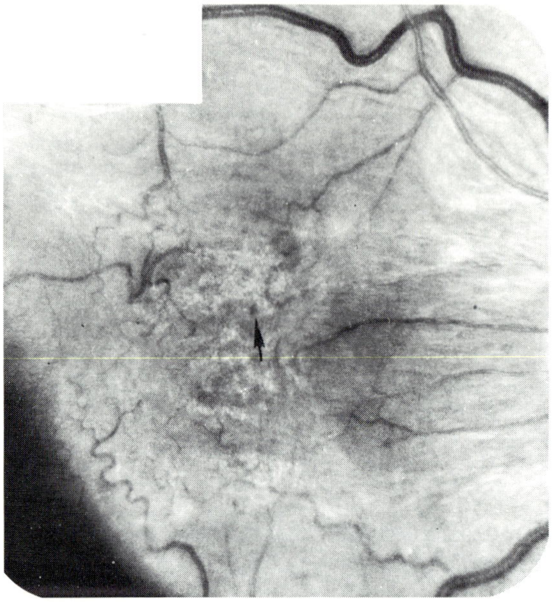

Fig. 14-15. Early preretinal macular fibrosis. The glinting light reflexes are due to deep retinal edema surrounding a small deep retinal hemorrhage **(arrow).** To the top and left note vascular distortion due to preretinal fibrosis.

Fig. 14-16. Early preretinal macular fibrosis. Note microcystic macular edema **(arrow)** and retinal traction lines with almost invisible preretinal fibrosis.

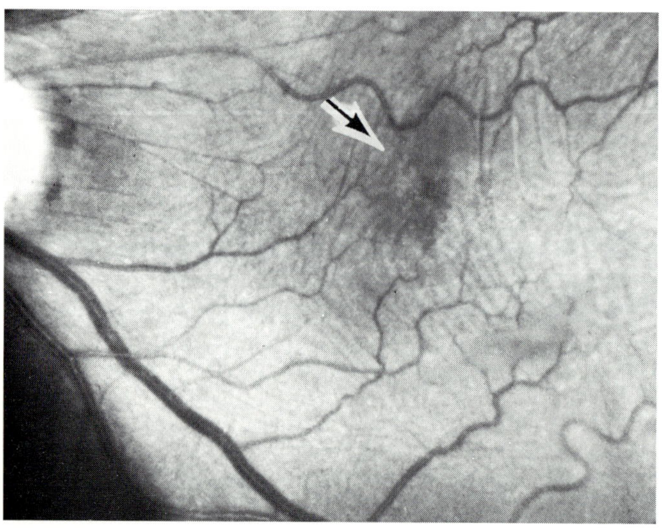

have observed only three with lesions beyond these limits—one above the superior temporal vessel arch; one just above and one just nasal to the disc. In the earliest stage there are no retinal traction lines, and if the fovea is uninvolved, it is free of edema and has a good reflex. In one eye we observed posterior vitreous detachment 1 year prior to the onset of macular disease. In this patient the posterior hyaloid was well away from the retina at the onset of macular edema. Most patients had posterior vitreous detachments at the time of discovery of the retinal lesion.

Even at this early stage, if the retinal veins of the two eyes are compared, a fullness and darkening of the veins in the involved eye can be seen. This change may be difficult to discern at first, but it becomes increasingly apparent as the disease progresses. With moderate advancement of the retinal lesion, dark, dilated, and increasingly tortuous veins become obvious. At this stage some patients show no venous pulsation at the disc, and one cannot be elicited by even moderate pressure on the globe. Others show spontaneous venous pulsation or a pulse readily apparent with the slightest pressure upon the eyeball.

Within several months fine traction lines can be seen on the retinal surface. These may occur in a single locus or in several areas (Fig. 14-16). So long as the fovea is not involved, central vision is good and the patient is still unaware of any difficulty. The traction lines may appear as a swathe, or more commonly radiate from one or more foci. With further development, delicate preretinal fibrosis becomes visible, usually lying closely adherent to the retinal surface. If the disease extends into the foveal area or if the traction lines distort the fovea, metamorphopsia and visual reduction occur. Near vision is more affected than distant acuity and the visual distortion is readily demonstrated with the Amsler grid. Most patients indicate a wavy irregularity of the grid lines, with only one of our patients having an actual scotoma.

Progression of the disease is highly variable. It may be rapid over the course of several months or progress very slowly during a number of years. One patient who has been observed for 10 years with parafoveal lesions in each eye has had no spread of her disease to either fovea, and the lesions have remained unchanged during this period of observation. Only three patients, all with mild disease, showed spontaneous regression of their lesions with disappearance of traction lines, edema, and metamorphopsia. In progressive cases vision seldom drops below 20/200, only two of our patients, the one having a central scotoma and another, being in this category.

Progressive cases show intermittent increase in the preretinal fibrosis and traction on the superficial retina (Fig. 14-17). Fine white spots, very small yellow fatty exudates, small blot hemorrhages, and microaneurysms are sometimes seen. A fluorescein angiogram taken at this stage of the disease will sometimes show a delayed and diffuse leakage from retinal capillaries (Fig. 14-18). Leakage is mild and usually occurs in the area of densest fibrosis (Fig. 14-19) although some cases with moderately advanced fibrosis show no leakage.

Strands of the fibrosis may extend well away from the major lesion along the retinal surface (Fig. 14-20). Others wave freely with eye movements in the thin fluid well behind the posterior face of the detached vitreous. Some of these occasionally bridge over normal retina and become attached to the retina several disc diameters away. Posterior vitreous attachment to the retinal lesions has not been observed in any of our patients.

In the presence of such obvious, early, deep retinal edema, one would expect to see microcystic macular edema more frequently. Perhaps it is hidden by the fibrosis, for it can be seen occasionally, and larger macular cysts have been observed. These are never round, as they usually appear, but are eliptical or slit-like due to distortion by the contracting fibrosis.

On several occasions we have observed fine new vessels in the preretinal fibroses. These are hard to differentiate from the distorted retinal vessels involved in the fibrous contracture.

Microaneurysms elsewhere in the retina, mild halo sheathing of venous segments away from the lesion, and macular pigment disturbance are all rare and have been seen only with the severer lesions. No localized retinal detachment has been observed.

Fig. 14-17. Progressive preretinal macular fibrosis. *A*, As seen in a 64-year-old female with vision of 20/70 and a lesion of 3 years' duration. *B*, As seen in a 66-year-old female with vision of 20/200 and a lesion of 5 years' duration.

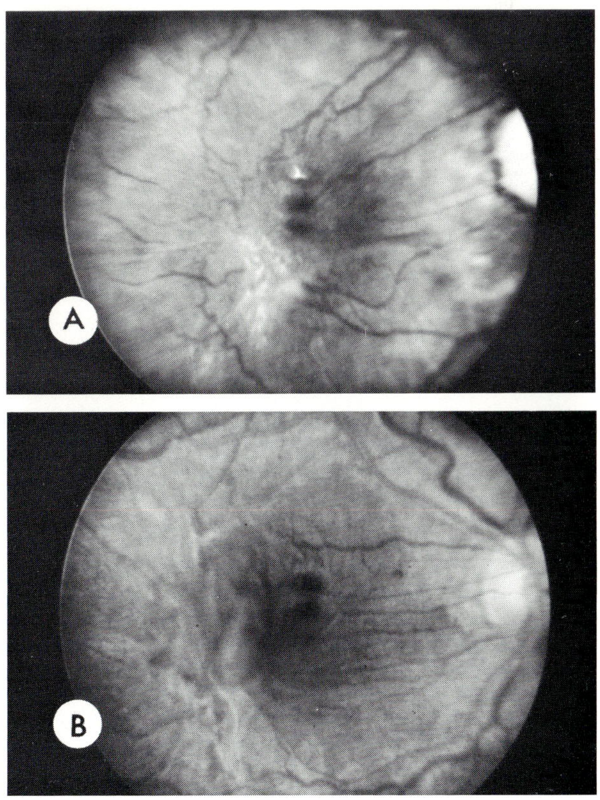

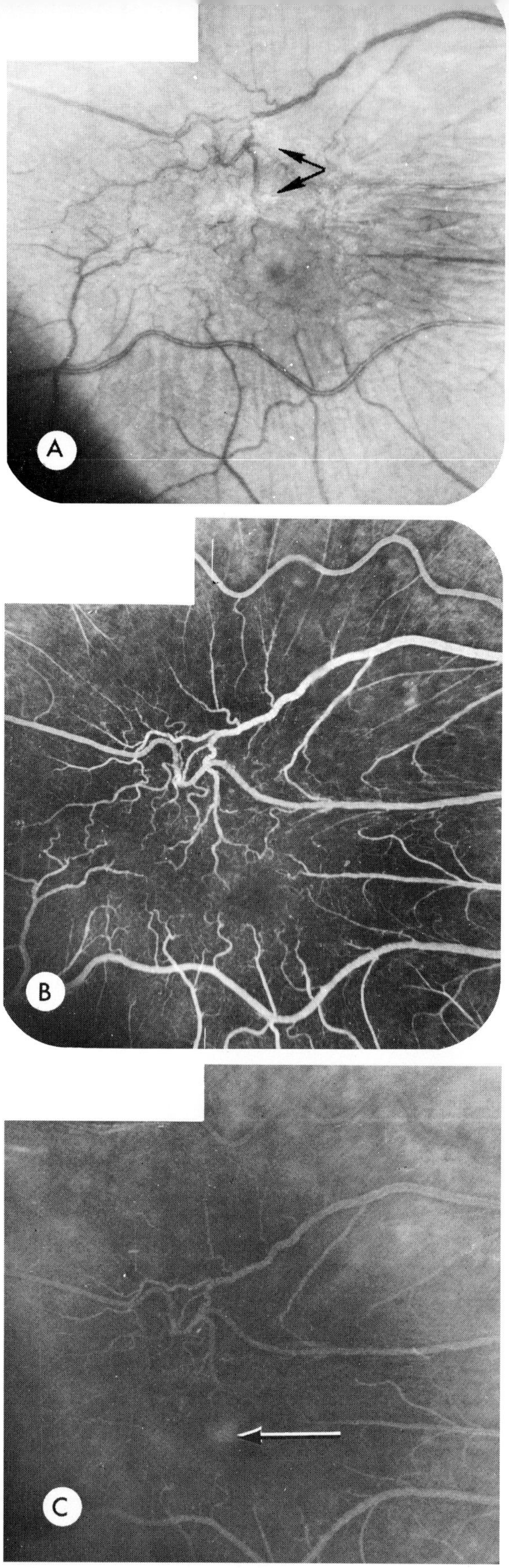

Fig. 14-18. *A*, Early preretinal macular fibrosis **(arrows)** with microcystic edema of the macula. *B*, Arteriovenous-phase fluorescein angiogram of *A*. *C*, Note late dye leakage from retinal perifoveal capillaries.

Fig. 14-19. *Opposite page. A*, Early preretinal macular fibrosis. Note the retinal traction lines, vascular distortion, and deep retinal hemorrhage **(arrow)**. *B*, Fluorescein angiogram of *A*. The superior vessels have filled before the inferior ones. Note beginning of leakage from retinal capillaries above the macula **(arrow)**. *C*, Later phase shows increased leakage **(arrow)**.

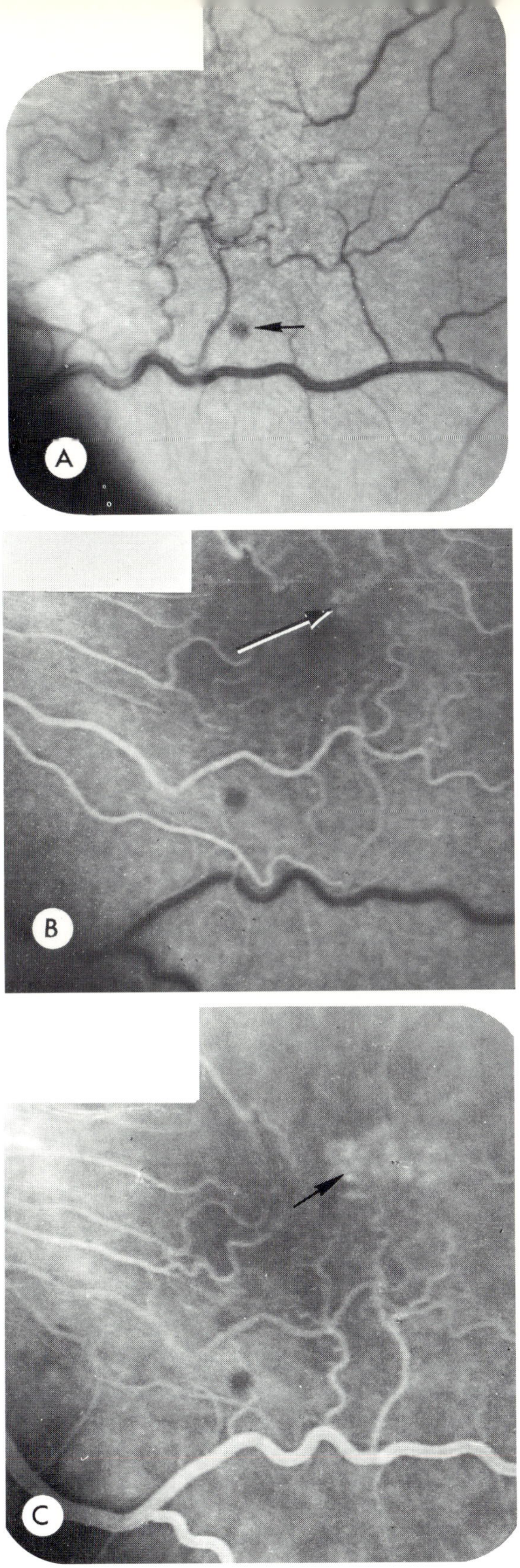

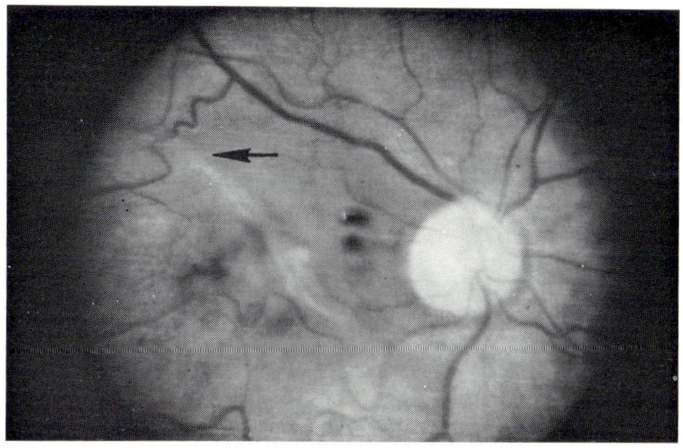

Fig. 14-20. *Above.* Preretinal macular fibrosis of about 2 years' duration in a 53-year-old female. Note retinal hemorrhage and the fibrosis extending well away from the major lesion **(arrow).**

Fig. 14-21. *Below.* Preretinal macular fibrosis in right eye following obstruction of a macular draining branch vein. Note deep retinal edema and retinal vascular distortion **(a),** preretinal macular fibrosis **(b),** and venous collaterals and microaneurysms temporal to the macula.

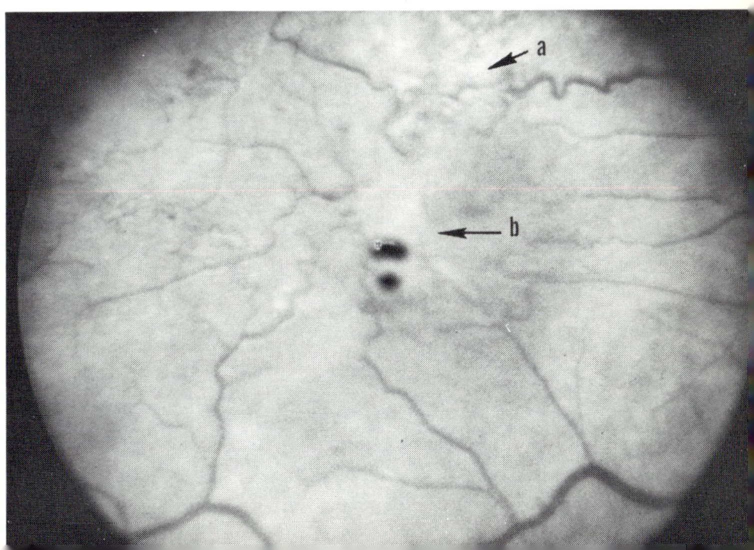

Kleinert's[118] is the earliest report of this condition which we have found in the literature. He has called it "primary retinal folds in the macular area." Red spots, radiating retinal folds, vascular distortion, and slowly increasing fibrosis were all seen in his 6 patients. The lesion has also been described as a manifestation of silent central retinal vein obstruction.[240] This concept of etiology is no longer held by the author. Maumenee[152] called the lesion "contraction" or "wrinkling" of the internal retinal surface. One case studied microscopically showed what was described as a split internal limiting membrane with a few cells between the two layers and wrinkling of the layer toward the retina.

DIFFERENTIAL DIAGNOSIS

Early nuclear cataract may reduce distant vision, make the macular area hard to see, and complicate proper early diagnosis. Nuclear cataract is usually associated with increasing myopia, normal visual acuity for near and a normal Amsler grid test.

Microcystic macular edema presents a honeycombed hillock at the macula with a larger central cyst at the fovea. There are no traction lines, distortion, or preretinal fibrosis. The fluorescein angiogram shows a late, characteristic, undistorted macular star pattern. The appearance of this microcystic macular edema following cataract extraction has been attributed to the tug of a vitreomacular adhesion.[184] Others have disputed the presence of such an adhesion in these cases.[84,244] The entirely different lesion of preretinal macular fibrosis, which may be discovered after cataract surgery, has been confused with this postoperative microcystic edema of the macula. In our opinion, the preretinal fibrosis in these patients had existed prior to surgery, and did not result from the operative procedure.

The Irvine syndrome[106] develops some time after cataract extraction. There is postoperative rupture of the vitreous face and the formation of a condensation band or "horse's tail" extending from the wound back through the pupil into the vitreous body. For months the eye is intermittently irritable with pain, photophobia, and lacrimation. The vitreous shrinks, vitreous opacities appear, and macular edema and degeneration (not described in detail by Irvine) ultimately develop. The visual acuity decreases and patients often note light flashes and a positive central scotoma.

This lesion was attributed to the tug of the anterior vitreous-wound adhesion, acting through the contracting vitreous body on the macula. A maculovitreous adhesion was thought necessary for its development. Irvine has stated, however, that the macular degeneration could result from an associated low-grade iridocyclitis.

Obstruction of any macular draining vein may be followed by preretinal macular fibrosis which cannot be differentiated from the preretinal macular fibrosis lesion under discussion (Fig. 14-21). If the vein has been a larger one, if the vein obstruction has been observed in its acute phase, or if there are sufficient remaining evidences of prior vein obstruction, then the etiologic diagnosis is obvious. On the other hand, mild and partial obstructions of one or more small macular draining veins may lead to preretinal macular fibrosis. These cases present a difficult problem in differential diagnosis.

ETIOLOGY

There are two major theories concerning the pathogenesis of preretinal macular fibrosis, one vitreal and the other retinal.

The vitreal concept assumes that the basic fault lies within the vitreous, which alters its state and undergoes shrinkage. Ultimately the posterior vitreous becomes detached from the optic disc, but for some reason an attachment of the vitreous to the macula persists. With ocular movements, a tug is exerted upon the macula due to the adhesion. The pull on the macula leads to macular edema, and a condensation and possibly proliferation of halocytes on the retinal surface.[107,215]

This concept probably arose from the widely held belief that vitreous retraction is primarily responsible for the fixed retinal folds occurring in cases of retinal detachment, especially postoperatively.[145] The star folds at the macula in such cases are very similar to the puckering of the macula produced in preretinal macular fibrosis. Klien[124] has demonstrated microscopically two cases of preretinal membranes with macular pucker which occurred following retinal detachment surgery. In both instances the preretinal membranes appeared to be retinal in origin, the vitreous being shrunken, detached, and well forward. There was no vitreomacular adhesion in either case. Both eyes showed retinal cellular elements extending along peripheral vitreous condensation bands. The tendency for proliferative retinopathy to adhere to an adjacent vitreous surface has been clearly demonstrated.[50]

Straatsma and Allen[214] have shown this same tendency for glial proliferation from the retina to extend along a condensation of vitreous at the edge of a liquified vitreous pocket overlying lattice degeneration. Wolter[247] has demonstrated fibrous and nuclear elements in the dense vitreous which overlay areas of paving-stone degeneration. The retinal vessels in these areas were hyalinized, and the fibrous structures were anchored firmly in the superficial retina, thus suggesting their retinal origin.

We believe in these cases that there is sufficient retinal vascular damage to induce fibrotic retinitis proliferans, and that the "vitreous condensations" or bands often contain fibrous and cellular elements derived from the retina secondary to its vascular derangement. As yet insufficient consideration has been given to the retinal circulation in cases of retinal detachment, especially those occurring after surgical procedures. Wood and Watzke[249] have demonstrated the ghosting of capillaries following photo- and laser coagulations of the retina. Retinal vascular damage also follows cryopexy.[248]

The retinal concept assumes a derangement leading to obstruction of retinal capillaries in the macular or paramacular area. This produces an indolent, predominantly fibrotic retinitis proliferans on the retinal surface. The contracture of the fibrosis leads to the inner retinal traction lines. As with so many retinovascular diseases, posterior vitreous detachment occurs at about the same time as the macular disease, but is unrelated to it.

The proponents of the vitreal theory do not see vitreomacular adhesions in all their patients, and some cases are progressive even after rupture of the adhesions.[107] The presence of an adhesiveness between the vitreous and the macula in the normal eye is very much disputed. In 100 cases of fresh, spontaneous, posterior vitreous detachments personally observed, no vitreomacular adhesion was noted in any case, and no macular pathology followed any detachment.

The presence of preretinal macular fibrosis after frank macular vein obstruction and its presence after signs suggesting indolent, chronic partial obstruction of small macular veins (dilated, dark, corkscrew veins distal to a crossing artery, and deep retinal edema) both imply some retinal capillary aberration in those cases in which macular vein obstruction cannot be determined. Finally, the presence of deep, retinal edema, prior to the development of traction lines strongly implicates the retinal circulation as the primary fault.

The presence or absence of delicate vitreomacular adhesions is a difficult determination to make even with contact lens and slit-lamp examination. This probably accounts for the diversity of opinion regarding their presence. The problem of etiology will remain unsettled until further microscopic material becomes available. Study of the early and delayed effects of retinal detachment surgery on the retinal circulation may also suggest etiologic clues.

TREATMENT

The treatment of this group of diseases often requires cooperation between internist and ophthalmologist. No attempt will be made to cover the systemic medical therapy. This section will be limited to those situations requiring no treatment, those requiring the guidance of the ophthalmologist, and those directly within his province.

Premature retinal arteriosclerosis without hypertension is often well tolerated by the eye for many years. In such patients, especially if they also have premature arcus senilis, it is well to alert the internist to the possibility of some lipid abnormality. Such patients may be carrying an elevated serum cholesterol or have some frank derangement of cholesterol metabolism such as ideopathic hypercholesteremia. Medical treatment of a prophylactic nature is indicated in these individuals.

Older patients with hypertensive retinopathy have some degree of associated arteriosclerosis. If there are hemorrhages and exudates or, in their absence, if the disease appears severe enough to suggest that the veins may be threatened in the future, the hypertension should be controlled. The treatment or nontreatment of hypertensive disease lies within the province of the internist, but a potentially threatening retinal situation could influence his decision.

There is no widely accepted regimen for the prevention of arteriosclerosis. As most present evidence suggests that elevated blood lipids play some part in its development, we suggest that these patients should avoid heavy fatty meals, take some form of regular mild exercise, and reduce any tendency to obesity. We have not observed the lipotropic drugs to be of value. Smoking should be avoided.

Central retinal artery occlusions due to arteriosclerosis cannot yet be prognosticated. The influence of arteriosclerosis on the veins at arteriovenous crossings or on the central vein at the lamina cribrosa, can either be directly visualized or be suggested by the retinal findings. Evidence of interference with venous drainage at any of these sites, such as the presence of Bonnet's prethrombosis sign or evidence of turbulence upon fluorescein angiography, does represent a potential source of trouble. Medical evaluation of such individuals is indicated. Any condition found such as diabetes, hypertension, hypercholesteremia, or polycythemia should be treated. An elevated hematocrit should be kept below 45 per cent. This is easily handled by periodic phlebotomy. Lowering the hematocrit alone has been observed to improve venous drainage in some cases.

Reasonable judgment is required, for crossing defects are commonly found, most of which will never create trouble. Only those defects in veins draining the macula represent a significant threat to vision. These patients should all be medically evaluated when there is significant evidence of venous insufficiency. (See section on Vein Obstruction Secondary to Arteriosclerosis.)

All patients seen after clinical or central retinal vein obstruction should have medical evaluation and treatment of those conditions which might have a bearing on the retinal situation. Once frank vein obstruction has occurred, anticoagulation should be considered. We have never advised this as prophylaxis against obstruction where signs of venous insufficiency were absent, nor do we now suggest anticoagulation in cases of branch vein obstruction. Our experience does suggest the value of anticoagulation in central retinal vein obstructions, especially in the incomplete obstructions or those seen shortly after onset. The reports of Klien and Olwin[128] and Klien,[119,127] and the statistical study of Vannas and Orma[220] are in agreement with this recommendation. The latter not only indicated less visual damage but also a lower incidence of late uncontrollable glaucoma in the anticoagulated cases.

The method and duration of anticoagulation therapy have varied considerably. Both heparin and the antiprothrombin group of drugs have been used and they have been given as long-term, short-term, and intermittent therapy. Short-term therapy of 10 days to 3 weeks' duration has been reported to be effective in some cases of stagnation thrombosis.[220] Long-term treatment may be started with heparin but is continued on an ambulant basis with one of the antiprothrombin drugs. The regimen and prothrombin levels are the same as those followed after coronary occlusion. This treatment should be handled medically and not by the ophthalmologist. It should be continued for a minimum of 6 months and, in some cases, may be necessary for 1 or 2 years. Reports[127,128,220] have suggested that long-term therapy is preferable and this is our own feeling. Bleeding is the only complication of this therapy. With properly selected cases, a competent laboratory, and a reliable patient, this complication can reasonably be risked.

In cases of central retinal vein obstruction, unrecognized chronic glaucoma should be excluded. If glaucoma is present in the eye with the vein obstruction, the second eye should be carefully watched for the development of glaucoma.[221]

Low molecular-weight dextran has been reported to be of value in the treatment of central retinal vein obstruction.[180] Due to its osmotic properties, dextran acts as a plasma expander, drawing fluid from the tissues into the vascular compartment. Both this and its de-aggregating effect on red blood cells tend to reduce the blood viscosity and improve the flow in the microcirculation. Dextran is also thought to have antithrombotic properties. This drug has had more use in general medicine than in ophthalmology and we have had no experience with it. It is not immediately excreted by the kidneys, does throw extra work upon the heart, and should not be given without careful medical supervision.

Fibrinolytic drugs have also had more use in general medicine than in ophthalmology. These drugs are not without side effects and are as yet of unproved value in the treatment of retinal vein occlusions.

Acute attacks of glaucoma with marked elevations of pressure should be vigorously and promptly treated. Sustained rises in pressure, even those of relatively short duration, can have a profoundly deleterious effect upon retinal and especially optic nerve vasculature. Every effort should be made to prevent glaucomatous cupping of the disc, for according to Dobree[54] cupping is more important than heights of pressure rise in the late central vein occlusions of chronic glaucoma.

In the inflammatory vein occlusions, treatment should be directed toward the primary inflammation rather than the secondary venous involvement. Steroids are of great value in some diseases such as sarcoidosis, nonspecific uveitis, and toxoplasmic retinochoroiditis. A relatively high dosage may be required, especially at first, but this can usually be reduced to manageable levels for more prolonged therapy, once the inflammation has shown signs of abating.

Elliot[67,68] has found that steroids administered subconjunctivally at intervals are of value in treating Eales's disease. Our experience with steroids administered either subconjunctivally or systemically in this disease has been disappointing. Donders[56] reported some success with surface diathermy over active areas of Eales's disease.

Where obvious sepsis has led to vein obstruction, as in orbital inflammations from the sinuses, vigorous antibiotic treatment is, of course, indicated.

The hyperviscosity diseases usually require medical treatment. The province of the ophthalmologist could be that of alerting the internist in suspected cases of macroglobulinemia, for here retinal changes are early and often marked.

In chronic leukemia significant infiltration of the optic nerve head should be treated with irradiation. One patient personally observed developed an elevated pale disc whose etiology and seriousness were not appreciated. This nerve ultimately became atrophic. When the same condition developed in the second eye, leukemic infiltration of the disc was presumed and the region was treated with irradiation. Clearing was rapid and vision was preserved in this eye.

Photocoagulation, introduced by Meyer-Schwickerath and best summarized in his book,[155] has already proved to be a most potent weapon against the newly formed vessels which develop following retinal venous and capillary obstructions of diverse etiologies. Neovascularization overlying the disc offers a serious problem with this form of treatment, but elsewhere throughout the retina, excepting in the macula, neovascular formations can be obliterated. Even the disc area may become treatable with further development of the argon laser.[140] Care must be exercised not to obliterate a brush of intraretinal collaterals, confusing them with preretinal neovascular formations. In cases of doubt, fluorescein angiography may aid in differentiating the two, for preretinal neovascularizations leak dye much more profusely than do intraretinal collaterals. Overtreatment must be avoided for it can lead to fibrosis, contracture, retinal traction lines, or local detachment. Bleeding from the fragile new vessels is another occasional complication of treatment. Fibrotic retinitis proliferans is a contraindication to treatment. Here, clinical judgment must be the guide, for minimal degrees of fibrosis among new vessels is amenable to photocoagulation.

In preretinal macular fibrosis, Wise and his colleagues[245] have reported limited success with laser photocoagulation. Treatment was undertaken to secure the edematous and thickened retina in closer apposition to its choroidal blood supply. It was also theoretically believed that destruction of the less visually important paramacular retinal elements would reduce the population of hypoxic retinal cells responsible for producing the preretinal fibrosis. In some cases the decrease in fibrosis over the untreated macula was observed and in one, all traction lines disappeared. Visual improvement, especially for near, was observed in some cases, and in these, metamorphopsia was less troublesome.

Treatment was carried out in a paramacular arc, approximately 1 dd in width and 0.75 dd from the fovea. Due to the distortion produced by the fibrosis, and the poor macular markings, great care in accurately locating the fovea before treatment must be exercised. Photographs of fluorescein angiograms should be at hand when treatment is undertaken. The papillomacular sector should be avoided. This report of only 7 patients is too small for definitive conclusions regarding this form of therapy.

Campbell and Wise[28] have successfully treated patients having peripheral choroiditis with photocoagulation and scleral depression. Welsh[233] has reported similar success in such cases with cryotherapy. The latter is much easier to perform, less likely to have such complications as iris burns, and is preferable. A combination of far peripheral cryosurgery and photocoagulation behind this has also been used.[28] Some patients require repeated treatments at intervals. In severe cases a course of steroids, while not completely suppressing the disease, will quiet it, clear the media to some extent, and possibly decrease the postoperative reaction. A decrease in the inflammation and clearing of microcystic macular edema with visual improvement occurs shortly after treatment. It is too soon for final evaluation of this form of therapy in such a chronic and stubborn disease.

REFERENCES

1. Ackerman, A. L.: The ocular manifestations of Waldenström's macroglobulinemia and its treatment. *Arch. Ophthal. 67:*701, 1962.
2. Allen, R. A., and Straatsma, B. R.: Ocular involvement in leukemia and allied disorders. *Arch. Ophthal. 66:*490, 1961.
3. Altschul, R.: *Endothelium, its Development, Morphology, Function and Pathology.* New York, MacMillan, 1954.
4. Anderson, B., and Samuelson, A.: A case of hyperglobulinemia with pronounced eye changes and acrocyanosis. *Acta Med. Scand. 117:*248, 1944.
5. Ashton, N.: Retinal microaneurysms in the non-diabetic subject. *Brit. J. Ophthal. 35:* 189, 1951.
6. Ashton, N.: Pathological basis of retrolental fibroplasia. *Brit. J. Ophthal. 38:*385, 1954.
7. Ashton, N.: Panel discussion. The prevention and management of retrolental fibroplasia *XVII.* Internat. Cong. Ophth. New York, September, 1954. Vol. I. p. 2.
8. Ashton, N.: Retrolental fibroplasia. *Amer. J. Ophthal. 39:*153, 1955.
9. Ashton, N.: *Pathogenesis and Aetiology of Eales's Disease.* 19th International Congress of Ophthalmology. New Delhi, India 1962. Ed. by Pandit, Y. K. Bombay, The Times of India Press 1962, Vol. *II,* p. 828.
10. Ashton, N.: Ocular changes in multiple myelomatosis. *Arch. Ophthal. 73:*487, 1965.
11. Ashton, N., and Cook, C.: Direct observation of the effect of oxygen on developing vessels. *Brit. J. Ophthal. 38:*433, 1954.
12. Ashton, N., and Cook, C.: Studies on developing retinal vessels *I.* Influence of retinal detachment. *Brit. J. Ophthal. 39:*449, 1955.
13. Ashton, N., Kok, D'A., and Foulds, W. S.: Ocular pathology in macroglobulinaemia. *J. Path. Bact. 86:*453, 1963.
14. Ashton, N., and Pedler, C.: Studies on developing retinal vessels *IX.* Reaction of endothelial cells to oxygen. *Brit. J. Ophthal. 46:*257, 1962.
15. Ashton, N., Ward, B., and Serpell, G.: Role of oxygen in the genesis of retrolental fibroplasia. *Brit. J. Ophthal. 37:*513, 1953.
16. Ashton, N., Ward, B., and Serpell, G.: Effect of oxygen on developing retinal vessels with particular reference to the problem of retrolental fibroplasia. *Brit. J. Ophthal. 38:* 397, 1954.
17. Ballantyne, A. J., and Michaelson, I. C.: *The Fundus of the Eye.* Baltimore, Md., Williams & Wilkins, 1962. p. 200.
18. Beck, A., Hutchings, M. W., Makay, A. R., and Tuck, I. M.: Infection with cryptococcus neoformans in man. Report of 2 cases. *Lancet 1:*535, 1955.
19. Behrman, S.: Retinal vein obstruction. *Brit. J. Ophthal. 46:*336, 1962.
20. Blatt, N.: Eye findings in malaria. *Klin. Mbl. Augenheilk. 80:*468, 1928.
21. Boniuk, M., and Burton, G. L.: Unilateral glaucoma associated with sickle-cell retinopathy. *Trans. Amer. Acad. Ophthal. Otolaryng. 68:*316, 1964.
22. Bonnet, P.: The prethrombosis sign observed in retinal vessels in arterial hypertension: its semeiologic value. *Arch. Ophtal.* (Paris) *11:*12, 1951.
23. Borgeson, E. J., and Wagener, H. P.: Changes in the eye in leukemia. *Amer. J. Med. Sci. 177:*663, 1929.
24. Braendstrup, P.: Central retinal vein thrombosis and hemorrhagic glaucoma. *Acta Ophthal. (Suppl. 35):*1, 1950.
25. Brockhurst, R. J., Schepens, C. L., and Okamura, I. D.: Uveitis *II.* Peripheral uveitis: clinical description, complications and differential diagnosis. *Amer. J. Ophthal. 49:*1257, 1960.

26. Brockhurst, R. J., Schepens, C. L., and Okamura, I. D.: Uveitis *III*. Peripheral uveitis: pathogenesis, etiology and treatment. *Amer. J. Ophthal. 51:*19, 1961.

27. Bruce, G. M., Denning, C. R., and Spalter, H. F.: Ocular findings in cystic fibrosis of the pancreas. *Arch. Ophthal. 63:*391, 1960.

28. Campbell, C. J., and Wise, G. N.: Unpublished data.

29. Campbell, K.: Intensive oxygen therapy as possible cause of retrolental fibroplasia: a clinical approach. *Med. J. Aust. 2:*48, 1951.

30. Carr, R. E., and Henkind, P.: Retinal findings associated with serum hyperviscosity. *Amer. J. Ophthal. 56:*23, 1963.

31. Chamberlain, W. P.: Ocular findings in scrub typhus. *Arch. Ophthal. 48:*313, 1952.

32. Cibis, P. A., and Yamashita, T.: Part *II*. Experimental aspects of ocular siderosis and hemosiderosis. *Amer. J. Ophthal. 48:* 465, 1959.

33. Coats, G.: Part *I*. Thrombosis of the central vein of the retina. *Roy. London Ophthal. Hosp. Rep. 16:*62, 1904.

34. Coats, G.: Part *IV*. Further cases of thrombosis of the central vein. *Roy. London Ophthal. Hosp. Rep. 16:*516, 1906.

35. Coats, G.: Part *III*. Forms of retinal disease with massive exudation. *Roy. London Ophthal. Hosp. Rep. 17:*440, 1908.

36. Coats, G.: Über Retinitis exsudativa (Retinitis hemorrhagica externa). *Arch. Ophth. 86:*275, 1912.

37. Coats, G.: Discussion on retinal vascular disease: Pathological aspects. *Trans. Ophthal. Soc. U.K. 33:*30, 1913.

38. Coats, G.: Der Verschluss der Zentralvene der Retina: Eine Übersich 36 pathologisch-anatomisch untersuchter Fälle. *Arch. Ophth. 86:*341, 1913.

39. Cogan, D. G.: Development and senescence of human retinal vasculature. *Trans. Ophthal. Soc. U.K. 83:*465, 1963.

40. Cogan, D. G., and Kuwabara, T.: Ocular pathology of the 13–15 trisomy syndrome. *Arch. Ophthal. 72:*246, 1964.

41. Cole, J. G., and Cole, H. G.: Incontinentia pigmenti associated with changes in the posterior chamber of the eye. *Amer. J. Ophthal. 47:*321, 1959.

42. Crick, R. P.: Ocular sarcoidosis. *Trans. Ophthal. Soc. U.K. 75:*189, 1955.

43. Cross, A. G.: Ocular sarcoidosis. *Trans. Ophthal. Soc. U.K. 75:*181, 1955.

44. Crosse, V. M., and Evans, P. J.: Prevention of retrolental fibroplasia. *Arch. Ophthal. 48:*83, 1952.

45. Culler, A. M.: War injuries of the eye. *U. S. Naval Med. Bull. 41:*1557, 1943.

46. Culler, A. M.: Fundus changes in leukemia. *Trans. Amer. Ophthal. Soc. 49:*445, 1951.

47. Cunha-Vaz, J. G.: Studies on the permeability of the blood-retinal barrier *III*. Breakdown of the blood-retinal barrier by circulatory disturbances. A topographical study of the vascular tree. *Brit. J. Ophthal. 50:* 505, 1966.

48. Curtin, V. T., Joyce, E. E., and Ballin, N.: Part *II*. Ocular pathology in the oculo-cerebro-renal syndrome of Lowe. *Amer. J. Ophthal. 64:*533, 1967.

49. Danis, M.: Ocular lesions in polycythemia. *Mem. Acad. Roy. Med. Belg. 1:*1, 1941.

50. Davis, M. D.: Vitreous contraction in proliferative diabetic retinopathy. *Arch. Ophthal. 74:*741, 1965.

51. Davis, T. S.: Malarial blindness, with a report of six cases. *New Orleans Med. Surg. J. 61:*501, 1908.

52. Delaney, W. V., Jr., and Liaricos, S. V.: Chorioretinal destruction in multiple myeloma. *Amer. J. Ophthal. 66:*52, 1968.

53. Dintenfass, L: Viscosity of the packed red and white blood cells. *Exp. Molec. Path. 4:* 597, 1965.

54. Dobree, J. H.: Venous obstruction and neovascularization at the disc in chronic glaucoma. *Trans. Ophthal. Soc. U.K. 77:*229, 1957.

55. Doherty, W. B.: Some of the most important ocular and orbital wounds in war. *Amer. J. Ophthal. 25:*135, 1942.

56. Donders, P. C.: Eales' disease. *Docum. Ophthal. 12:*1, 1958.

57. Donnelly, E. J.: Ocular complications of multiple myelomatosis. *Amer. J. Ophthal. 47:*211, 1959.

58. Dudgeon, L. S.: A case of malignant malaria. *Trans. Ophthal. Soc. U. K. 41:*236, 1921.

59. Duke, J. R., Wilkinson, C. P., and Sigelman, S.: Retinal microaneurysms in leukemia. *Brit. J. Ophthal. 52:*368, 1968.

60. Duke-Elder, S.: *System of Ophthalmology.*

Congenital Deformities. London, Kimpton, 1964, Vol. III, pt. 2, p. 488.

61. Duke-Elder, S.: *System of Ophthalmology. Congenital Deformities,* London, Kimpton, 1964, Vol. III, pt. 2, p. 634.
62. Duke-Elder, S.: *System of Ophthalmology. Diseases of the Retina.* London, Kimpton, 1967, Vol. X, p. 114.
63. Duke-Elder, S.: *System of Ophthalmology. Diseases of the Retina.* London, Kimpton, 1967, Vol. X, p. 189.
64. Duke-Elder, S.: *System of Ophthalmology. Diseases of the Retina.* London, Kimpton, 1967, Vol. X, pp. 221–222.
65. Duke-Elder, S.: *System of Ophthalmology. Diseases of the Retina.* London, Kimpton, 1967, Vol. X, p. 384.
66. Eales, H.: Cases of retinal hemorrhage associated with epistaxis and constipation. *Birmingham Med. Rev. 9:*262, 1880.
67. Elliot, A. J.: Recurrent intraocular hemorrhage in young adults (Eales' disease). *Trans. Amer. Ophthal. Soc. 52:*811, 1954.
68. Elliot, A. J.: Recurrent intraocular hemorrhage in young adults (Eales' disease) with continuous subconjunctival therapy with hydrocortisone. *Trans. Amer. Ophthal. Soc. 56:*383, 1958.
69. Ennema, M. C., and Zeeman, W. P.: Venous occlusions in the retina. *Ophthalmologica 126:*329, 1953.
70. Evans, P. J.: Retrolental fibroplasia. *Trans. Ophthal. Soc. U. K. 71:*613, 1951.
71. Fahey, J. L., Barth, W. F., and Solomon, A.: Serum hyperviscosity syndrome. *JAMA 192:*464, 1965.
72. Faris, B. M., and Brockhurst, R. J.: Retrolental fibroplasia in the cicatricial stage. The complication of rhegmatogenous retinal detachment. *Arch. Ophthal. 82:*60, 1969.
73. Fenton, R. H., and Easom, H. A.: Behçet's syndrome. A histopathologic study of the eye. *Arch. Ophthal. 72:*71, 1964.
74. Ferguson, R. H., and Paris, J.: Sarcoidosis: study of twenty-nine cases with a review of splenic, hepatic, mucous membrane, retinal and joint manifestations. *Arch. Intern. Med. 101:*1065, 1958.
75. Fine, M., and Flocks, M.: Bilateral acute neuroretinitis with sarcoidosis treated with corticotropin and cortisone. *Arch. Ophthal. 50:*358, 1953.
76. Fink, A. I., Tsunematsu, M., and Kaplan, D.: Conjunctival blood flow in cryoglobulinemia. *Arch. Ophthal. 71:*787, 1964.
77. Fisher, J. H.: Connective tissue on the central part of the retina in a patient who has suffered from malaria, the organization having taken place in all probability in a film of blood extravasated from an obstructed retinal vein. *Trans. Ophthal. Soc. U. K. 41:*235, 1921.
78. Foggitt, K. D.: Ocular disease due to brucellosis. *Brit. J. Ophthal. 38:*273, 1954.
79. Franceschetti, A., and Babel, J.: La choriorétinite en "taches de bougie" manifestation de la maladie de Besnier-Boeck. *Ophthalmologica 118:*701, 1949.
80. Friedenwald, H.: Über jugendliche Netzhaut und Glaskörper-blutungen durch sichtbare. Netzhautvenenerkraukungen bedingt: *Centrabl. Prakt. Augenheilk. 20:*33, 1896.
81. Friedenwald, J. S.: Symposium: Retrolental fibroplasia pathology. *Trans. Amer. Acad. Ophthal. Otolaryng. 59:*11, 1955.
82. Friedenwald, J. S., Owens, W. C., and Owens, E. N.: Retrolental fibroplasia in premature infants: III. Pathology of the disease. *Trans. Amer. Ophthal. Soc. 49:*207, 1952.
83. Fuchs, E.: Ueber veranderungen des Schnerven bei ektogener intraokularer Entzündung. *Arch. Ophth. 91:*1, 1915.
84. Gass, J. D. M., and Norton, E. W. D.: Fluorescein studies of patients with macular edema and papilledema following cataract extraction. *Trans. Amer. Ophthal. Soc. 64:* 232, 1966.
85. Gates, R. F., and Richards, R. D.: Macroglobulinemia with unusual vascular changes. *Arch. Ophthal. 64:*77, 1960.
86. Geeraets, W. J., and Guerry, D. III: Angioid streaks and sickle-cell disease. *Amer. J. Ophthal. 49:*450, 1960.
87. Geeraets, W. J., and Guerry, D. III: Elastic tissue degeneration in sickle-cell disease. *Amer. J. Ophthal. 50:*213, 1960.
88. Gibson, G. G., and Smith, L. W.: Retinal phlebosclerosis. *Arch. Ophthal. 26:*840, 1941.
89. Gilbert, W.: Concerning periphlebitis and endovasculitis of the retinal vessels, also remarks on sclerotic, tuberculous and septicemic choroidal disease. *Klin. Mbl. Augenheilk. 94:*335, 1935.
90. Goldberg, S., and Newell, F. W.: Sarcoidosis

with retinal involvement. *Arch. Ophthal. 32:*93, 1944.

91. Goodman, G., von Sallman, L., and Holland, M. G.: Ocular manifestations of sickle-cell disease. *Arch. Ophthal. 58:*655, 1957.
92. Gould, H. L., and Kaufman, H. E.: Boeck's sarcoid of the ocular fundus. *Amer. J. Ophthal. 52:*633, 1961.
93. Gould, H., and Kaufman, H. E.: Sarcoid of the fundus. *Arch. Ophthal. 65:*453, 1961.
94. Gyllensten, L. J., and Hellström, B. E.: Retrolental fibroplasia: animal experiments – the effect of intermittently administered oxygen on the post-natal development of the eyes of fullterm mice; a preliminary report. *Acta Paediat. 41:*577, 1952.
95. Gyllensten, L. J., and Hellström, B. E.: Experimental approach to the pathogenesis of retrolental fibroplasia. *Amer. J. Ophthal. 39:*475, 1955.
96. Gyllensten, L. J., and Hellström, B. E.: Experimental approach to the pathogenesis of retrolental fibroplasia. III. Changes in the eye induced by exposure of newborn mice to general hypoxia. *Brit. J. Ophthal. 39:*409, 1955.
97. Hager, H.: Thromboangiitis obliterans and the eye. *Klin. Mbl. Augenheilk. 114:*238, 1949.
98. Harrell, G. T.: Rocky mountain spotted fever. *Medicine 28:*333, 1949.
99. Hayreh, S. S.: Occlusion of the central retinal vessels. *Brit. J. Ophthal. 49:*626, 1965.
100. Heath, P.: Retrolental fibroplasia as a syndrome. *Arch. Ophthal. 44:*245, 1950.
101. Heath, P.: Pathology of the retinopathy of prematurity: retrolental fibroplasia. *Amer. J. Ophthal. 34:*1249, 1951.
102. Hogan, M. J., and Kimura, S. J.: Cyclitis and peripheral chorioretinitis. *Arch. Ophthal. 66:*667, 1961.
103. Hook, E. W., and Cooper, G. R.: The clinical manifestations of sickle-cell hemoglobin C disease and sickle-cell anemia. *Southern Med. J. 51:*610, 1958.
104. Hope-Robertson, W. J.: Thrombosis of the central retinal vein following injury: report of two cases. *Trans. Ophthal. Soc. N.Z. 6:*22, 1952.
105. Hunter, W. S., and Zimmerman, L. E.: Unilateral retinal dysplasia. *Arch. Ophthal. 74:*23, 1965.
106. Irvine, S. R.: A newly defined vitreous syndrome following cataract surgery. *Amer. J. Ophthal. 36:*599, 1953.
107. Jaffe, N. S.: Macular retinopathy after separation of vitreoretinal adherence. *Arch. Ophthal. 78:*585, 1967.
108. Jebejian, R., and Kalfayan, B.: Le syndrome oculo-bucco-génital. *Ann. Oculist. 179:*481, 1946.
109. Jefferson, M., and Cloake, P. C. P.: Nervous manifestations in Eales' disease. *Brit. J. Ophthal. 36:*143, 1952.
110. Jensen, V. A.: Clinical studies of tributary thrombosis in the central retinal vein. *Acta Ophthal. (Suppl. X):*1, 1936.
111. Jones, B. R.: Acute retinal periphlebitis associated with infectious mononucleosis. *Trans. Ophthal. Soc. U.K. 74:*119, 1954.
112. Kahán, A., Kahán, I. L., Benko, A., and Mindszenti, S.: Erythrocytic anomalies in hereditary vitreo-retinal degeneration (degeneratio hyaloidoretinalis). *Brit. J. Ophthal. 47:*620, 1963.
113. Kearns, T. P.: Changes in the ocular fundus in blood diseases. *Med. Clin. N. Amer. 40:*1209, 1956.
114. Kiep, W. H.: Ocular complications occurring in malaria. *Trans. Ophthal. Soc. U.K. 42:*394, 1922.
115. Kimura, S. J., Carriker, F. R., and Hogan, M. J.: Retinal vasculitis with intraocular hemorrhage. Classification and results of special studies. *Arch. Ophthal. 56:*361, 1956.
116. Kimura, S. J., and Hogan, M. J.: Chronic cyclitis. *Arch. Ophthal. 71:*193, 1964.
117. Kinsey, V. E., and Hemphill, F. M.: Symposium: retrolental fibroplasia. Etiology of retrolental fibroplasia and preliminary report of cooperative study of retrolental fibroplasia. *Trans. Amer. Acad. Ophthal. Otolaryng. 59:*15, 1955.
118. Kleinert, H.: Primäre Netzhaut-fältelung im Maculaberrich. *Arch. Ophth. 155:*350, 1954.
119. Klien, B. A.: Anticoagulant therapy of occlusion of central vein of the retina in relation to pathogenesis and differential diagnosis. *Arch. Ophthal. 29:*699, 1943.
120. Klien, B. A. Personal communication.
121. Klien, B. A.: Obstruction of the central retinal vein. *Amer. J. Ophthal. 27:*1339, 1944.
122. Klien, B. A.: Prevention of retinal venous occlusion. *Amer. J. Ophthal. 33:*175, 1950.

123. Klien, B. A.: Occlusion of the central retinal vein: clinical importance of certain histopathologic observations. *Amer. J. Ophthal. 36:*316, 1953.

124. Klien, B. A.: Concerning the pathogenesis of retinal holes. *Amer. J. Ophthal. 40:*515, 1955.

125. Klien, B. A.: Retinal lesions associated with uveal disease.: Part *I. Amer. J. Ophthal. 42:*831, 1956.

126. Klien, B. A.: Spontaneous vascular repair. *Amer. J. Ophthal. 50:*691, 1960.

127. Klien, B. A.: Sidelights on retinal venous occlusion. *Amer. J. Ophthal. 61:*25, 1966.

128. Klien, B. A., and Olwin, J. H.: A survey of the pathogenesis of retinal venous occlusion. *Arch. Ophthal. 56:*207, 1956.

129. Knapp, A.: Retinal periphlebitis in the course of acute exudative choroiditis. *Arch. Ophthal. 26:*750, 1941.

130. Knapp, H.: Emolie eines Zweiges der Netzhautarterie mit hämorrhagischem drefarkt in der Netzhaut. *Arch. Ohr. Kehlkopfheilk. 1:*29, 1869.

131. Kopp, W. L., Bevine, G. J., and Burns, R. O.: Hyperviscosity syndrome in multiple myeloma. *Amer. J. Med. 43:*141, 1967.

132. Kornzweig, A. L., Eliasoph, I., and Feldstein, M.: The retinal vasculature in macular degeneration. *Arch. Ophthal. 75:*326, 1966.

133. Krause, A. C.: Congenital encephalo-ophthalmic dysplasia. *Arch. Ophthal. 36:*387, 1946.

134. Kroll, A. J.: Experimental central retinal artery occlusion. *Arch. Ophthal. 79:*453, 1968.

135. Kuwabara, T., and Aiello, L.: Leukemic miliary nodules in the retina. *Arch. Ophthal. 72:*494, 1964.

136. Kuwabara, T., Carroll, J. M., and Cogan, D. G.: Retinal vascular patterns: Part III. Age, hypertension, absolute glaucoma and injury. *Arch. Ophthal. 65:*708, 1961.

137. Lagrange, F.: *Fractures of the Orbit and Injuries to the Eye in War.* London, Univer. of London Press, 1918, p. 134.

138. Landau, J.: Vasculitis retinae in leprosy. *Amer. J. Ophthal. 51:*831, 1961.

139. Landers, P. H.: Vitreous lesions observed in Boeck's sarcoid. *Amer. J. Ophthal. 32:*1740, 1949.

140. L'Esperance, F. A.: An ophthalmic argon laser photocoagulation system: design, construction and laboratory investigations. *Trans. Amer. Ophthal. Soc. 66:*827, 1968.

141. Lester, A., and Zwink, F. B.: The course of thrombosis of the retinal veins. *Trans. Ophthal. Soc. U.K. 73:*55, 1953.

142. Levitt, J. M.: Boeck's sarcoid with ocular localization. *Arch. Ophthal. 26:*358, 1941.

143. Lieb, W. A., Geeraets, W. J., and Guerry, D. III: Sickle-cell retinopathy. *Acta Ophthal. (Suppl. 58)* 1959.

144. Lieb, W. A., and Guerry, D. III: Fundus changes in incontinentia pigmenti. *Amer. J. Ophthal. 45:*265, 1958.

145. Lincoff, H. A., and McLean, J. M.: Cryosurgical treatment of retinal detachment. Part II. *Amer. J. Ophthal. 61:*1227, 1966.

146. Locke, J. C.: Retrolental fibroplasia. *Arch. Ophthal. 51:*73, 1954.

147. Loewenstein, A., Michaelson, I. C., and Hill, J.: Retinal vasculitis of the young: a pathological report. *Trans. Ophthal. Soc. U.K. 66:*211, 1946.

148. MacDonald, A. E.: Boeck's sarcoid of the retina-miliary form. *Trans. Amer. Ophthal. Soc. 41:*200, 1943.

149. Manschot, W. A.: Etiology of retrolental fibroplasia. *Arch. Ophthal. 52:*833, 1954.

150. Mann, I.: *Developmental Abnormalities of the Eye.* Philadelphia, Lippincott, 1958.

151. Mamo, J. G., and Baghdassarian, A.: Behçet's disease. A report of 28 cases. *Arch. Ophthal. 71:*4, 1964.

152. Maumenee, A. E.: Fluorescein angiography in the diagnosis and treatment of lesions of the ocular fundus. *Trans. Ophthal. Soc. U.K. 88:*529, 1968.

153. Mavioğlu, H.: Behçet's recurrent disease. Analytical review of the literature. *Missouri Med. 55:*1209, 1958.

154. Merriam, G. R., Jr.: Retinoblastoma. Analysis of seventeen autopsies: one case reported at 16 years of age. *Arch. Ophthal. 44:*71, 1950.

155. Meyer-Schwickerath, G.: *Light Coagulation.* (Tr. by Drance, S.). St. Louis, Mosby, 1960.

156. Michaelson, I. C.: Traversing intraocular foreign bodies with retinal detachment. *Trans. Ophthal. Soc. U.K. 66:*193, 1946.

157. Michaelson, I. C.: *Retinal Circulation in Man and Animals.* Springfield, Ill. Thomas, 1954.

158. Michaelson, I. C., and Kraus, J.: War injuries of the eye: traumatic proliferative choroiditis due to double penetrating foreign body. *Brit. J. Ophthal. 27:*448, 1943.

159. Miller, M., Robbins, J., Fishman, R., Medenis, R., and Rosenthal, I.: A chromosomal anomaly with multiple ocular defects. *Amer. J. Ophthal. 55:*901, 1963.

160. Mortada, A., and Imam, I. Z. E.: Virus aetiology of Behçet's syndrome. *Brit. J. Ophthal. 48:*250, 1964.

161. Motegi, A., Kan, I., Kó, S., and Syú, S.: Ophthalmological observations of 100 cases of patients with malaria. *Klin. Mbl. Augenheilk. 92:*797, 1934.

162. Munro, S., and Walker, C.: Ocular complications in sickle-cell hemoglobin C disease. *Brit. J. Ophthal. 44:*1, 1960.

163. Myerson, R. M., Harrison, E., and Lohmuller, H. W.: Incidence and significance of abnormal hemoglobins. *Amer. J. Med. 26:* 543, 1959.

164. Nagy, F.: Changes in the fundus caused by polycythemia. *Brit. J. Ophthal. 34:*380, 1950.

165. Owens, W. C., and Owens, E. N.: Retrolental fibroplasia in premature infants. *Amer. J. Ophthal. 32:*1, 1949.

166. Parker, A. E. P.: Complete thrombosis of retinal veins followed by recovery of vision. *Trans. Ophthal. Soc. U.K. 59:*420, 1939.

167. Parsons, H. J.: Partial thrombosis of the central vein. *Trans. Ophthal. Soc. U.K. 27:* 121, 1907.

168. Paton, D.: Angioid streaks and sickle-cell anemia. *Arch. Ophthal. 62:*852, 1959.

169. Paton, R. T.: Recurrent retinal and vitreous hemorrhages in the young-Eales' disease. *Arch. Ophthal. 20:*276, 1938.

170. Payne, B. F.: Ocular contusions in national emergencies. *JAMA 142:*243, 1950.

171. Patz, A.: Oxygen studies in retrolental fibroplasia. *Amer. J. Ophthal. 38:*291, 1954.

172. Patz, A.: Symposium: Retrolental fibroplasia. Experimental studies. *Trans. Amer. Acad. Ophthal. Otolaryng. 59:*25, 1955.

173. Patz, A.: Role of oxygen in retrolental fibroplasia. *Trans. Amer. Ophthal. Soc. 66:*940, 1968.

174. Patz, A., Eastham, A., Higginbotham, D. A., and Kleh, T.: Oxygen studies in retrolental fibroplasia. *Amer. J. Ophthal. 36:*1511, 1953.

175. Patz, A., Hoeck, L. E., and de la Cruz, E.: Studies on the effect of high oxygen administration in retrolental fibroplasia. *Amer. J. Ophthal. 35:*1248, 1952.

176. Pietruschka, G.: Ueber Klinische Beobachtungen bei Iridozyklitis, insbesondere hinsichlich der Fundus-veränderungen. *Klin. Mbl. Augenheilk. 124:*309, 1954.

177. Presley, G. D.: Fundus changes in Rocky Mountain spotted fever. *Amer. J. Ophthal. 67:*263, 1969.

178. Raab, E. L., Leopold, I. H., and Hodes, H. L.: Retinopathy in Rocky Mountain spotted fever. *Amer. J. Ophthal. 68:*42, 1969.

179. Rabinowicz, I. M., Litman, S., and Michaelson, I.C.: Branch venous thrombosis – a pathological report. *Trans. Ophthal. Soc. U.K. 88:*191, 1968.

180. Radnot, M., and Follmann, P.: Rheo-macrodex (dextran) in the treatment of the occlusion of the central retinal vein. *Ann. Ophthal. 1:*58, 1969.

181. Reese, A. B.: Persistent hyperplastic primary vitreous. *Amer. J. Ophthal. 40:*317, 1955.

182. Reese, A. B.: Telangiectasia of the retina and Coats' disease. *Amer. J. Ophthal. 42:*1, 1956.

183. Reese, A. B., Blodi, F. C., and Locke, J. C.: The pathology of early retrolental fibroplasia. *Amer. J. Ophthal. 35:*1407, 1952.

184. Reese, A. B., Jones, I. S., and Cooper, W. C.: Macular changes secondary to vitreous traction. *Trans. Amer. Ophthal. Soc. 64:*123, 1966.

185. Reese, A. B., King, M. J., and Owens, W. C.: A classification of retrolental fibroplasia. *Amer. J. Ophthal. 36:*1333, 1953.

186. Reese, A. B., and Straatsma, B. R.: Retinal dysplasia. Part II. *Amer. J. Ophthal. 45:*199, 1958.

187. Reimann, H. A.: Hyperproteinemia as a cause of auto-hemagglutination. *JAMA 99:* 1411, 1932.

188. Rosen, E. S., Simmons, A. V., and Warnes, T. W.: Retinopathy of Waldenström's macroglobulinemia: photographic assessment. *Amer. J. Ophthal. 65:*696, 1968.

189. Rudd, C., Evans, P. J., and Peeney, A. L. P.: Ocular complications in thalassemia minor. *Brit. J. Ophthal. 37:*353, 1953.

190. Salzmann, M.: Part 4. Prepapillary proliferation of connective tissue in glaucoma

and its relation to retinitis proliferans. *Arch. Ophth. 140:*629, 1939.

191. Samuels, B.: Chronic post-operative or post-traumatic retinitis (retinitis serosa). *Amer. J. Ophthal. 19:*493, 1936.

192. Sanders, M. D., and Hoyt, W. F.: Hypoxic ocular sequellae of carotid-cavernous fistulae. *Brit. J. Ophthal. 53:*82, 1969.

193. Sanders, T. E., Podos, S. M., and Rosenbaum, L. J.: Intraocular manifestations of multiple myeloma. *Arch. Ophthal. 77:*789, 1967.

194. Scheie, H. G.: Ocular changes associated with scrub typhus. *Arch. Ophthal. 40:*245, 1948.

195. Schmid, A. E.: The relation of periphlebitis retinae and recurrent juvenile vitreous hemorrhages to thromboangiitis obliterans (Buerger's disease). *Ophthalmologica 110:* 259, 1945.

196. Schmid, A. E., and von Albertini, A. V.: Conditions of the ocular vessels in endarteritis obliterans (Winiwater-Buerger). *Ophthalmologica 113:*129, 1947.

197. Schwab, P. J., Okun, E., and Fahey, J. L.: Reversal of retinopathy in Waldenström's macroglobulinemia by plasmapheresis. A report of two cases. *Arch. Ophthal. 64:*515, 1960.

198. Sezer, F. N.: The isolation of a virus as the cause of Behçet's disease. *Amer. J. Ophthal. 36:*301, 1953.

199. Sezer, N.: Further investigations on the virus of Behçet's disease. *Amer. J. Ophthal. 41*:41, 1956.

200. Seidel, E.: Zur Entstehung des Krankheitsbildes der Thrombose der Vena centralis retinae. *Arch. Ophth. 141:*151, 1939.

201. Seitz, R.: *The Retinal Vessels.* (Tr. by Blodi, F. C.) St. Louis, Mo., Mosby, 1964.

202. Shakib, M.: Personal communication.

203. Shikano, S.: A histopathological study of Behçet's disease. *Jap. J. Ophthal. 5:*54, 1961.

204. Shikano, S., and Shimizu, K.: *Atlas of Fluorescence Fundus Angiography.* Philadelphia, Saunders, 1968, p. 136.

205. Shimkin, N. I.: Ophthalmic injuries in war. *Brit. J. Ophthal. 24:*265, 1940.

206. Sifverskiöld, R. P.: Retinal periphlebitis associated with paraplegia. *Arch. Neurol. Psychiat. 57:*351, 1947.

207. Solanes, M. Puig, Heatley, J., Arenas, F., and Ibarra, G. G.: Ocular complications in brucellosis. *An. Soc. Mex. Oftal. 23:*223, 1949.

208. Somer, T.: The viscosity of blood, plasma, and serum in dys- and paraproteinemia. *Acta Med. Scand.* (*Suppl. 456*), 1966.

209. Sorsby, A.: *Systemic Ophthalmology.* St. Louis, Mo., Mosby, 1951. p. 573.

210. Sorsby, A., Klien, M., Gann, J. H., and Siggins, G.: Unusual retinal detachment, possibly sex-linked. *Brit. J. Ophthal. 35:* 1, 1951.

211. Spalter, H. F.: Abnormal serum proteins and retinal vein thrombosis. *Arch. Ophthal. 62:*868, 1959.

212. Spalter, H. F., and Bruce, G. M.: Ocular changes in pulmonary insufficiency. *Trans. Amer. Acad. Ophthal. Otolaryng. 68:*661, 1964.

213. Stern, H. J.: Thrombosis of central retinal vein. *Brit. J. Ophthal. 28:*643, 1944.

214. Straatsma, B. R., and Allen, R. A.: Lattice degeneration of the retina. *Amer. Acad. Ophthal. Otolaryng. 66:*600, 1962.

215. Tanenbaum, H. L., Schepens, C. L., Elzeneiny, I., and Freeman, H. M.: Macular pucker following retinal surgery: a biomicroscopic study. *Canad. J. Ophthal. 4:*20, 1969.

216. Terry, T. L.: Fibroblastic overgrowth of persistent tunica vasculosa lentis in infants born prematurely. *Trans. Amer. Ophthal. Soc. 40:*262, 1942.

217. Toussaint, D., and Danis, P.: Retinopathy in generalized *Loa loa* filariasis. *Arch. Ophthal. 74:*470, 1965.

218. Tyner, J. S., and Frayer, W. C.: Clinical and autopsy findings in early retrolental fibroplasia: report of a case. *Arch. Ophthal. 46:* 647, 1951.

219. Unsworth, A. C.: Retrolental fibroplasia. A preliminary report. *Arch. Ophthal. 40:* 341, 1948.

220. Vannas, S., and Orma, H.: Experience of treating retinal venous occlusion with anticoagulant and antisclerosis therapy. *Arch. Ophthal. 58:*812, 1957.

221. Vannas, S., and Tarkkanen, A.: Retinal vein occlusion and glaucoma. Tonographic study of the incidence of glaucoma and of its prognostic significance. *Brit. J. Ophthal. 44:*583, 1960.

222. Veirs, E. R.: Periphlebitis retinalis associ-

ated with intracranial manifestations. *Amer. J. Ophthal. 31:*168, 1948.

223. Verhoeff, F. H.: Obstruction of the central retinal vein. *Arch. Ophthal. 36:*1, 1907.

224. Verhoeff, F. H.: Effect of chronic glaucoma on the central retinal vessels. *Arch. Ophthal. 42:*145, 1913.

225. Verhoeff, F. H.: Retinoblastoma. Report of a case in a man aged forty-eight. *Arch. Ophthal. 2:*643, 1929.

226. Verhoeff, F. H.: Discussion of MacDonald, A. E.: Heparin in the treatment of complete thrombosis of the central retinal vein. *Arch. Ophthal. 24:*1058, 1940.

227. Verhoeff, F. H.: Discussion of Maucall, I. T.: Occlusion of the central retinal vein. *Arch. Ophthal. 46:*668, 1951.

228. Verhoeff, F. H., and Simpson, G. V.: Tubercle within central vein. *Arch. Ophthal. 24:* 645, 1940.

229. von Michel, J.: Die spontane thrombose der vena centralis des opticus. *Arch. Ophth. 24(2):*37, 1878.

230. Wagener, H. P., and Rucker, C. W.: Lesions of the Retina and Optic Nerve in Association with Blood Dyscrasias, *Modern Trends in Ophthalmology,* ed. by Sorsby, A. London, Butterworth, 1948, Vol. II, p. 300.

231. Walsh, F. B.: Ocular importance of sarcoid. *Arch. Ophthal. 21:*421, 1939.

232. Warburg, M.: Norrie's disease. *Acta Ophthal.* (*Suppl.* 89), 1966.

233. Welch, R. B.: The use of cryosurgery in the treatment of fundus lesions other than detachment. *Trans. Amer. Acad. Ophthal. Otolaryng. 73:*1035, 1969.

234. Welch, R. B., and Goldberg, M. F.: Sickle-cell hemoglobin and its relation to fundus abnormality. *Arch. Ophthal. 75:*353, 1966.

235. Welch, R. B., Maumenee, A. E., and Wahlen, H. E.: Peripheral posterior segment inflammation, vitreous opacities, and edema of the posterior pole. Pars planitis. *Arch. Ophthal. 64:*540, 1960.

236. Wells, R. E., and Merrill, E. W.: The variability of blood viscosity. *Amer. J. Med. 31:* 505, 1961.

237. Weskamp, L. R., Rogue, A. M., and Peirotti, M. J.: Complicaciones oculares en la brucellosis. *Arch. Oftal. B.Air. 18:*666, 1943.

238. White, R. H. R.: The aetiology and neurological complications of retinal vasculitis. *Brain 84:*262, 1961.

239. Wise, G. N.: Retinal neovascularization. *Trans. Amer. Ophthal. Soc. 54:*729, 1956.

240. Wise, G. N.: Macular changes after venous obstruction. *Arch. Ophthal. 58:544, 1957.*

241. Wise, G. N.: Arteriosclerosis secondary to retinal vein obstruction. *Trans. Amer. Ophthal. Soc. 56:*361, 1958.

242. Wise, G. N.: Uveitis with secondary retinal arteriosclerosis. *Amer. J. Ophthal. 51:*797, 1961.

243. Wise, G. N.: Factors influencing retinal new vessel formation. *Amer. J. Ophthal. 52:*637, 1961.

244. Wise, G. N.: Discussion of Gass, J. D. M., and Norton, E. W. D.: Fluorescein studies of patients with macular edema and papilledema following cataract extraction. *Trans. Amer. Ophthal. Soc. 64:*245, 1966.

245. Wise, G. N., Campbell, C. J., Wendler, P. F., and Rittler, M. C.: Photocoagulation of vascular lesions of the macula. *Amer. J. Ophthal. 66:*452, 1968.

246. Wise, G. N., and Horava, A.: Coats' disease. *Amer. J. Ophthal. 56:*17, 1963.

247. Wolter, J. R.: Degeneration of the peripheral retina. *Amer. J. Ophthal. 47:*153, 1959.

248. Wood, L. W., and Watzke, R. C.: Effects of cryopexy upon the retinal vasculature. *Arch. Ophthal. 81:*254, 1969.

249. Wood, L. W., and Watzke, R. C.: The effects of photo- and laser coagulation on the retinal vasculature. *Arch. Ophthal. 82:*499, 1969.

250. Yanoff, M., Frayer, W. C., and Scheie, H. G.: Ocular findings in a patient with 13–15 trisomy. *Arch. Ophthal. 70:*372, 1963.

251. Yanoff, M., Rahn, E. K., and Zimmerman, L. E.: Histopathology of juvenile retinoschisis. *Arch. Ophthal. 79:*49, 1968.

252. Zacharias, L., Chisholm, J. F., and Chapman, R. B.: Visual and ocular damage in retrolental fibroplasia. *Amer. J. Ophthal. 53:* 337, 1962.

253. Zeavin, B. H., King, M. J., and Gohd, R. S.: A case of Behçet's disease. *Amer. J. Ophthal. 41:*55, 1956.

254. Zeeman, W. P. C.: Ueber Netzhaut und Schnervenleiden bei Iridocyclitis. *Arch. Ophth. 112:*152, 1923.

255. Zimmerman, L.: "Discussion" in *Symposium on Glaucoma: Transactions of the New Orleans Academy of Ophthalmology, 1966.* C. V. Mosby, 192, 1967.

256. Zimmerman, L. E.: Histopathologic basis for ocular manifestations of congenital rubella syndrome. *Amer. J. Ophthal. 65:*837, 1968.

chapter 15

Diabetic Retinopathy

The earliest known description of diabetic retinopathy was by von Jaeger in 1856. His patient was a young gardner aged 22 with glycosuria whose retinal features included dilated veins, striate extravasations, and flecks of light yellow or orange material.[45] During the following years many case reports appeared and these were reviewed by Leber in 1876.[65] At this stage there was still some confusion between the retinal appearances in diabetes and Bright's disease as both groups of patients often had proteinuria. Ashton has suggested that retinal microaneurysms were recognized as early as 1854 by Bowman.[5] MacKenzie's paper of 1879 is a classic, the first in which retinal microaneurysms were recognized and associated with diabetes.[70] MacKenzie's clinical description included dilated veins, punctate and blot hemorrhages, and white spots of various sizes in the eyes of a patient with glycosuria. His patient died in diabetic coma and an eye was examined microscopically by Nettleship who found minute aneurysms on retinal capillaries and illustrated them by a drawing. He suggested that the vitreous hemorrhages that the patient had suffered might derive from the aneurysms. This observation was forgotten and it was 64 years later that the retinal microaneurysms of diabetes were rediscovered by Ballantyne and Lowenstein.[6,7]

A series of illustrated articles by Hirschberg in 1890[41] clarified the main clinical features of simple diabetic retinopathy, and separated the features of diabetes from those found in Bright's disease.

Nettleship[73] was probably the first to describe the histology of proliferative diabetic retinopathy. His patient, a 48-year-old drayman with a clinical history suggesting diabetes of 4 years' duration, had no proteinuria, but did have diabetic neuropathy with a perforating ulcer of the foot. The right eye contained hemorrhages and blood vessels in the vitreous. It is interesting to note the infrequency of reports of proliferative retinopathy in papers written before the discovery of insulin by Banting and Best in 1922. In that era patients did not usually live long enough to develop severe retinopathy or become blind from their disease. In 1930 less than 1 per cent of newly reported cases of blindness in the United States were due to diabetes while in 1960 the figure had risen to 15 per cent.[72,75] In the 1930s an incidence of proliferative retinopathy of about 1 per cent was reported[90] but by 1959, Root, Mirsky, and Ditzel have noted that more than 8 per cent of diabetics had proliferative changes.[79]

The increase in the absolute numbers of patients with diabetic retinopathy because of their long survival, the increased incidence of proliferative retinopathy and of blindness have made diabetic retinopathy a major clinical problem.

CLINICAL FEATURES

Diabetes causes varied and bizarre changes in the retinal circulation.[63,64] The earliest change is the appearance of a few microaneurysms at the posterior pole of the retina. These aneurysms are rounded in contour and the color of the blood in them varies from the dark shade of veins up to the pale pink of arterial blood. They are often accompanied by hemorrhages which are darker, more irregular and transient than the aneurysms (Fig. 15-1). The half-life of aneurysms varies from a few months up to years while that of hemorrhages is much less. Some of the aneurysms become hyalinized and appear as circular whitish spots sometimes with a red center.

Hard fatty exudates are often an early feature, beginning as discrete white or yellowish flecks but later becoming confluent into larger yellowish patches. These larger aggregates of fatty material often form a partial or complete circle around an area of abnormal capillaries and aneurysms and are sometimes referred to as "circinate retinopathy" (Fig. 15-2). Even larger confluent patches of fatty exudates may form and if these surround the macula, vision is seriously impaired. In many cases some or all of these features are present at one time. Changes in retinal vessels occur both in arteries and veins. General dilatation of veins is a difficult clinical sign to appreciate unless it is gross. An irregular beaded appearance of the veins is a more distinctive characteristic, but is not common (Fig. 15-3). Arterial abnormalities are frequent in longstanding cases; sclerotic changes with wall thickening, irregular caliber, and crossing changes occur in many eyes with diabetic retinopathy, particularly those with proliferative changes. More severe arterial disease with whitish pipe-stem sheathing of minute branches is common in areas of capillary nonperfusion. These areas of nonperfusion, particularly around the macula, may be recognized by a yellowish tint instead of the normal uniform pink.

Cotton-wool spots occur in at least 5 per cent of diabetic patients with retinopathy, particularly those with arterial disease, and are not confined to diabetics with an elevated blood pressure.[58,69] In diabetics, cotton-wool spots are often less distinct than in other conditions and may have a faint grayish white color (Fig. 15-4).

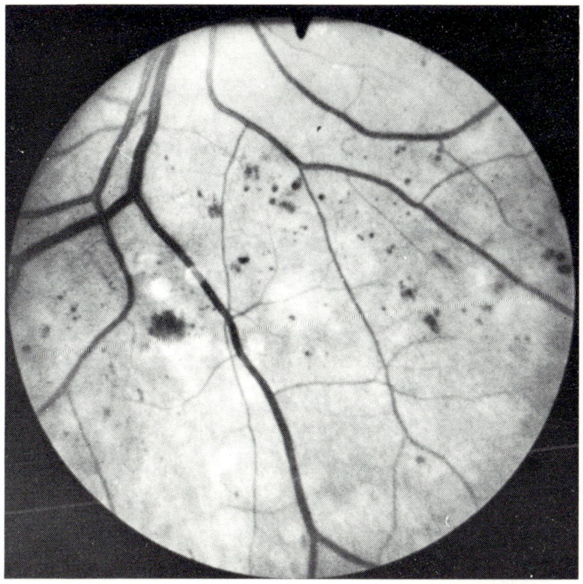

Fig. 15-1. Diabetic retinopathy with multiple small discrete rounded or oval microaneurysms and larger irregular blot hemorrhages. (From Oakley et al.[74])

Fig. 15-2. Circular (circinate) rings of fatty exudate with central hemorrhages and microaneurysms in a patient with diabetic retinopathy.

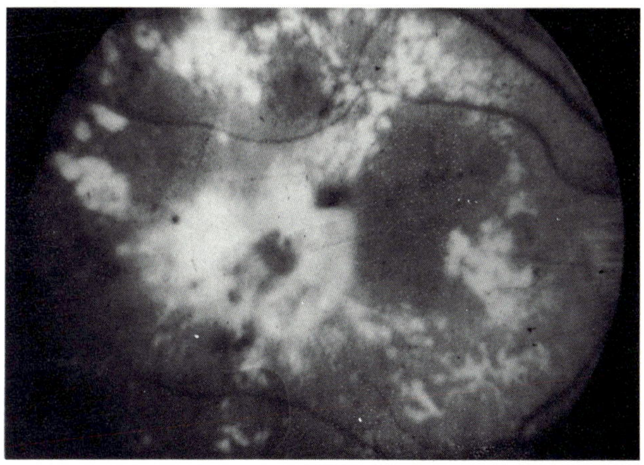

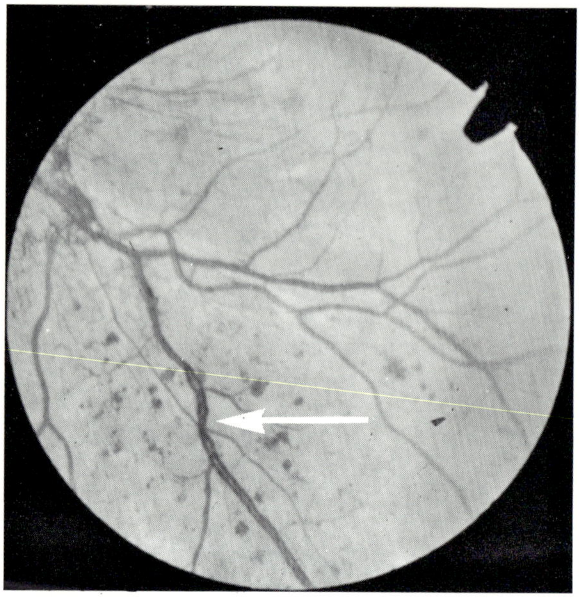

Fig. 15-3. Irregular beading of a large retinal vein **(arrow)** in a patient with severe diabetic retinopathy.

Fig. 15-4. Faint, grayish white, cotton-wool spots in the nasal retina of a diabetic patient. (From Kohner and Dollery[58]: *Diabetes 18:*691, 1969.)

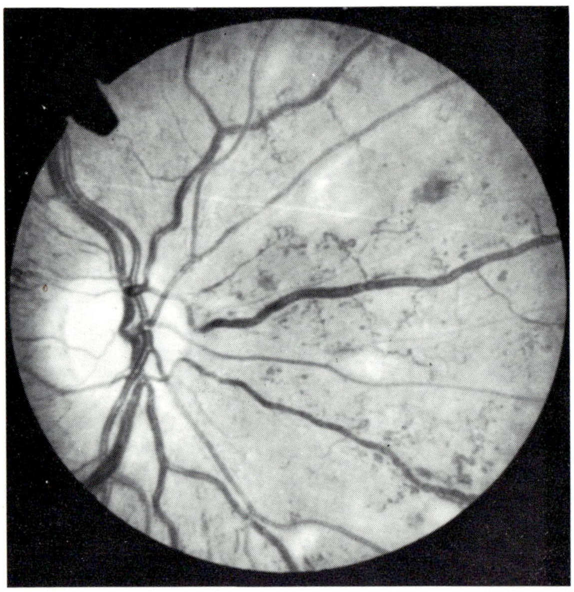

Proliferative vascular changes affect one-third of patients whose diabetes begins in childhood or adolescence and who survive into middle age.[96] Proliferative changes may begin as areas of dilated vascular arcades, as rosettes of tightly packed capillaries, or as abnormal vessel loops connected to veins[28] (Fig. 15-5). A cloud-like condensation of connective tissue appears around these new vessels as they get larger and later this condenses into bands. Common situations for new vessels are on the optic disc or as crescents along the main vessel groups (Fig. 15-6). Hemorrhages are common around and among these vessels but do not precede them, as is often stated. Later, the vascularity of the proliferating tissue decreases and it becomes whiter. Contraction of the tissue may then cause gross disorganization of the retina and retinal detachment.

Discussion of these features involves classification into categories. From the standpoint of pathophysiology it is convenient to divide them into three groups; (*1*) capillary and venous changes, (*2*) arterial changes, and (*3*) proliferative changes. The most important clinical distinction is between eyes with aneurysms, hemorrhages, exudates, and those with venous changes and new vessel proliferation. Some authors refer to the first type as "simple" diabetic retinopathy and the second as "malignant." The distinction is a valid one but the terminology is unfortunate and it seems best to categorize diabetic eyes according to the different clinical features.

MEASURING SEVERITY

It would be convenient both from the standpoint of clinical description and for assessing natural history and response to treatment if there were some method of measuring the severity of diabetic retinopathy. Two grading systems have been published,[36,66] and in 1966 a meeting was held in Airlie House, Virginia to obtain the cooperation of a number of research groups in the use of a standard system for grading various features of diabetic retinopathy.[36] The workers at this meeting agreed that hemorrhages and microaneurysms, hard exudates, cotton-wool spots, venous abnormalities, new vessels, and fibrosis should be graded by comparing color photographs of the individual patient with a standard set. For capillary and arterial lesions fluorescein pictures would be used. Clinical examination would be used to determine whether retinitis proliferans and new vessels were within or anterior to the retina and what their relationship was to the vitreous body.

The progress of diabetic retinopathy can be followed by comparing fluorescein and color photographs taken over a period. If several sets of fluorescein pictures are available of the same area the rate of appearance and disappearance of microaneurysms can be measured.[57]

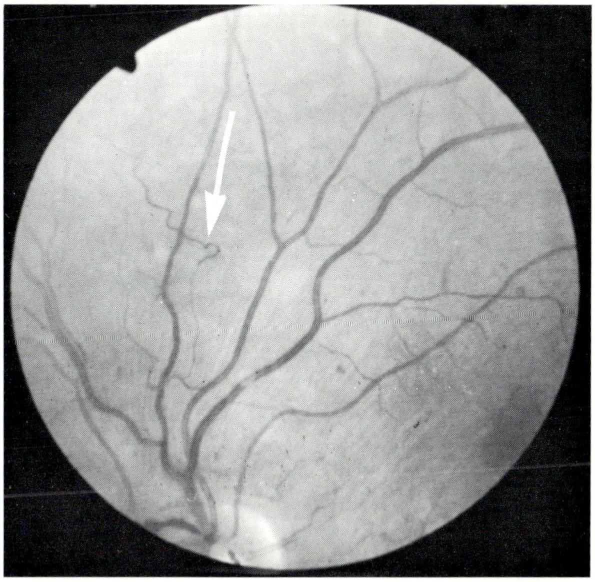

Fig. 15-5. An early new vessel system loops over the vein with which it is connected (**arrow**).

PATHOPHYSIOLOGY AND MORPHOLOGY OF THE RETINAL VASCULAR BED IN DIABETES

The clinical study of diabetic retinopathy has been facilitated by the development of fluorescein angiographic techniques. Injection, digest, and electron microscopic methods in pathologic examination have added greatly to our knowledge of morphology.

Fig. 15-6. A crescent of preretinal neovascularization sweeps down from the optic disc toward the inferior temporal vessels.

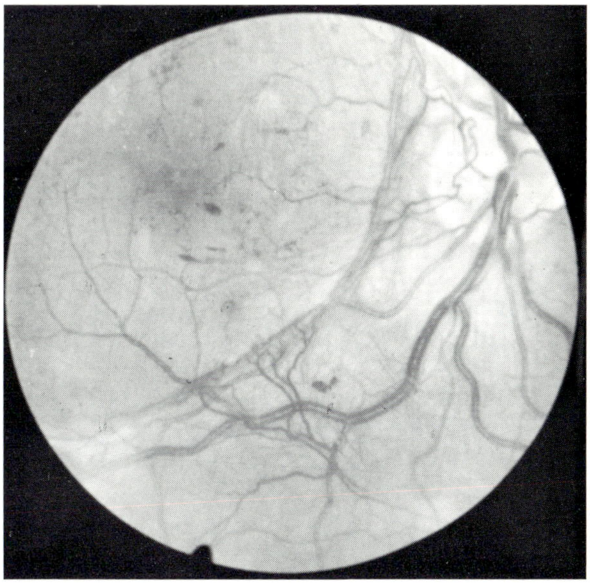

CHANGES IN CAPILLARIES AND VEINS

Normal retinal capillaries are approximately 5 μ in diameter and are clearly visible on high-definition fluorescence angiograms. In clinically normal retinae of pa-

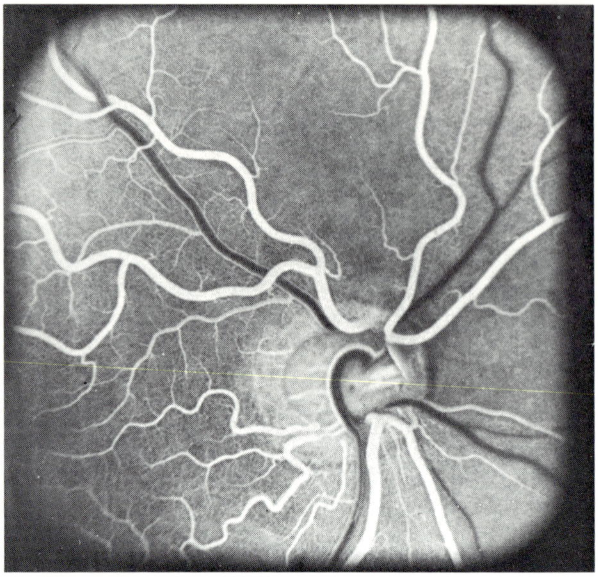

Fig. 15-7. Normal fluorescence angiogram in a patient with long-standing diabetes who had no clinical evidence of retinopathy.

tients with diabetes the capillaries appear normal (Fig. 15-7) on angiographic examination, although electron microscopy[88] may show a thicker, irregular and reduplicated basement membrane with broken layers, in retinal capillaries. Microaneurysms are the earliest clinically demonstrable vascular abnormality in diabetic patients.[35,60] They appear much more numerous on fluorescein angiograms than on ophthalmoscopic examination.[60] For example, over 200 aneurysms were found in one retinal photograph where fundoscopic examination revealed only a few (Fig. 15-8). Besides the localized globular microaneurysms on one side of a capillary, fusiform or general dilatation of capillary loops often occurs. Dilated capillaries frequently form hairpin loops, sometimes with a local dilatation at the bend of the hairpin. Capillary aneurysms are particularly prominent around the edge of areas of nonperfused capillaries (Fig. 15-9). Small areas of nonperfused capillaries are found in patients with early diabetic retinopathy.

Most microaneurysms range between 15 and 50 μ in diameter but occasionally very large ones up to 100 μ are seen, particularly around the edges of areas of capillary closure. Friedenwald[34] states that aneurysms are most often located at capillary bifurcations, but Bloodworth[11] who examined over

Fig. 15-8. *A*, From a color transparency of the right disc of a patient with mild diabetic retinopathy. There are a few scattered blot-and-dot hemorrhages. *B*, Fluorescence angiogram of the same area as shown in *A*. Many microaneurysms and dilated capillaries are present which are not seen on the color transparency. (From Kohner et al.[60]: *Diabetes 16*:1, 1967.)

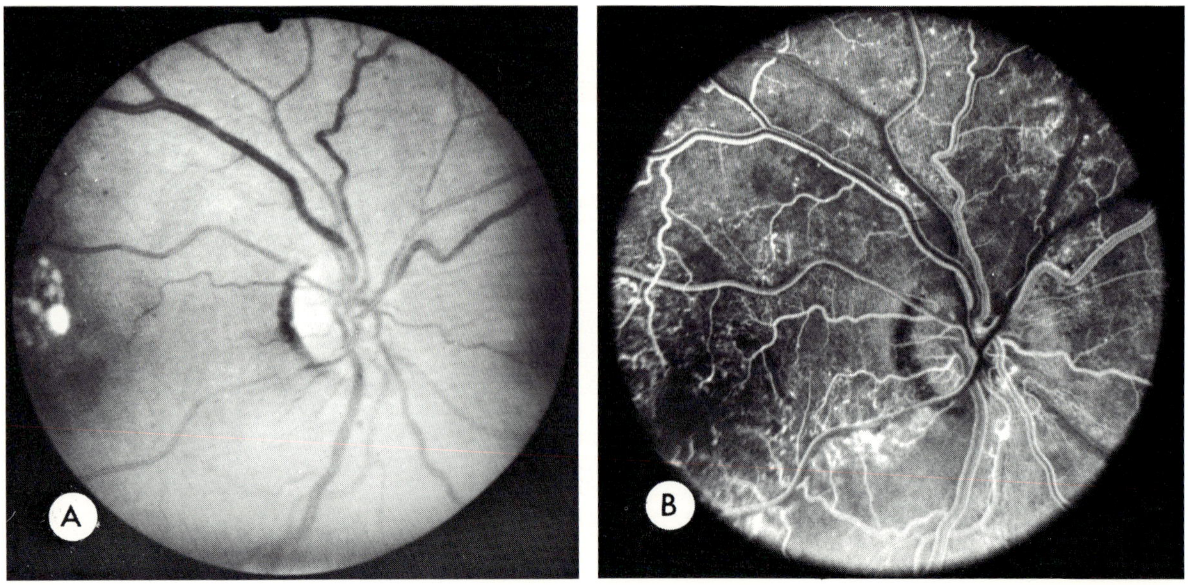

300 diabetic eyes, found this to be an uncommon site. Ashton[2,4] reported that the majority of aneurysms occurred on the venous side of the circulation. Bloodworth found that nearly half were in the superficial capillary layer and he commented that the only vessels free of them were arterioles. Fluorescein studies show that microaneurysms are distributed on capillaries around terminal arterioles as well as on venules (Fig. 15-10). In mild retinopathy they are more common on the venous side but in severe cases they are seen with about equal frequency on the arterial and venous side.

Fluorescein often empties from aneurysms more slowly than from normal capillaries showing that blood flow through aneurysms is slow in relation to their volume (Fig. 15-11). This is not surprising as the aneurysm is many times the diameter of a normal capillary, but the vessel on which it is located probably has no more than the normal capillary flow. Microaneurysms commonly leak fluorescein into the surrounding retina in contrast to normal capillaries (Fig. 15-12).

Histologic examination shows that most diabetic microaneurysms are thin-walled, but some are hyalinized with a thick wall which gives an intense PAS-positive reaction. The latter may have many lamellae of PAS-positive material laid down within them.[12]

Cogan, Toussaint, and Kuwabara, using the digest technique, have reported that abnormalities of intramural pericytes are common in diabetes and these cells may be either lost or necrotic giving a smudgy staining reaction. They found that abnormalities of "mural cells" (intramural pericytes) were particularly common on capillaries containing microaneurysms.[21]

De Oliveira,[75] although agreeing that areas with selective loss of pericytes occur in diabetes, has found the reverse situation of more severe damage to endothelial cells to

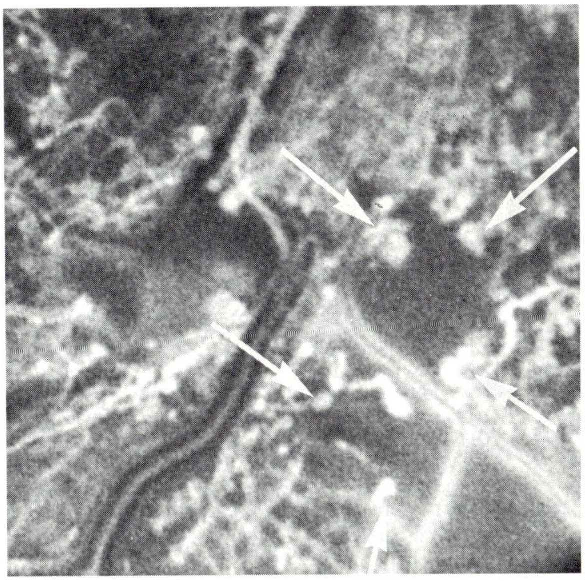

Fig. 15-9. Large capillary aneurysms surround an area of capillary closure **(arrows).**

Fig. 15-10. *A*, Arterial- and capillary-phase fluorescence angiogram of a patient with diabetic retinopathy. Some microaneurysms are connected to a branch artery **(arrows).** *B*, Venous-phase fluorescence angiogram taken 3 seconds later than *A*. Some aneurysms are seen to be connected to terminal venous radicals.

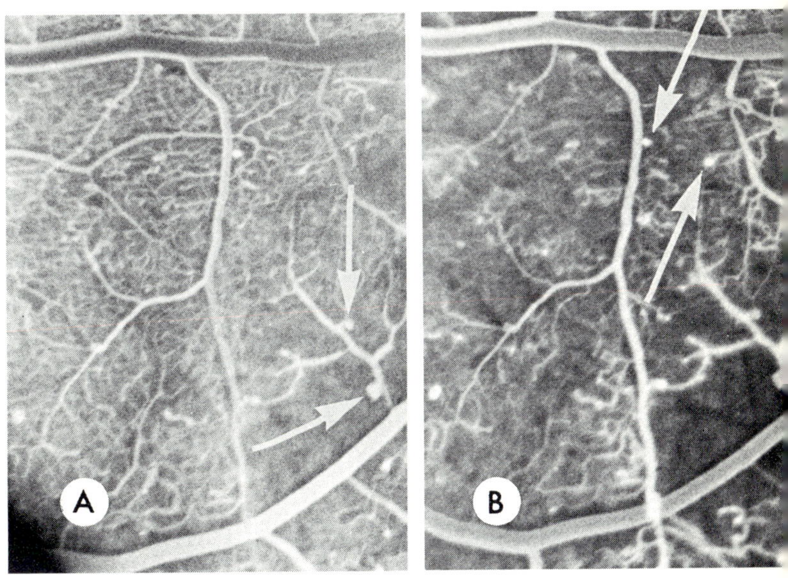

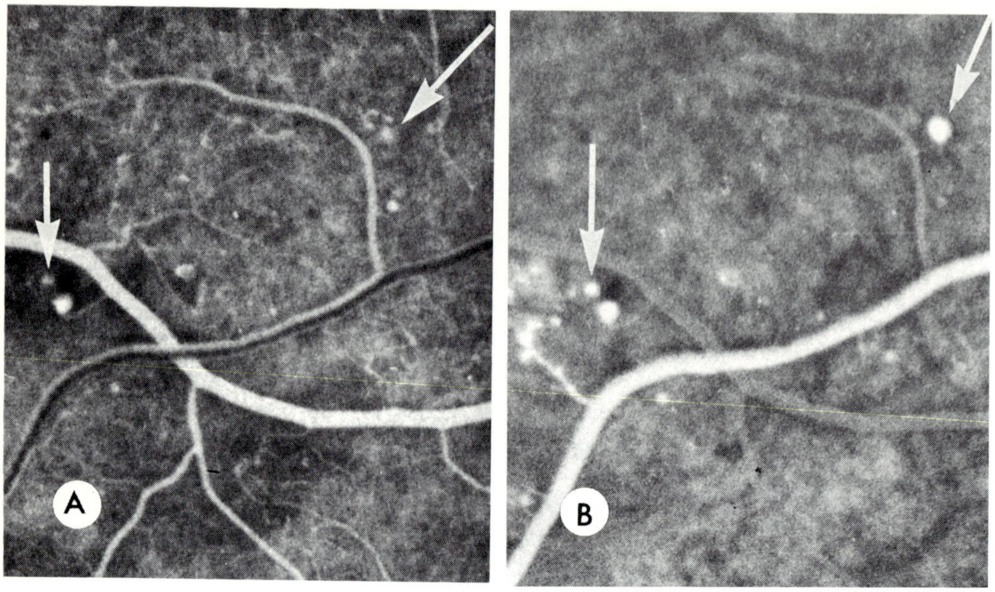

Fig. 15-11. *A*, Arterial-phase fluorescein angiogram of a patient with multiple aneurysms. Filling of two large aneurysms is incomplete (**arrows**). *B*, Venous-phase fluorescence angiogram taken 10 seconds later. Capillaries have emptied but the large aneurysms still contain dye (**arrows**).

Fig. 15-12. *A*, Capillary-phase fluorescein angiogram of a diabetic patient shows microaneurysms. *B*, In the late venous phase the position of the aneurysms can be seen because of leakage of dye through their walls.

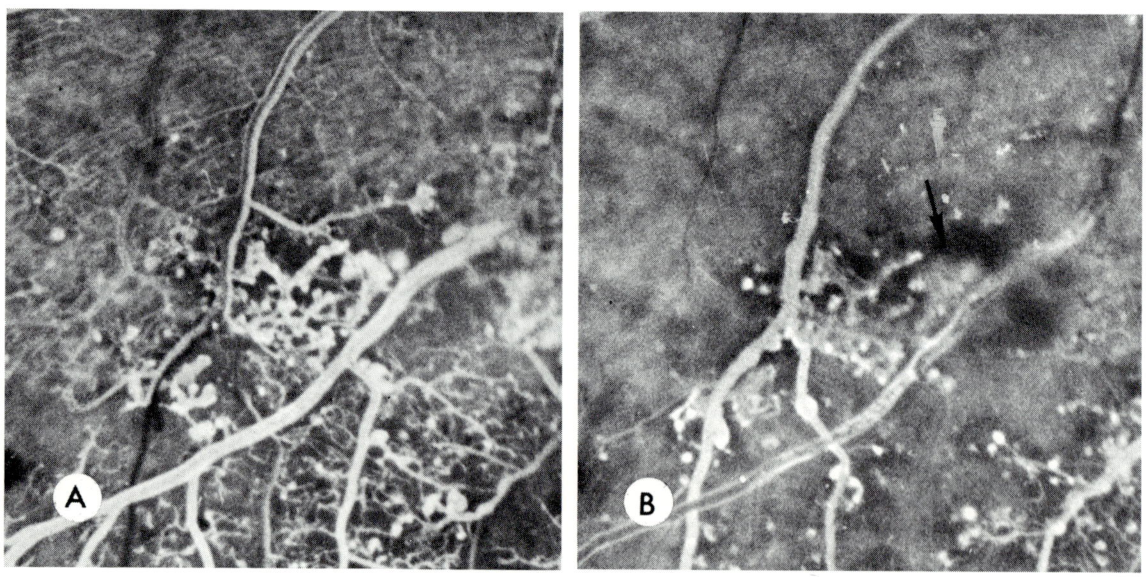

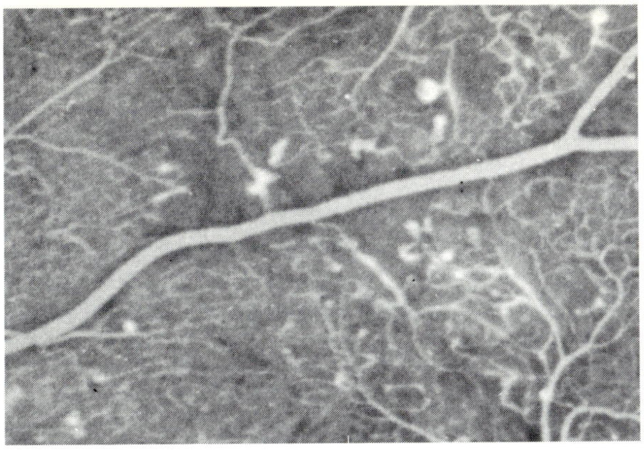

Fig. 15-13. Fluorescein angiogram shows areas of capillary closure in a diabetic retina.

be even more common. He illustrated capillaries with microaneurysms which had intramural pericytes at their caps. However, Yanoff[100] and Speiser, Gittlesohn, and Patz[84] have carried out cell counts and obtained strong quantitative evidence of a selective loss of pericytes in diabetes. In normal retinal capillaries the mean ratio of the number of endothelial cell nuclei to intramural pericyte nuclei was 1.1 while in diabetic retinopathy it was between 4.2 and 3.6.

Yamashita and Rosen[99] have studied the electron microscopic features and found that thin-walled aneurysms had a thin and structureless basement membrane containing some dense osmophilic deposits and were lined by a thin layer of endothelial cell cytoplasm. The thick wall of hyalinized aneurysms contained a thick laminated basement membrane and the lumen was lined with degenerated endothelial cells.

There are many theories concerning the origin of microaneurysms. Ashton[2] has suggested that they represented an abortive attempt at neovascularization with budding of the wall, but the histology is not consistent with this theory, and Ashton[4] now has withdrawn it. Kuwabara and Cogan[62] believed that a local weakness of the capillary wall is caused by loss of the intramural pericyte while Bloodworth[11] felt that disease of the basement membrane is primary. Wolter[98] has suggested that traction strands in the retina, demonstrated by silver staining, may play a role.

Fig. 15-14. *A*, From a color transparency of a patient with diabetic retinopathy showing the macular area with microaneurysms, blot hemorrhages, and cotton-wool spots. *B*, Fluorescein angiogram in the capillary phase of the same area as *A*. A large area of capillaries in the macular area is not perfused.

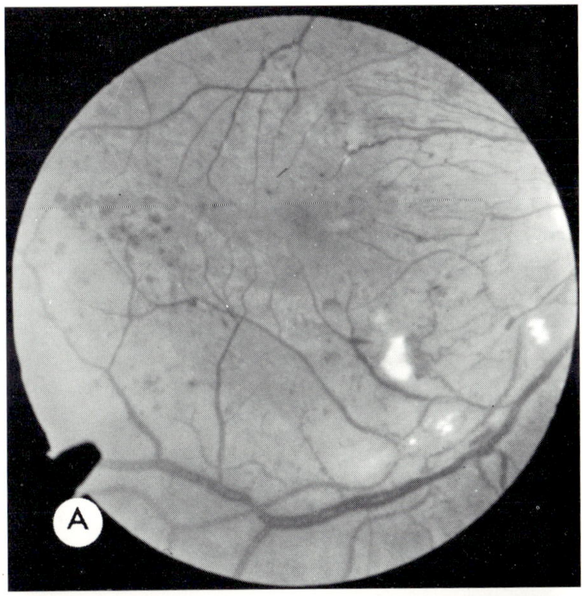

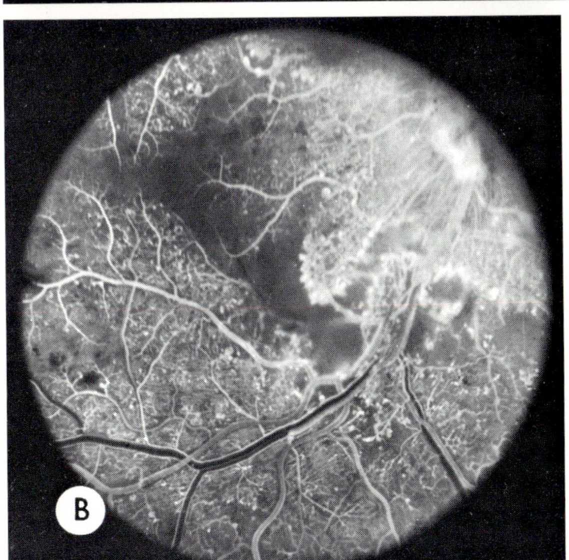

The life cycle of retinal microaneurysms is poorly documented. Recent studies on their half-life show that it may vary from a few months to years.[57] It is not known whether the process of obliteration relies on hyalinization and deposition of material in the wall, thrombosis, or on gradual remodeling.

CAPILLARY CLOSURE

Clinical studies with the fluorescein technique[60] show that small areas of capillary closure up to about 100 μ in diameter are common (Fig. 15-13) even in patients with early diabetic retinopathy. Much larger areas of closure are found in severe cases (Fig. 15-14). Some of these areas, up to 1 mm in diameter, are the site of cotton-wool spots, but others are not. Very large areas, up to 5 mm in diameter, are found in the macular and surrounding retina in some patients with severe diabetic retinopathy.

Other vascular abnormalities are common in the vicinity of areas of capillary closure. Dilated capillaries and larger aneurysms facing in towards the nonperfused zone often form a ring surrounding the area. Larger areas of capillary closure are often traversed by arteriovenous "shunt vessels" which are larger in diameter than normal capillaries, linking an artery directly to a vein. In some instances these vessels appear to act as high-flow shunts putting an early lamina of dye into the draining vein (Fig. 15-15). More often they fill slowly, sometimes more slowly than surrounding normal capillaries. Shunt vessels sometimes appear after an area of capillary closure has formed. Arteries crossing a large area of capillary closure frequently show abnormalities including fluorescein staining of their walls and localized out-pouching which probably represent pruned-off side branches.

Cogan and Kuwabara[20] have been impressed by the prominence of shunt vessels on digest preparations and have suggested that these vessels are important in the pathogenesis of capillary closure (Fig. 15-16). They believe that these vessels can carry a sufficiently high flow to drain blood away from the surrounding capillaries. There are several reasons for rejecting this explanation in most cases of capillary closure. Firstly, shunt vessels are often absent (Fig. 15-17*A*). Secondly, when present they fill so sluggishly that it is evident that they could not be acting as a high-flow shunt (Fig. 15-16). Thirdly, the resistance of these vessels is unlikely to be less than the many capillaries of the bed which they have replaced. Finally, they may appear after the capillary bed has closed (Fig. 15-17*B*).[60]

Digest studies[11,20,21] show that the capillaries in areas of closure are acellular tubes which have lost both endothelial cells and intramural pericytes (Fig. 15-18). Large areas of capillary closure usually remain closed over periods of study lasting many months. However, a few may reopen when the area of closure was the site of a cotton-wool spot. In this case capillary nonperfusion may have resulted from external compression. It is not known whether the endothelial cells and intramural pericytes can recolonize a vascular ghost.

RETINAL VEINS IN DIABETES

Dilatation of retinal veins is often recorded during clinical examination of early diabetic retinopathy. Lundbaeck[69] found that the veins had a blurred outline and were dilated in 61 per cent of diabetics less than 30 years old but in only 8 per cent of older ones. There are dangers of bias in a purely clinical assessment but Jutte[50] has attempted a more quantitative approach. He found that 17 of 70 juvenile-onset diabetics had dilated retinal veins and that retinal vein dilatation appeared to reach a maximum after 10 years of diabetes.

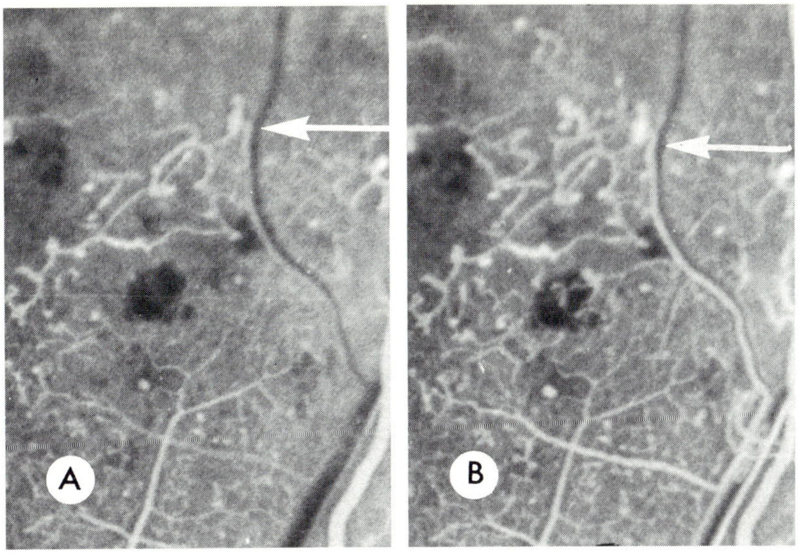

Fig. 15-15. *A*, Rapid passage of dye across the shunt vessels in an area of capillary closure has placed an early layer of fluorescein in the draining vein before the normal capillaries fill **(arrow).** *B*, As the normal capillaries fill, a thick layer of dye runs down the vein fed by the shunt **(arrow).**

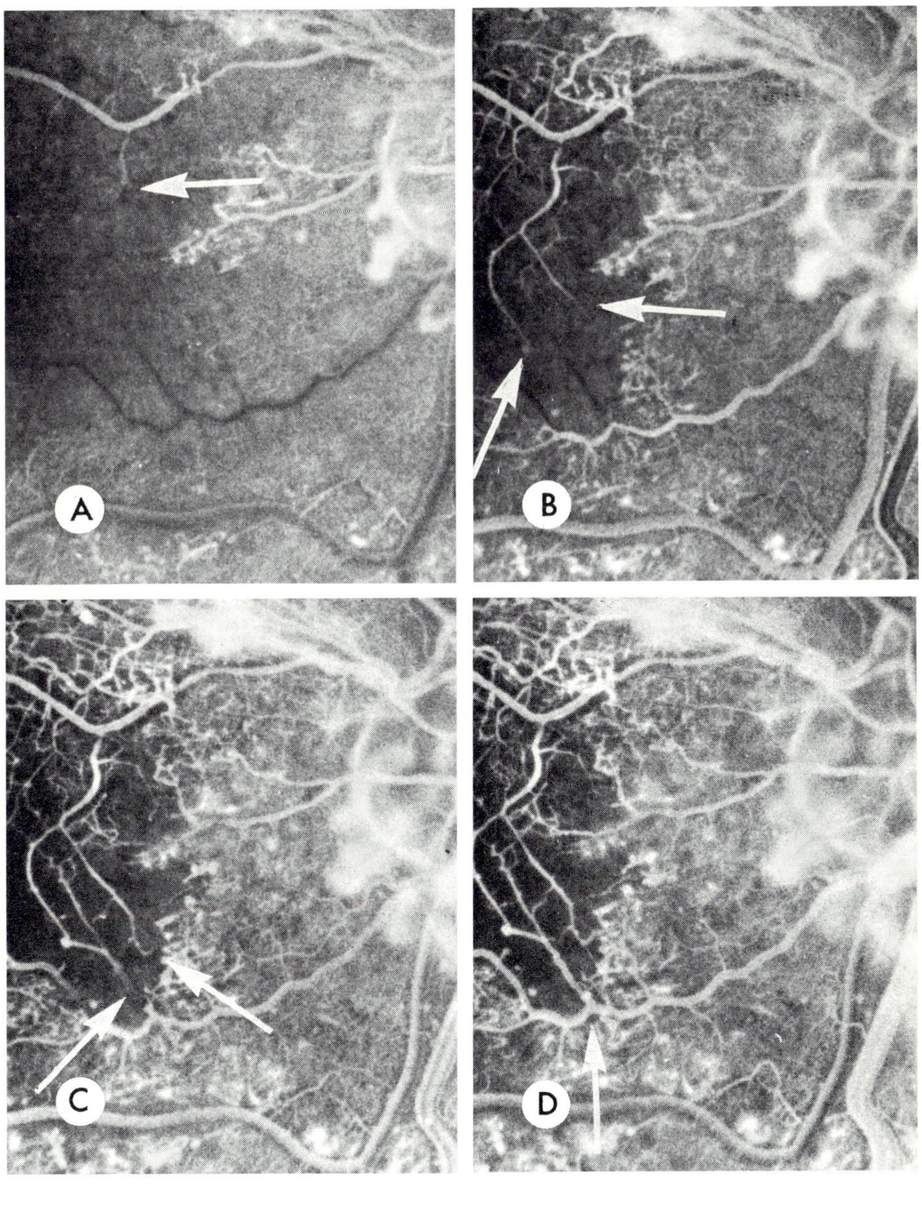

Fig. 15-16. *A*, Arterial-phase fluorescein angiogram of a patient with an area of capillary closure at the macula crossed by "shunt vessels." The shunt is beginning to fill **(arrow).**

B, One second later: fluorescein has flowed part of the way through the shunt **(arrows).** Surrounding capillaries have filled in more normal areas.

C, Two seconds after *A*. Dye is still passing through the vessel but has not yet reached its venous end **(arrows).**

D, After 3 seconds the dye front in the shunt has reached its venous end **(arrow).**

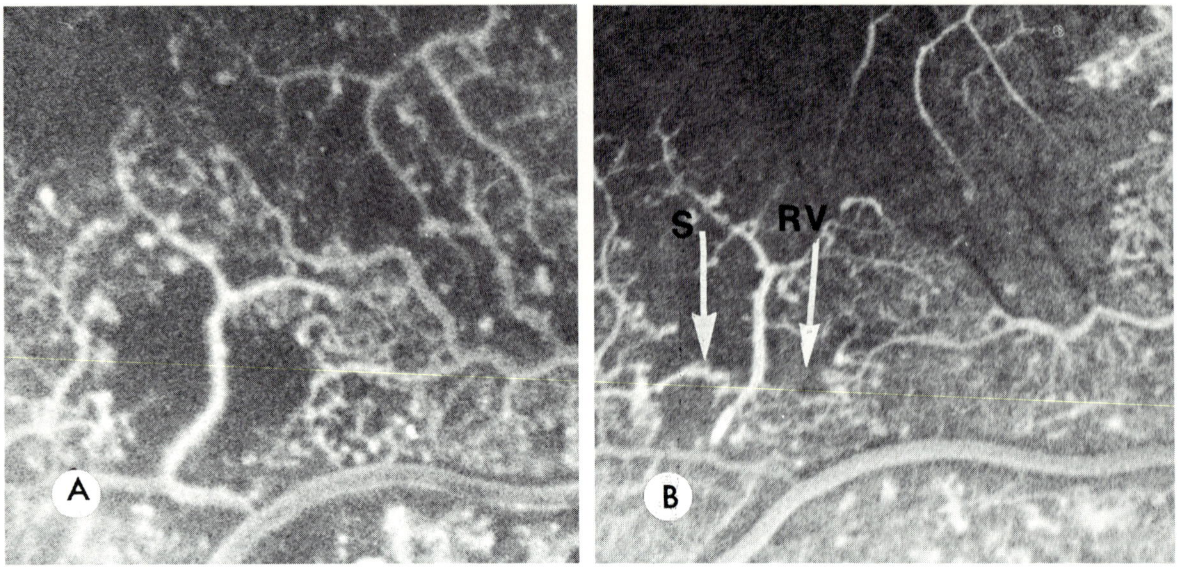

Fig. 15-17. *A*, Two areas of capillary closure in a diabetic patient without "shunt vessels." *B*, The same patient as seen in *A*, but 6 months later. A shunt vessel has formed across one of the areas of capillary closure **(arrow S)**. The second area of capillary closure has become partly revascularized **(arrow RV)**.

Fig. 15-18. Digest preparation of a diabetic retina. Many capillaries have lost their endothelial cells and pericytes and appear as acellular tubes. (PAS and Hematoxylin, ×75.)

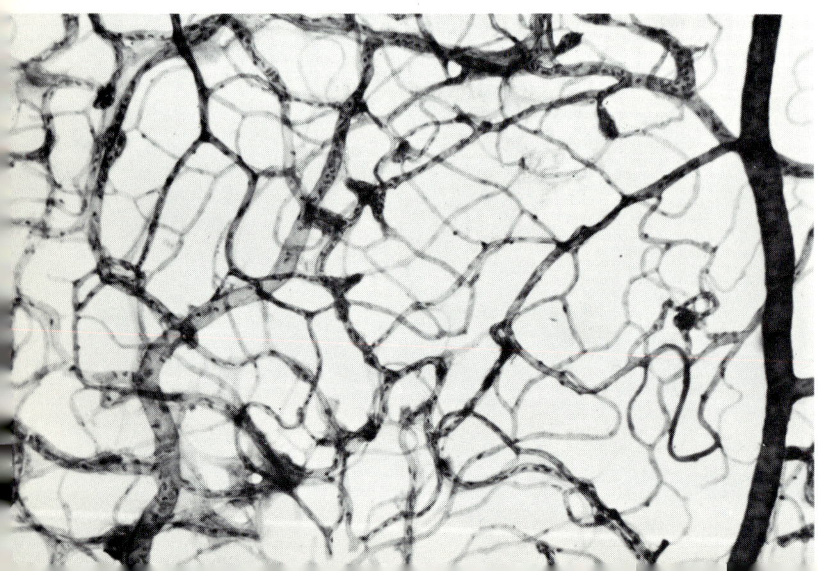

Tortuosity, localized constriction, beading, aneurysmal dilatation, and halo sheathing of the veins are common in diabetes. Kornerup[61] has found that 2 per cent of diabetics without other evidence of retinopathy had changes in the veins, 10 per cent of those with hemorrhages had venous changes and 78 per cent of those with proliferative retinopathy had venous abnormalities. Davis[25] has illustrated many of the extraordinary abnormalities of veins that are seen in patients with proliferative retinopathy. These include beading, narrowing, reduplication of the lumen, hairpin loops on large venous channels, and grossly abnormal venous branches draining areas of new vessel proliferation (Fig. 15-19). Reduplication of the lumen and formation of hairpin loops suggests the formation of collaterals. One patient that we investigated (Fig. 15-19) had severe capillary abnormalities upstream to a hairpin venous loop and while there may have been obstruction at that point in the past, there was none at the time of the study. The walls of the abnormal veins often leak fluorescein (Fig. 15-19) while normal veins do not.

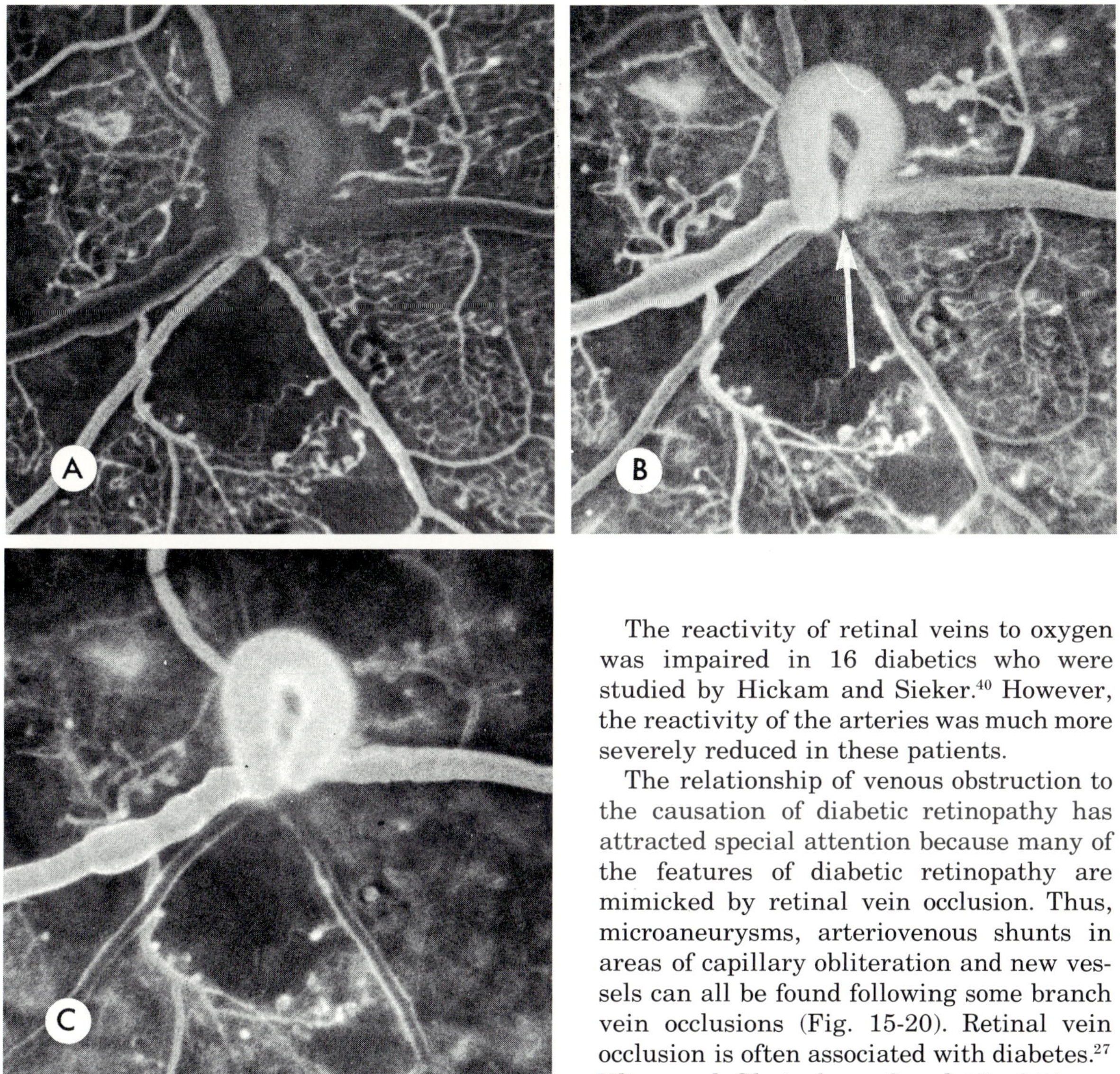

Fig. 15-19. *A*, Capillary-phase fluorescein angiogram of an area of retina containing a venous loop. Capillary changes are more severe upstream to the left of the loop. *B*, Venous phase of the same area shown in *A*. The lumen of the main venous channel is interrupted at the site of the loop (**arrow**) and flow takes place through the loop which acts as a collateral. *C*, Late phase of the same area as seen in *A* and *B*. Dye is leaking from the abnormal venous loop.

The reactivity of retinal veins to oxygen was impaired in 16 diabetics who were studied by Hickam and Sieker.[40] However, the reactivity of the arteries was much more severely reduced in these patients.

The relationship of venous obstruction to the causation of diabetic retinopathy has attracted special attention because many of the features of diabetic retinopathy are mimicked by retinal vein occlusion. Thus, microaneurysms, arteriovenous shunts in areas of capillary obliteration and new vessels can all be found following some branch vein occlusions (Fig. 15-20). Retinal vein occlusion is often associated with diabetes.[27] Klien and Olwin have found 12 of 74 patients with retinal vein occlusion had diabetes.[55] However, the majority of diabetic retinae show no evidence of acute occlusion of branch veins. Bloodworth,[11] in his extensive study of diabetic eyes, did not find evidence of obstruction in retinal veins by either degenerative changes or thrombosis. However, it is possible that such occlusions need only be transient and, for example, obstruction of branch retinal veins in monkey eyes need persist for only a few days to

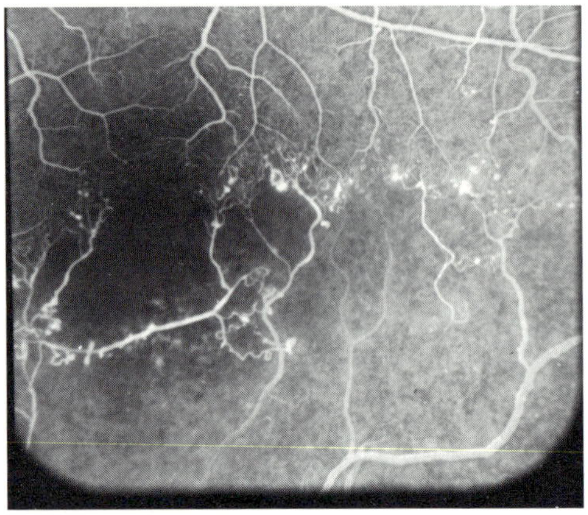

Fig. 15-20. Fluorescein study of a patient 3 months after a branch retinal vein occlusion. In the territory of the obstructed vein (*top*) there is extensive capillary closure. Collaterals cross to link with patent venous branches *below* and there are microaneurysms in the capillary bed at the junction between the blocked and patent vein.

Fig. 15-21. Fluorescein study of the retina of a monkey with a branch retinal vein occlusion occurring 5 weeks after photocoagulation **(arrow).** Upstream to the vein occlusion there are extensive areas of capillary closure.

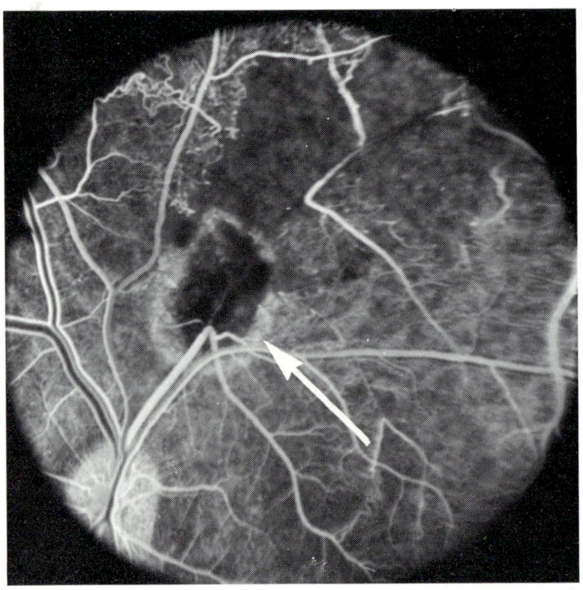

cause permanent damage to the capillary bed (Fig. 15-21).[59]

The evidence does not suggest that obstruction of retinal veins plays a significant part in the pathogenesis of diabetic retinopathy although the point is not entirely settled. It is obvious that the veins are seriously involved in patients with extensive diabetic retinopathy, particularly those with proliferative changes. In theory the vein wall could be damaged either by humoral factors in the blood flowing through or changes in the surrounding retina. It is not certain which of these factors is the more important, but it is tempting for one to speculate that products of the disordered retinal metabolism in diabetes are carried by the draining veins and damage them.

RETINAL ARTERIES IN DIABETIC RETINOPATHY

It is often assumed that the retinal arteries are not involved in diabetic retinopathy. This may be true, in early cases, but it is not true in severe diabetic retinopathy. Wagener, Dry, and Wilder[90] have drawn attention to the presence of arteriolar sclerosis and cotton-wool spots, which they have attributed to angiospasm in some patients with diabetes and subsequent work has shown that these changes can occur in normotensive diabetics. Wendland[92] has studied the extent of retinal arteriolar sclerosis in 217 diabetic patients and an equal number of controls using four grades of severity of arterial damage. Among the controls, 78 per cent had no arteriolar sclerosis, 21 per cent fell in the first grade, and 1 per cent in the second. Among the diabetics, 60 per cent had no sclerosis, 24 per cent were in Group I, 15 per cent in Group II, and 1 per cent in Group III. Waite and Beetham[91] have reported that 26 per cent of diabetics had normal arteries, 23 per cent an increased light reflex, 33 per cent had both increased light reflex and loss of translucency of the wall, 15 per cent had arteriovenous crossing changes, and 1.4 per cent had sheathing of arteries.

Hickam and Sieker [40,82] have found that the degree of narrowing of retinal arteries during oxygen breathing averaged 3.0 per cent in 16 patients with severe diabetes. Comparable figures for normals were 13.6 per cent and for hypertensives 3.2 per cent. Thus, the diabetics had as marked a reduction of arterial reactivity as hypertensive patients. The loss of reactivity is probably explained by the arteriosclerosis described by Ashton.[3]

Damage to small arteries is a prominent feature of patients with severe diabetic retinopathy. Clinical examination may show obliteration of small arterial branches, particularly in the macular area.[83] Arteriosclerosis sometimes with pipe-stem sheathing is particularly common in relation to areas on nonperfused capillaries. Kohner and her colleagues [60] have shown that arteries of 25 to 50 μ in diameter which crossed areas of capillary closure often showed leakage of fluorescein into the vessel wall, and localized out-pouchings which probably represented pruned-off side branches (Fig. 15-22). Ashton [4] has drawn attention to a similar appearance in injected specimens and has suggested that the capillary perfusion ceased because of the arterial involvement. It seems somewhat more probable that closure of the capillaries supplied by the artery was the primary process and the remaining stumps of pruned-off branches support this explanation.

Other arteries may show severe narrowing and/or leakage on fluorescence photographs and Ashton [3] has reported a corkscrew appearance of small arterial branches in more advanced cases. Leaking points on minute arteries are sometimes found in relation to cotton-wool spots in diabetic retinopathy.

Thus, there is firm evidence for involvement of arteries in more advanced cases of diabetic retinopathy. It is noteworthy that the greatest damage to small and medium-sized arteries occurs in areas where capillary bed destruction is also severe. This suggests that the metabolic abnormalities responsible for damage to capillaries may also affect the arteries. It has also been suggested that retinal arterial obstruction by lipid emboli may be the primary cause of diabetic retinopathy.[19,23] The authors do not explain why these emboli should have a predilection for the eye and fluorescein studies have not disclosed evidence of transitory arterial obstruction such as is seen with other malleable emboli.

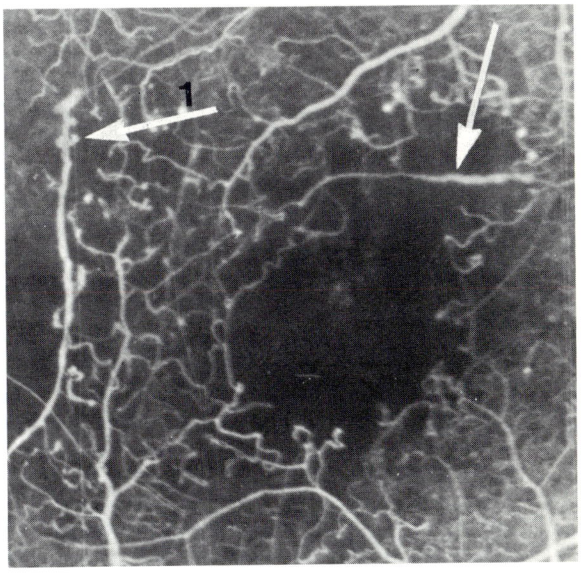

Fig. 15-22. Fluorescein angiogram in the arterial phase of the macular area of a patient with diabetic retinopathy. Two small arteries show loss of side branches **(arrows)**. One has out-pouchings which may be pruned-off side branches **(arrow 1)**.

PROLIFERATIVE RETINOPATHY

The increase in the incidence of proliferative retinopathy and the number of patients who suffer blindness as a result of it makes this one of the most dreaded complications of diabetes.

The incidence of retinitis proliferans among diabetics has risen steeply since the 1930s when it was only about 1 per cent. In their retrospective study of the Oxford diabetic clinic, Burditt, Caird, and Draper[16] have found proliferative retinopathy in only 2 per cent of all diabetic patients and in 6 per cent of those with retinopathy. Kornerup, in 1958,[61] examined 1402 patients and found that 117 or 8.4 per cent had proliferative retinopathy. The majority had diabetes which began in childhood, in 67 of the 117 before their fourteenth year. In a few patients proliferative changes were the first feature of diabetic retinopathy to be noted.

Proliferative retinopathy is rare under the age of 20, but as diabetics whose disease began in childhood survive into adult life the incidence of proliferative retinopathy begins to rise steeply. Root, Mirsky, and Ditzel[79] have studied 1072 patients attending the Joslin Clinic who had developed diabetes before their fifteenth birthday and survived for 20 or more years. Retinitis proliferans was present in 28.7 per cent of patients between 20 and 29 years, in 53.1 per cent between 30 and 39 years, and in 58.4 per cent of patients between 40 and 49 years of age. In all patients with proliferative retinopathy the average duration of diabetes prior to discovery of retinitis proliferans was 17 years in patients up to 39 years, 10 years in those between 40 and 59 years, and 4 years in those over 60. The survival of patients who develop retinitis proliferans is relatively poor. The average survival time from the appearance of proliferative lesions was only 5.4 years. The incidence of diabetic retinopathy continues to rise with duration of the disease and White[96] found that among 478 patients whose disease began in childhood, 90 per cent had retinopathy 30 years later. Of these, one-third had proliferative retinopathy.

PATHOPHYSIOLOGY

The pathophysiology of new vessel growth and fibrous proliferation is incompletely understood. The first visible change is a brush of abnormal capillaries, often with an exaggerated hairpin loop pattern (Fig. 15-23) lying in an area where the normal capillary bed is damaged or destroyed. On fluorescein angiograms these vessels often empty more slowly than surrounding normal capillaries and tend to leak fluorescein (Fig. 15-23). Unless they can definitely be seen as preretinal it is difficult to determine the point at which they cease to be abnormal capillaries and can properly be termed new vessels. As they begin to grow, these vessels push forward through the internal limiting membrane and extend along the surface of the retina behind the vitreous. Rapid forward growth of new vessels is particularly prone to occur when these vessels arise from the optic nerve head (Fig. 15-24) and Wise[97] has suggested this occurs because the internal limiting membrane is absent over the optic disc.

As the new vessel system expands the draining veins tend to dilate and at this stage the vascular inflow appears to arise from the capillary bed itself (Fig. 15-25). Later distinct arterial connections can be visualized with fluorescein angiograms (Fig. 15-26). On clinical examination the vessels appear to be bare, although later a thin, cloudy film of fibrous tissue surrounds

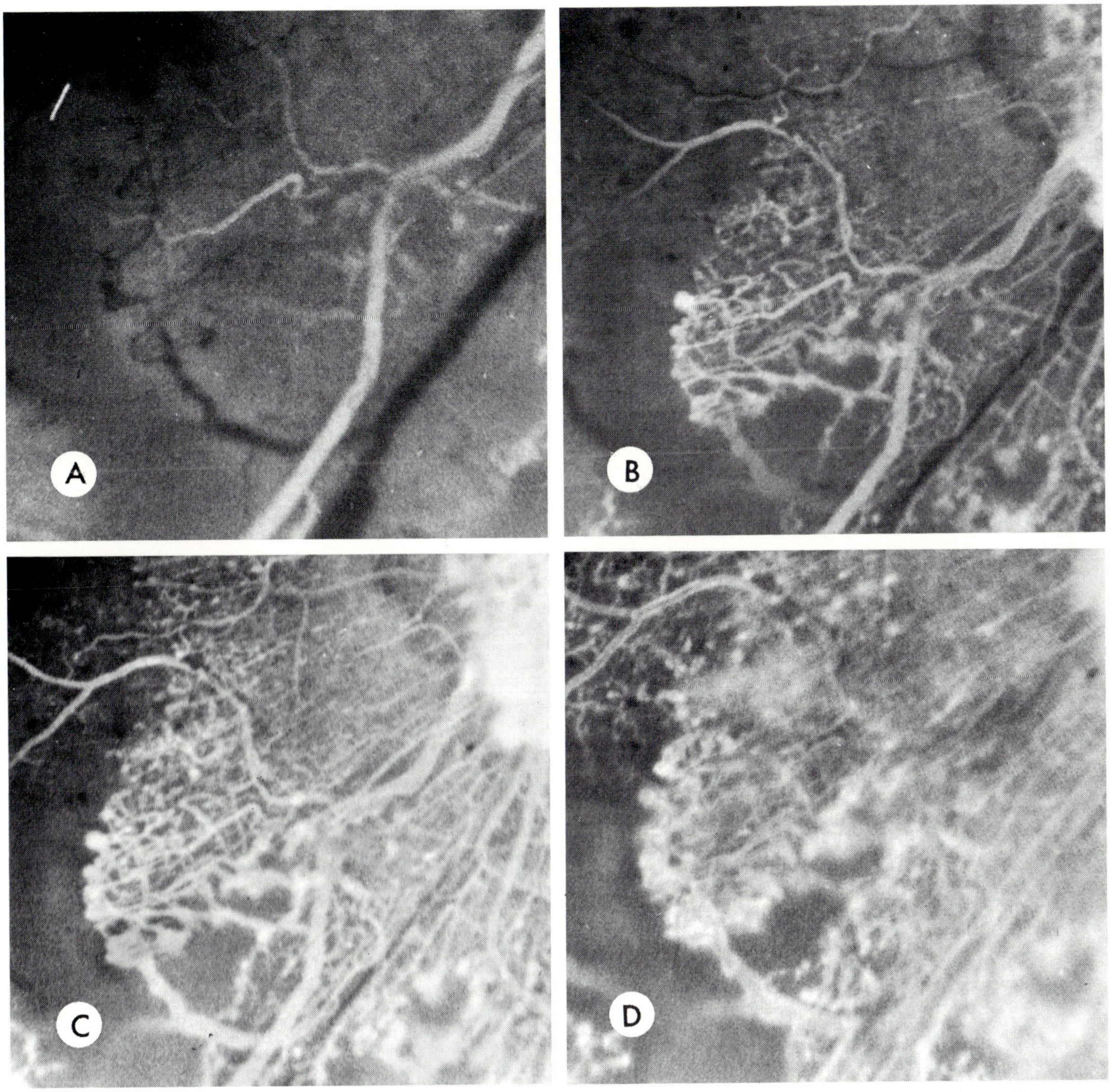

Fig. 15-23. *A*, Arterial-phase fluorescein angiogram in a patient with a brush of abnormal capillaries at the edge of an area of capillary closure. *B*, Taken 1 second later than *A*. Note that the capillary loops are filling and there are large microaneurysms along the edge of the area of closure. *C*, At 2 seconds the capillary loops have filled completely and there is early leakage of dye. *D*, At 3 seconds there is a diffuse leakage of dye from the dilated capillary loops.

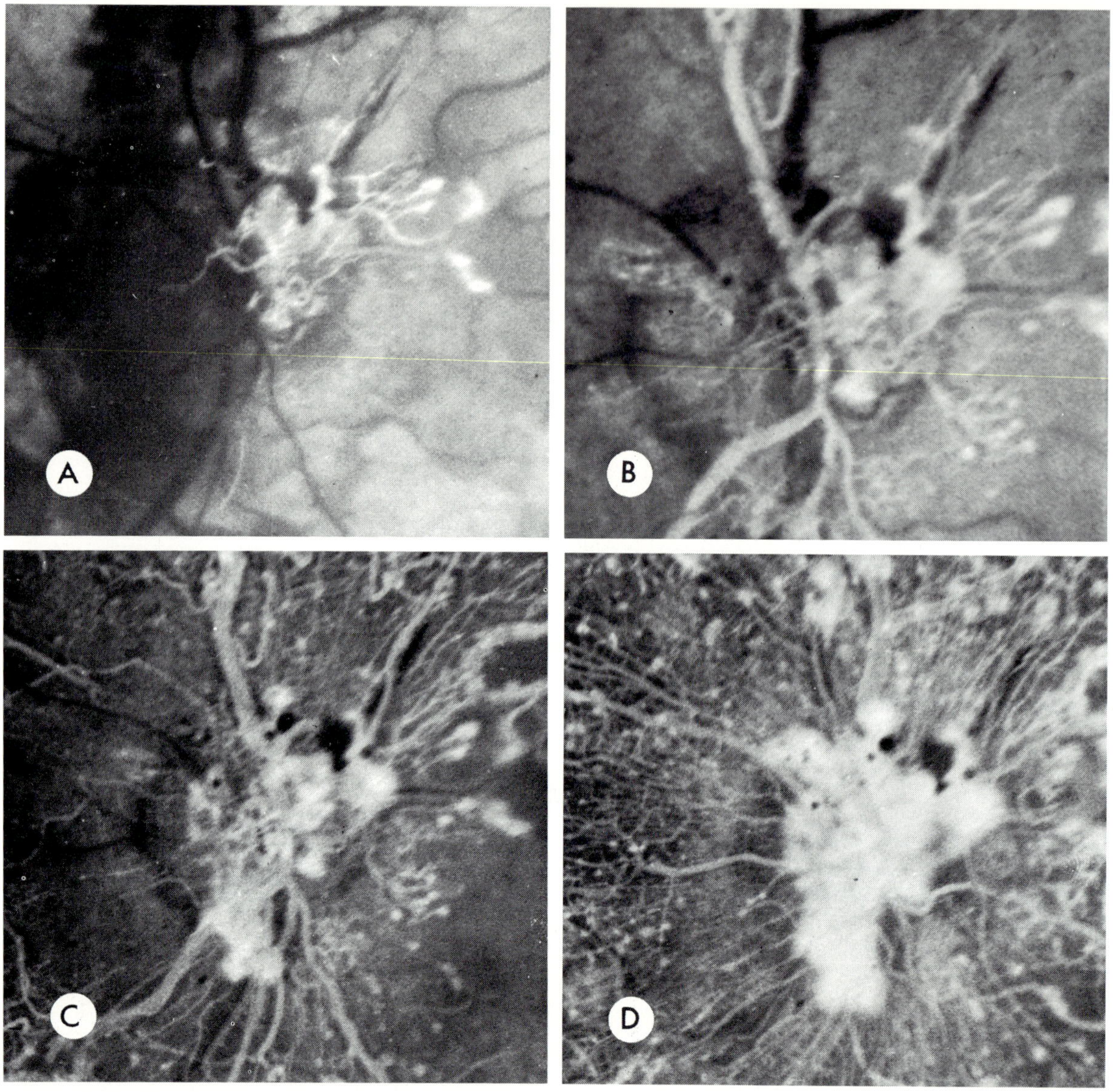

Fig. 15-24. *A*, Early-arterial phase of a fluorescein angiogram in a patient with a leash of new vessels arising from the optic nerve head. Some of the new vessels have filled although there is no dye in the retinal vessels. *B*, One second after *A* the fronds of the new vessel system are filled while only the main retinal arteries contain fluorescein. *C*, After 2 seconds the retinal capillaries have filled and dye is beginning to spread out from the new vessels on the papilla as it leaks through their wall. *D*, At 3 seconds there is diffuse leakage from the mass of new vessels on the papilla.

argue that bleeding from new vessels is an important cause of visual deterioration in diabetic patients.

Recently a much more widespread type of photocoagulation treatment has been applied by Wetzig and others.[93] In this technique the aim is to photocoagulate wide areas of the retina at low dosage to destroy small blood vessels along each of the four main vessel groups but sparing the macula. Wetzig has even photocoagulated abnormal vessels springing from the disc or overlying the papillomacular bundle, without necessarily causing permanent damage to vision. It has been claimed that vascular abnormalities may be improved in areas not directly subjected to the photocoagulating beam.

There is an urgent need for these methods of photocoagulation to be subjected to a randomized controlled trial so that their place in therapy can be established. Causing such severe retinal damage with the light coagulator must be justified by showing that the long-term prognosis for vision is improved.[14]

EFFECT OF DIABETIC CONTROL ON RETINOPATHY

Many authors have suggested that there is a relationship between diabetic control and the incidence of diabetic retinopathy.[15,16,22,38,44,52,80,85] In 1949, Jackson and his colleagues reported a study of 75 juvenile diabetics with disease of at least 10 years' standing and in 1956 the same group expanded the numbers to 132 patients.[38,44] There was a significant inverse relationship ($r = 0.65$) between the diabetic control and the severity of the retinal lesions.

Spoont, and his co-workers[85] have used a glycosuria score of zero to 4 to assess diabetic control and divided their patients into two groups, with a score of less than 25 per cent of maximum and those with more. The former group, "well-controlled," had only 4 of 25 individuals with diabetic retinopathy while the latter contained 17 individuals with retinopathy out of 25. The age and insulin requirements were different: the well-controlled group averaged 63 years of age and had 23 units of insulin daily while the poorly controlled group averaged 56 years of age and had 39 units of insulin daily. Of 9 patients who had at least one episode of diabetic acidosis there were 6 who had retinal lesions.

Schlesinger and his colleagues studied 47 patients with long-term diabetes. Of 18 well-controlled patients, 4 had escaped retinopathy, while of 23 poorly controlled patients all had retinopathy.[80]

Colwell reviewed the literature in 1966.[22] Of 373 patients having well-controlled diabetes of more than 15 years' duration, he found that about 53 per cent had retinopathy while of the 292 with poor control about 75 per cent had retinopathy. He pointed out the difficulty of interpreting data on incidence during the period of 5 to 15 years after onset of diabetes when the incidence of diabetic retinopathy is rising steeply. It may be that good diabetic control only slows down the onset of retinopathy so that studies made on the steeply rising part of the curve are more likely to show a significant difference than those made later when both groups have a high incidence. This view is supported by the data of Burditt, Caird, and Draper[16] who have used a system of scoring glycosuria percentage (percentage of occasional urine containing 2 per cent of sugar) and divided the patients into groups, with scores above and below 20 per cent. In patients over 60 there was no difference in the incidence of retinopathy between those with good or poor control but in younger age groups there was a consistent difference (Fig. 15-31). Thus for diabetics of 15 to 19 years' duration, 63 per

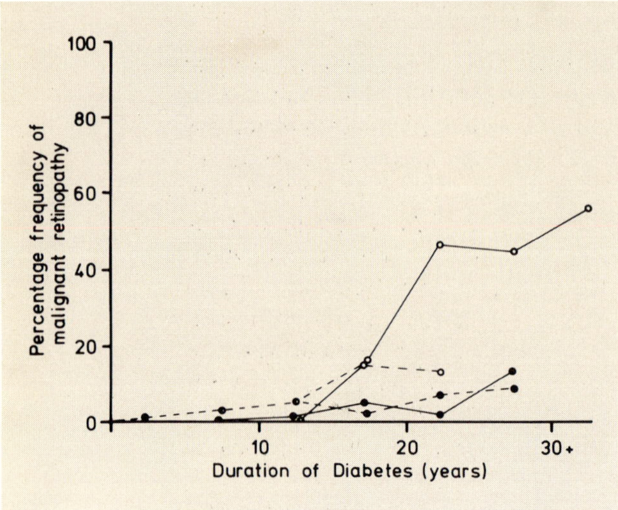

Fig. 15-31. The incidence of proliferative diabetic retinopathy versus the duration of diabetes from a number of published series. (From Burditt, Caird, and Draper.[16])

Fig. 15-32. *A*, Fluorescein angiogram in a girl with badly controlled diabetes. There are multiple abnormal capillary loops and aneurysms. *B*, After 9 months of strict diabetic control the capillary bed had almost returned to normal. (From Dollery and Oakley[29]: *Diabetes 14:*121, 1965.)

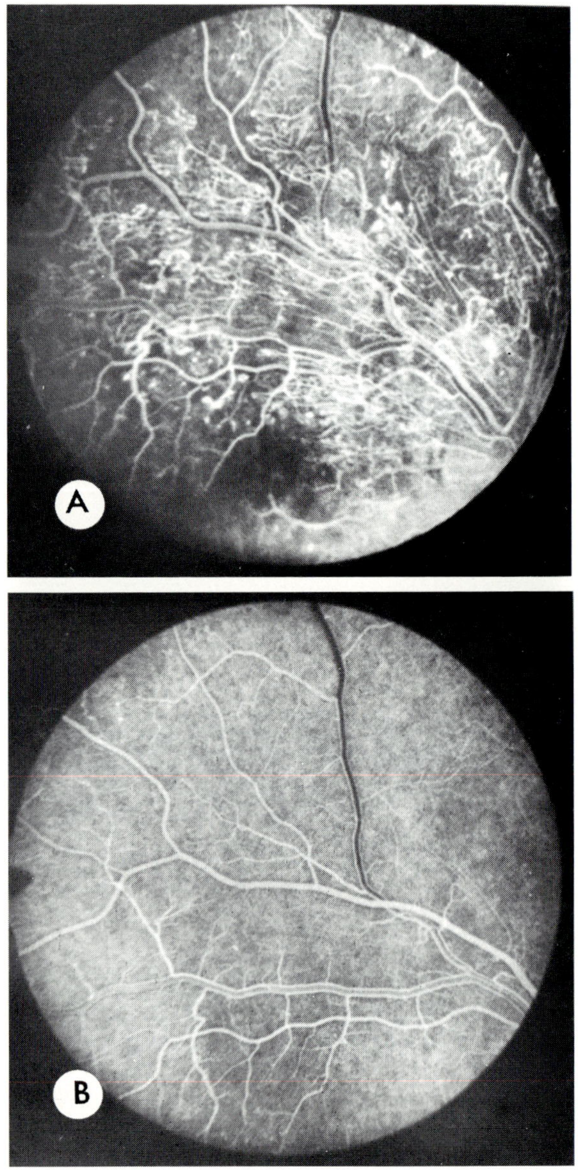

cent of those under 29 years with good control had retinopathy while 77 per cent of those with poor control were so affected. Similar figures for the same duration, for those between the ages of 30 to 59 were 52 per cent among those with good control and 72 per cent among those with poor control. Caird and his colleagues have plotted the incidence of retinopathy versus duration of disease and found a linear relationship up to 20 years with the incidence of retinopathy in the well-controlled group running slightly lower than the others.

Those patients with the lower incidence of glycosuria had a 50 per cent chance of developing retinopathy after 14.4 years of diabetes while the group with heavier glycosuria reached the same point after 12.9 years. The difference is small, but statistically significant. In all these studies which relate the severity of complications to diabetic control it is possible that there are differences in the underlying diabetes which are responsible for both the higher incidence of complications and the difficulty in controlling the blood sugar.

SPONTANEOUS IMPROVEMENT

One of the problems of assessing treatment of diabetic retinopathy is that spontaneous improvement can occur, sometimes associated with improvement in diabetic control. Burditt, Caird, and Garrett[16] esti-

TABLE 15-1
Retinal Changes in Diabetic Animals

Species	Type of Diabetes	Retinal Changes
Dog	Spontaneous	Microaneurysms, degeneration of intramural pericytes, nonfunctioning capillaries
	Pancreatectomy	Hemorrhages
Cat	Spontaneous	Nonfunctioning capillaries, ghost cells
Rat	Alloxan	Retinal hemorrhages, dilated vessels
	Alloxan and cortisone	Tortuous capillaries
	Alloxan and testosterone and estrogen	Hemorrhages and exudates
	Pancreatectomy	Hyaline changes of arterioles, microaneurysms
Hamster	Cortisone and growth hormone	Dilated vessels
Rabbit	Alloxan	Hemorrhages
	Alloxan and fatty diet	Fusiform aneurysms of vessels
	Alloxan and hypoxia	Vasodilatation and tortuous vessels
	Cortisone and growth hormone	Microaneurysms and venous distension

Adopted from Table 14 of Toussaint.[87] In many instances the changes reported have been minimal and have not been confirmed by other workers.

mated the chance of spontaneous clearing might be as high as 30 per cent in younger patients with microaneurysms but their study was carried out from written clinical records and may prove to be an overestimate. Dobree[28] has found four eyes in three patients with new vessels that showed spontaneous regression and Davis[25] has reported a similar patient. Dollery and Oakley[29] have reported a girl with severe and poorly controlled diabetes who showed complete regression of masses of dilated hairpin capillary loops and fatty exudates during a period when her diabetic control was improved (Fig. 15-32).

The possibility of spontaneous improvement emphasizes the need to carry out properly designed, controlled trials of any form of therapy.[51]

EXPERIMENTAL DIABETIC RETINOPATHY

Bloodworth and Molitor[12] have studied the retinal changes in dogs made diabetic either by treatment with bovine growth hormone or alloxan. There was diffuse but irregular involvement of the capillary basement membrane, and a number of thin-walled microaneurysms were found. Except for the out-pouching, the aneurysm wall was identical with that of nearby capillaries.

Patz and Maumenee[77] have reported a study of a 12-year-old cocker spaniel dog that developed spontaneous diabetes at the age of 9. The animal was treated with both insulin and tolbutamide at different times and had two episodes of acidosis. The retina contained several microaneurysms and the capillaries showed some loss of intramural pericytes and cell ghosts. The glomeruli contain PAS-positive material but not typical Kimmelstiel-Wilson nodules.

Becker[8] felt he had produced aneurysms in alloxan-diabetic rabbits given ACTH, but Engerman, Meyer, and Buesseler[31] were unable to reproduce this observation. Hausler, Sibay, and Stachowska[39] have produced arterial and capillary dilatation in the retinae of Chinese hamsters made diabetic with cortisone and growth hormone.

There does not seem any doubt that microaneurysms have been produced in diabetic dogs and probably in other species.[12,31,77,87] Retinitis proliferans may occur occasionally in alloxan-diabetic rats.[87] Toussaint recently reviewed the literature (see Table 15-1).

REFERENCES

1. Armstrong, J. K., Daily, R. K., Dobson, H. L., and Girard, L. J.: The incidence of glaucoma in diabetes mellitus. *Amer. J. Ophthal. 50:*55, 1960.
2. Ashton, N.: Diabetic retinopathy. *Proc. Roy. Soc. Med. 44:*747, 1951.
3. Ashton, N.: Arteriolar involvement in diabetic retinopathy. *Brit. J. Ophthal. 37:*282, 1953.
4. Ashton, N.: Studies of retinal capillaries in relation to diabetic and other retinopathies. *Brit. J. Ophthal. 47:*521, 1963.
5. Ashton, N.: Bowman, attributed to by. In: The blood-retinal barrier and vaso-glial relationships in retinal disease. *Trans. Ophthal. Soc. U.K. 85:*199, 1965.
6. Ballantyne, A. J.: The state of the retina in diabetes mellitus. *Trans. Ophthal. Soc. U.K. 65:*503, 1945.
7. Ballantyne, A. J., and Loewenstein, A.: The pathology of diabetic retinopathy. *Trans. Ophthal. Soc. U.K. 63:*95, 1943.
8. Becker, B.: Diabetic retinopathy. *Ann. Intern. Med. 37:*273, 1952.
9. Beetham, W. P.: Visual prognosis of proliferating diabetic retinopathy. *Brit. J. Ophthal. 47:*611, 1963.
10. Berkow, J. W., Shugarman, R. L., Maumenee, A. E., and Patz, A.: A retrospective study of blind diabetic patients. *JAMA 193:*867, 1965.
11. Bloodworth, J. M. B.: Diabetic retinopathy. *Diabetes 11:*1, 1962.
12. Bloodworth, J. M. B., and Molitor, D. L.: Ultrastructural aspects of human and canine diabetic retinopathy. *Invest. Ophthal. 4:*1037, 1965.
13. Bradley, R. F., Rees, S. B., and Fager, C. A.: Pituitary ablation in the treatment of diabetic retinopathy. *Med. Clin. N. Amer. 49:*1105, 1965.
14. Brockhurst, R. J.: Diabetes and photocoagulation. *Arch. Ophthal. 75:*305, 1966.
15. Brown, I. K., and Jones, A. T.: Retinopathy and diabetic control. *Brit. J. Ophthal. 48:* 148, 1964.
16. Burditt, A. F., Caird, F. I., and Draper, G. J.: The natural history of diabetic retinopathy. *Quart. J. Med. 37:*303, 1968.
17. Caird, F. I., Burditt, A. F., and Draper, G. J.: Diabetic retinopathy. A further study of prognosis for vision. *Diabetes 17:*121, 1968.
18. Caird, F. I., and Garrett, C. J.: Prognosis for vision in diabetic retinopathy. *Diabetes 12:* 389, 1963.
19. Chester, E. M., and Barker, B. Q.: The role of lipid thrombi in the pathogenesis of diabetic retinopathy. *Arch. Intern. Med. 120:* 397, 1967.
20. Cogan, D. G., and Kuwabara, T.: Capillary shunts in the pathogenesis of diabetic retinopathy. *Diabetes 12:*293, 1963.
21. Cogan, D. G., Toussaint, D., and Kuwabara, T.: Studies of retinal vascular patterns. IV. Diabetic retinopathy. *Arch. Ophthal. 66:* 366, 1961.
22. Colwell, J. A.: Effect of diabetic control on retinopathy. *Diabetes 15:*497, 1966.
23. Cook, C. A. G.: Role of fat emboli in diabetic retinopathy. *Brit. J. Ophthal. 41:*741, 1957.
24. Cristiansson, J.: Intraocular pressure in diabetes mellitus. *Acta Ophthal. 39:*155, 1961.
25. Davis, M. D.: "Natural Course of Diabetic

Retinopathy," in *Vascular Complications of Diabetes Mellitus*. Ed. Kimura, S. J., and Caygill, W. M. St. Louis, Mo., Mosby, 1967, pp. 139–169.

26. Deckert, T., Simonsen, S. E., and Poulsen, J. E.: Prognosis of proliferative retinopathy in juvenile diabetics. *Diabetes 16:*728, 1967.
27. Ditzel, J., and White, P.: Central vein occlusion in diabetes. *J. Chron. Dis. 3:*205, 1956.
28. Dobree, J. H.: Proliferative diabetic retinopathy: Evolution of the retinal lesions. *Brit. J. Ophthal. 48:*637, 1964.
29. Dollery, C. T., and Oakley, N. W.: Reversal of retinal vascular changes in diabetes. *Diabetes 14:*121, 1965.
30. van Eck, W. F.: The effect of a low-fat diet on the serum lipids in diabetes and its significance in diabetic retinopathy. *Amer. J. Med. 27:*196, 1959.
31. Engerman, R. L., and Bloodworth, J. M. B.: Experimental diabetic retinopathy in dogs. *Arch. Ophthal. 73:*205, 1965.
32. Engerman, R. L., Meyer, R. L., and Buesseler, J. A.: Effects of alloxan diabetes and steroid hypertension on retinal vasculature. *Amer. J. Ophthal. 58:*965, 1964.
33. Field, R. A., Schepens, C. L., Sweet, W. H., and Appels, A.: Effect of hypophyseal stalk section on advancing diabetic retinopathy. *Diabetes 11:*465, 1962.
34. Friedenwald, J. S.: Diabetic retinopathy. *Amer. J. Ophthal. 33:*1187, 1950.
35. Gass, J. D. M.: A fluorescein angiographic study of macular dysfunction secondary to retinal vascular disease. IV. Diabetic retinopathy. *Arch. Ophthal. 80:*583, 1968.
36. Goldberg, M. F., and Fine, S. L. (Ed.): *Symposium on Treatment of Diabetic Retinopathy.* Washington, D.C., U.S. Dept. of Health, Education and Welfare, 1969.
37. Hanum, S.: Diabetes retinitis. *Acta Ophthal. Suppl.* 16, 1938.
38. Hardin, R. C., Jackson, R. L., Johnston, T. L., and Kelly, H. G.: The development of diabetic retinopathy: Effects of duration and control of diabetes. *Diabetes 5:*397, 1956.
39. Hausler, H. R., Sibay, T. M., and Stachowska, B.: Observations of retinal microaneurysms in a metahypophyseal diabetic Chinese hamster. *Amer. J. Ophthal. 56:*242, 1963.
40. Hickam, J. B., and Sieker, H. O.: Retinal vascular reactivity in patients with diabetes mellitus and with atherosclerosis. *Circulation 22:*243, 1960.
41. Hirschberg, J.: Ueber diabetische netzhautentsundung. *Deutsch. Med. Wschr. 51:*1181, 1890; and *51:*1236, 1890.
42. Houssay, B. A., and Biasotti, A.: Pankreasdiabetes und Hypophyse beim Hund. *Arch. Ges. Physiol. 227:*664, 1931.
43. Ireland, J. T., Cullen, J. F., and Oliver, M. F.: A study of the effect of Atromid therapy in exudative diabetic retinopathy. *J. Atheroscler. Res. 3:*70, 1963.
44. Jackson, R. L., Hardin, R. C., Walker, G. L., Hendricks, A. B., and Kelly, H. G.: Degenerative change in young diabetic patients in relationship to level of control. *Pediatrics 5:*959, 1950.
45. von Jaeger, E.: *Beitrage sur Pathologie des Auges.* Wien, Kaiserlich Koniglichen hof und Staatsdruckerei, 1855.
46. Jain, I. S., and Luthra, C. L.: Diabetic retinopathy. Its relationship with intraocular pressure. *Arch. Ophthal. 78:*198, 1967.
47. Jain, I. S., Luthra, C. L., and Das, T.: Diabetic retinopathy and its relation to errors of refraction. *Arch. Ophthal. 77:*59, 1967.
48. Joplin, G. F., Fraser, R., Hill, D. W., Oakley, N. W., Scott, D. J., and Doyle, F. H.: Pituitary ablation for diabetic retinopathy. *Quart. J. Med. 34:*443, 1965.
49. Joplin, G. F., Oakley, N. W., Hill, D. W., Kohner, E. M., and Fraser, R.: Diabetic retinopathy. II. Comparison of disease remission induced by various degrees of pituitary ablation by Y^{90}. *Diabetologia 3:*406, 1967.
50. Jutte, A.: Gefassweiterungmessungen am augenhintergrund bein jugendlichen diabetikern. *Ber. Deutsch. Ophthal. Ges. 63:*419, 1960.
51. Keen, H., and Smith, R.: Vitamin B_{12} and the course of diabetic retinopathy. *Lancet 1:*849, 1959.
52. Keiding, N. R., Root, H. F., and Marble, A.: Importance of control of diabetes in prevention of vascular complications. *JAMA 150:* 964, 1952.
53. Kempner, W.: Radical dietary treatment of hypertensive and arteriosclerotic vascular disease, heart and kidney disease, and vascular retinopathy. *GP 9:*71, 1954.
54. King, R. C., Dobree, J. H., Kok, D. A., Foulds, W. S., and Dangerfield, W. G.: Exudative diabetic retinopathy: Spontaneous

changes and effects of a corn oil diet. *Brit. J. Ophthal. 47*:666, 1963.

55. Klien, B. A., and Olwin, J. H.: A survey of the pathogenesis of retinal vein occlusion. *Arch. Ophthal. 56*:207, 1956.
56. Kohner, E. M.: "Diabetic Retinopathy: Cause, Treatment and Prognosis." (M.D. Thesis, University of London, 1969.)
57. Kohner, E. M., and Dollery, C. T.: The rate of formation and disappearance of retinal microaneurysms in diabetes. *Europ. J. Clin. Invest. 1*:167, 1970.
58. Kohner, E. M., Dollery, C. T., and Bulpitt, C. J.: Cotton-wool spots in diabetic retinopathy. *Diabetes 16*:691, 1969.
59. Kohner, E. M., Dollery, C. T., Shakib, M., Henkind, P., Paterson, J. W., de Oliveira, L. N. F., and Bulpitt, C. J.: Experimental retinal branch vein occlusion. *Amer. J. Ophthal. 69*:778, 1970.
60. Kohner, E. M., Dollery, C. T., Paterson, J. W., and Oakley, N. W.: Arterial fluorescein studies in diabetic retinopathy. *Diabetes 16*:1, 1967.
61. Kornerup, T.: Retinopathia diabetic proliferans. *Acta Ophthal. 36*:87, 1958.
62. Kuwabara, T., and Cogan, D. G.: Retinal vascular patterns. VI. Mural cells of the retinal capillaries. *Arch. Ophthal. 69*:492, 1963.
63. Larsen, H-W.: Atlas of diabetic retinopathy. *Acta Ophthal. Suppl. 55,* 1959.
64. Larsen, H-W.: Diabetic retinopathy. *Acta Ophthal. Suppl. 60,* 1960.
65. Leber, T. H.: Ueber die Erkraukungen des Auges bei Diabetes Mellitus. *Graefe Arch. Ophthal. 31(3)*:206, 1875.
66. Lee, P., McMeel, J. W., Schepens, C. L., and Field, R. A.: A new classification of diabetic retinopathy. *Amer. J. Ophthal. 62*:207, 1966.
67. Luft, R.: The use of hypophysectomy in juvenile diabetes mellitus with vascular complications. *Diabetes 11*:461, 1962.
68. Luft, R., Olivecrona, H., Ikkos, D., Kornerup, T., and Ljunggren, H.: Hypophysectomy in man. Further experience in severe diabetes mellitus. *Brit. Med. J. 2*:752, 1955.
69. Lundbaeck, K.: Ocular manifestations of diabetic angiopathy. J. *Roy. Coll. Surg. I. 1*:28, 1963.
70. MacKenzie, S.: A case of glycosuric retinitis, with comments. *Ophthal. Hosp. Rep. 9*:134, 1879.
71. Meyer-Schwickerath, G. R. E., and Schott, K.: Diabetic retinopathy and photocoagulation. *Amer. J. Ophthal. 66*:597, 1968.
72. Mooney, A. J.: Diabetic retinopathy—a challenge. *Brit. J. Ophthal. 47*:513, 1963.
73. Nettleship, E.: Chronic retinitis with formation of blood vessels in the vitreous in a patient with diabetes. Results of chronic iritis accompanied by the formation of large vessels in the iris. *Trans. Ophthal. Soc. U.K. 8*:159, 1888.
74. Oakley, N. W., Hill, D. W., Joplin, G. F., Kohner, E. M., and Fraser, R.: A grading system for diabetic retinopathy. *Diabetologia 3*:402, 1967.
75. Okun, E., and Cibis, P.: The role of photocoagulation in the therapy of proliferative diabetic retinopathy. *Arch. Ophthal. 75*:337, 1966.
76. de Oliveira, L. F. N.: Pericytes in diabetic retinopathy. *Brit. J. Ophthal. 50*:134, 1966.
77. Patz, A., and Maumenee, A. E.: Studies on diabetic retinopathy. I. Retinopathy in a dog with spontaneous diabetes mellitus. *Amer. J. Ophthal. 54*:532, 1962.
78. Poulsen, J. E.: Recovery from retinopathy in a case of diabetes with Simmonds' disease. *Diabetes 2*:7, 1953.
79. Root, H. F., Mirsky, S., and Ditzel, J.: Proliferative retinopathy in diabetes mellitus. *JAMA 169*:903, 1959.
80. Schlesinger, F. G., Franken, S., van Lange, L. Th. P., and Schwarz, F.: Incidence and progression of retinal and vascular lesions in long-term diabetes. *Acta Med. Scand. 168*:483, 1960.
81. Scott, D. J., Dollery, C. T., Hill, D. W., Hodge, J. V., and Fraser, R.: Fluorescein studies of diabetic retinopathy. *Brit. Med. J. 1*:811, 1964.
82. Sieker, H. O., and Hickam, J. B.: Normal and impaired vascular reactivity. *Circulation 7*:79, 1953.
83. Speakman, J. S., Mortimer, C. B., Briant, T. D. R., Ezrin, C., Lougheed, W. M., and Clarke, W. T. W.: Pituitary ablation for diabetic retinopathy. *Canad. Med. Ass. J. 94*:627, 1966.
84. Speiser, P., Gittelsohn, A. M., and Patz, A.: Studies on diabetic retinopathy. *Arch. Ophthal. 80*:332, 1968.
85. Spoont, S., Dyer, W. W., Day, R., and Blazer, H.: Incidence of diabetic retinopathy rela-

tive to the degree of diabetic control. *Amer. J. Med. Sci. 221:*490, 1951.

86. Sprague, R. G.: Comments on reports of the effect of hypophysectomy, of hypophyseal stalk section, and of adrenalectomy on diabetic retinopathy. *Diabetes 11:*491, 1962.
87. Toussaint, D.: "Contribution a l'etude Anatomique et Clinique de la retinopathie Diabetic chez l'homme et animaux," in *Pathologia Europa* (*Quarterly*). Brussels, Press Academy European, 1968.
88. Toussaint, D., and Dustin, P.: Electron-microscopy of normal and diabetic retinal capillaries. *Arch. Ophthal. 70:*96, 1963.
89. Valdorf–Hansen, F., Hoyer, I., and Larsen, H–W.: Long-term anticoagulant therapy in diabetic retinopathy. *Acta Ophthal. 42:*579, 1964.
90. Wagener, H. P., Dry, T. J. S., and Wilder, R. M.: Retinitis in diabetes. *New Eng. J. Med. 211:*1131, 1934.
91. Waite, J. H., and Beetham, W. P.: The visual mechanism in diabetes mellitus. *New Eng. J. Med. 212:*367, 1935.
92. Wendland, J. P.: Retinal arteriosclerosis in age, essential hypertension and diabetes mellitus. *Trans. Amer. Ophthal. Soc. 64:*735, 1966.
93. Wetzig, P. C., and Jepson, C. N.: Treatment of diabetic retinopathy by light coagulation. *Amer. J. Ophthal. 62:*459, 1966.
94. Wetzig, P. C., and Worlton, J. T.: Treatment of diabetic retinopathy by light-coagulation. *Brit. J. Ophthal. 47:*539, 1963.
95. White, P.: Natural cause and prognosis of juvenile diabetes. *Diabetes 5:*443, 1956.
96. White, P.: Childhood diabetes, its course and influence on the second and third generations. *Diabetes 9:*345, 1960.
97. Wise, G. N.: Retinal neovascularisation. *Trans. Amer. Ophthal. Soc. 54:*729, 1956.
98. Wolter, J. R.: Diabetic capillary microaneurysms of the retina. *Arch. Ophthal. 65:*107, 1961.
99. Yamashita, T., and Rosen, D. A.: Electron-microscopic study of diabetic capillary aneurysms. *Arch. Ophthal. 67:*875, 1962.
100. Yanoff, M.: Diabetic retinopathy. *New Eng. J. Med. 274:*1344, 1966.

Disciform Macular Diseases

A number of macular diseases, at some time during their course, develop a disc-like elevated mound at the macula. At this stage, diseases of diverse etiology may have such similar clinical appearances that differential diagnosis is difficult.

In the course of their natural history, some disciform diseases have such a varied morphology that specific stages of a single condition have been described as separate entities.

This section is devoted to the natural course of these disciform macular lesions.

GENERAL PRINCIPLES

One of the most important contributions toward understanding the disciform macular diseases has been the demonstration in them of fluorescein leakage from the choroid into the subretinal fluid.[50] Interpretation of this finding necessarily involves a consideration of the factors that normally control penetration of fluorescein from the choriocapillaris into the subretinal tissues.

The blood-retinal barrier to fluorescein exists at two sites. First, between the lumen of the retinal vessels and the retinal tissues at the level of the endothelial cells lining these vessels.[10] Second, the barrier of concern in the disciform diseases lies between the lumen of the choroidal capillaries and the retinal neuroreceptors. There are three structures between the choroidal capillary blood and the retina, the wall of the choroidal capillaries, Bruch's membrane, and the pigment epithelium. Studies with colored dyes such as trypan blue and fluorescein all show that these substances escape readily from the choroidal capillaries so that this is an unlikely site of the chorioretinal barrier.[59,67]

Bruch's membrane is not apt to constitute the site of blockage for it is acellular. The blood-retinal barrier for fluorescein appears to depend upon active cellular transport of the dye which can be inhibited by enzyme poisons.[10] Thus, the most likely location of the choriocapillary blood-retinal barrier is the pigment epithelium.

VISIBILITY OF CHOROIDAL FLUORESCENCE WITHOUT LEAKAGE

In a normal eye the pigment epithelium screens most of the choroidal fluorescent light and it is only visible as a back-lighting effect seen immediately before the retinal vessels fill with dye. In patients whose pigment epithelium has a local or more widespread reduction in pigment as with drusen, fundus flavimaculatus, and retinitis pigmentosa, the choroidal fluorescence is clearly visible as bright spots or patches against the generally darker background of normally pigmented areas (Fig. 16-1).[25,40,55] Although the choroidal fluorescence is clearly visible in these conditions, no leakage takes place from the choroid into the subretinal space. In those conditions in which choroidal fluorescence is abnormally visible but no leakage occurs, the layer of pigment epithelial cells is intact, although the cellular pigment content in places is partly or wholly lost. Thus, in drusen an amorphous granular material accumulates within and beneath the epithelial cells often elevating them from contact with Bruch's membrane, but not interrupting their con-

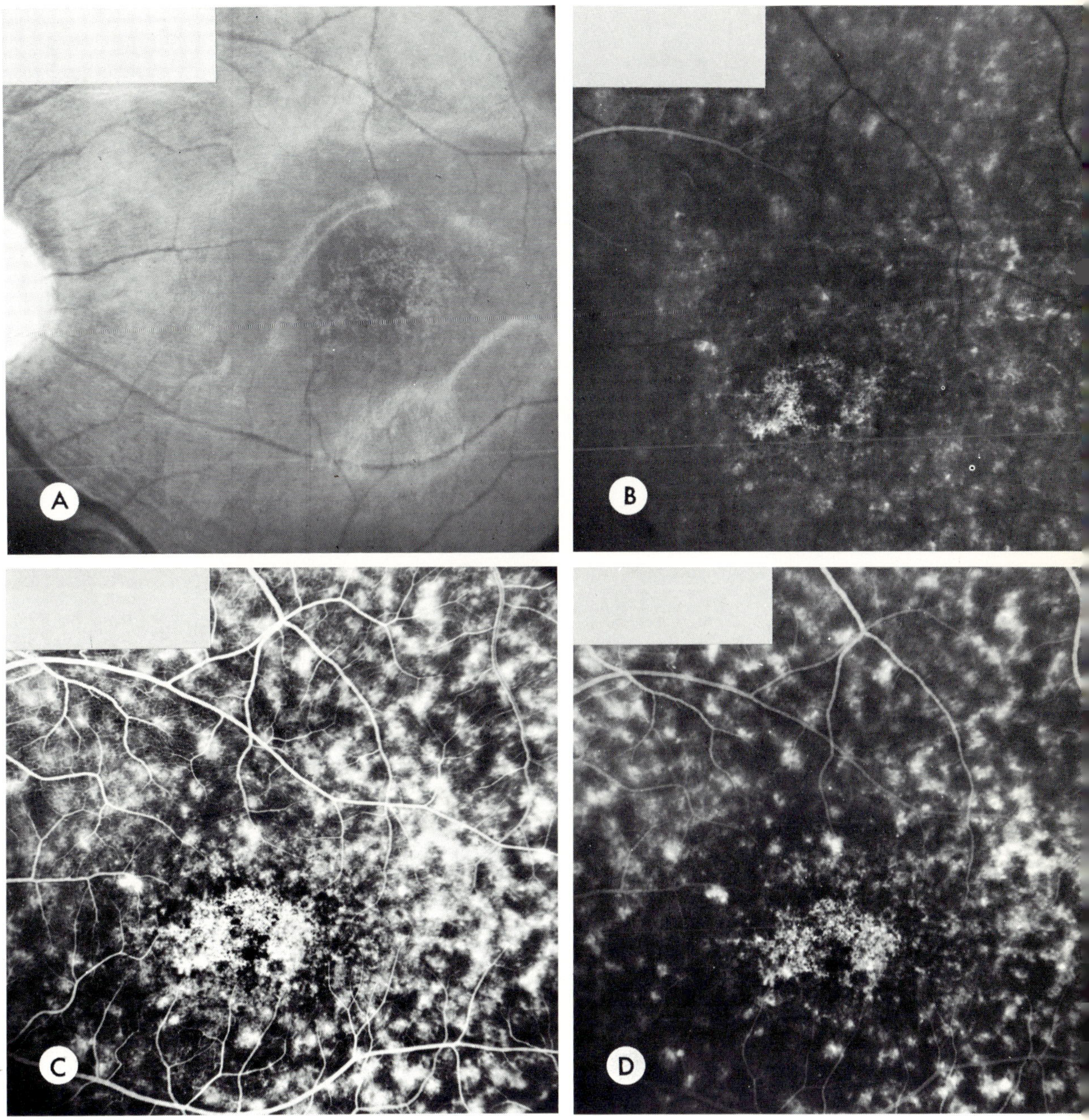

Fig. 16-1. *A*, Fundus flavimaculatus. The retinal highlights are more prominent than the disturbance of pigment epithelium. *B*, Fluorescein angiogram of *A* shows early arterial phase. *C*, Arteriovenous phase shows much more disturbance of the pigment epithelium than is seen clinically in *A*. *D*, A later phase shows decreasing choroidal fluorescence and no leakage.

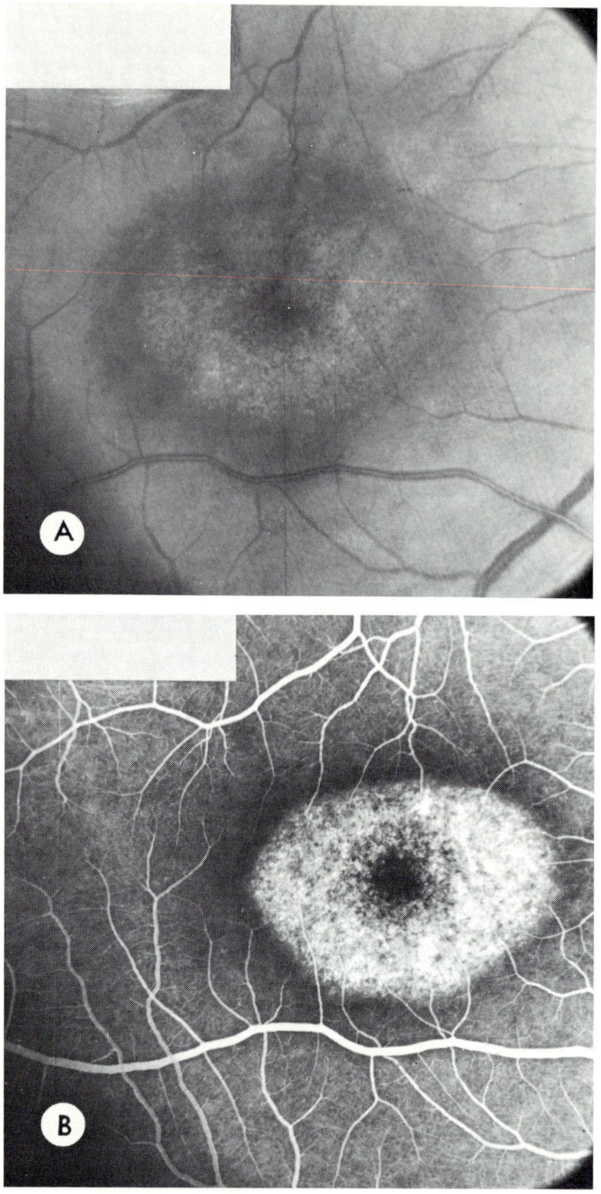

Fig. 16-2. *A*, Macular bullseye in chloroquine retinopathy. *B*, Fluorescein angiogram of *A*.

tinuity.[30] The same is true of fundus flavimaculatus in which a continuous pigment epithelium remains but there is marked variation in the size and pigment content of the cells.[40] In retinitis pigmentosa those areas where the pigment epithelium is lost have a very sclerosed and partly obliterated underlying choriocapillaris. In other areas the pigment epithelium is present but has lost some of its pigment.[16] In chloroquine retinopathy, the pigment is lost from the pigment epithelium around the macula but the cells remain intact. In such areas there is visible fluorescence in the choroid without leakage of dye (Fig. 16-2).

In the absence of macular degeneration, breaks in Bruch's membrane without interruption of the pigment epithelium, such as are seen in the angioid streaks of pseudoxanthoma elasticum, are associated with abnormally visible choroidal fluorescence without dye leakage into the subretinal space (Fig. 16-3).

Thus, abnormal visibility of choroidal fluorescence without leakage requires an intact layer of pigment epithelium with a reduced or entirely lost pigment.

CHOROIDAL LEAKAGE

Leakage of dye from the choroid is a prominent feature following retinal exposure to minimally damaging doses of high-intensity light.[41] The pigment is much more severely damaged than other tissues by such light exposure and dye leakage probably occurs because the cells forming the barrier are damaged. Injection of glass microspheres into the carotid artery causes leakage of fluorescein from retinal vessels at points where the spheres lodge and traumatize the vascular endothelium.[14] Such emboli rarely cause leakage through the chorioretinal barrier although this has been observed to occur on several occasions. Multiple embo-

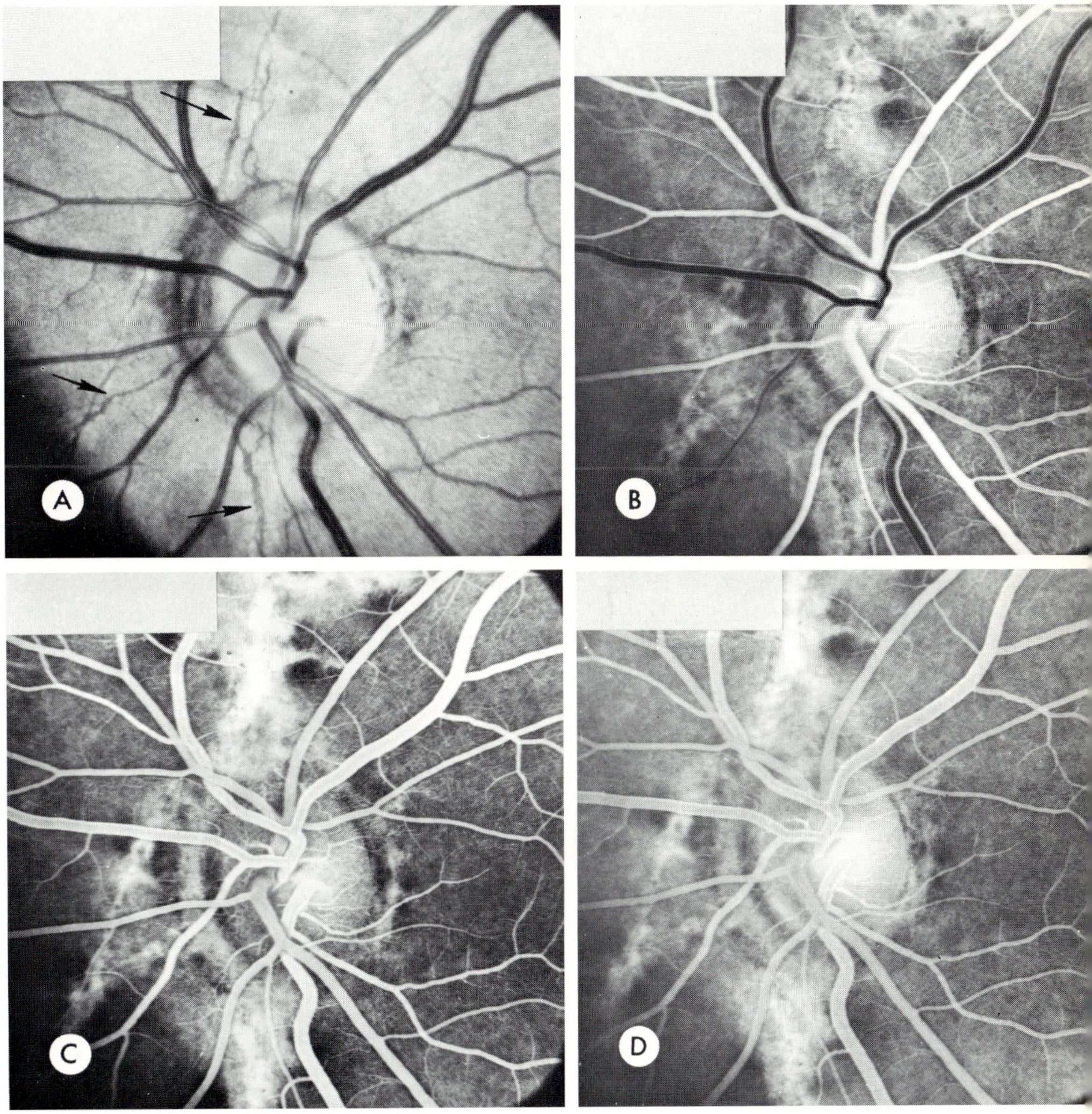

Fig. 16-3. *A*, Angioid streaks **(arrows)** in pseudoxanthoma elasticum. *B*, Arterial-phase fluorescein angiogram. *C*, Arteriovenous-phase fluorescein angiogram. Note prominent fluorescence in regions of angioid streaks. *D*, Later phase showing decreasing fluorescence in regions of angioid streaks and no leakage.

lization of the richly anastomosing choriocapillaris is probably required before sufficient ischemia is produced to impair the viability of the pigment epithelium.

Dye leakage from choroid into the retina appears to require either a break in the continuity of the pigment epithelium or cellular damage such as is caused by exposure to high intensity light or enzyme poisons which inhibit the ability of the cell to pump fluorescein from retina into choroid. Leaking points in diseases such as central serous retinopathy probably represent a break in the continuity of the pigment epithelium. A physically intact epithelium locally damaged by metabolic factors could probably initiate the same process. The blood-retinal barrier presumably exists to control the environment of the retinal cells and protect them from certain materials, possibly organic anions, which would damage them.

REVERSIBLE CENTRAL SEROUS RETINOPATHY

Through the years this lesion has been called by many names, the most common of which are: central serous retinopathy, angiospastic central retinopathy, idiopathic flat detachment of the macula, juvenile macular degeneration, and serous detachment of the pigment epithelium and macula. The term central serous retinopathy is the most widely accepted designation, is still the most descriptive title, and, until exact etiology is available, seems the most useful.

Some patients with central serous retinopathy recover completely without treatment while others show progression to irreversible retinal damage with a macular scar and a corresponding scotoma. For the purposes of discussion central serous retinopathy has been divided into reversible and progressive types although this division does not imply any differences in their etiology. This division can be compared with Klien's [38,39] classification into retinal and chorioretinal central serous retinopathies. Since leakage occurs from the choroid in both types at the onset of the condition, the latter division no longer appears appropriate.

THE CHORIORETINAL LESION

Reversible central serous retinopathy affects young and middle aged men more often than women. Its etiology is unknown and few microscopic studies are available. The disease is acute in onset, may involve one or both eyes, and can be so mild that the patient is unaware of its presence. It is not unusual for the disease to be discovered during a general ocular examination. Vision is often only slightly impaired with a haziness due to increased hyperopia or a slight distortion due to metamorphopsia or micropsia. Central field examination may reveal a relative scotoma or some distortion of the Amsler grid. Macular recovery time following bright light exposure is prolonged [4,48,49] and may remain prolonged after the retina has returned to its normal position.

The typical lesion appears as a sharply demarcated, round or oval elevation of the retina centered at or near the fovea (Fig. 16-4). Typical lesions have been seen without foveal involvement. Extramacular foci are usually found within the boundary of the temporal vessel arcades, but they can occur anywhere at the posterior pole, even nasally to the disc. Such lesions, often called "satellites" (Fig. 16-5), are usually seen in conjunction with central involvement. They may be single or multiple and of varying sizes, but are always smaller than the central mound.

Central lesions range in size from less than 1 dd to large elevations extending from

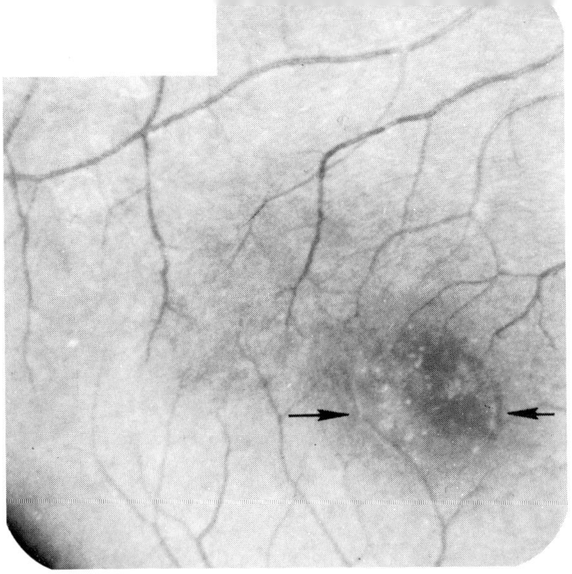

Fig. 16-4. Typical reversible central serous retinopathy. The serous detachment of the retina is well circumscribed **(arrows).** The central white spots lie on the under surface of the retina and on the pigment epithelium.

Fig. 16-5. *Below. A*, Large reversible central serous retinopathy with a satellite lesion **(s)** below; **(f)** is just off the fovea at 5 o'clock; **(p)** points to the pigment epithelial leak of the large lesion just outside of the frame; and the smooth, rounded border of the primary lesion is indicated by **arrows.** *B*, fluorescein angiogram of *A*. Late phase, shows the pigment epithelium leak **(p)** of the primary lesion; the fovea **(f),** and the satellite leak **(s).**

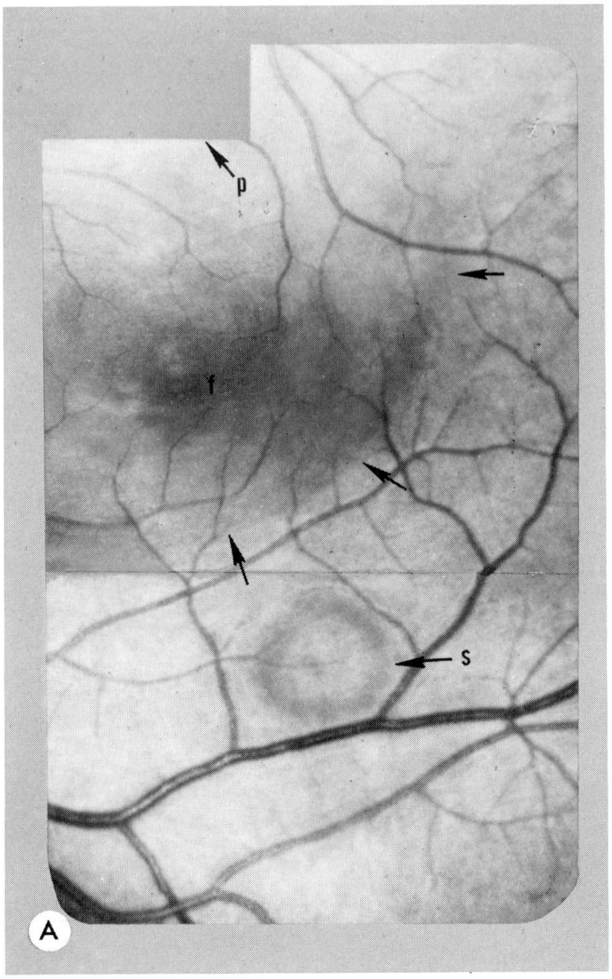

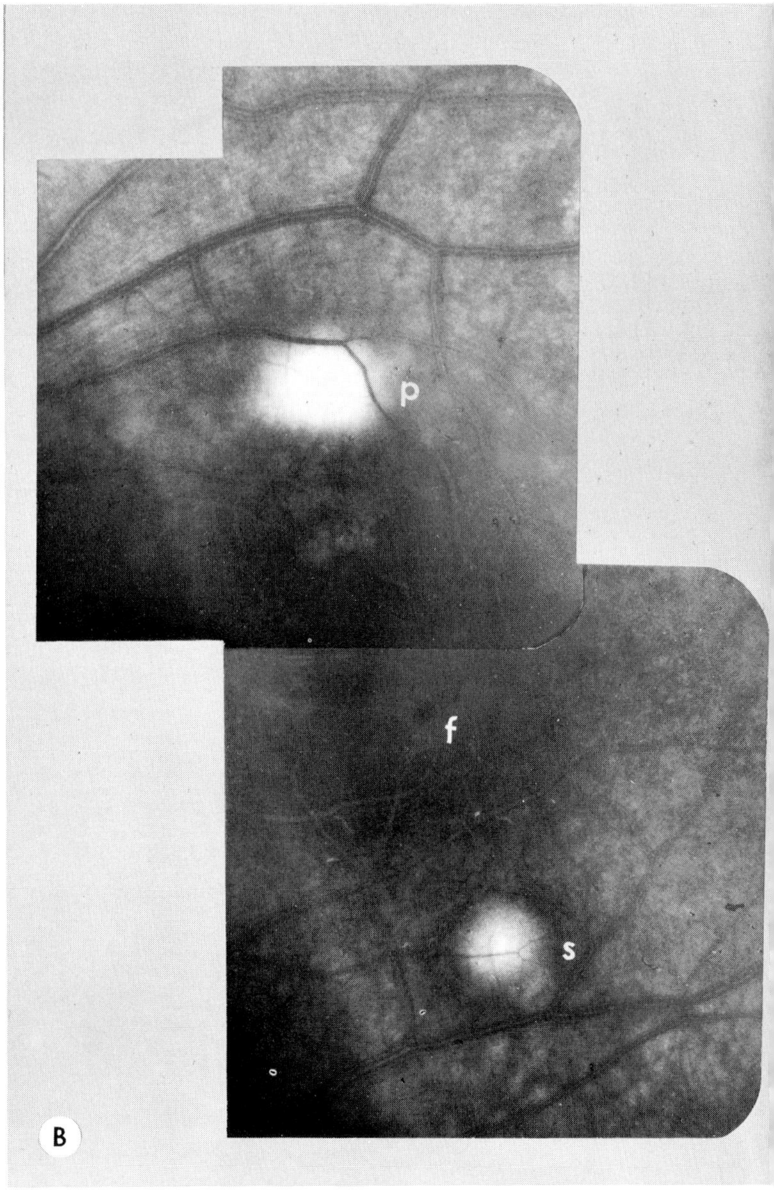

the disc margin temporally to well beyond the fovea. Relatively flat, large lesions may be difficult to delineate because some portion of their rim may not be clearly outlined.

When centrally located, there is a round, hazy appearance at the macula and the foveal reflex is absent. As the light of the ophthalmoscope is moved across the fundus, retinal highlights dance about, but at the border of the lesion they run around its rim and clearly outline its extent. The elevated retina is smooth and appears noncystic when examined by retroillumination. The retinal vessels cast a shadow on the underlying pigment epithelium, the distance between vessel and shadow being greater at the center than at the periphery of the lesion. The clear space between the vessel and its underlying shadow denotes the degree of retinal elevation. This finding, together with an early absence of any microcystic appearance of the retina, places the fluid subretinally between the neuroepithelium and pigment cell layer.

The pigment epithelium beneath the elevated retina shows one or more defective areas (Fig. 16-6). These spots vary, some showing the mildest pigment granularity and others demonstrating more severe pigment clumping or absence or a mixture of the two. Dirty yellow white spots are sometimes noted. Small serous detachments of the pigment epithelium have been reported[21] but in our experience these are not common. It is difficult to predict which, if any, of the areas of pigment disturbance will show leakage on fluorescein angiography. Often a faint granular spot will leak whereas a more obvious defect will not. A clinically visible defect in the pigment epithelium is always present at a point of fluorescein leakage.

FLUORESCEIN ANGIOGRAPHY

Fluorescein angiography shows one or more punctate leaks from the choroid. The leak becomes visible during the venous phase of the angiogram, has fuzzy borders, and spreads with increasing intensity into the subretinal space long after the dye has left the retinal vessels (Fig. 16-7). An occasional leak has been located just outside of the retinal elevation but the vast majority occur somewhere beneath its dome. Some leaks diffuse upward producing a mushroom appearance (Fig. 16-8). Rarely, intermittent leakage from a single point during the course of an attack is suggested by a positive fluorescein test, then a negative test in the presence of good retinal filling, and a subsequent positive test, again at the original leaking site. This observation demonstrates the need of a second fluorescein angiogram, if the first is negative in the presence of a clinically observable lesion. Satellite lesions show similar but milder choroidal leaks.

CLINICAL COURSE

Following the serous elevation, discrete white dots may collect either on the pigment epithelium or the undersurface of the detached retina. Such dots may represent agglomerates of proteinaceous material formed from the subretinal serum. A larger, fuzzy yellowish aggregate may be present beneath the center of the mound. This is generally seen later in the course of the disease, may represent an exaggeration of the previous phenomenon, and is thought to contain a lipid component.

Although they are usually smaller, satellite lesions have similar clinical features and course to those located centrally.

Reversible central serous retinopathy with mild fluctuations in the size and elevation of the mound may persist for several months without causing permanent visual loss (macular function, as determined by macular recovery time may be abnormal even if vision returns to normal). In the vast majority of patients spontaneous recovery

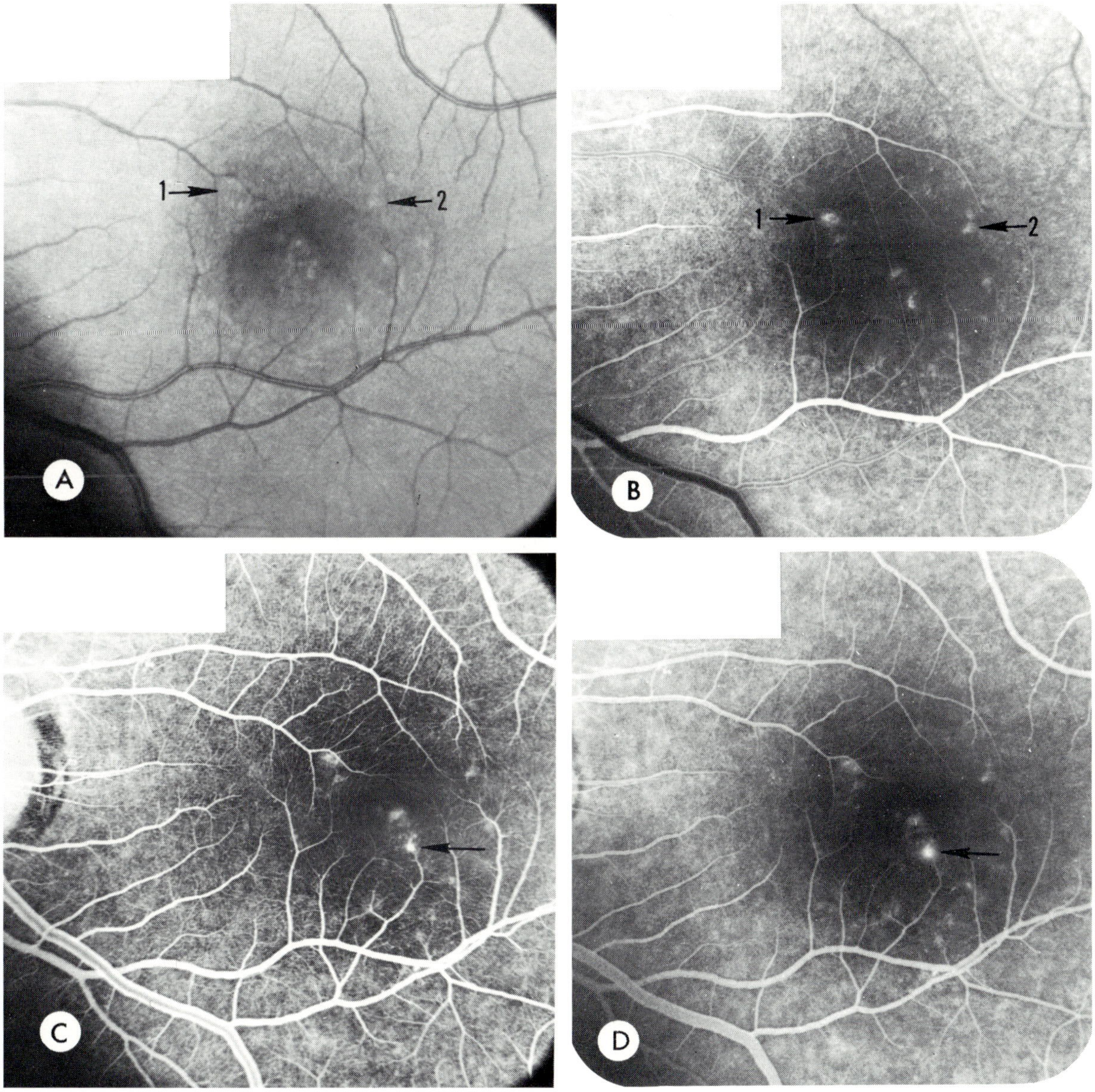

Fig. 16-6. *A*, Reversible central serous retinopathy. Note areas of mild pigment disturbance (**1** and **2**) and compare with *B*. *B*, Fluorescein angiogram of *A*. Arterial phase shows increased prominence of dye at same areas of mild pigment disturbance (**1** and **2**) shown in *A*. *C*, Arteriovenous-phase fluorescein angiogram shows an early single point of leakage **(arrow)**. *D*, A later phase shows increasing leakage **(arrow)**.

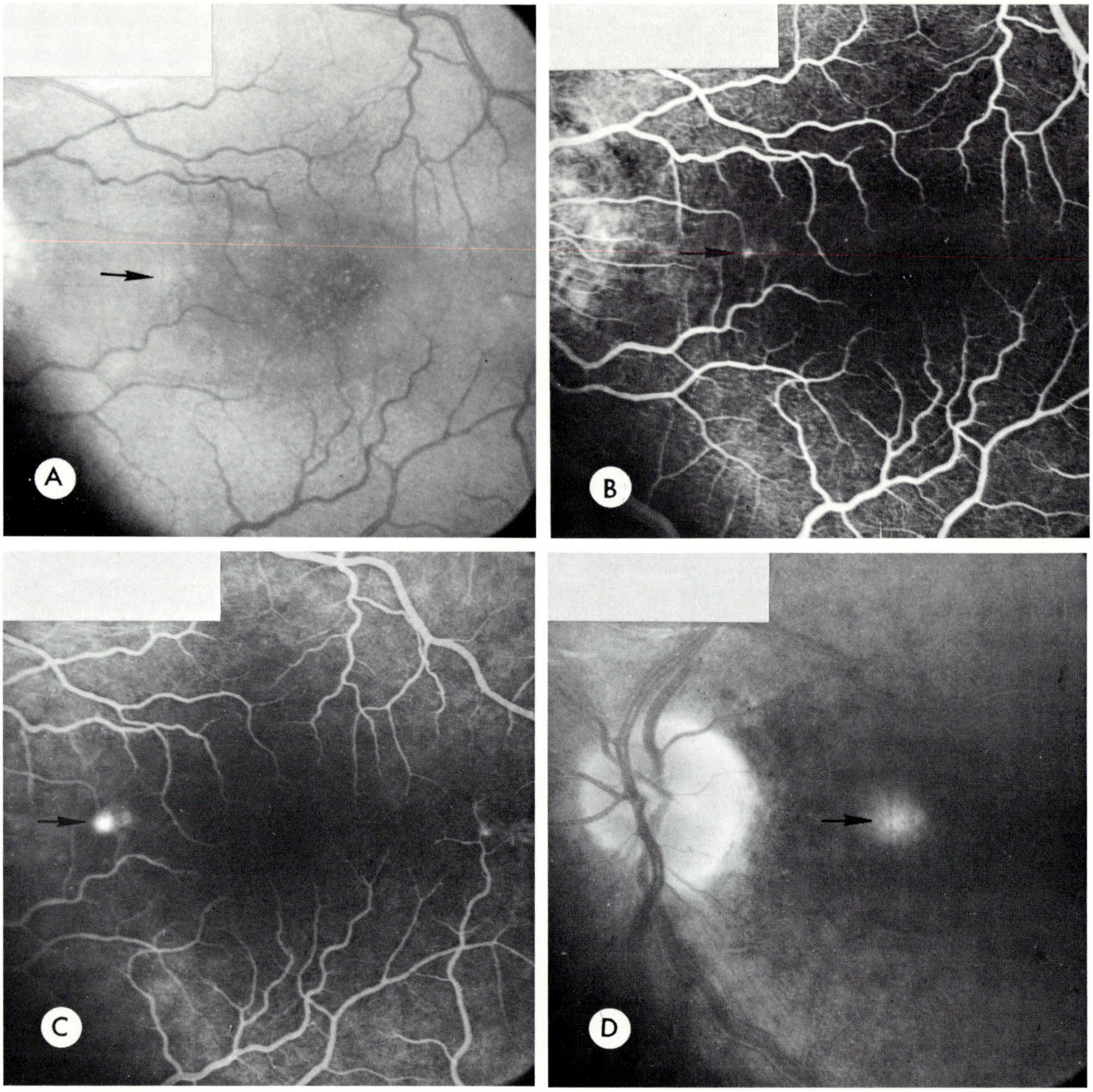

Fig. 16-7. *A*, Reversible central serous retinopathy. Note how difficult it may be to determine the point of leakage (**arrow**) clinically. *B*, Fluorescein angiogram of *A*. Minimal leakage (**arrow**) in arteriovenous phase. *C*, Later phase shows increasing leakage (**arrow**). *D*, Late phase after all dye has left the retinal circulation. Note the spreading dye (**arrow**) beneath the serous detachment of the macula.

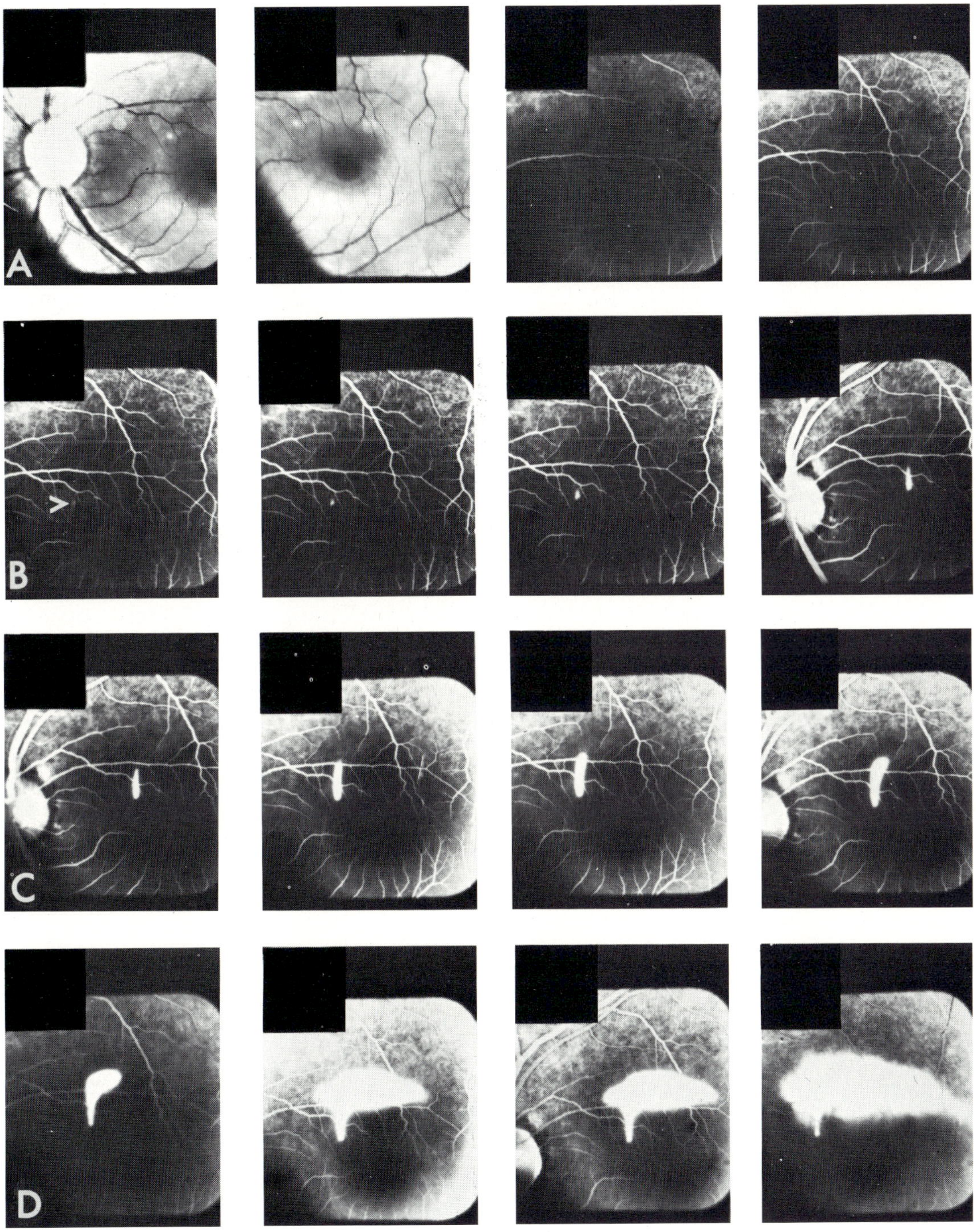

Fig. 16-8. Photographic series shows the upward spread of the dye beneath a large serous detachment of the macula. First leakage shown in column *1*, line *B* **(arrowhead).**

occurs within a few months, and complete recovery has been seen even after 5 months. Just how long the retina can remain elevated without permanent damage is unknown, but cases persisting for several years and then responding to treatment have had variable permanent visual loss. Clinically, these cases could show no more residual retinal pathology than others with full visual recovery.

When recovery begins, there is lessening of the hyperopia and improvement in vision with decreasing distortion and scotoma. Objectively, the retinal mound begins to flatten and fluorescein leakage decreases. When recovery is complete, vision and refraction return to their normal level and all symptoms disappear; the retina returns to its normal position against the pigment epithelium and the foveal reflex reappears. At this stage the fluorescein angiogram shows no leakage. If previously present, the fuzzy yellow central spot disappears, but the discrete white subretinal dots and the blemishes of the pigment epithelium remain as the only evidence of a prior attack. Eventually, even the white dots disappear.

Repeated attacks of this disease do occur, and multiple attacks may occur in a single eye with spontaneous recovery in each instance with no permanent visual loss. Recurrent attacks appear to result from a new leaking point rather than a releak from the original site.

TREATMENT

Many forms of therapy have been tried in cases of central serous retinopathy. Among the more popular recent ones are steroids, carbonic anhydrase inhibitors, and vasodilators. None of these has proved valuable.

So far, photocoagulation has proved to be a dramatic and highly effective means of closing the choroidal leak and aborting individual attacks of the disease. All cases with leaking sites more than 0.5 dd from the fovea are treatable, and laser coagulation has been preferable in our hands. Such treatment requires accurate localization of leaking sites by fluorescein angiography with photography and adequate treatment of all leaks.[78]

As most cases of reversible central serous retinopathy spontaneously regress, they should remain under observation without treatment. Lesions persisting for 5 months and those showing signs of progressive disease (see under Progressive Central Serous Retinopathy) should have laser therapy.

PROGRESSIVE CENTRAL SEROUS RETINOPATHY

SIGNS OF PROGRESSION

Instead of resolving spontaneously, central serous retinopathy may progress and produce an irreversible lesion. Signs suggesting this progressive nature include: increasing turbidity of the subretinal fluid, progressive deposition of opaque subretinal yellowish material, hemorrhagic detachment of the pigment epithelium, proliferation of pigment epithelium, subretinal hemorrhage, intraretinal blot hemorrhages around the mound, and fatty exudation into the midretinal layers around the elevation. Associated with these changes there is progressive loss of visual acuity and increasing density of the central scotoma. The development of fibrosis beneath the elevated retina is a late sign of irreversibility.

The nature of the turbid fluid is unknown but it probably represents altered transudate from the choriocapillaris. The denser, yellowish material in this subretinal fluid tends to accumulate on the pigment epithe-

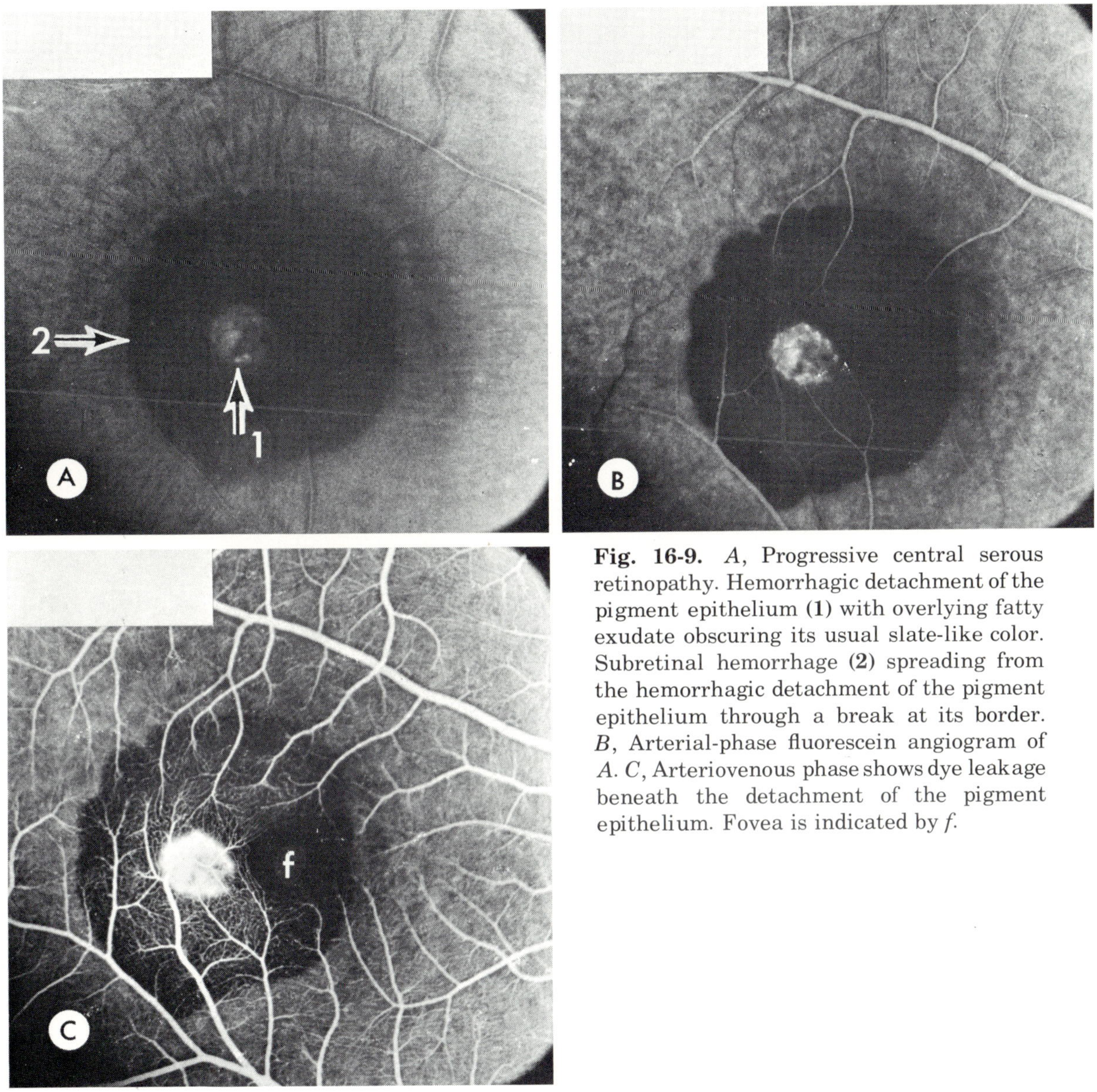

Fig. 16-9. *A*, Progressive central serous retinopathy. Hemorrhagic detachment of the pigment epithelium **(1)** with overlying fatty exudate obscuring its usual slate-like color. Subretinal hemorrhage **(2)** spreading from the hemorrhagic detachment of the pigment epithelium through a break at its border. *B*, Arterial-phase fluorescein angiogram of *A*. *C*, Arteriovenous phase shows dye leakage beneath the detachment of the pigment epithelium. Fovea is indicated by *f*.

lium and to heap up at the edges of the retinal elevation. There is often a zone of relatively clear fluid between this exudate and the detached retinal dome.

Hemorrhagic detachment of the pigment epithelium appears as a dark blister somewhere under the retinal elevation. While the pigment epithelium may maintain its continuity for some time, breaks often occur. These usually take place at the edge of the elevated blister (Fig. 16-9). When the break develops blood seeps out beneath the neural retina and forms a curved border around the edge of the blister. Blood beneath the intact

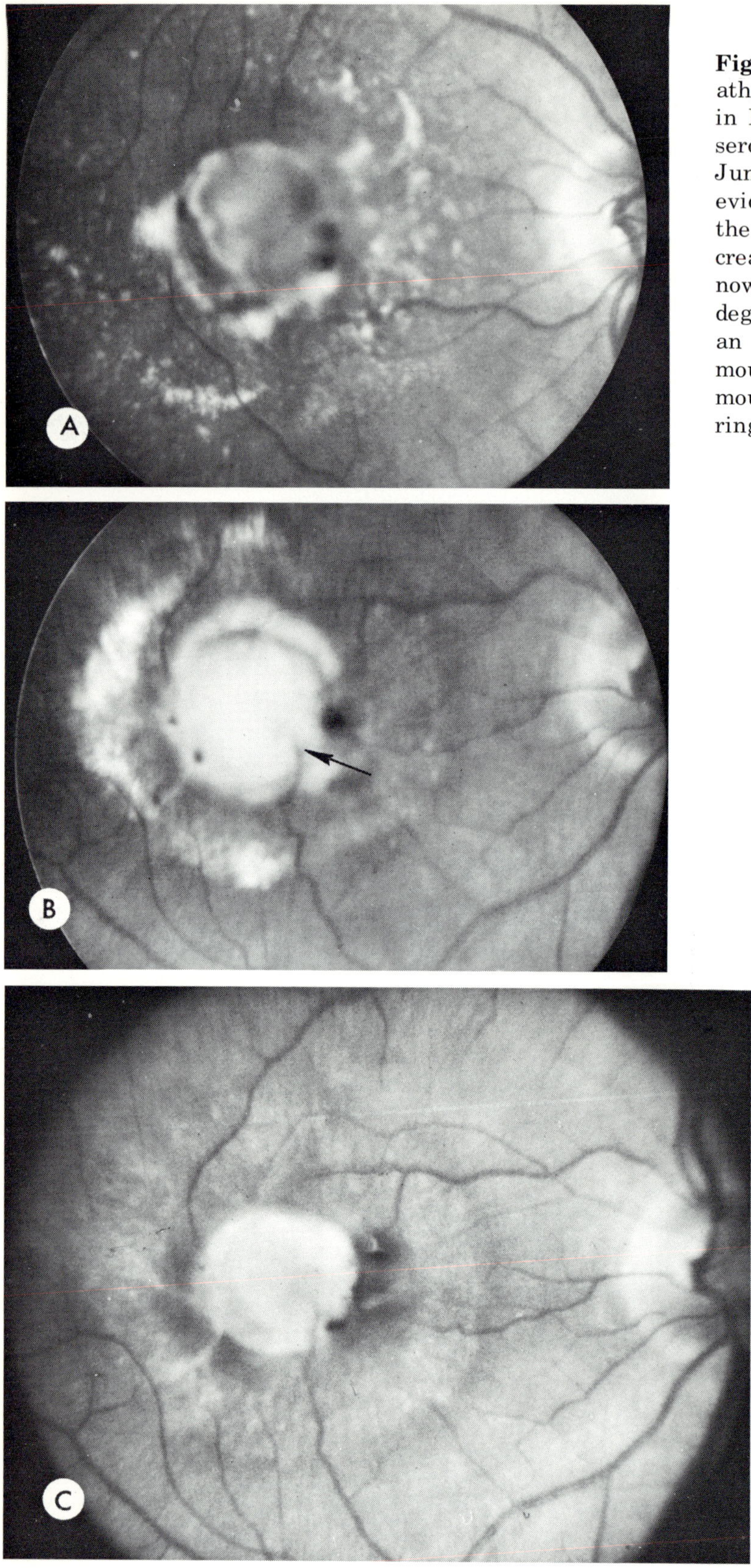

Fig. 16-10. Progressive central serous retinopathy in a 35-year-old male. *A*, This lesion started in February 1956 as a typical reversible central serous retinopathy. The photograph was taken in June 1956 some time after progression became evident. Note the early fatty exudate ring around the central mound. *B*, January 1957. Note increasing fatty exudate in the mound and ring. This now has the appearance of a disciform macular degeneration. Note the retinal vein dipping into an umbilication **(arrow)** near the apex of the mound. *C*, March 1958. Shows contracture of the mound and disappearance of the fatty exudate ring.

pigment epithelium has a light to dark, slate-like color with no red value. Subretinal blood has a bright red, or dark red color and may appear as a thin red line to one side of the pigment epithelium detachment. Later, hemorrhage may extend more extensively beneath the retina. Blot hemorrhages from the deep retinal capillary bed appear on the slope of the retinal elevation, or just beyond its border.

Proliferation of the pigment epithelium appears as a hyperpigmented ring at the border of the subretinal fluid, or as an independent pigmented clump beneath the retinal elevation. This may develop prior to any evidence of hemorrhage.

Fatty exudates are deposited in some cases in a zone just beyond the edge of the detached retina (Fig. 16-10). These exudates lie in the outer plexiform layer, and while scattered at first, they may increase to form a complete circinate figure around the mound.

CLINICAL COURSE

Many cases show signs of progressive disease from their onset. These start with hemorrhagic detachment of the pigment epithelium, or one or more serous detachments of the pigment epithelium, one of which shortly becomes darker and hemorrhagic. There is an accompanying serous detachment of the overlying retina and exudation appears early and is more profuse.

From onset to quiescence, the lesion may take months or years. The mound reaches its height with maximum hemorrhagic and exudative features, and then slowly subsides, with flattening, absorption of hemorrhage and exudate, and the formation of a pigmented, fibrosed, subretinal scar. In the later stages, it is not unusual to see one or more neovascular extensions from the smaller macular radicals—usually veins—dipping into the umbilicated crest of the

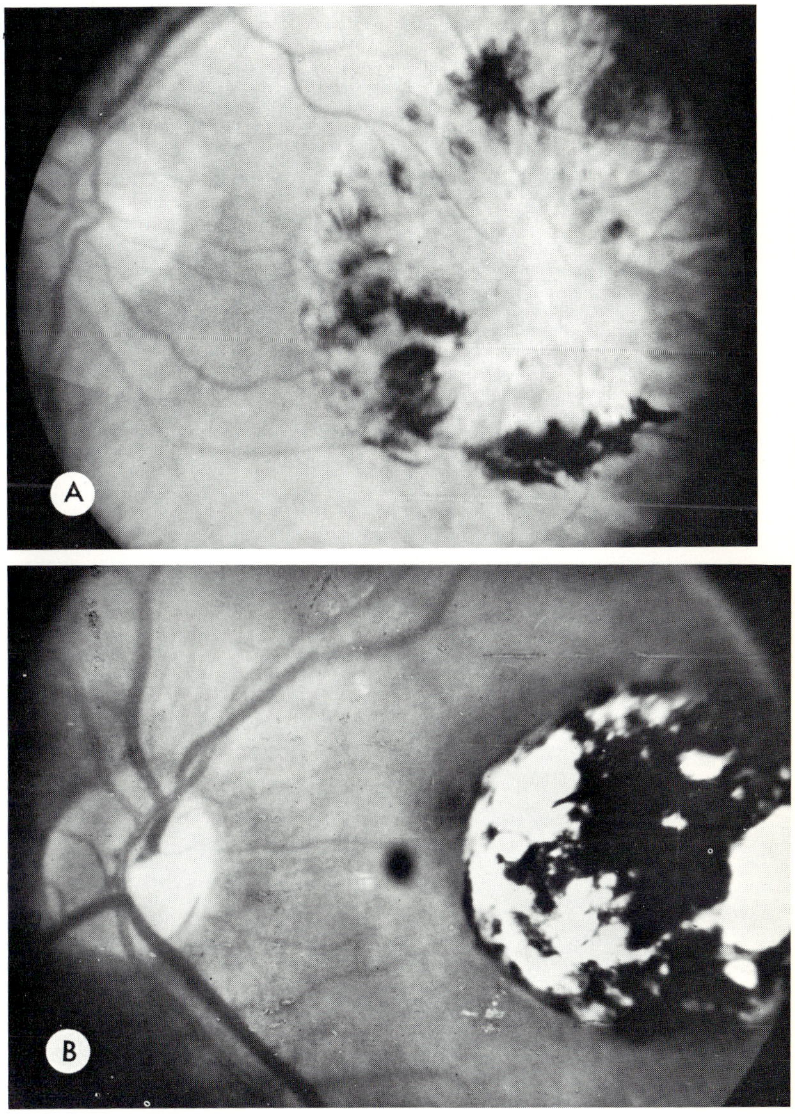

Fig. 16-11. *A*, Old healed macular scar due to disciform macular degeneration. Note absence of temporal disc pallor. *B*, Old healed toxoplasmic macular retinochoroiditis. Note temporal disc pallor.

mound, and connecting with the subretinal vascularized scar (Fig. 16-10).

Progressive central serous retinopathy need not go through all of these stages. Resolution may proceed at any point, but invariably some permanent scar and visual loss remain.

Satellite lesions seldom progress in this manner and paramacular lesions sometimes subside with only mild macular damage. Progressive involvement of the macular zone is the usual course, however.

The overlying retina is clinically intact during the early stages of all central serous retinopathies. With prolonged detachment, the overlying retina may later show signs of intraretinal microcystic edema. The ganglion cell and nerve fiber layer are never involved in the disease, for irrespective of its severity, late temporal pallor of the disc does not occur. This is a helpful differential diagnostic point in separating the old flattened pigmented macular scars of this disease from healed central chorioretinitis which usually shows temporal disc pallor (Fig. 16-11).

At no stage of central serous retinopathy are inflammatory signs present. The vitreous remains clear, and the hazy retinal whiteness of active chorioretinitis is not seen. Except for the later overlying microcystic edema of the macula, there is no accompanying retinal reaction; and except for the late penetration of new vessels from the retina into the mound, the retinal vessels remain clinically uninvolved.

Microscopically, progressive central serous retinopathy shows the same changes seen in senile disciform macular degeneration, although often of a milder degree.[19,37,81] (See under Senile Disciform Macular Degeneration).

FLUORESCEIN ANGIOGRAPHY

Fluorescein angiography of these patients shows a leak similar to that seen in reversible central serous retinopathy, but the site of leak is usually larger and the leakage more profuse. Leakage invariably occurs beneath a hemorrhagic detachment of the pigment epithelium. In these instances it first appears at the rim of the blister where the screening blood layer is thinnest. Later it diffuses throughout the entire blister and beneath the retina as well.

TREATMENT

As in reversible central serous retinopathy, there has been no treatment of proved value for the progressive disease. Photocoagulation of leaking sites is presently being attempted with some apparent success, but follow-up periods are too short for its final evaluation and double-blind studies are not available. If photocoagulation is to be attempted, it should be undertaken at the earliest sign of progressive disease. More intensive burns are usually required and more extensive areas must be treated than in reversible central serous retinopathy.

Technically, laser treatment near the fovea must be very exact for in this disease the fovea is often hard to identify accurately. A photograph of the leaking site should be at hand during treatment. Using small macular vessels as landmarks, the leaking point is first located on the photograph, then in the patient's fundus, and only then is treatment attempted.[78]

SEROUS DETACHMENT OF THE MACULA ASSOCIATED WITH CONGENITAL PITS IN THE OPTIC NERVE HEAD

A number of macular changes have been reported in association with congenital pits in the optic disc. Among these are macular edema, cyst or hole, pigmentary irregularities, and serous detachment of the macular retina.[17,42] In Kranenburg's[42] review of 123 patients with congenital pits in the optic disc reported in the literature, one-fourth had serious macular disease. This is probably not an accurate incidence of macular pathology associated with this disc lesion. Congenital holes in the optic disc are not unduly rare, yet we have observed only one such case with a macular lesion. Undoubtedly, many cases of congenital pits without other pathology are not considered worthy of report.

CLINICAL APPEARANCE OF THE MACULAR LESION

The serous detachment of the macular retina associated with congenital holes in the optic disc can closely simulate central serous retinopathy.[17,22,42,69] The disc pit is always located temporally and may be of variable size. The disc itself may be of about normal size or considerably enlarged. The mound of detached retina is commonly pear-shaped with its narrowest portion at the disc border adjacent to the pit (Fig. 16-12). The borders of the retinal elevation are smooth and rounded. Subretinal white dots as described in central serous retinopathy may be seen. Some cases show cystic change in the detached retina but this is not described in all. A yellowish material on the under surface of the detached retina has been noted occasionally.[22] The pigment alteration beneath the mound increases with the duration of the retinal detachment and for this reason Gass[22] has suggested its secondary nature.

FLUORESCEIN ANGIOGRAPHY

Fluorescein angiography in several of Gass's cases[22] and one of our own failed to demonstrate a leak from the hole in the optic disc (Fig. 16-12*E*). The hole area and sometimes spots at the temporal border of the disc fluoresce brightly but do not leak fluid; nor has any leak through Bruch's membrane, as in central serous retinopathy, been demonstrated. Thinking that ocular rotations and the tug of the optic nerve at the site of the hole might induce leakage, we had our patient constantly and forcefully rotate her eye during and for several minutes after her fluorescein injection. Still, no leakage occurred.

SOURCE OF SUBRETINAL FLUID

The source of the subretinal fluid in this lesion is unknown. It has been suggested that the fluid is either cerebrospinal fluid leaking from the subvaginal space through the loose tissue of the pit wall into the subretinal space or that it is aqueous passing from the vitreous cavity through the neuroepithelium and pit wall into this space.[22] Diffusion from the choroid around the end of Bruch's membrane is an equally likely source. The frequent association of cilioretinal arteries with these congenital holes in the disc suggests the possibility of such a route.

Whatever the source of the subretinal fluid in these cases, efforts to treat them by light coagulation of the pit and disc border area have been unsuccessful in two of Gass's patients and one of our own.

HISTOPLASMOSIS

Some cases of progressive central serous retinopathy have other scattered lesions in the fundus. These vary in number from several to many and are most common in the

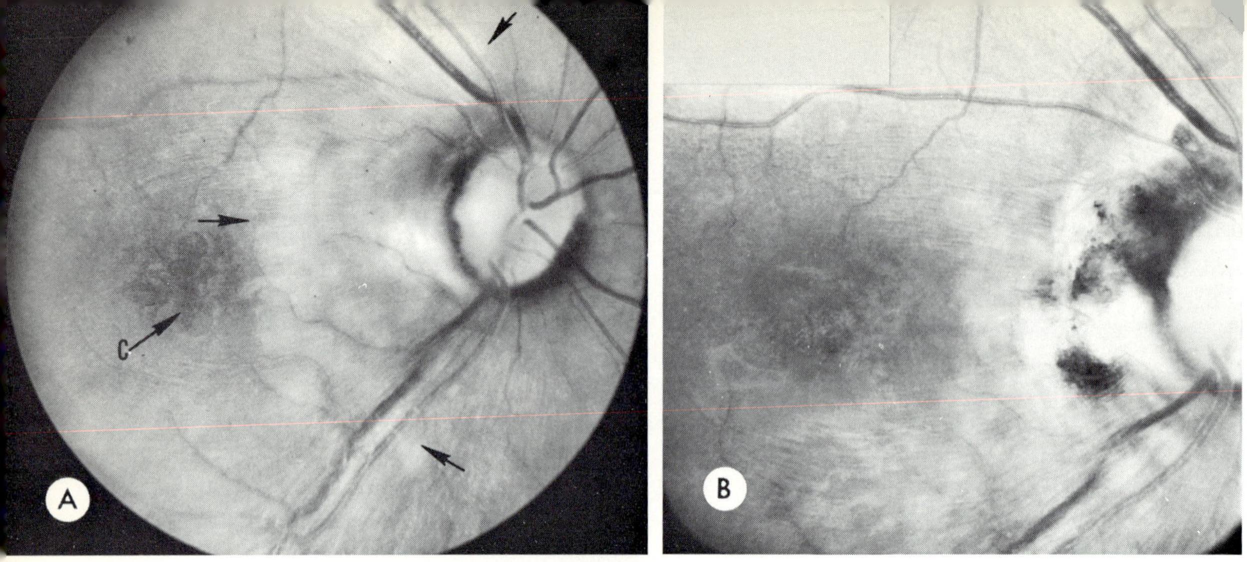

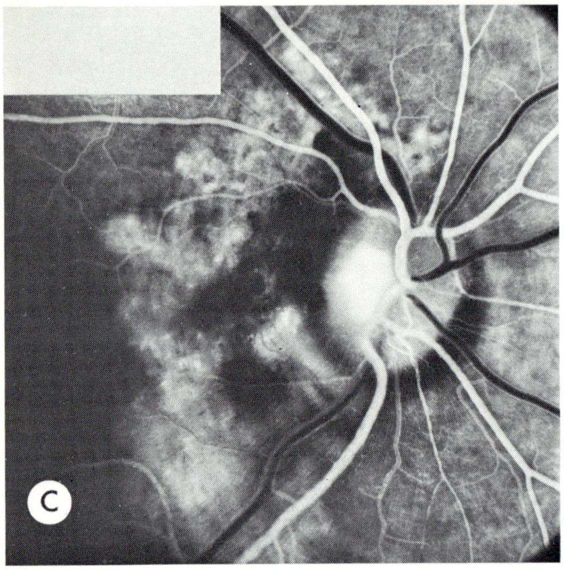

Fig. 16-12. Coloboma of the disc with serous detachment of the retina extends from the disc border and includes the macula. Vision is 20/100. *A*, Photograph of fundus taken immediately after photocoagulation temporal to the disc. **C,** indicates the cystic, detached macula. **Arrows** outline the treatment area. *B*, Same eye 4 years later. The serous retinal detachment has persisted. The pigmented treatment scars are temporal to the disc. *C*, Arterial-phase fluorescein angiogram of *B*. *D*, Later phase shows maximal fluorescence in the disc coloboma and choroid. *E*, Very late phase shows decreasing fluorescence without leakage. Ocular rotations during this procedure failed to induce fluorescein spread beneath the macula.

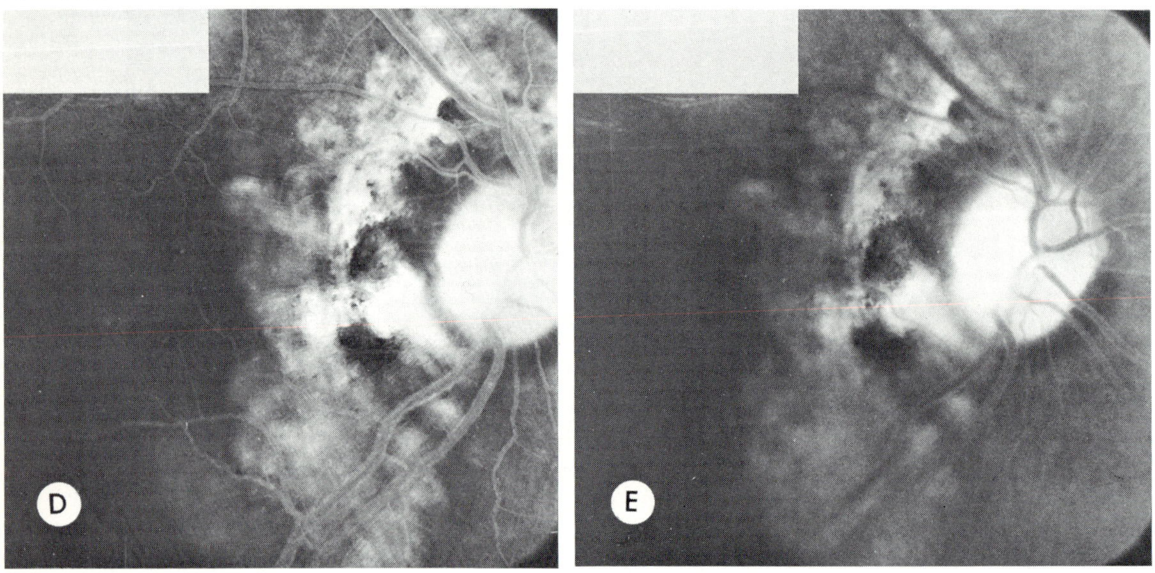

periphery and about the posterior pole, where small lesions adjacent to the disc are frequently seen. The onset and development of these spots have been carefully described.[43] They start as deep, yellow white dots, with disturbed overlying pigment epithelium, slowly enlarge over weeks or months, and when full size, are seldom larger than the disc and usually are much smaller. The borders are punched-out and pigment epithelium shows a ragged proliferation at the edges, a clumping within the lesion, or there is heavy pigment proliferation throughout. The spots are discrete and have a grayish white or yellowish granular base where pigment is absent. (Fig. 16-13). When numerous they can suggest old, healed disseminated chorioretinitis, but choroidal vessels are seldom visible within their boundaries and at no time during their development do they show the usual inflammatory signs of chorioretinitis; nor do they leak fluorescein as would a true inflammatory focus (Fig. 16-13). There is no serous elevation of the retina over these so-called "histo spots" nor any reaction within the retina itself.

Histo spots may be present in one or both eyes, be about equal in number in each eye or predominate in one, and either eye or both can have macular involvement. Macular involvement in one eye may be followed by macular disease in the other months, or years, later. The macular lesion can be minute, parafoveal and subside spontaneously without loss of foveal vision, or proceed as a typical progressive central serous retinopathy.

Woods and Wahlen [79] have studied patients showing these histo spots associated with macular disease and have found an increased incidence of positive histopolasmin skin reactions among them. They have proposed that the histo spots result from healed uveitis occurring during the initial phase of benign systemic histoplasmosis and consider the macular lesion to be a later hypersensitivity phenomenon. As the widespread incidence of histoplasmosis became apparent, it was recognized as being endemic in certain geographical areas—notably in mid-central United States.[60] Although there were exceptions, most reported ocular cases came from these same regions. The diagnosis of presumed ocular histoplasmosis now rests on the typical fundic appearance in a patient usually residing in an endemic area of the disease, who has a positive skin reaction to histoplasmin and anergy to tuberculin. X-ray evidence of pulmonary calcifications would constitute further diagnostic evidence.

Systemic histoplasmosis produces granulomatous lesions as do all other fungi.[6,28,51] The only proved case of ocular histoplasmosis [29] was one of a granulomatous endophthalmitis. Although searched for, *Histoplasma capsulatum* has not been identified in the few eyes with presumed ocular histoplasmosis which have been available for microscopic study.

In a histoplasmosis survey of 1417 individuals from an endemic area of the disease, Asbury [1] has concluded that the concept of ocular histoplasmosis based solely on the correlation of positive skin test results and histo spots was not supported. Others have reported ocular cases showing little evidence suggestive of systemic involvement and clinically typical cases having negative skin reactions.[43]

Spaeth [68] has found no record of presumed ocular histoplasmosis in a review of 134 patients with culturally or histologically proved systemic histoplasmosis. Because of these findings, he has questioned the propriety of using an antifungal drug as toxic as amphotericin B in suspected ocular cases. Giles and Falls [26] have found the use of amphotericin B has failed to favorably influence the course of the disease in most of their cases of presumed ocular histoplasmosis.

While most agree that the cases of presumed ocular histoplasmosis do constitute a characteristic clinical group, the evidence

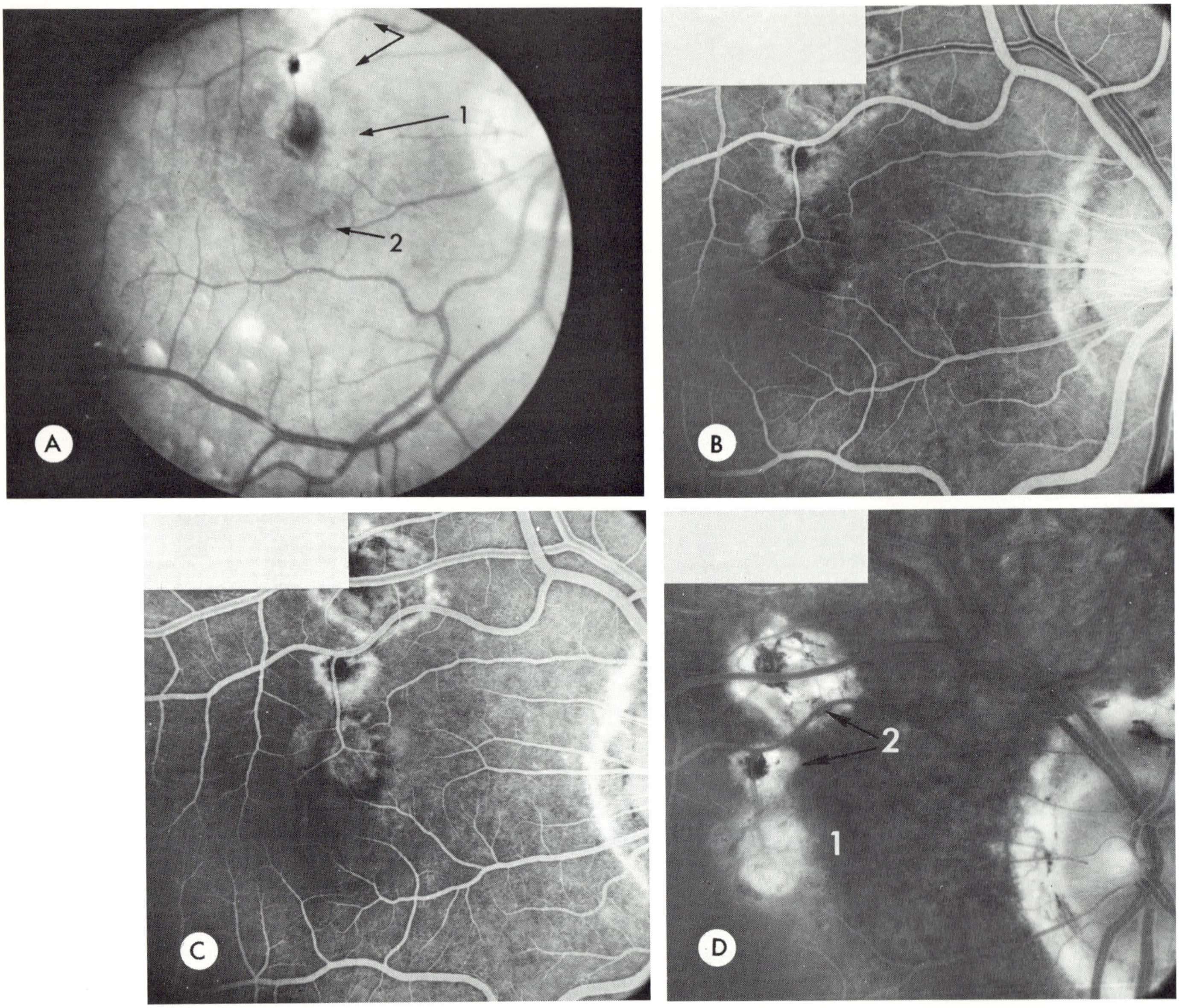

Fig. 16-13. *A*, Presumed histoplasmosis. Note hemorrhagic detachment of the pigment epithelium **(1)** serous detachment of the retina **(2)** and quiescent histo spots **(arrows).** *B*, Arterial-phase fluorescein angiogram. *C*, Arteriovenous-phase fluorescein angiogram. *D*, Late-phase fluorescein angiogram shows dye leakage at the detachment of the pigment epithelium **(1)** and no leakage at quiescent histo spots **(2).** Note the appearance at the disc border often found in presumed histoplasmosis.

incriminating *Histoplasma capsulatum* as their etiologic agent appears unproved.

Fluorescein angiography reveals the typical choroidal leak in the macular lesions as is seen in other progressive central serous retinopathies (Fig. 16-13). In addition, all histo spots and many other areas of clinically minimal pigment epithelial alteration light up brightly with choroidal filling, but none of these show leakage. Treatment is the same as in progressive central serous retinopathy. (Fig. 16-14).

AMEBIASIS

On the basis of finding *Entamoeba histolytica* in the stools of several patients with the clinical picture of progressive central serous retinopathy, and because ocular improvement followed oral antiamoebic therapy, the ocular lesion has been ascribed to this etiology.[7,35]

An ocular *Entamoeba histolytica* has never been demonstrated histologically in such cases, and the ocular lesions as described have shown no inflammatory signs. Both intestinal and hepatic amebiasis are chronic granulomatous inflammations. A noninflammatory ocular lesion, therefore, seems hard to equate with this intestinal parasite, which remains an unproved cause of progressive central serous retinopathy.

VITELLIFORM MACULAR DEGENERATION

Vitelliform macular degeneration is a rare hereditary disease with autosomal dominant transmission sometimes showing reduced penetrance. It was first described by Best[5] and was formerly called by his name. Both eyes are affected and usually have a similar appearance, although Velzeboer[71] has reported a patient with one practically normal macula. The progress from onset to quiescent macular scarring has not been traced in an individual patient, but some concept of this sequence has been gained from observations of family members of different ages, all of whom were affected.[8]

The early stage of the disease irrespective of age at onset is similar in each case. Clinical pathology is limited to the macular areas which show round or oval cystic yellow elevations about 1 to 2 dd in size. Although there are no detailed descriptions of the lesion as observed with the slit lamp and contact lens, some illustrations[45] show the characteristic ring of retinal highlights about the rim of the mound as is common in central serous retinopathy. This, with the fluid level of the yellow material shown in other pictures, suggests that it has a subretinal position in front of the pigment epithelium. The early typical state of the disease is associated with no visual symptoms. Its appearance has been likened to a "fried egg, sunny side up."

With the onset of visual disturbance the egg is said to become "scrambled" in appearance. From this point on the yellow material becomes scattered and decreases as pigment proliferation and macular scarring increase. The disease becomes quiescent with the retinal clinicopathology limited to the pigmented macular scars and a permanently reduced central vision.

The nature of this disease is not clear. Krill et al.[44] have placed the yellow material in Bruch's membrane or between this structure and the pigment epithelium. The abnormal electro-oculograms in the three patients tested suggested a diffuse disease at the pigment epithelium—Bruch's membrane level and supported this hypothesis.[18] Deutman[13] has studied five families having the disease and all 24 ophthalmoscopically

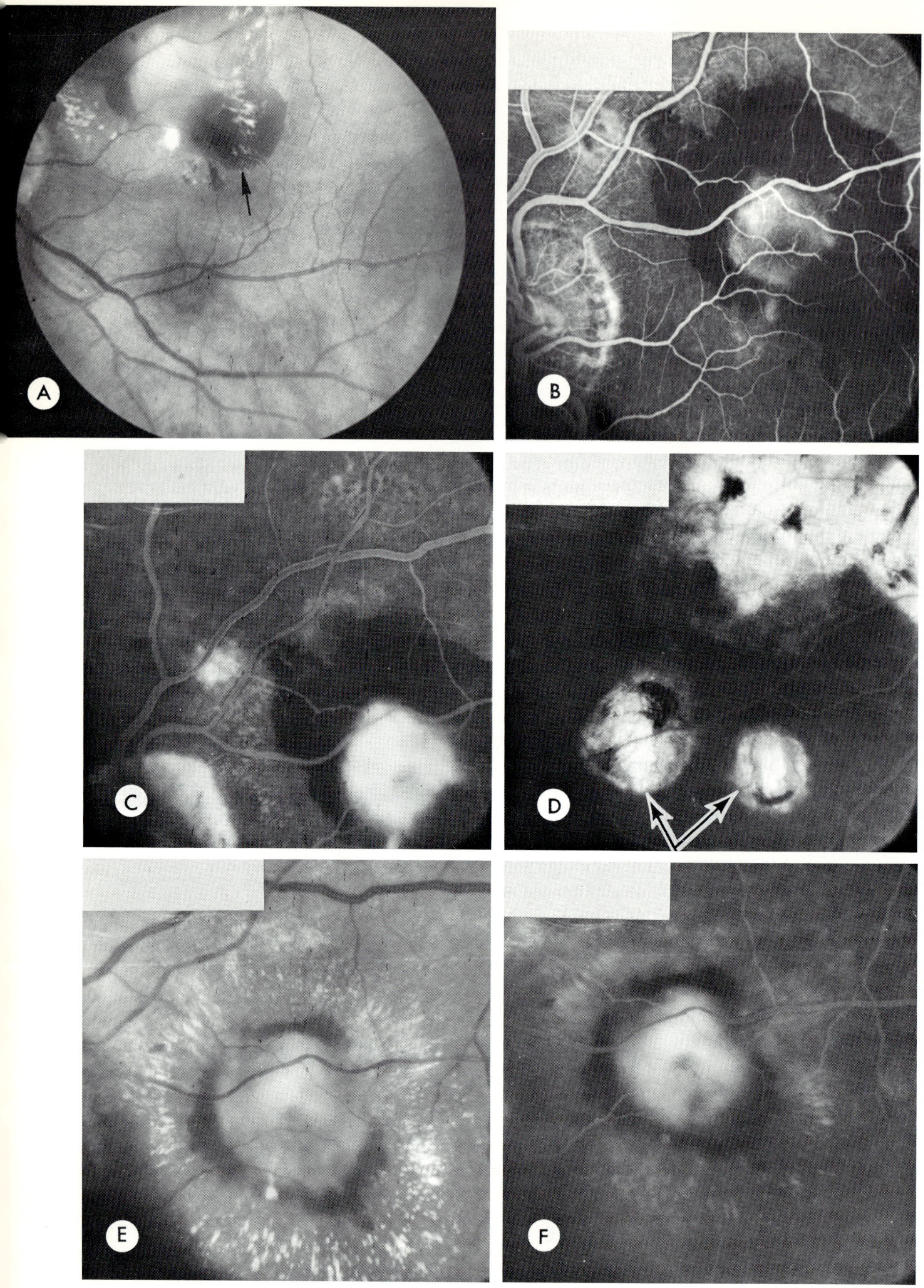
A
B
C
D
E
F

Fig. 16-14. Presumed histoplasmosis in a 67-year-old woman with bilateral macular involvement. Her vision was 1/200 in both eyes.

A, Fundus photograph of the left eye shows an acentric disciform lesion encroaching on the fovea **(arrow).**

B, Fluorescein angiogram of *A* shows leakage beneath the mound.

C, Late-phase fluorescein angiogram shows increased leakage.

D, The right eye shows old scar involving the macula and satellite histo spots **(arrows).** There is another similar peripheral spot.

E, Fundus photograph of *A* taken 2 months after photocoagulation.

F, Fluorescein angiogram shows persisting leakage.

G, Visual field and corrected vision of this eye, 14 months after a second photocoagulation. The mound was contracting although fluorescein leakage was still present.

H, Clinical photograph taken 1 year after *G*. This vision was unchanged although the lesion still showed activity.

I, Fluorescein angiogram of *H* shows persistent leakage.

J, Late-phase fluorescein angiogram.

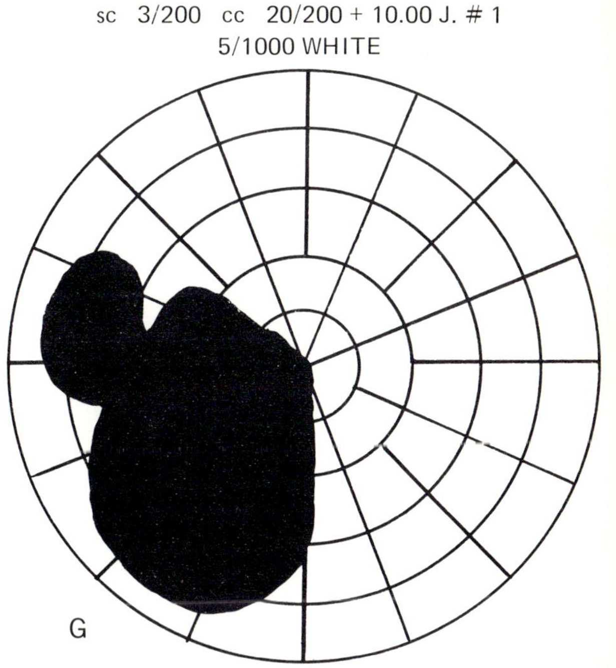

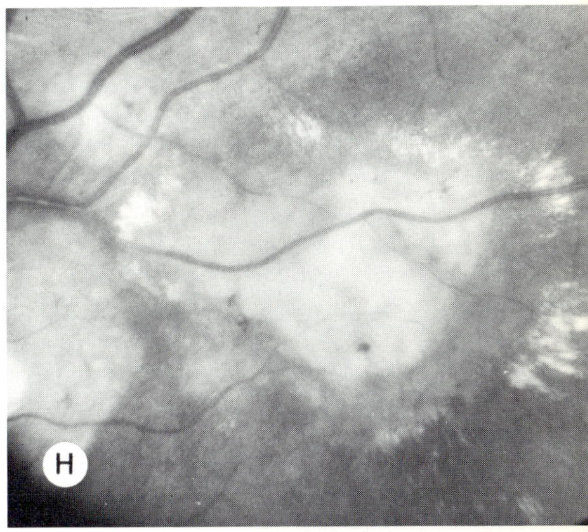

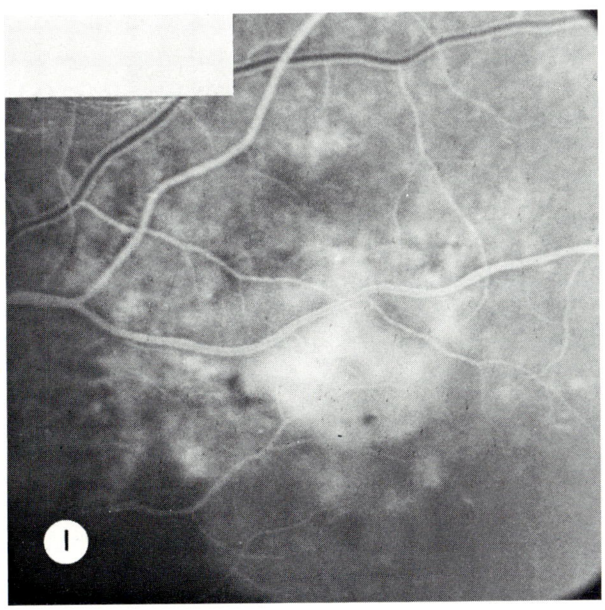

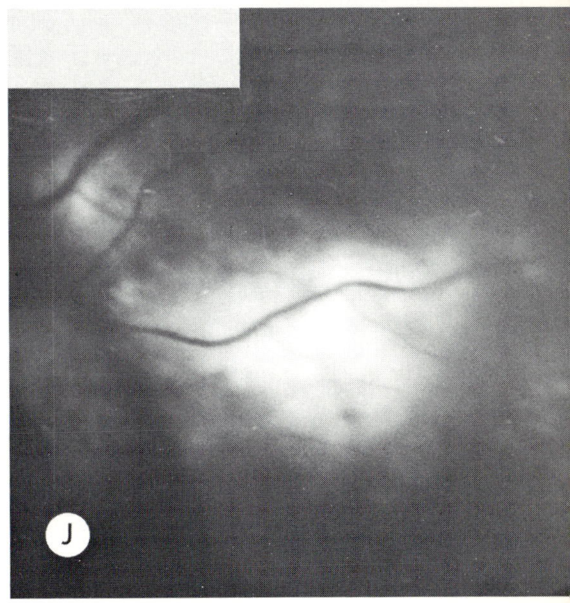

affected individuals had pathologic electro-oculograms. Carriers showed pathologic light/dark ratios of their electro-oculograms even though their fundi were clinically normal. Three of his patients also showed multiple vitelliform lesions about the macula.

Fluorescein studies by Curry and Moorman[11] have demonstrated no choroidal leaks nor visible choroidal fluorescence at the macula in early cases and visible choroidal fluorescence without leakage in the older cases. These findings indicate a clinically intact pigment epithelium in the early disease stages. These findings have been confirmed by Morse and MacLean.[53]

No treatment has been of any proved value in these patients. Some end with marked visual impairment; some have little permanent visual defect. Rare patients have shown some visual improvement during the active phase of the disease.

SENILE DISCIFORM MACULAR DEGENERATION

Oeller[57] first used the term disciform macular degeneration in 1903, but Pagenstecher[58] probably published the first anatomic report of such a case in 1875. Fuchs's retinitis circinata, in 1893 is undoubtedly a description of this same entity. Junius and Kuhnt[34] and Coppez and Danis[9] both in 1926 independently described this disease and since then it has often been called Kuhnt-Junius disciform macular degeneration.

This is a common lesion of older people and varies markedly in its mode of onset, and the kaleidoscopic clinical manifestations it presents during the various stages throughout its course. This great variability has led to much confusion, some stages of the disease having been described as separate entities: retinitis circinata,[20] macular exudative retinitis,[12] and hematomas under the pigment epithelium.[64]

PREDISCIFORM PHASE

Senile disciform macular degeneration usually starts with yellowish white, deep retinal spots in the macular area (Fig. 16-15). These spots are almost universally called drusen, although they are not drusen and, if at all numerous, can usually be differentiated from drusen clinically. They multiply and enlarge slowly over months, have fuzzy borders, a dull light reflection and tend to become confluent when numerous. Careful stereoscopic view with the slit lamp and contact lens reveals their varying but deep position. Those actually lying on the pigment epithelium may show a fringe of increased pigment at their borders, but those even slightly above this level have no associated pigment. When large and of some duration, these spots develop crystals (Fig. 16-16), a change which drusen never undergo. Drusen are all at one level, usually have a fringe of increased pigment at their borders, are more apt to be discrete, with sharper margins and a brighter light reflex (Fig. 16-17). In the later predisciform stage, these yellow spots become so numerous that if they were drusen any section passing through the area should demonstrate them microscopically. However, in a study of 78 cases of senile disciform macular degeneration at the Armed Forces Institute of Pathology, Wangvivat and Wise[74] found only two containing drusen in the macular area and in both cases they were few in number. Gass[21] also failed to find drusen in his patients, but described eosinophilic bodies lying on the under surface of the retina or on the pigment epithelial layer. He thought

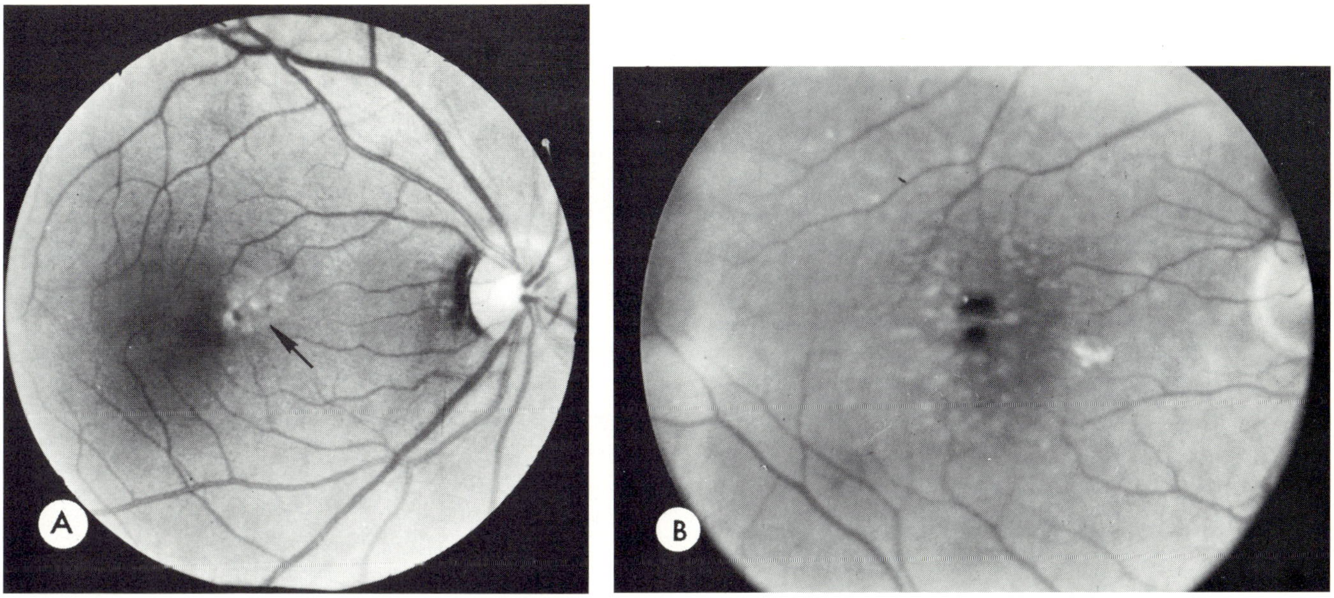

Fig. 16-15. *A*, Early predisciform phase of senile disciform macular degeneration as seen in patient with disciform macular degeneration other eye. Note fatty exudates **(arrow).** *B*, A later stage of the predisciform phase in another patient. Note increased fatty exudates.

Fig. 16-16. Predisciform macular degeneration with multiple fatty exudates, some of which contain crystals **(arrows).** Note serous detachment of the pigment epithelium **(1).**

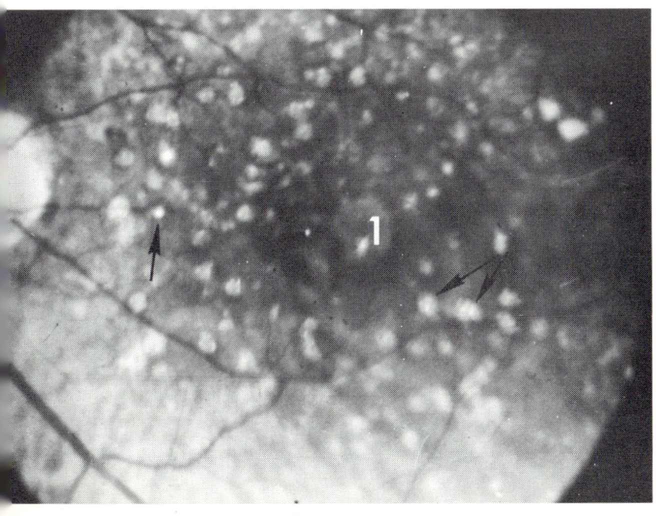

that these bodies represented the yellow spots seen clinically. Their clinical appearance, course, and sometimes crystalline content strongly suggest a lipid component and they are, therefore, probably comparable to other fatty exudates.

These fatty exudates are not necessarily limited to the immediate macular area. While usually more numerous toward the fovea, they may be widely distributed as large clumps with free intervening spaces throughout the zone encompassed by the temporal vessel arcades, and even appear nasally to the disc. Their presence is quite compatible with normal macular function for months, or even several years, so long as they do not involve the fovea.

Usually after the fatty exudates have been present for some time, deep translucent serous detachments of the pigment epithelium appear scattered among them (Fig. 16-18). These are best seen by retroillumination, which also best demonstrates a pigment rarefaction and the fine clumping overlying the blisters. In spite of the fact that there are small blisters of the pigment epithelium, there is no demonstrable fluorescein leak. So long as no blister lies directly under the fovea, no visual symptoms occur.

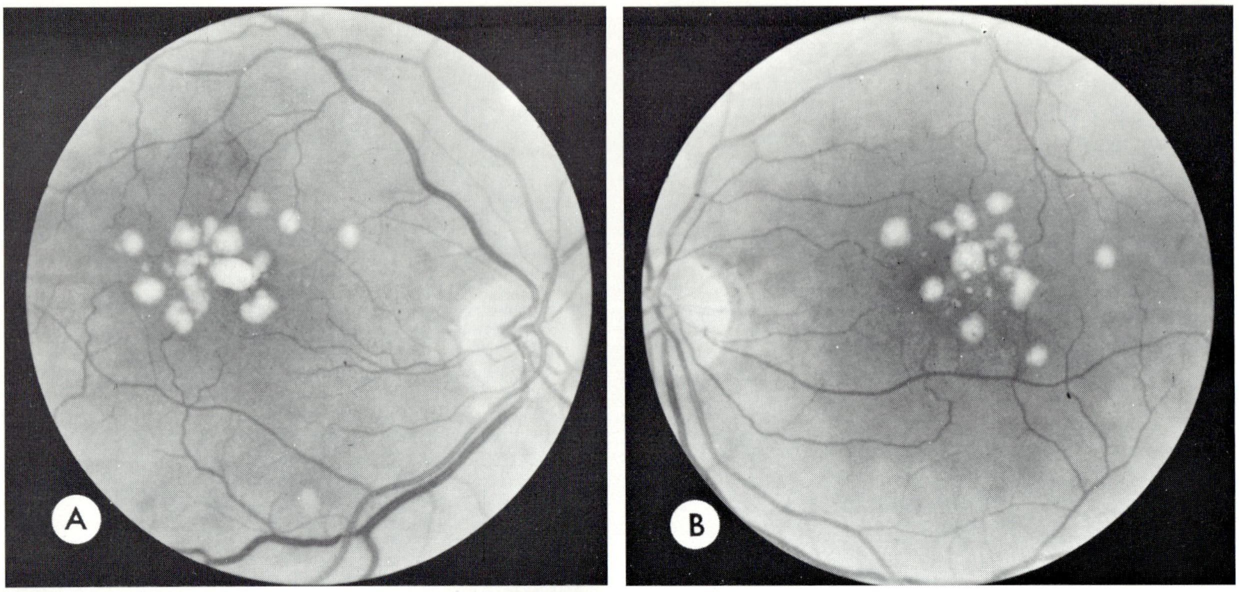

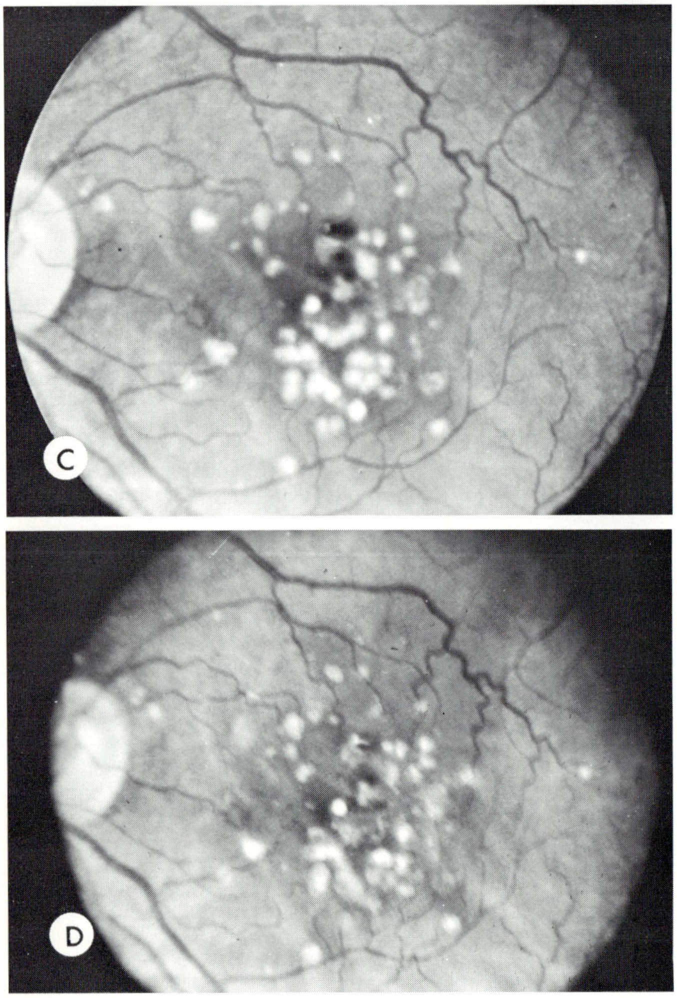

Fig. 16-17. *A*, Giant drusen at the macula. Patient's vision is 20/20. *B*, other eye of patient shown in *A*. Vision is 20/20. *C*, Another patient with giant drusen at the macula. Vision is 20/20. *D*, Same patient as *C*, 4 years later. Vision is 20/20. Note stability of fundic appearance and vision.

PROGRESSIVE PHASE

Two changes occur next, heralding a more rapid phase of the disease process: (*1*) Serous detachment of the overlying retina (Fig. 16-19); and (*2*) hemorrhage beneath one or more of the serous blisters (Fig. 16-20).

Hemorrhagic detachments of the pigment epithelium are usually single or few in number at onset. In the latter case they shortly fuse into a single dome. These are slate colored or darker to direct view, do not transmit light on retroillumination, and screen choroidal fluorescence with angiography. Serous fluid leaks through the pigment epithelium and begins to detach the overlying retina. Accompanying retinal detachment, small vascular twigs traversing the retinal elevation can be seen by slit-lamp fundoscopy to cast a shadow on the deeper pigment epithelium. With involvement of the fovea, any previously present foveal reflex disappears, metamorphopsia and visual loss occur, and Amsler grid testing shows a macular field defect. Fluorescein angiography now shows leakage from the choroid (Fig. 16-21).

From this stage on the subretinal fluid increases, at first forming a relatively clear, well-outlined macular mound. The serum becomes increasingly turbid and hemorrhagic detachments of the pigment epithelium appear beneath the retinal mound. These are prone to rupture at their borders and blood seeping through such gaps forms a curved border at the edge of the pigment blister and spreads out beneath the retina for varying distances as a red, sheet-like subretinal hemorrhage (Fig. 16-22). The shape of this subretinal hemorrhage abutting on the rising slope of the detached mound of pigment epithelium is a characteristic feature of this disease. Outlying midretinal blot hemorrhages develop from the deep retinal capillary bed about the eleva-

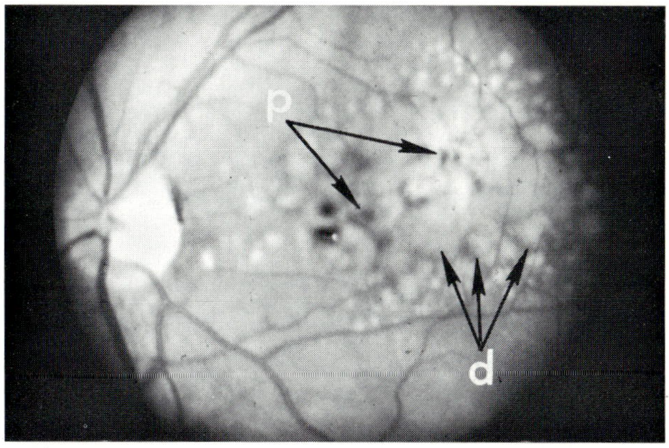

Fig. 16-18. The predisciform phase of senile disciform macular degeneration. Note the multiple, coalescing, serous detachments of the pigment epithelium **(d)** and the clumps of migrated and proliferated pigment epithelium **(p)** part of which lies in superficial retinal layers. Some of the outlying spots are fatty exudates.

Fig. 16-19. The progressive phase of senile disciform macular degeneration. The central, coalescent, serous detachment of the pigment epithelium **(arrow)** underlies a serous detachment of the macular retina. Note the outlying, deep, fatty exudates.

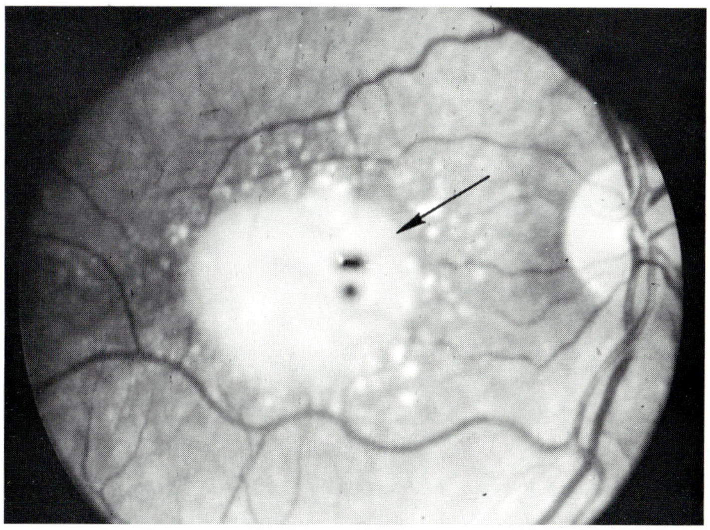

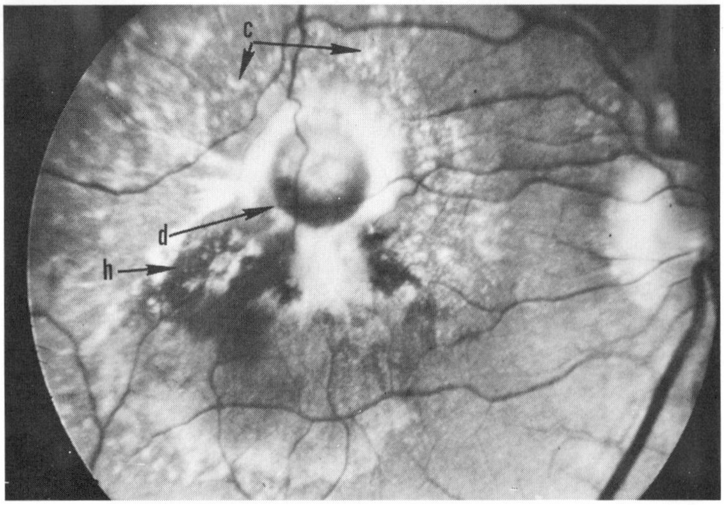

Fig. 16-20. *Left.* The progressive phase of senile disciform macular degeneration. The central, dome-shaped, hemorrhagic detachment of the pigment epithelium **(d)** has some overlying fatty exudate, heavier exudate around it, and scattered intraretinal fatty exudates further out are beginning to form a circinate figure **(c).** Subretinal hemorrhage **(h)** has leaked through a break in the pigment epithelium from under the dome in the region indicated by the point of the **arrow d.**

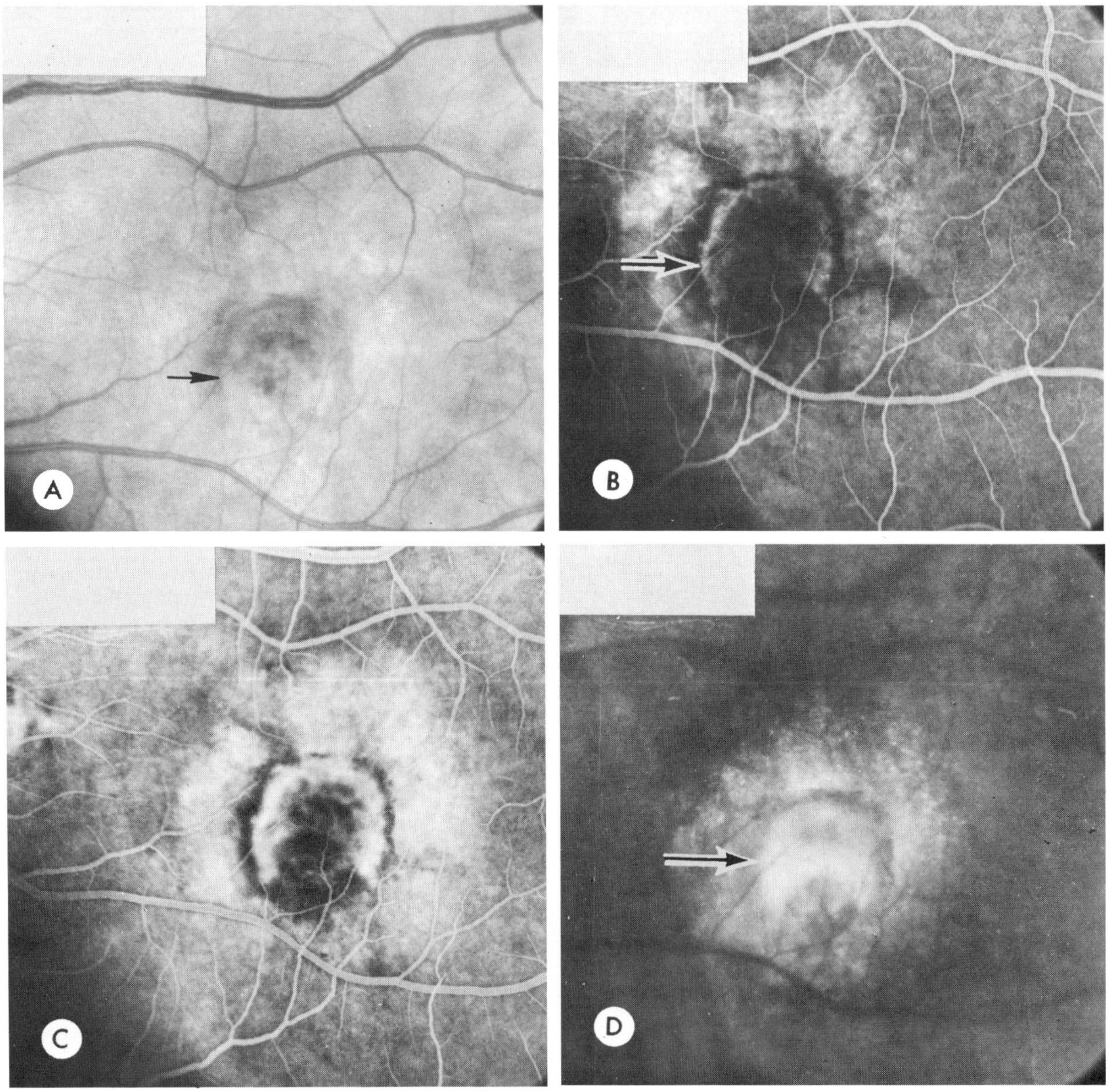

Fig. 16-21. *Opposite page. A*, Early senile disciform macular degeneration. Hemorrhagic detachment of the pigment epithelium is indicated by **arrow.** *B*, Arteriovenous-phase fluorescein angiogram of *A*. Early dye leakage is seen beneath the detached pigment epithelium **(arrow).** *C*, Late-phase fluorescein angiogram shows increasing dye leakage. *D*, A later phase shows diffusion of the dye beneath the detached pigment epithelium **(arrow).**

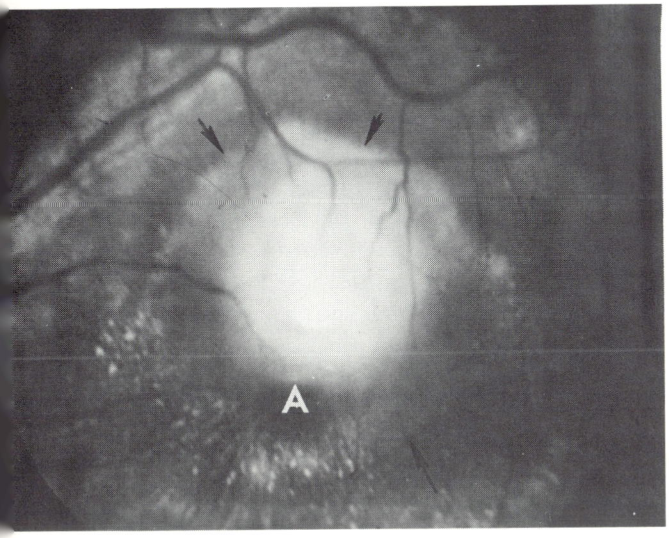

Fig. 16-22. *Left.* Senile disciform macular degeneration. The subretinal hemorrhage underlying **(A)** has broken through the edge of the hemorrhagic detachment of the pigment epithelium at the point indicated by the apex of the letter. Overlying fatty exudate obscures the dome of the hemorrhage beneath the pigment epithelium. Fatty exudate is also collecting at the border **(arrows)** of the overlying serous detachment of the retina.

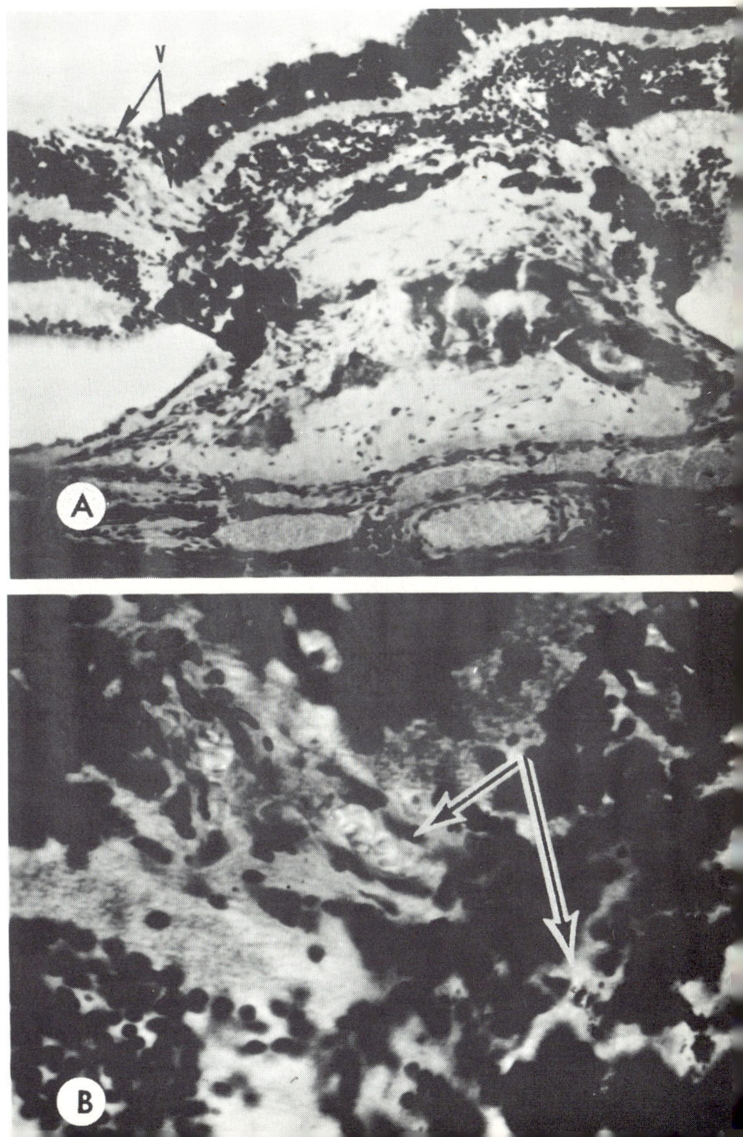

Fig. 16-23. *A*, Microscopic section of the late stage of scarring in disciform macular degeneration. An enlarged retinal vein (*V*) extends down into subretinal fibrovascular scar. (Courtesy of the Armed Forces Institute of Pathology, Washington, D.C.) *B*, A high-power view of *A* shows the same vessel **(arrows)** containing red blood cells and partially hidden by proliferated pigment epithelium in the scar. (Courtesy of the Armed Forces Institute of Pathology.)

tion, fatty exudation spreads over the base of the mound accumulating at its border or as a circinate figure around it (Fig. 16-22), and fibrosis and pigment proliferation progress under the dome on the inner surface of Bruch's membrane. These changes are very similar to those in progressive central serous retinopathy, but considerably magnified.

Slowly, over a number of years, the lesion first swells up, then ultimately settles with absorption of hemorrhages, exudation, and subretinal fluid, to end in a contracted, pigmented macular scar with a permanent central scotoma (Fig. 16-11*A*). The latter is often larger at the height of the disease than at its conclusion. Often in the later stages of this sequence, retinal vessels—veins much more commonly than arteries—dip into an umbilication near the crest of the mound and pass to its base, contributing to the terminal subretinal vascular fibrosis of the end stage. (Fig. 16-23).

The macular tributaries from which this neovascular subretinal growth proceeds become at first dilated, and then as the mound contracts and absorption of hemorrhage, fluid, and exudate proceeds, they narrow to one-half, or one-third of their maximum size. As in progressive central serous retinopathy and irrespective of the severity of the disease, there is never temporal pallor of the disc.

VARIATIONS IN THE CLINICAL PICTURE

No disease shows more variability from start to finish than senile disciform macular degeneration.

Many patients at an early stage show multiple serous detachments of the pigment epithelium intermingled with relatively few deep fatty exudates and little or no subretinal fluid. Such an appearance may persist for weeks without alteration in visual acuity or with only mild fluctuations in vision and variable metamorphopsia.

Sudden hemorrhage beneath the macular pigment epithelium with rapid visual loss is a rarer mode of onset. Such cases with little or no exudation, no predisciform yellow spots and no break in the pigment epithelium have been mistaken for choroidal melanoma. Persistent bleeding with rupture of the pigment epithelium dome produces a characteristic subretinal hemorrhage[64] which points to the correct diagnosis. This type of onset suddenly reduces vision and such cases usually have a more rapid course of mound development.

Occasionally, the disease starts as a reversible central serous retinopathy with a few deep-lying fatty exudates and spots of mild pigment mottling under the retinal dome. Slow but steady enlargement of the retinal mound with little other change creates a picture suggestive of a huge macular retinal cyst (Fig. 16-24). Later, fatty exudation forms a sheet over the pigment epithelium base and piles up intraretinally as a yellow ring at the edge of the retinal elevation. Both intraretinal and subretinal hemorrhages may be minimal in such cases. After months with little change, new blood vessels growing from macular tributaries, dip into the summit of the mound, dimpling the mound and ramifying subretinally. There is often a clump of migrated pigment superficially in the retina at this dimple (Fig. 16–24*D*).

Hemorrhage in senile disciform macular degeneration can vary tremendously. Extensive sheet-like subretinal hemorrhages sufficiently thick in places as to appear almost black may be present. Profuse intraretinal hemorrhages from the deep capillary bed around the mound may also occur. Rarely, massive hemorrhages will break through the retina into the vitreous. On the other hand, overt hemorrhage may be completely subordinate and minimal. Well-developed lesions can occur with only the most minimal intraretinal bleeding and sub-

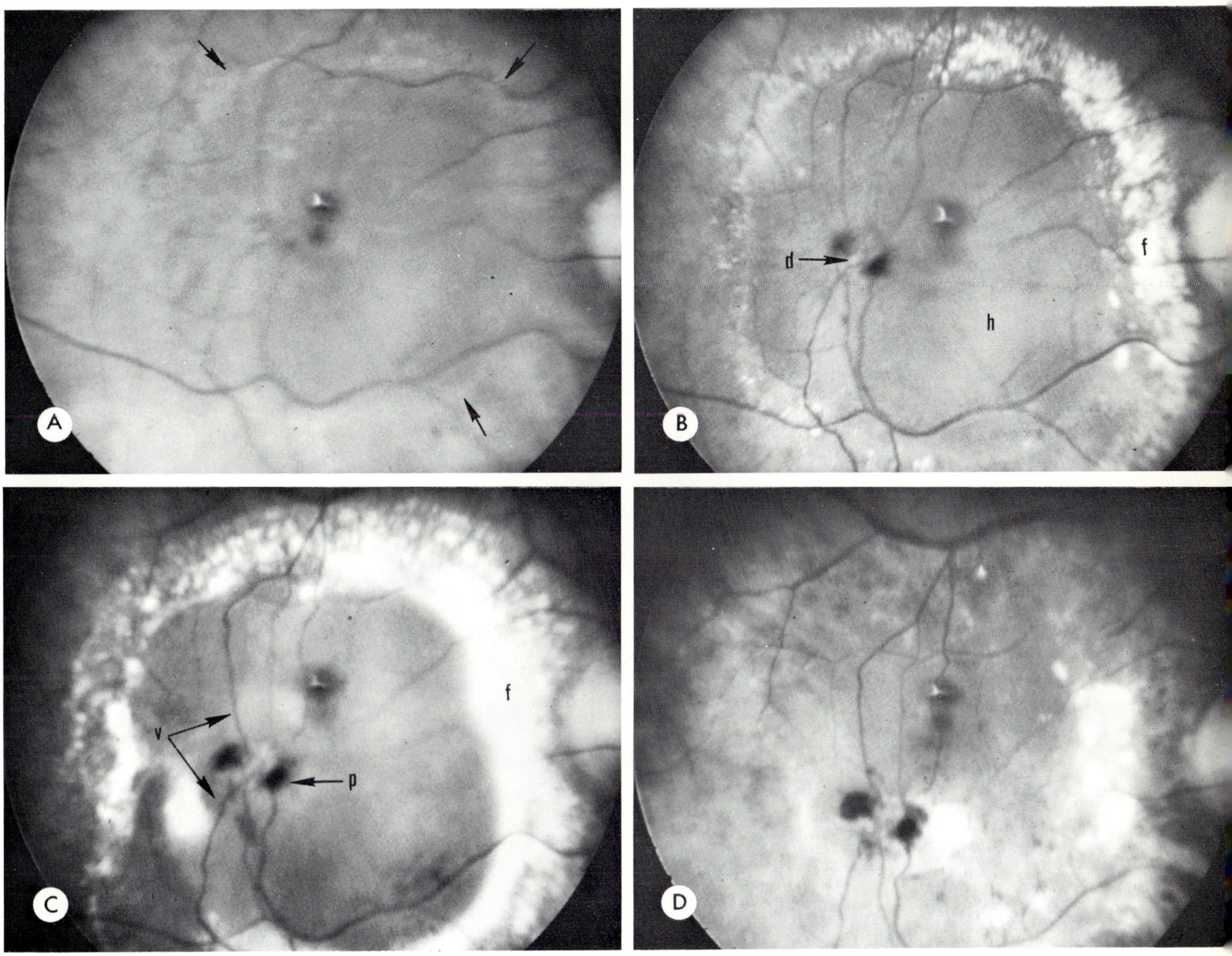

Fig. 16-24. A typical senile disciform macular degeneration in a 66-year-old woman. *A*, As seen on July 10, 1961, the huge, highly elevated serous detachment of the macular retina has only slightly hazy subretinal fluid. The pigment epithelium at the base shows mild mottling with a few scattered overlying fatty exudates. The mound border is indicated by **arrows.** Her vision is 20/200. *B*, Same eye as seen on March 22, 1962. Note increased fatty exudates at the mound border **(f),** increasing haze of subretinal fluid **(h),** and retinal arterial and venous branches dipping into a dimple in the mound at **(d).** Vision is 7/200. *C*, On October 10, 1962, heavy fatty exudation **(f)** can be seen at the border of the mound; pigment epithelium **(p)** has migrated into the superficial retina and clumped near the increasingly turgid retinal vessels **(v)** dipping into the mound. Vision is 3/200. *D*, On April 13, 1964, the retinal mound is settling, the ring of fatty exudates absorbing, and the retinal vessels dipping into the mound are less dilated than when the mound was at its height as in *C*. Patient now is able to count fingers at 3 feet.

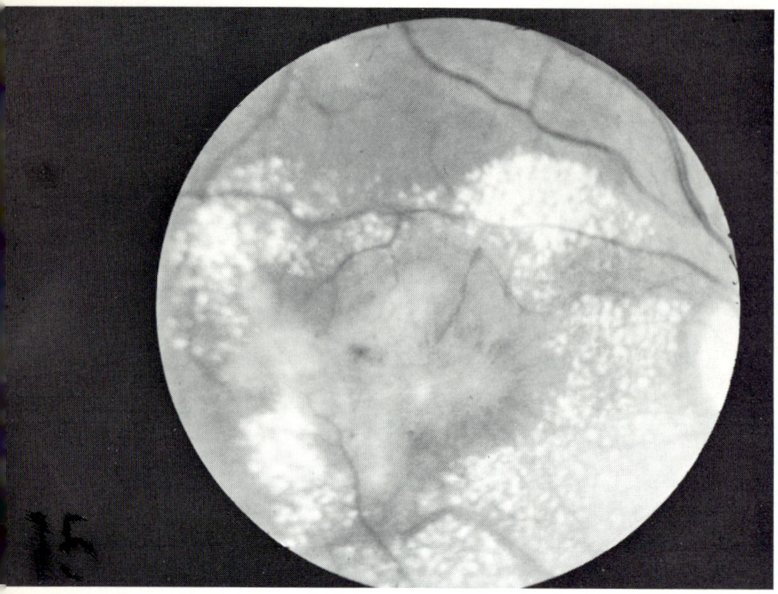

Fig. 16-25. Senile disciform macular degeneration with a ring of intraretinal fatty exudates around the mound.

pigment epithelial or subretinal hemorrhage may be absent.

Fatty exudation may be mild and restricted to the base of the mound, with a slight increase at its periphery, or there may be an accompanying discrete, circinate figure surrounding the dome (Fig. 16-25). Other patients may never exhibit this ring of fatty exudates. More commonly, the exudative feature of the disease is pronounced and may completely predominate. Exudation may be extensive within the mound area, profuse in the surrounding retina, extending around the disc out beyond the vessel arcades, or as the tail of a kite toward the periphery. In rare cases exudation proceeds throughout large regions of the retina producing, eventually, the picture of Type 1 Coats's disease. Aging exudates tend to develop cholesterin crystals. This is especially true where exudation is profuse. Commonly, blood and exudation beneath or around the mound become mixed. Such a mixture has a dirty, mottled, rusty color.

Changes in the pigment epithelium may be minimal well into the disease sequence, or there may be mottling, rarefaction, and clumping at an early phase. Pigment dispersal and proliferation is always a feature of the late scarring state. A few patients who have developed a concomitant choroidal sclerosis may show extensive areas of absent pigment epithelium about a smaller residual scar.

Finally, lesions are uncommonly macular-centered at the start. Paramacular onset, or early elevation somewhere within the bounds of the disc border and vessel arcades is the rule. Rarely, a mound will develop well away from the fovea and only involve the latter in its developing stages. One such case never invaded the macula. Satellite lesions seldom occur because the early individual elevations tend to coalesce into one large mound.

Although rare cases remain unilateral, the disease is usually bilateral. Both eyes may become involved at the same time, or years apart. It has been the observation of the early predisciform stage of the disease in these second symptomless eyes that has led to a more complete understanding of its pathogenesis. In spite of the lesions' variable appearance at onset, once the stage of retinal elevation is reached, all pass inexorably through a similar sequence, which is modified only in degree.

SUBRETINAL NEOVASCULARIZATION AND HEMORRHAGE

The neovascular formations in disciform macular disease have generally been dismissed with the statement that they take part in organizing the preexistent subretinal hemorrhage into the final fibrotic macular scar. Only Verhoeff and Grossman[73] have questioned this interpretation. In a microscopic study of disciform macular degeneration, they wondered why the new vessels from the choroid organized the blood under the central mound, but failed to grow and organize direct subretinal extensions of this same hemorrhage beyond the mound border.

Microscopic study of disciform macular disease has usually shown a break in Bruch's membrane somewhere under the fibrotic macular scar. New vessels and fibrous tissue have grown from the choroid through this opening into the subretinal space. In some cases, the neovascular fibrosis has entered through a break in Bruch's membrane outside the mound area and rarely has it grown around the disc border of Bruch's membrane, whose continuity is undisturbed.[21,64,80] In both instances, once inside of Bruch's membrane, the fibrovascular tufts tend to grow toward the submacular area. They have a predilection for extension between Bruch's membrane and its adjacent pigment epithelium. Such fibrovascular membranes in this position may be innocuous for on occasion they have been found unexpectedly in the posterior aspects of older globes subjected to routine microscopic examination.[27,73]

Clinically, neovascular growths beneath the pigment epithelium cannot be visualized. In a number of instances, where they pierce both Bruch's membrane and the pigment epithelium and extend along the inner surface of this layer, they can be seen. A careful search for instances of this phenomenon has shown it to be more frequent than expected, and what is more important, to appear much earlier than anticipated. The clinically visible vessels lie somewhere near the macula or, if they pierce Bruch's membrane and the pigment epithelium at a more distant site, tend to grow toward it. New vessels may be well developed at a stage prior to any subretinal or subpigment epithelial hemorrhage. They have been seen at the beginning stage of a disciform mound (early progressive phase) and may be well developed under a more advanced stage of mound formation. In one instance of the latter, they formed orderly arborizing arcs of new vessels, lying on the pigment epithelium and bounded by the borders of the mound. In this patient there was no hemorrhage beneath the retina or pigment epithelium (Fig. 16-26).

Early neovascularization from retinal vessels into the subretinal area of the mound has never been observed. This is fairly common as a later phenomenon where extensions from small macular tributaries contribute to the subretinal scar. Neovascular extensions from veins are much more common than from arteries, although both have been observed. Klien[37] has described a case in which the retinal neovascular growth made up the subretinal fibrovascular scar, a distant neovascularization from the choroid not having as yet reached the subretinal mound zone.

The assumption that the subretinal hemorrhage in disciform macular disease is due

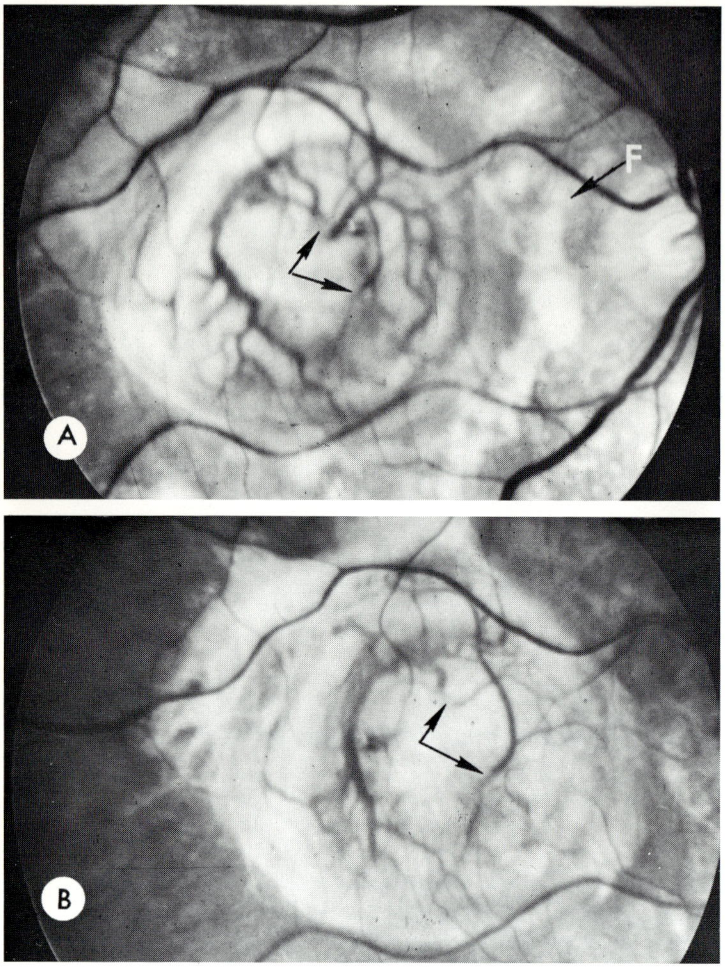

Fig. 16-26. *A*, Senile disciform macular degeneration in a 75-year-old female seen on October 1, 1959. Note the arching subretinal vessels lying just above the pigment epithelium. Their points of entrance from the choroid are marked by **arrows.** **(F)** is the intraretinal fatty exudate ring around the mound. *B*, Same as in *A* as seen on June 26, 1961. Note the absorption of the fatty exudate ring and the changed pattern and caliber of the subretinal vessels entering from the choroid at the **arrows.**

to the rupture of Bruch's membrane is without real foundation. This hemorrhage commonly occurs between the pigment epithelium and Bruch's membrane, a potential space normally devoid of blood vessels. Were the blood in a hemorrhagic detachment of the pigment epithelium to arise from a ruptured choriocapillary vessel and break through Bruch's membrane, it should also rupture the pigment epithelium and spread at least in part through the choroid at the same time. Rupture of the pigment epithelium usually occurs later, and choroidal hemorrhage has not been seen clinically, nor reported microscopically in this disease. Although it is unproved, some evidence suggests that the subpigment epithelial hemorrhages in disciform macular disease arise from preexistent neovascular growths derived from the choroid which are clinically quiescent until the time of bleeding. If this be so, the sequence of events here would be comparable to that of retinitis proliferans.

FLUORESCEIN ANGIOGRAPHY

In the predisciform state of this disease fluorescein angiograms show no choroidal leak. With the onset of progressive mound formation choroidal leakage can be demonstrated. Leaks under detachments of the pigment epithelium are similar to those seen in progressive central serous retinopathy. More commonly there is widespread sievelike leakage beneath the mound beginning in the early venous phase of the angiogram (Fig. 16-27). This leakage, mild at first, becomes profuse as the disease progresses and fluorescence may persist for several hours in a well-developed mound.

TREATMENT

There is no satisfactory treatment for this disease. The successful closure of leaks in central serous retinopathy by photocoagu-

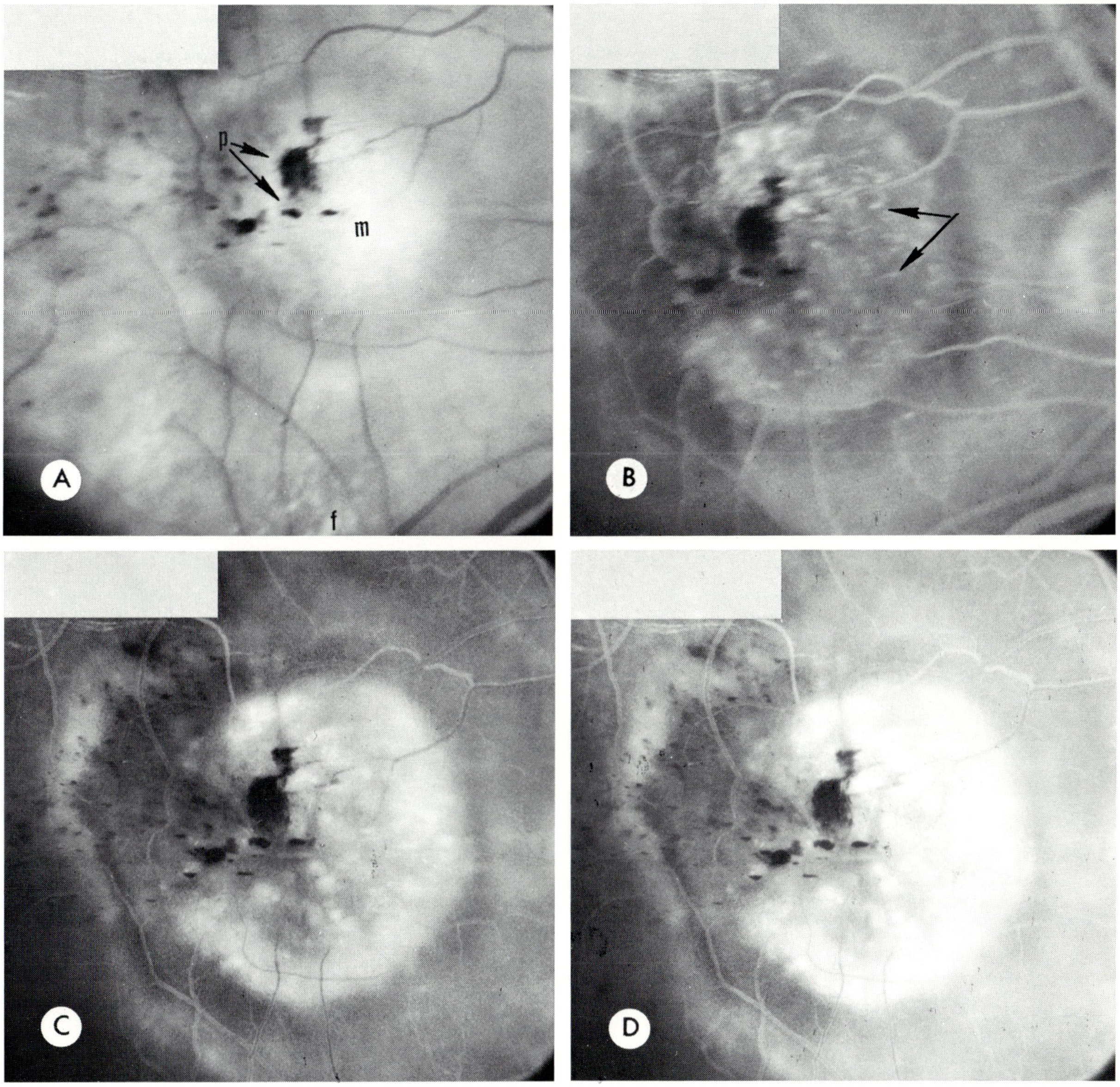

Fig. 16-27. Senile disciform macular degeneration. *A*, Note the central mound **(m)**; migrated clumps of pigment epithelium **(p)**; circinate fatty exudates **(f)**. *B*, A fluorescein angiogram of *A*. Note sieve-like leakage **(arrows)** beneath the mound. *C*, late-phase fluorescein angiogram shows increasing leakage. *D*, Later-phase fluorescein angiogram shows profuse leakage with diffusion under the retina.

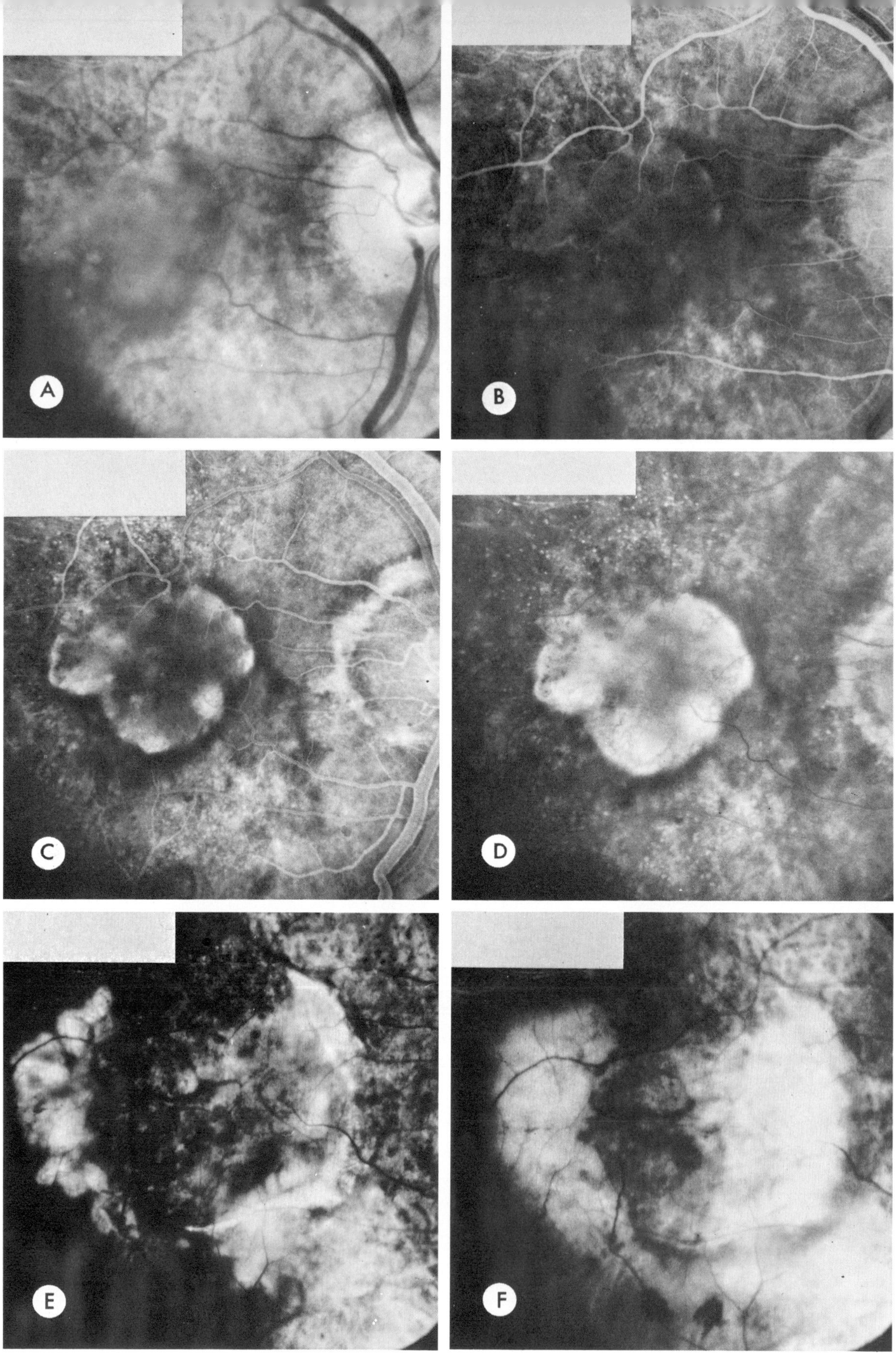
A
B
C
D
E
F

Fig. 16-28. *Opposite page.* Disciform macular degeneration in the second eye of a 67-year-old woman with an old disciform macular scar in left eye. Vision: counts fingers at 1 foot.

A, Fundic photograph of right eye shows hemorrhagic detachment of the pigment epithelium and serous elevation of the retina. Vision is 20/200.

B, Arterial-phase fluorescein angiogram of *A* shows very early leakage beneath the detached pigment epithelium.

C, Late-venous phase fluorescein angiogram shows increasing leakage.

D, Very late phase fluorescein angiogram. Following perifoveal photocoagulation the original leaks were sealed.

E, Fluorescein angiogram made 4 months after treatment showing diffuse new leakage at the outer border of the original leaks.

F, Late-phase fluorescein angiogram. Treatment has failed to control the progression of this disease.

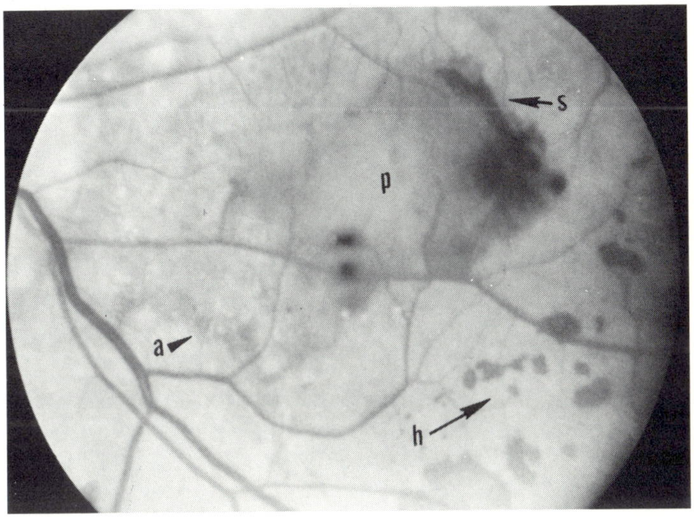

Fig. 16-29. Pseudoxanthoma elasticum and angioid streaks in a 47-year-old woman. Patient had angioid streaks (**a**) with normal vision for many years. Vision suddenly was reduced to 20/100 2 weeks prior to photograph. Note hemorrhagic detachment of the pigment epithelium (**p**) with a corona of subretinal hemorrhage (**s**) at its border and the outlying deep retinal hemorrhages (**h**).

lation suggested this same mode of treatment for senile disciform macular degeneration. Early results had suggested some promise[33,75,78] but longer observation has proved to be disappointing. Closure of leaks with the laser beam in those cases with leakage far enough from the fovea to be treatable have required more intensive burns and more extensive treatment areas (Fig. 16-28). Frequently, patients have required repeated burns to close effectively the leaks and interpretation of the fluorescein angiograms subsequent to treatment was much more difficult. Following treatment, hemorrhages and exudates may rapidly absorb and the retina may begin to settle, only to have leakage occur at the same, or some other site. With leakage beneath the fovea, further treatment is impossible. The ultimate value of this form of treatment is still to be determined and at present it seems limited.

MACULAR DEGENERATION IN ANGIOID STREAKS

Angioid streaks have been described most commonly in pseudoxanthoma elasticum and Paget's disease of the bone.[27,36,62,66,70,72] They have also been reported in sickle cell disease.[23,24,61] Rarely, they may be seen in idiopathic familial hyperphosphatemia,[52] senile elastosis of the skin, and fibrodysplasia hyperelastica of Ehlers-Danlos.[15] While ill-defined macular changes have been observed in those patients with sickle cell disease,[23] only in pseudoxanthoma elasticum and Paget's disease have actual macular degenerations been seen. Until macular involvement occurs the patient is unaware of any visual difficulty (Fig. 16-29). While both eyes are likely to be involved in the macular degeneration, the latter appears late in the disease and one eye may follow the second with an interval of as long as 21 years.

We have traced four patients having this macular lesion from their inception. All had extensive typical angioid streaks in both fundi. Three patients had pseudoxanthoma elasticum and one had Paget's disease. When visual impairment was first noted, subretinal fluid was present, and visible shadows could be seen in the macular area. Mottled areas of pigment epithelium were present under the macular zone. At first, the region of subretinal fluid was ill defined, but as it increased producing a retinal mound, the margin became well defined, smooth, and oval, encompassing the fovea. From this point on the lesion passed through the typical stages of development and quiescence seen in senile disciform macular degeneration. There were hemorrhages beneath the pigment epithelium, in front of it and about the mound in the midretina; fatty exudation within the mound and in a circinate zone about it (Fig. 16-30); a welling up and slow settling with absorption of hemorrhages, exudation, and subretinal fluid; and finally, the formation of a pigmented, subretinal fibrovascular scar with a permanent central scotoma. Oeller's *Atlas*[56] shows a typical hemorrhagic detachment of the macular pigment epithelium at the start of disciform macular degeneration in angioid streak retinopathy. Published in 1900, this may be the first recorded case of this development. Fluorescein angiography and microscopic study[36,39] have shown the typical findings of senile disciform macular degeneration.

The disciform macular degenerations associated with angioid streaks had no predisciform phase. The angioid streaks varied greatly in length and profusion prior to macular involvement. In one such case, they were traced almost to the equator. In no case was there leakage from a distant streak with spread to the macula. In all cases, the macula seemed directly involved from the onset of leakage. From the beginning of choroidal leakage, proliferation and migration of pigment epithelium was prominent. The exudation, hemorrhagic features, and mound size were moderate in all cases. Final scarring contained masses of proliferated pigment (Fig. 16-31).

THE MACULAR LESION IN TEMPORAL ANGIOMA

Sufficiently large temporal retinal angioma produce fatty exudation at the macula (see Chapter 10, under section on Exaggerated Macular Response to Retinal Disease and Chapter 11, under section on Cerebrovascular Anomalies and Retinal Angioma). This lesion starts with intraretinal macular edema and the deposition of fatty exudate in Henle's layer. Fatty exudate accumulates progressively, filling in the foveal area and becoming a continuous mass obliterating the star figure from the center outward. When it passes the peripheral border of Henle's fibers, the serrate border is converted into a smoothly rounded one. The lesion may become elevated as much as 4D and always produces a central scotoma. If seen at this stage, it can be mistaken for an exudative disciform macular

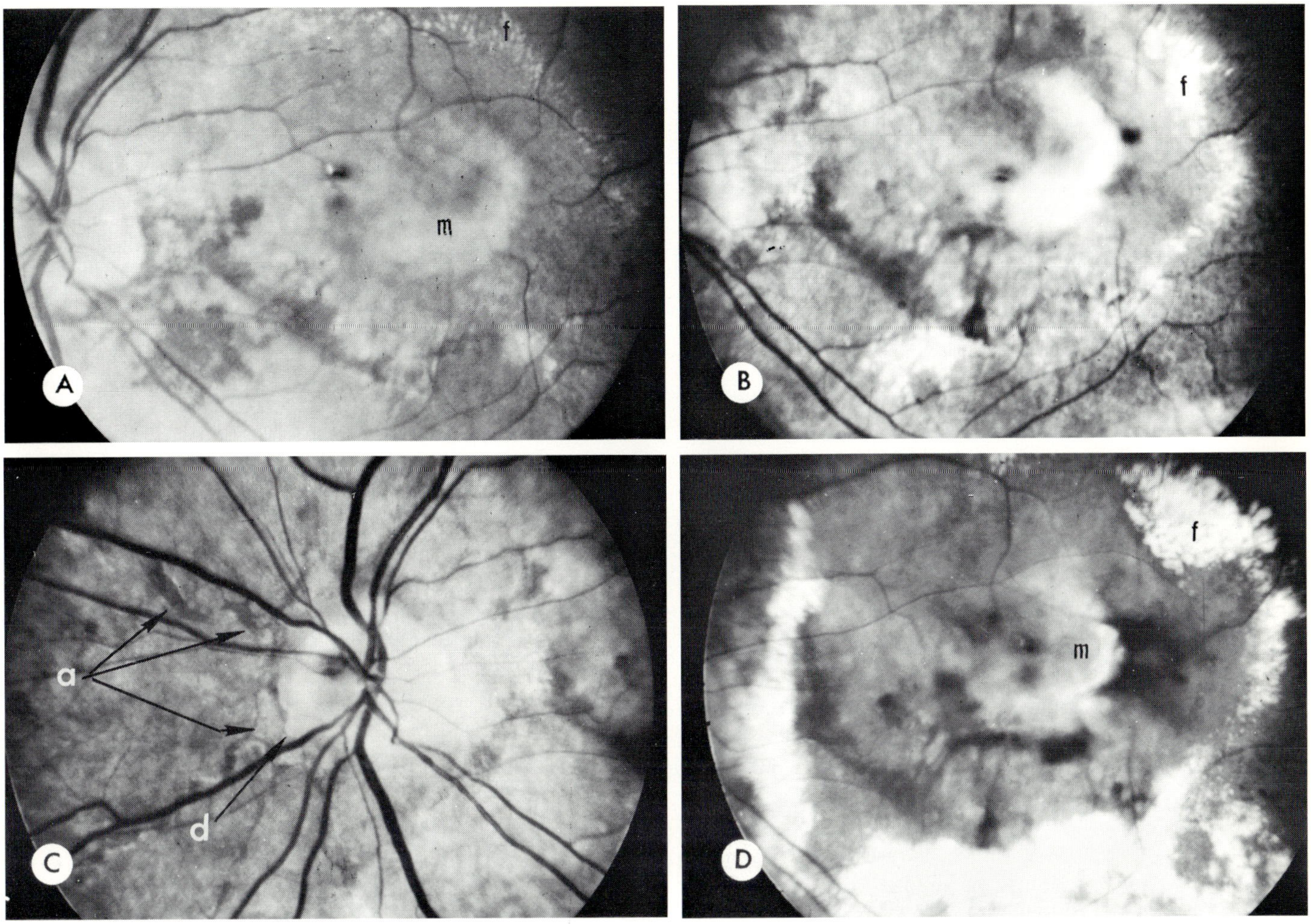

Fig. 16-30. Pseudoxanthoma elasticum and angioid streaks in a 50-year-old woman who developed disciform macular degeneration in the first eye 23 years previously. First visual difficulty in this eye began 2½ years ago.

A, Picture taken September 9, 1960 shows macular area 2½ years after first visual difficulty in the second eye. Note mound **(m)** and circinate fatty exudates **(f)**.

B, Picture taken October 8, 1962 of same eye. Note increasing fatty exudate ring **(f)**.

C, At the same time disc area shows angioid streaks **(a)**. Drusen of the disc **(d)** was an unrelated finding.

D, As seen on April 6, 1964, the overlying detached retina is cystic. The subretinal serous fluid is relatively clear. The underlying mound **(m)** of detached pigment epithelium is flattening and partially obscured by fatty exudate. The intraretinal fatty exudate ring **(f)** is still increasing.

degeneration (see Fig. 10-35b). Hemorrhage is not a constituent of the lesion, nor is there a circinate figure around the mound. The latter has a solid appearance, and there is no choroidal leak of fluorescein beneath it.

If the angioma is obliterated, the macular exudate slowly absorbs over months to several years. It leaves in its wake a variable degree of pigment mottling (rarefaction and proliferation) and a few inspissated, yellowish spots of exudate. Visual recovery may be remarkable.

THE MACULAR LESION DUE TO TOXOCARA

That *Toxocara canis* can produce a retinal lesion has only recently been recognized.[3,32,54,76] The incidence of the disease, its systemic manifestations, and mode of transmission are not yet fully known; nor has the highly similar parasite *T. cati* yet been identified as a cause of human illness.

The parasite, commonly affecting children, is thought to come from a pet dog, especially a puppy, and pass via the alimentary tract and blood stream to the lungs, where it produces a transient, ill-defined pneumonitis with low grade fever and eosinophilia. Some time after recovery from the acute manifestation, a *T. canis* larva reaches the eye and produces a granulomatous retinal reaction.

The ocular larva has a propensity to settle at the posterior pole of the eye, usually at the macula or slightly toward the disc, and to lie between the retina and the pigment epithelium. Migration of larva does occur,[65] Hogan, Kimura and O'Connor having reported a *Toxocara* larva at the ora serrata.[31]

Clinical descriptions of the early phases of the retinal lesion are unavailable and clinical descriptions of cases not subjected to microscopic study are still somewhat suspect, as absolute identification in our present state of knowledge can only be made in this manner.

The limitation imposed by retrospective utilization of clinical descriptions in histologically proved cases leaves certain gaps in our knowledge. There is, however, sufficient data to include this lesion among the disciform macular diseases. In one instance (Ref. 3, Case 2), a case was described both clinically and, at first, microscopically, as juvenile disciform macular degeneration.

Well-developed retinal toxocara lesions have the following clinical similarities to disciform macular disease:

1. A predilection for the macular area
2. A solitary elevated lesion with minimal inflammatory signs
3. The yellowish white color of the umbilicated mass (Ref. 3, Case 1)
4. The retinal vessels dipping into the mound at its umbilication (Ref. 3, Case 1)
5. The absence of temporal disc pallor in the presence of well-developed disease (Ref. 3, Cases 1 and 2)
6. The sheet-like, deep hemorrhage adjacent to the rim of the lesion (Ref. 3, Case 2)
7. The transparent and gelatinous superficial aspect of the tumor and its opaque white deeper portion (Ref. 3, Case 2)
8. The exudates in the outer plexiform layer adjacent to the mass (Ref. 3, Case 2), and the ring of fatty exudates around the mound in a circinate distribution (Ref. 3, Case 1 which has subsequently been proven to be *toxocara*)

The appearance of a posterior retinal *toxocara* lesion is so similar to other disciform macular mounds that it cannot be clinically diagnosed with certainty. It only differs in always being unilateral. So far, a fluorescein angiogram in a proved case has not been reported. A disciform lesion near the macula in a child or young person with a history of recent pneumonitis and a pet dog would be suggestive of *toxocara*.

In spite of its clinical similarities to other disciform macular diseases, microscopic identification of the parasite with the eosinophilic reaction about it, and the associated giant cells clearly distinguishes this lesion. Numerous sections through the mass must be studied as the parasite may appear on only two or three slides and is, therefore, easily overlooked.[76]

DISCIFORM MACULAR SYNDROME[77]

The exact mechanism by which each of these diseases is initiated is unknown. Although quite different in the beginning, a number of them in their later stages become clinically and microscopically more and more alike. It seems likely, therefore, that, irrespective of their possible diverse etiologies, at some point in their development, they share a common pathologic mechanism.

Reversible central serous retinopathy starts with early focal serous leakage from the choriocapillaris through Bruch's membrane and the pigment epithelium. Minute change in the choriocapillary wall and perivascular tissue and a few round cells found in some patients have suggested an initial inflammatory choriocapillary defect.[21] If this were a focal inflammation in the usual sense of focal superficial chorioretinitis, one would expect to find clinically a fuzzy, white, edematous lesion in the choroid and outer retina as might be seen in a single locus of miliary tuberculosis. Inflammatory chorioretinal lesions do not show a clear serous leakage elevating the retina, but rather a diffuse leakage into the inflamed areas as has been demonstrated by fluorescein angiography in acute chorioretinitis. The retina remains adherent to the choroid at the site of inflammation and eventually forms a chorioretinal scar with some destruction of overlying retinal elements and choroid.

Generally speaking a pathologic alteration in the microcirculation can come from a stimulus anywhere in its milieu. Thus, a stimulus from the outer retina, pigment epithelium, or Bruch's membrane could equally well produce an abnormal focal dilatation of the underlying choriocapillaris and the minute microscopic changes seen in the latter be interpreted as a part of the reparative process in this so often self-limited disease. The absence of pathologic change in the retina and its normal fluorescein pattern make it an unlikely exciting source. The early serous detachment of the overlying pigment epithelium, with retention of the intercellular adhesiveness and the lack of discernable pigmentary change within the cells, as is seen *early* in some cases, make this layer also an unlikely source of initial stimulus. On the other hand, a defect in the pigment epithelium without detachment at the point of fluorescein leakage as is seen *early* in many cases does suggest an initial pigment epithelial defect. In either case, the pigment epithelium very shortly becomes defective as is demonstrated by fluorescein leakage beneath the retina. Bruch's membrane itself cannot be excluded as an initiating factor.

Irrespective of its pathogenesis, once the retina is elevated by serous fluid, the outer retina becomes removed from its normal choriocapillary blood supply. If the retina does not remain elevated too long and repair takes place, leakage ceases, subretinal fluid is absorbed, and the retina returns to its normal position and resumes normal function. This is the course of events in reversible central serous retinopathy.

With progressive disease there would be continued leakage into the subretinal space and thickening of the fluid with fatty exudation and often hemorrhage. This would produce increased retinal ischemia leading to retinal capillary dilatation, fluid leakage, and the microcystic macula seen clinically at this stage. It is this increasing retinal ischemia and the reactions to it that become irreversible and represent the pathologic sequence shared by those eyes demonstrating this disciform macular syndrome.

Progressive central serous retinopathy would include all cases not fully reversible. As healing can take place at any stage of the disease, not all patients will develop the full syndrome. The amount of residual scarring will depend upon the duration of the disease and the extent of the changes before healing begins. The course of events in presumed histoplasmosis would be entirely comparable. The effect of aging on the vascular system, pigment epithelium, and Bruch's membrane must be a pertinent one, for younger patients with progressive central serous retinopathy, or presumed histoplasmosis are more likely to have healing at an early stage, or with full development of the syndrome, to end with a smaller mound, residual scar, and final scotoma. Older patients almost invariably progress through the full syndrome once the disease begins and the exudative and hemorrhagic features, mound formation, residual scar, and scotoma are regularly more extensive.

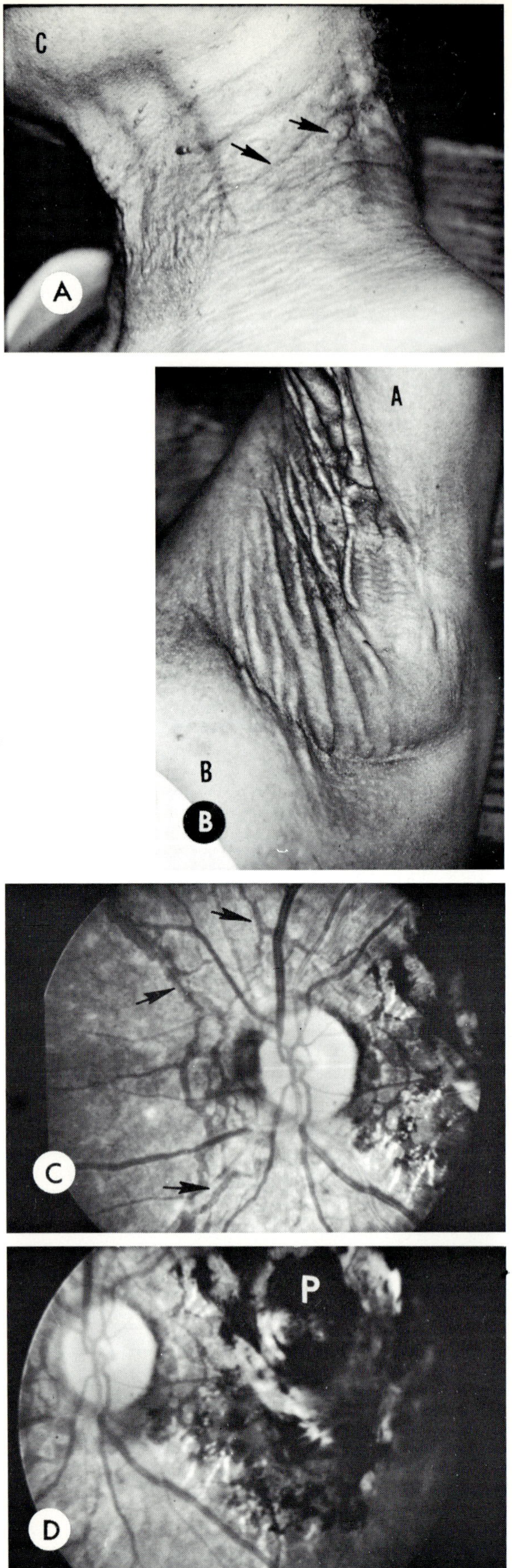

Fig. 16-31. *A*, Pseudoxanthoma elasticum showing papillary and striae-like neck lesions. **(C)** indicates the chin. *B*, Same patient showing exaggerated axillary skin changes. **(A)** indicates the raised arm and **(B)** the breast. *C*, Same patient. Disc area shows angioid streaks **(arrows)**. *D*, Same eye shows the heavy pigment proliferation **(P)** in the late scar stage of the disciform macular degeneration. Note absence of any temporal disc pallor.

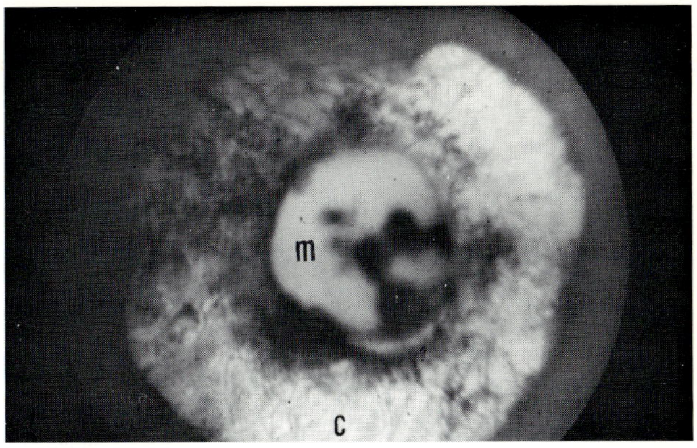

Fig. 16-32. Old disciform macular degeneration shows disc-sized macular mound **(m)** and surrounding choroidal sclerosis **(c).**

In senile disciform macular degeneration, aging changes in Bruch's membrane [30] may well contribute to initiating the disease and are apt to be partly responsible for the sieve-like fluorescein leakage seen. Aging changes in the perimacular retinal capillaries (loss of endothelial and mural cells and obliteration of capillary lumens) [46,47] would make the macular retina more vulnerable to interference with its normal choriocapillary blood supply.

It would be helpful to know exactly at what stage new vessels begin to grow through Bruch's membrane or around its disc border toward the macula in senile disciform macular degeneration. Their early development from the choroid toward the macula would suggest an early serious vascular insufficiency of the macular retina. The early deep fatty exudation of this disease is another indirect evidence of vascular insufficiency.

Thus, one could postulate that in senile disciform macular degeneration, where aging has already compromised both Bruch's membrane and the retinal perimacular capillary bed, an insidious further alteration in Bruch's membrane develops. This embarrasses nutrient exchange between a relatively normal choriocapillaris and its dependent overlying retina. Eventually, serous leakage through Bruch's membrane lifts the retina from the choroid, the vicious circle is initiated and the disciform macular syndrome becomes inevitable. Rupture of preformed new vessels produces hemorrhage first beneath the pigment epithelium and then subretinally, if the pigment layer does not hold. Blood and increasing fatty exudation beneath the mound produce further retinal ischemia. The resulting retinal capillary dilatation leads to microcystic macular edema at the summit of the mound and midretinal hemorrhages at its periphery. Later, if new vessels from the choroid are insufficient to appease the subretinal vasoformative stimulus, new vessels grow down subretinally into the mound from the retinal surface. From this point on the process can be considered purely reparative with increasing subretinal fibrosis and pigment proliferation, absorption of hemorrhage serous fluid and exudation, and decreasing vascularity.

Macular choroidal sclerosis was formerly thought to be a forerunner of disciform macular degeneration. This disease, readily apparent in its early stages because of the prompt migration of overlying pigment, is a rare feature in early senile disciform macular degeneration. When it does occur in the predisciform phase of the disease, serous leakage beneath the retina is absent or minimal and typical mound formation has not been seen. When it is present late in the disease around the mound, the latter is always small, sometimes no larger than the disc (Fig. 16-32). Choroidal sclerosis not only obliterates choriocapillary channels, but also leads to death and disappearance of overlying outer retinal elements.[2] Since both a reasonably functional choriocapillaris and viable outer retinal cells are necessary for the development of the disciform macular syndrome, the damping effect of coincident choroidal sclerosis is understandable.

The development of the disciform macular syndrome in angioid streaks is entirely comparable to the course of events just described. The fact that such a macular lesion develops in pseudoxanthoma elasticum, a systemic disease attacking the elastic tissue of Bruch's membrane, lends considerable weight to the importance of this membrane in initiating the disciform macular syndrome.

Just why disciform lesions have such a propensity for macular involvement is not clear. The lesions of progressive central serous retinopathy are always severest at the macula, satellite lesions commonly being benign and reversible. Nonmacular histo spots and angioid streaks show no fluorescein leakage, nor do they develop the disciform syndrome except at the macula. The macula appears to be more sensitive than other retinal areas in a number of retinal diseases but the physiologic basis of this sensitivity is still unknown (see Chapter 10, under section on Exaggerated Macular Response to Retinal Disease).

REFERENCES

1. Asbury, T.: The status of presumed ocular histoplasmosis: Including a report of a survey. *Trans. Amer. Ophthal. Soc. 64:*371, 1966.
2. Ashton, N.: Central areolar choroidal sclerosis. A histopathological study. *Brit. J. Ophthal. 37:*140, 1953.
3. Ashton, N.: Larval granulomatosis of the retina due to *toxocara. Brit. J. Ophthal. 44:* 129, 1960.
4. Batra, D. V., and Paul, S. D.: Macular illumination tests in central serous retinopathy. *Amer. J. Ophthal. 63:*146, 1967.
5. Best, F.: Über eine hereditäre Macula-affektion. Beitrage zur Verebungslehre. *Z. Augenheilk. 13:*199, 1905.
6. Bonatti, W. D., Jaeger, E. A., and Frayer, W. C.: Endogenous fungal endophthalmitis. *Arch. Ophthal. 70:*772, 1963.
7. Braley, A. E., and Hamilton, H. E.: Central serous choroidosis associated with amebiasis. *Arch. Ophthal. 58:*1, 1957.
8. Braley, A. E., and Spivey, B. E.: Hereditary vitelline macular degeneration. *Arch. Ophthal. 72:*743, 1964.
9. Coppez, H., and Danis, M.: Rétinite exudative maculaire sénile et rétinite circinée. *Arch. Ophtal. 43:*461, 1926.
10. Cunha-Vaz, J. G., and Maurice, D. M.: The active transport of fluorescein by the retinal vessels and the retina. *J. Physiol. 191:*467, 1967.
11. Curry, H. F., and Moorman, L. T.: Fluorescein photography of vitelliform macular degeneration. *Arch. Ophthal. 79:*705, 1968.
12. Davenport, R. C.: Senile macular exudative retinitis. *Trans. Ophthal. Soc. U.K. 46:*137, 1926.
13. Deutman, A. F.: Electro-oculography in families with vitelliform dystrophy of the fovea. *Arch. Ophthal. 81:*305, 1969.
14. Dollery, C. T., Henkind, P., Paterson, J. W., Ramalho, P. S., and Hill, D. W. Focal retinal ischaemia. Part I. Ophthalmoscopic and circulatory changes in focal retinal ischaemia. *Brit. J. Ophthal. 50:*285, 1966.
15. Duke-Elder, S.: *System of Ophthalmology. Diseases of the Uveal Tract.* London, Kimpton, 1966, Vol. IX, p. 726.
16. Duke-Elder, S.: *System of Ophthalmology. Diseases of the Retina.* London, Kimpton, 1967, Vol. X, p. 601.
17. Ferry, A. P.: Macular detachment associated with congenital pit of the optic nerve head. *Arch. Ophthal. 70:*346, 1963.
18. François, J.: Vitelliform degeneration of the macula. *Bull. N.Y. Acad. Med. 44:*18, 1968.
19. Frayer, W. C.: Elevated lesions of the macular area. *Arch. Ophthal. 53:*82, 1955.
20. Fuchs, E.: Retinitis circinata. *Arch. Ophth. 39:*229, 1893.

21. Gass, J. D. M.: Pathogenesis of disciform detachment of the neuroepithelium. *Amer. J. Ophthal. 63:*573, 1967.

22. Gass, J. D. M.: Serous detachment of the macula secondary to congenital pit of the optic nerve head. *Amer. J. Ophthal. 67:*821, 1969.

23. Geeraets, W. J., and Guerry, D.: Angioid streaks and sickle-cell disease. *Amer. J. Ophthal. 49:*450, 1960.

24. Geeraets, W. J., and Guerry, D.: Elastic tissue degeneration in sickle-cell disease. *Amer. J. Ophthal. 50:*213, 1960.

25. Geltzer, A. I., and Berson, E. L.: Fluorescein angiography of hereditary retinal degenerations. *Arch. Ophthal. 81:*776, 1969.

26. Giles, C. L., and Falls, H. F.: Amphotericin B. Therapy in the treatment of presumed histoplasma chorioretinitis: A further appraisal. *Trans. Amer. Ophthal. Soc. 65:*136, 1967; *Amer. J. Ophthal. 66:*101, 1968.

27. Hagedoorn, A.: Angioid streaks. *Arch. Ophthal. 21:*746, 935, 1939.

28. Harley, R. D., and Mishler, J. E. Endogenous intraocular fungus infection. *Trans. Amer. Acad. Ophthal. Otolaryng. 63:*264, 1959.

29. Hoefnagels, K. L. J., and Pijpers, P. M.: *Histoplasma capsulatum* in a human eye. *Amer. J. Ophthal. 63:*715, 1967.

30. Hogan, M. J.: Bruch's membrane and disease of the macula. Role of elastic tissue and collagen. *Trans. Ophthal. Soc. U.K. 87:*113, 1967.

31. Hogan, M. J., Kimura, S. J., and O'Connor, G. R.: Peripheral retinitis and chronic cyclitis in children. *Trans. Ophthal. Soc. U.K. 85:* 33, 1965.

32. Irvine, W. C., and Irvine, A. R.: Nematode endophthalmitis: Part II. *Toxocara canis. Amer. J. Ophthal. 47:*185, 1959.

33. Jepson, C. N., and Wetzig, P. C.: Photocoagulation in disciform macular degeneration. *Amer. J. Ophthal. 67:*920, 1969.

34. Junius, P., and Kuhnt, H.: *Die Scheibenförmige Entartung der Netzhautmitte (Degeneratio Maculae Luteae Disciformis).* Berlin, Karger, 1926.

35. King, R. E., and Praeger, D. L.: Amebic choroidosis. *Arch. Ophthal. 72:*16, 1964.

36. Klien, B. A.: Angioid streaks: A clinical and histopathologic study. *Amer. J. Ophthal. 30:* 955, 1947.

37. Klien, B. A.: Macular lesions of vascular origin. *Amer. J. Ophthal. 34:*1279, 1951.

38. Klien, B. A.: Macular lesions of vascular origin: II. Functional vascular conditions leading to damage of the macula lutea. *Amer. J. Ophthal. 36:*1, 1953.

39. Klien, B. A.: Symposium: Macular diseases. *Trans. Amer. Acad. Ophthal. Otolaryng. 69:* 614, 1965.

40. Klien, B. A., and Krill, A. E.: Fundus flavimaculatus. *Amer. J. Ophthal. 64:*3, 1967.

41. Kohner, E. M., Dollery, C. T., Henkind, P., Paterson, J. W., and Ramalho, P. S. Retinal vascular changes following exposure to high-intensity light. *Amer. J. Ophthal. 63:*1748, 1967.

42. Kranenburg, E.: Crater-like holes in the optic disc and central serous retinopathy. *Arch. Ophthal. 64:*912, 1960.

43. Krill, A. E., Chishti, M. I., Klien, B. A., Newell, F. W., and Potts, A. M.: Multifocal inner choroiditis. *Trans. Amer. Acad. Ophthal. Otolaryng. 73:*222, 1969.

44. Krill, A. E., Morse, P. A., Potts, A. M., and Klien, B. A.: Hereditary vitelliruptive macular degeneration. *Amer. J. Ophthal. 61:* 1405, 1966.

45. Krill, A. E., Newell, F. W., and Chishti, M. I.: Fluorescein studies in diseases affecting the retinal pigment epithelium. *Amer. J. Ophthal. 66:*470, 1968.

46. Kornzweig, A. L.: The Retinal Vasculature in Macular Degeneration, *Proceedings of the XXth International Congress of Ophthalmology* (Munich, August, 1966). Nijmegen, MacDonald, 1967.

47. Kornzweig, A. L., Eliasoph, I., and Feldstein, M.: The retinal vasculature in macular degeneration. *Arch. Ophthal. 75:*326, 1966.

48. Locke, J. C.: After-image scotometry: A method of functional examination of the eye. *Trans. Amer. Ophthal. Soc. 61:*682, 1963.

49. Magder, H.: Test for central serous retinopathy. *Amer. J. Ophthal. 49:*147, 1960.

50. Maumenee, A. E.: Discussion of Gass, J. D. M.: Disciform macular degeneration. Presented at the Wilmer Residents Meeting in Baltimore, Md., April, 1964.

51. McLean, J. M.: Oculomycosis. *Trans. Amer. Acad. Opthal. Otolaryng. 67:*149, 1963.

52. McPhaul, J. J., and Engel, F. L.: Heterotopic calcification, hyperphosphatemia and an-

gioid streaks of the retina. *Amer. J. Med. 31:*488, 1961.

53. Morse, P. H., and MacLean, A. L.: Fluorescein fundus studies in hereditary vitelliruptive macular degeneration. *Amer. J. Ophthal. 66:*485, 1968.

54. Nichols, R. L.: The etiology of visceral larva migrans. I. Diagnostic morphology of infective second-stage *Toxocara* larvae. *J. Parasit. 42:*349, 1956.

55. Norton, E. W. D., and Gutman, F.: Diabetic retinopathy studied by fluorescein angiography. *Ophthalmologica 150:*5, 1965.

56. Oeller, J.: Atlas seltener ophthalmoskopischer. Befunde Zugleich Ergänzungstafeln zu dem Atlas der Ophthalmoskopie. Wiesbaden, Bergmann, 1900, C. Tab. VI.

57. Oeller, J.: Atlas seltener ophthalmoskopischer. Befunde Zugleich Ergänzungstafeln zu dem Atlas der Ophthalmoskopie. Wiesbaden, Bergmann, 1900–1905, C. Tab. XII.

58. Pagenstecher, H., and Genth, C.: *Atlas of Pathological Anatomy of the Eye.* Wiesbaden, Kreidel, 1875, Plate XVI.

59. Palm, E.: On the occurrence in the retina of conditions corresponding to the blood-brain barrier. *Acta. Ophthal. 25:*29, 1947.

60. Palmer, C. E.: Nontuberculous pulmonary calcification and sensitivity to histoplasmin. *Public Health Rep. 60:*513, 1945.

61. Paton, D.: Angioid streaks and sickle cell anemia. *Arch. Ophthal. 62:*852, 1959.

62. Percival, S. P. B.: Angioid streaks and elastorrhexis. *Brit. J. Ophthal. 52:*297, 1968.

63. Reese, A. B.: Massive retinal fibrosis in children. *Amer. J. Ophthal. 19:*576, 1936.

64. Reese, A. B., and Jones, I. S.: Hematomas under the pigment epithelium. *Amer. J. Ophthal. 53:*897, 1962.

65. Rubin, M. L., Kaufman, H. E., Tierney, J. P., and Lucas, H. C.: An intraretinal nematode. (A case report.) *Trans. Amer. Acad. Ophthal. Otolaryng. 72:*855, 1968.

66. Scheie, H. G., and Freeman, N. E.: Vascular disease associated with angioid streaks of the retina and pseudoxanthoma elasticum. *Arch. Ophthal. 35:*241, 1946.

67. Sollom, A. W.: Ocular tissue staining in the rabbit after fluorescein injection. *Exp. Eye Res. 7:*551, 1968.

68. Spaeth, G. L.: Absence of so-called *Histoplasma* uveitis in 134 cases of proven histoplasmosis. *Arch. Ophthal. 77:*41, 1967.

69. Sugar, H.: Congenital pits in the optic disc with acquired macular pathology. *Amer. J. Ophthal. 53:*307, 1962.

70. Terry, T. L.: Angioid streaks and osteitis deformans. *Trans. Amer. Ophthal. Soc. 32:*555, 1934.

71. Velzeboer, C. M. J.: Hereditary degenerative macular lesions with inflammatory signs and late visual disturbance. *Brit. J. Ophthal. 47:*641, 1963.

72. Verhoeff, F. H.: Histological findings in a case of angioid streaks. *Brit. J. Ophthal. 32:*531, 1948.

73. Verhoeff, F. H., and Grossman, H. P.: Pathogenesis of disciform degeneration of the macula. *Arch. Ophthal. 18:*561, 1937.

74. Wangvivat, Y., and Wise, G. N.: Unpublished data from a study of the pathology of senile disciform macular degeneration conducted at the Armed Forces Institute of Pathology, May, 1965.

75. Watzke, R. C., and Snyder, W. B.: Light coagulation for hemorrhagic disciform degeneration of the macula. *Trans. Amer. Acad. Ophthal. Otolaryng. 72:*389, 1968.

76. Wilder, H. C.: Nematode endophthalmitis. *Trans. Amer. Acad. Ophthal. Otolaryng. 55:*99, 1950.

77. Wise, G. N.: The concept of the disciform macular syndrome has been presented at the following meetings: Dec. 4–5, 1964, N.Y. State Univ. Post Grad. Review Course, Syracuse, N.Y.; Nov. 8, 1965, Brooklyn Ophth. Soc., N.Y., N.Y.; Jan. 19, 1966, New England Ophth. Soc., Boston, Mass.; April 27–28, 1967, Virginia Eye, Ear, Nose & Throat Soc., Hot Springs, Va.

78. Wise, G. N., Campbell, C. J., Wendler, P. F., and Rittler, M. C. Photocoagulation of vascular lesions of the macula. *Amer. J. Ophthal. 66:*452, 1968.

79. Woods, A. C., and Wahlen, H. E.: The probable role of benign histoplasmosis in the etiology of granulomatous uveitis. *Amer. J. Ophthal. 49:*205, 1960.

80. Zimmerman, L. E.: Personal communication, March 1960.

81. Zimmerman, L. E.: Symposium macular diseases. Differential diagnosis. *Trans. Amer. Acad. Ophthal. Otolaryng. 69:*623, 1965.

chapter 17

Experimental Retinal Vascular Diseases

In order to understand human retinal vascular disease it is often necessary to design and conduct experiments which duplicate clinical situations. In many cases the experimental procedure and its results barely resemble the human condition, but in a few instances the picture is virtually identical to that found in man. Furthermore, experiments permit us to study vascular alterations from their inception to their conclusion, and this is almost impossible in human disease. For example, experimental models have demonstrated the significance of oxygen in retrolental fibroplasia; the course of both arterial and venous occlusion; the cause, pathology, and natural history of cotton-wool spots; the effect of altered intraocular and systemic blood pressure on the retinal circulation; the relationship between degeneration of the outer retinal elements and retinal capillary degeneration; and the effect of cryosurgery on retinal vasculature. Other studies have revealed the pharmacologic effect of various agents on retinal circulation, and the significance of the blood-retinal barrier in health and disease. As the conditions dealt with in this chapter are varied, we have included a separate reference list for each section.

ARTERIAL OCCLUSION

In man most retinal vascular disease involves all components of the vascular tree, and it is often impossible to ascertain whether the initial pathology was centered in the arteries, capillaries, or veins. Embolization of the arteries is one situation in which the injurious agent can be localized to a specific portion of the retinal vascular bed.

Attempts to embolize retinal arteries in experimental animals date back to the nineteenth century. In the past various agents including oil dye,[10,18] mercury,[2] soot in liquid paraffin,[17] fat,[3] cholesterol,[12] uric acid,[12] atheromatous plaque crystals,[12] pumice stone,[12] chopped fetal hair,[11] latex particles,[6] glass balls,[1] fibrin,[14] and platelet emboli[15] have been used. Hollenhorst, Lensink, and Whisnant,[12] in a series of acute experiments using dogs and monkeys, have injected cholesterol into the carotid artery and produced bright intra-arterial plaques similar to those seen in retinal arteries of humans with carotid artery disease. Gay, Goldor, and Smith[6] have injected latex microspheres 7 to 28 μ in diameter into the infraorbital artery of dogs and produced both choroidal and retinal vascular occlusions. Occlusion of small vessels in the nerve fiber layer of the retina resulted in cytoid body lesions, while blockade of the choriocapillaris led to overlying retinal ischemia with subsequent atrophy and necrosis of the external layers of the retina. In a long-term study, Goldor and Gay[7] reported that occlusion of large choroidal vessels with larger latex spheres (up to 50 μ in diameter) resulted in diffuse atrophy of all retinal layers, including the inner layers presumably fed by patent retinal vessels.

In a series of reports[1,4,5,8,9,16] the effects of embolizing the retinas of cats, monkeys, and pigs with glass spheres were documented. Changes were observed both in the blood vessels and the surrounding retina.

VASCULAR CHANGES

The glass microspheres which entered the retinal vessels were clearly visible (Fig. 17-1). Sometimes they could be seen as sparkling dots rushing down the center of large vessels and vanishing into the periphery. Usually they were noted at arterial bifurcations or within small branch arteries. On occasion, an embolus lodged in the mouth of a small branch artery with most of its surface still within the main channel. In this case the glass sphere might become dislodged back into the main trunk.

Immediately after embolization the blood column distal to the embolus broke into segments, and the blood became darker than that in adjacent patent arteries (Fig. 17-2). The blood column was rarely stationary and frequently small packets of red blood cells could be seen moving slowly in retrograde fashion towards the obstruction. This sludging or "cattle trucking" persisted for various lengths of time, often lasting more than a week. The larger the caliber of vessel occluded, the more prominent was the sludging and retrograde flow. Though venules were not occluded, sludging of venous blood, particularly in cats, was observed in several instances. This was most obvious in cases where the arteries were heavily embolized and blood flow was thereby greatly diminished (Fig. 17-3). Clinically it is known that embarrassment of arterial inflow will cause retinal venous changes including venous stasis.

In cats collateral arterial channels were observed within several hours to several days after embolization. Appearing initially as little more than dilated and tortuous capillaries, the anastomotic channels broadened and became less sinuous over a period of several days to weeks. Occasionally they attained a diameter almost as large as the blocked vessel (Fig. 17-4). Such large caliber collaterals persisted, but a number of

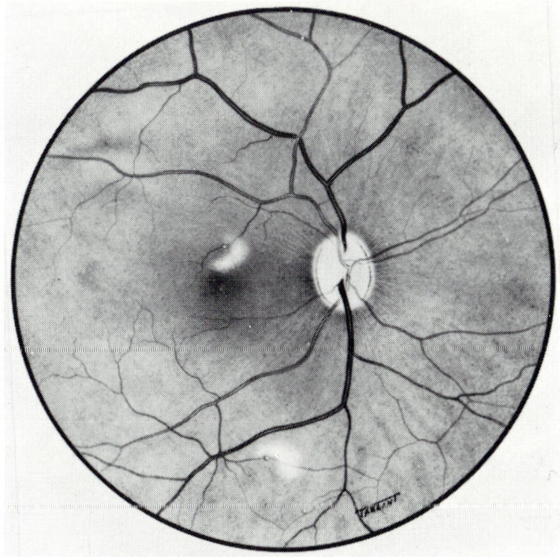

Fig. 17-1. Fundus painting of a rhesus monkey made 24 hours after embolization shows glass emboli within retinal arteries. Edema is present around two balls, one in the macular region and another beneath the inferior temporal vein. (From Henkind.[8a])

Fig. 17-2. Fundus photograph of a cat shortly after embolization. There is segmentation of blood within a retinal artery **(arrow).** (Courtesy of Drs. R. and B. Klein.)

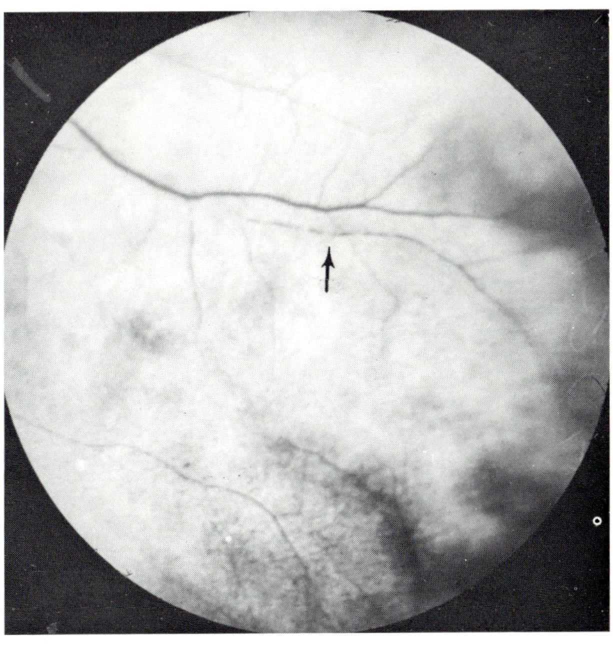

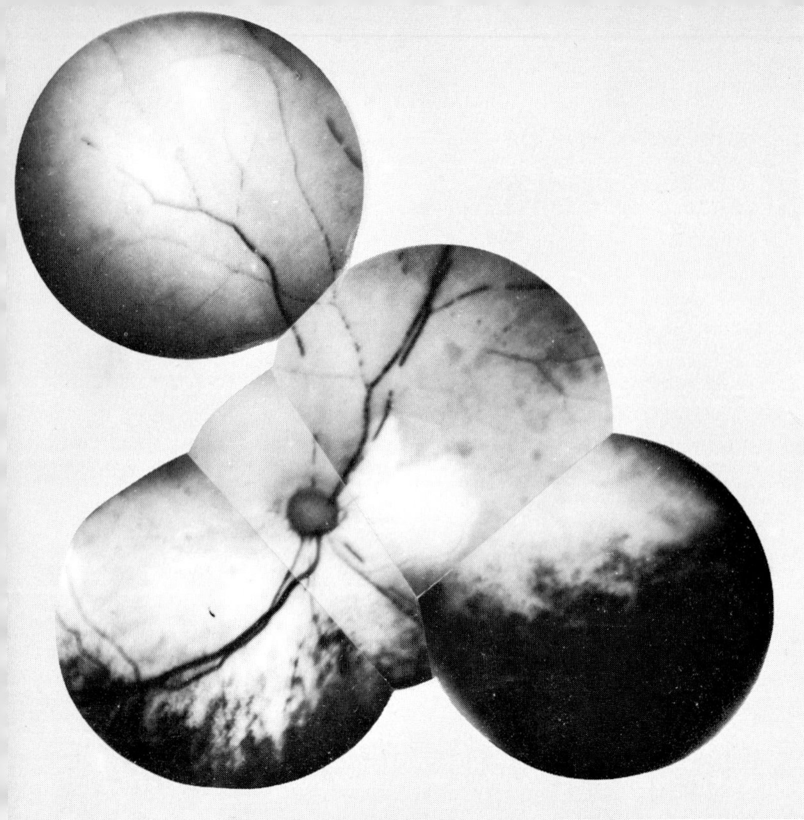

Fig. 17-3. Photomontage of a cat fundus 24 hours after embolization. Most of the arteries are embolized. There is sludging and segmentation of blood both in retinal arteries and veins. The retina appears edematous except in the nasal peripapillary region **(white area).** (From Henkind.[8a])

Fig. 17-4. Fundus photograph of a cat 21 days after embolization with glass balls. **Arrow** points to an arterial collateral. (From Henkind. *Brit. J. Ophthal. 50:*482, 1966. By permission of the Editor and Publisher.)

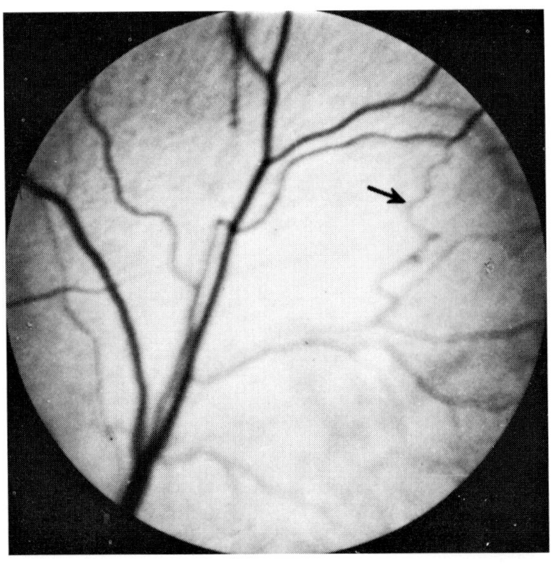

smaller ones regressed and even disappeared. The collaterals were of two types: the first and least frequent was a small tortuous channel which bypassed a visible embolus and joined the distal nonperfused segment with the patent portion of the artery, these were found mainly at the posterior pole; collaterals of the second type were larger and more prominent and linked the blocked vessel with an adjacent patent artery (Fig. 17-5*A*). This type was noted most often near the equator, usually at some distance from a visible embolus. Either type of collateral was often first noted as a dilated and tortuous small caliber channel within a patch of retinal haze or opacity. Digest preparations showed that the collateral arteries developed a cellular coat resembling that of the occluded artery (Fig. 17-5*B*). There was a suggestion that the long-standing collaterals had developed a muscularis.

India-ink studies of embolized retinas showed that the vascular bed downstream to the embolus was inked in a patchy fashion. This finding showed that blood could enter the territory of the obstructed vessel by an alternative pathway, through capillary links with surrounding vessels (Fig. 17-6).

Angiographic studies with fluorescein revealed that the vascular bed beyond the obstruction did not fill at the same time as the surrounding area. When the surrounding capillaries filled the ischemic area was clearly demonstrated and appeared empty (Fig. 17-7*A*). In the succeeding few seconds capillary twigs could be seen slowly filling in at the periphery of the ischemic zone (Fig. 17-7*B*). Flow derived from these capillary collaterals passed first into minute arteries and then back down the main stem of the blocked vessel. Blood passing back down the main trunk supplied the central part of the ischemic zone through smaller proximal branches (Fig. 17-7*C*). As a result capillaries in the center of the area filled later and the number of perfused capillaries ap-

Fig. 17-5. *A*, Retinal vessels of a cat injected with india ink show a tortuous interarterial anastomosis bypassing the segment of artery occluded by a glass ball. Shown 16 days after embolization. (From Ashton and Henkind. *Brit. J. Ophthal. 49:*225, 1965. By permission of the Editor and Publisher.)

B, Retinal digest preparation of a cat 56 days after embolization. Collateral channels **(arrows)** link an embolized artery **(E)** with a patent one (not seen in picture). PAS and hematoxylin, ×110. (From Henkind. *Brit. J. Ophthal. 50:*482, 1966. By permission of the Editor and Publisher.)

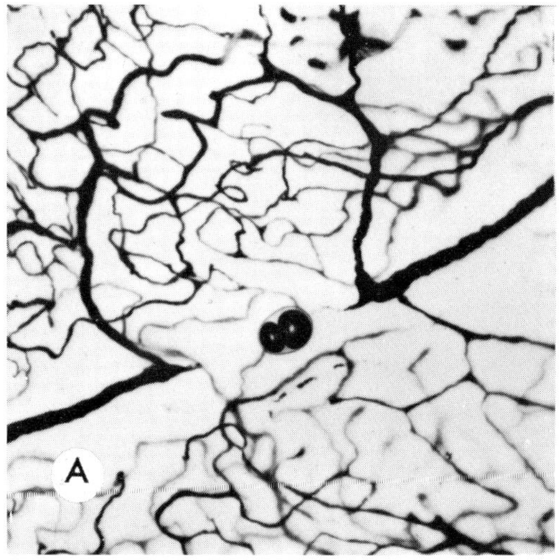

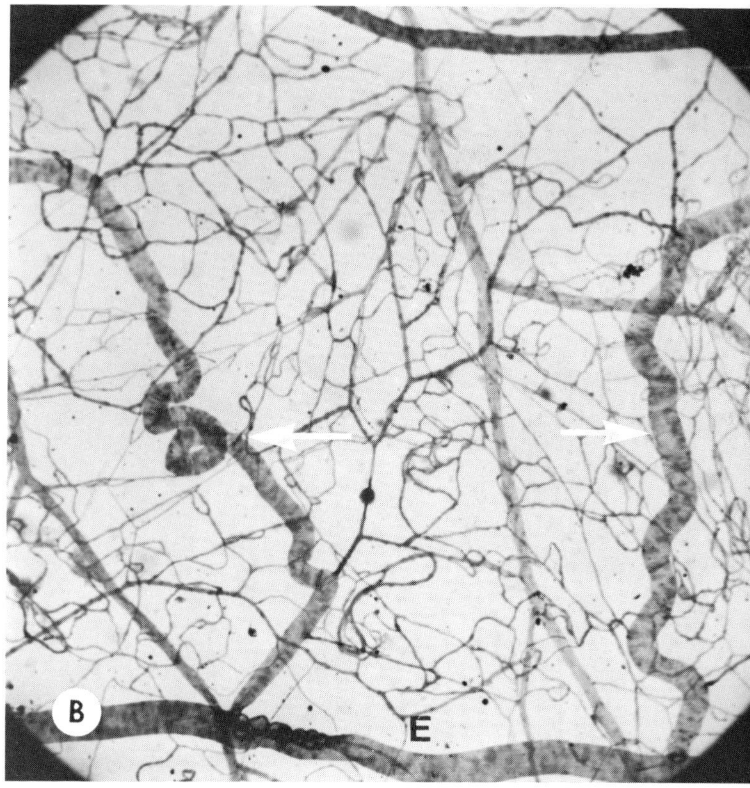

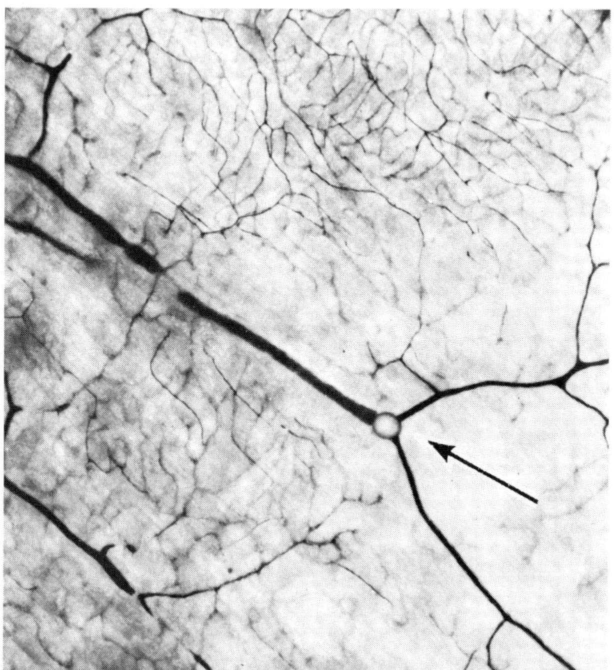

Fig. 17-6. India-ink study prepared 1 hour after embolization in a pig. Ink fills the occluded artery in a retrograde fashion via collaterals. **Arrow** points to embolus. (From Dollery et al. *Brit. J. Ophthal. 50:*285, 1966. By permission of the Editor and Publisher.)

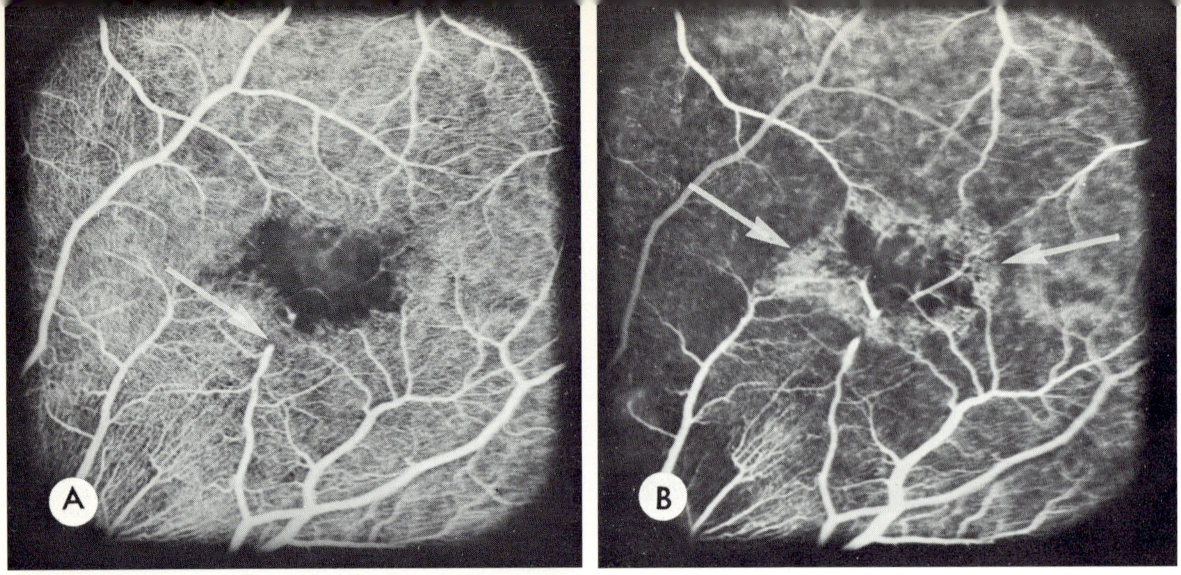

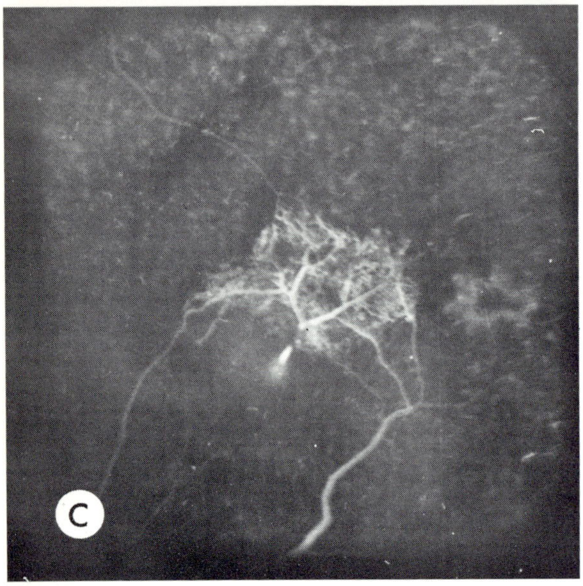

Fig. 17-7. *A*, Arterial-phase fluorescein angiogram of a pig 35 minutes after an artery had been obstructed by a glass microsphere **(arrow).** The capillary bed downstream to the block has not filled. *B*, Same view as in *A* but 1.2 seconds later. There is early filling of the obstructed capillary bed via collaterals at the edge of the ischemic area **(arrows).** *C*, Same view as in *A* but 4 seconds later. The main divisions of the artery downstream to the embolus have filled through capillary collaterals.

Fig. 17-8. *A*, Arterial-phase fluorescein angiogram made 7 days after embolization. A collateral **(arrow)** bridges the blocked segment. *B*, Fluorescein angiogram made 2 seconds later than *A*. The distal part of the blocked vessel beyond the embolus is filled via the collateral. (From Dollery et al. *Brit. J. Ophthal. 50:*285, 1966. By permission of the Editor and Publisher.)

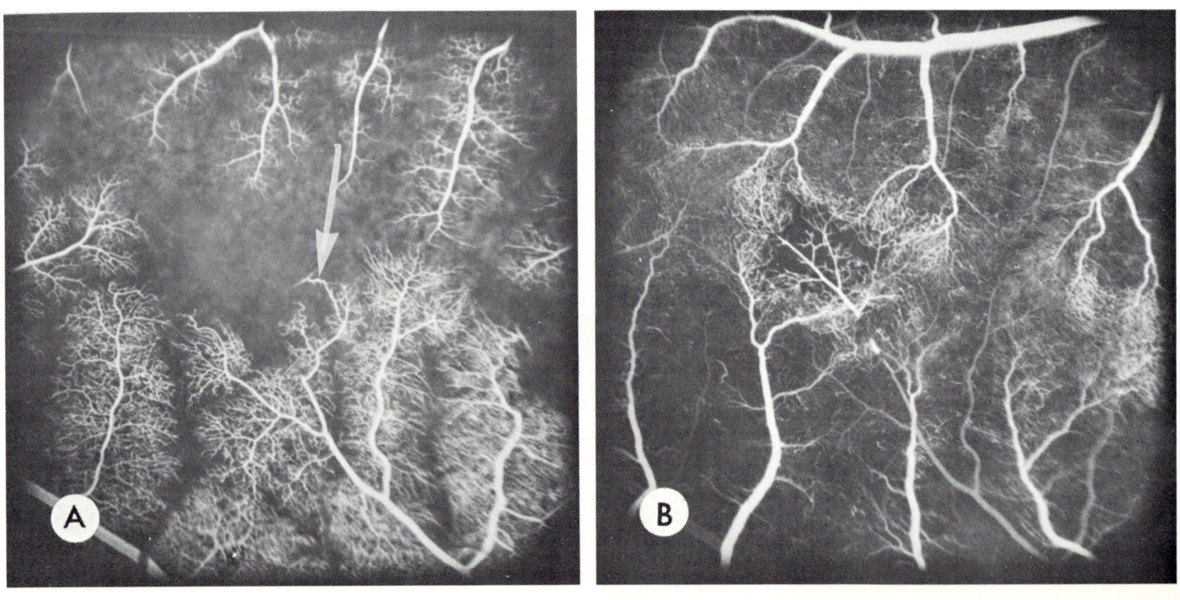

peared less than in control angiograms of the same area.

Capillary collateral flow depends upon the number of capillary linkages which exist around the circumference of the territory of the blocked vessel. The blood flow requirement must depend upon the total area supplied by that vessel. Thus, the ratio circumference per area is a measure of the adequacy of collateral flow and must be less favorable the larger the vessel involved. Experimental observations confirmed that the collateral supply through capillaries was more effective to smaller areas than larger ones.

Cineangiographic studies of pig retina immediately following embolization showed that the retrograde flow fed from capillary collaterals was relatively small. Arteries of about 50 μ diameter had a normal forward-flow velocity of about 20 mm per second and the retrograde flow following obstruction varied between 0.05 and 0.6 mm per second. Even these low values overstate the nutritional supply to the retina because blood flowing through capillary collaterals has already passed through a relatively ischemic bed and is venous in composition.

The most striking late change which influenced the collateral blood flow pattern was the development of larger-diameter channels linking the obstructed segment of the artery with surrounding normal arteries. Such collaterals were first visible 4 days after vascular occlusion in pigs. Two patterns of development of large-diameter collaterals could be distinguished. The first arose by dilatation of capillary bridges at the arterial end of the capillary network, when a side branch of the blocked artery ran parallel to a side branch of the same artery immediately before the block. This produced a large-diameter collateral of short-path length linking the proximal and distal parts of the blocked artery (Fig. 17-8). The second type arose as a dilatation of the capillaries at the periphery of the ischemic zone, and linked the blocked segment with surrounding uninvolved arteries (Fig. 17-9). Both types of collateral channels can develop within the human retina and have been reported in the literature.[8] The experiments demonstrate how they evolve. The conclusions that may be drawn from the work are as follows: (*1*) capillary collateral flow occurs immediately after branch artery occlusion; (*2*) larger-caliber channels usually develop to improve flow to the ischemic area; (*3*) such collaterals or anastomoses arise from the preexistent vascular bed of the retina, and are not "new" vessels; and (*4*) the collaterals develop in spite of the fact that the retina in the involved area may have lost its function. Study of retinal collateral vessel formation may be of value to workers concerned with other portions of the vascular system which are less accessible to direct observation. As yet unstudied are questions concerning the possible effects of various agents on the development and function of collaterals.

Retinitis proliferans was produced in a single kitten that was embolized 8 days after birth.[1] This was the only instance of true neovascularization and it occurred at the retinal periphery where the vessels were in an immature state of development.

EXTRAVASCULAR CHANGES

In cats two distinct types of retinal opacification were seen. The first was a grayish haze which appeared deep within the retinal tissue a few minutes after embolization. The borders were irregular and there were usually no ballotini in the immediate vicinity of the opacity (Fig. 17-10). They became more dense over a period of an hour, and then faded leaving no obvious sequelae. The deep location of these opacities, their lack of relation to retinal arterial emboli, and their transient nature all suggested that these lesions were due to temporary occlusion of choroidal arteries or the choriocapil-

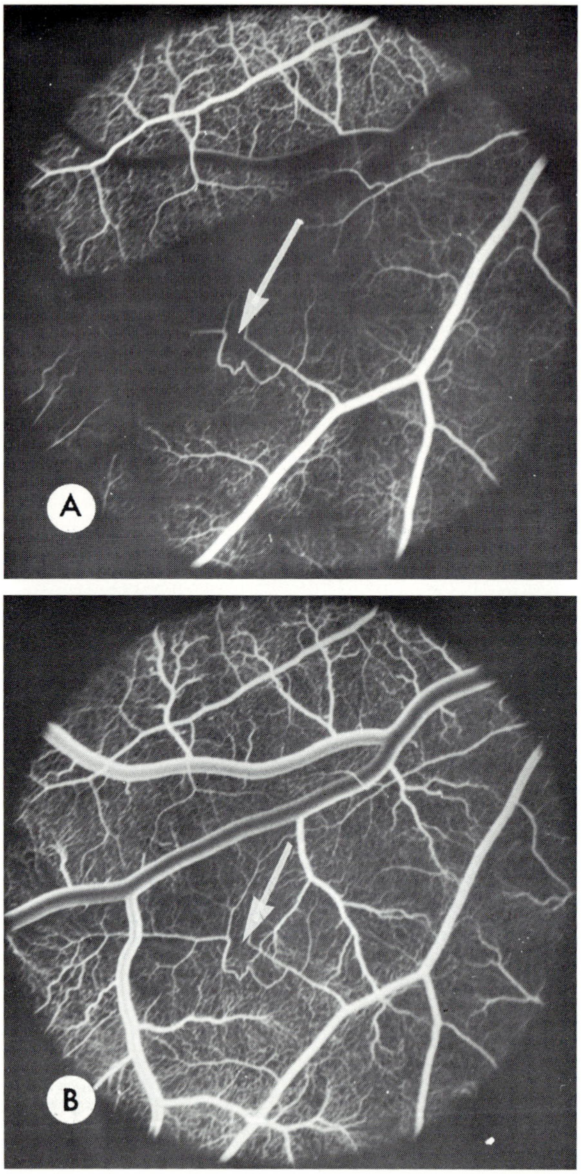

Fig. 17-9. *A*, Fluorescein angiogram made 14 days after embolization. A collateral is present, bypassing the blocked segment of the vessel **(arrow).**

B, In the capillary phase there is no delay in filling beyond the block. (From Dollery et al. *Brit. J. Ophthal. 50:*285, 1966. By permission of the Editor and Publisher.)

laris. In several instances fluorescein angiograms showed areas of choroid which filled more slowly than normal but these could not be related to particular emboli in the choroid because these were invisible with the ophthalmoscope. On one occasion profuse leakage of dye occurred from the choroid into the retina probably as a result of ischemic damage to the retinal pigment epithelium following embolization. The second type of opacity was much more common and in most instances could be specifically related to an intra-arterial embolus. These lesions ranged from 0.5 to 3 to 4 dd in size, they were irregular in shape, their borders often appeared feathery, and they often obscured small vessels running through them (Fig. 17-11). They appeared from 70 minutes to several hours after injection as a faint haze involving the inner retinal layers, and the nerve fibers often appeared spread apart. Within a few hours the lesion became denser and almost "creamy" in appearance, and in some instances resembled the cotton-wool patches found in man (Fig. 17-12). The lesions resolved within 1 to 2 weeks leaving thinned atrophic-looking areas in their place. The size of the opacity seemed to be related to the size of the vessel that was occluded, the larger the vessel the bigger the opacity.

A more detailed study of these retinal changes was undertaken in the pig. In this species it was possible to correlate fundic lesions with fluorescein angiographic flow studies. Several minutes after embolization there were alterations in the color of the fundus in ischemic areas. This varied from a barely perceptible gelatinous gray to a prominent grayish-white discoloration of the normally transparent retina (Fig. 17-13*A*). This discoloration was reversible for, in several instances, emboli moved further downstream and restored flow to the area in which case the normal transparency was regained within a few minutes. When the eyes were examined between 1 and 4 days

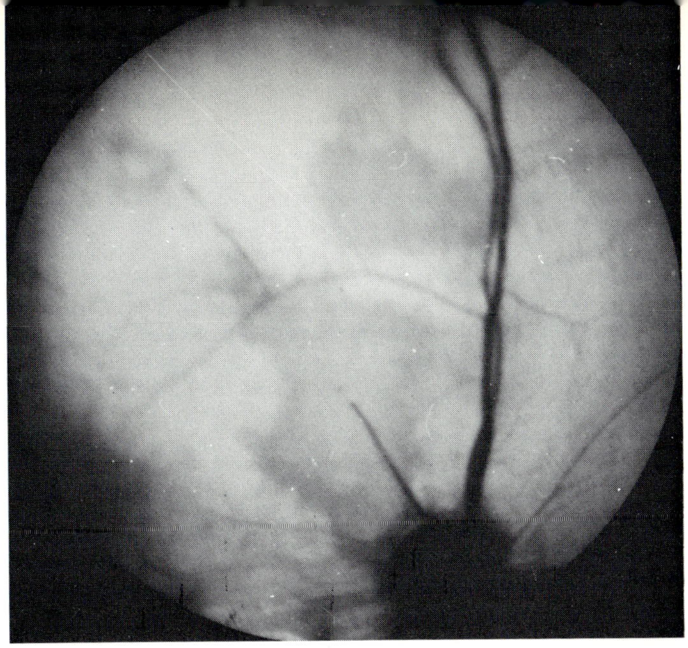

Fig. 17-10. Fundus photograph of a cat taken 1 hour after embolization. Geographic retinal opacities appear deep to the retinal vessels. These areas are not related to occluded retinal arteries, although a blocked retinal artery can be seen above the largest patch of opacity which extends outward from the disc. (From Henkind.[8a])

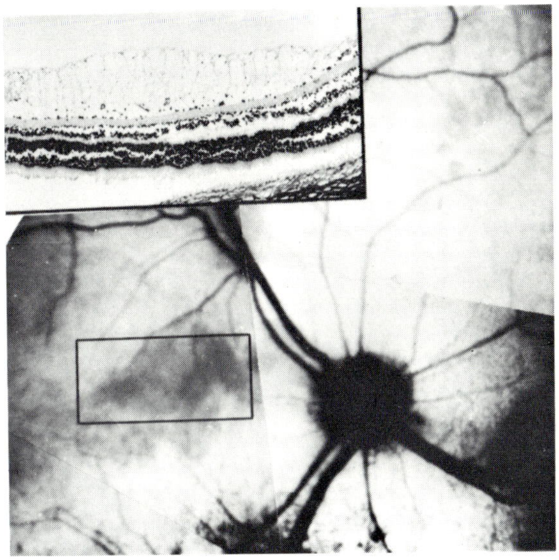

Fig. 17-11. Fundus photograph of a cat 24 hours after embolization. The superficial retinal opacity appears nasal to the disc. **Inset** is a low-power photomicrograph of a section through the lesion which demonstrates the marked swelling of the inner retinal layers.

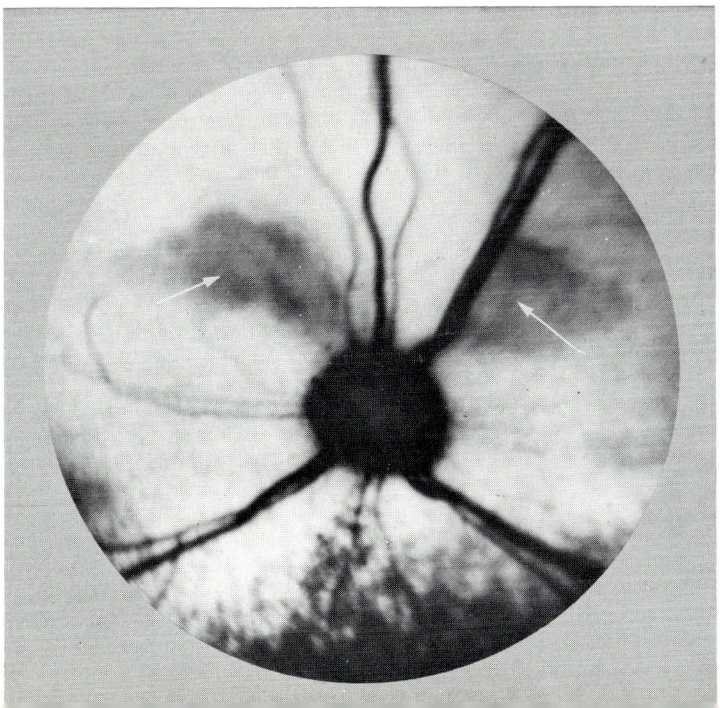

Fig. 17-12. Fundus photograph of a cat 48 hours after embolization. Two areas resembling cotton-wool patches **(arrows)** are seen above the disc. (From Ashton and Henkind. *Brit. J. Ophthal.* *49*:225, 1965. By permission of the Editor and Publisher.)

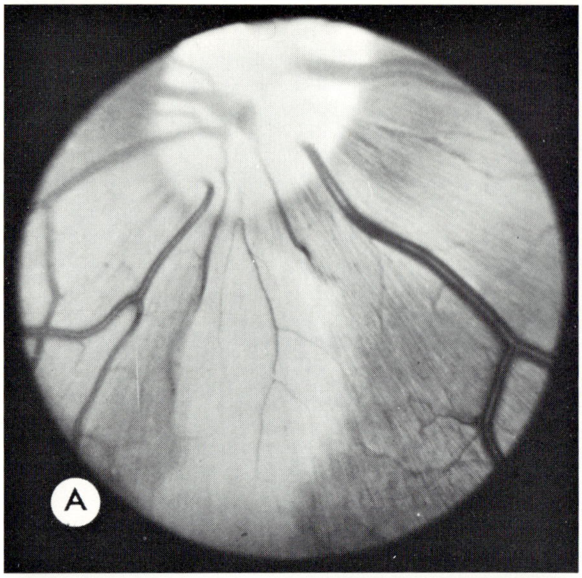

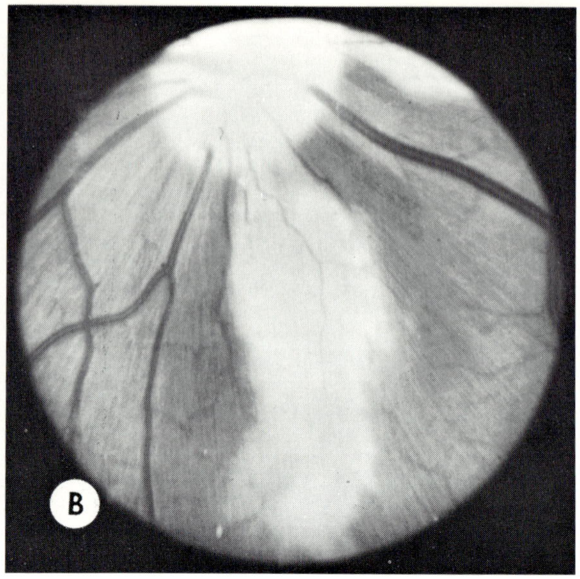

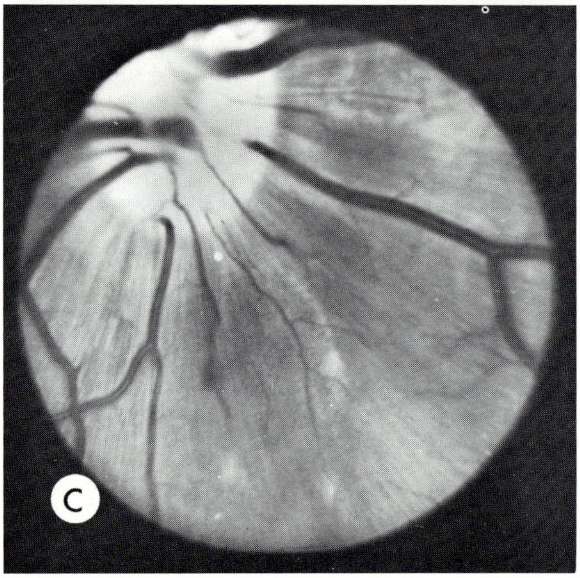

Fig. 17-13. *A*, Twenty-seven minutes after embolization of a small artery on the optic disc of a pig. The retina downstream has become grayish white. *B*, Same view as *A* but 2 days later. A cotton-wool spot occupies the area of the grayish-white color in the earlier study. *C*, Same view as *A* but 10 days later. Only a few white flecks remain in the area of the cotton-wool patch. (From Dollery et al. *Brit. J. Ophthal.* *50*:285, 1966. By permission of the Editor and Publisher.)

after embolization, white patches which closely resembled cotton-wool spots of humans were seen in the distribution of occluded arteries (Fig. 17-13*B*). One week later the cotton-wool spots had largely faded, leaving only a granular whitish appearance. Some granularity was still apparent some 2 weeks later (Fig. 17-13*C*). Angiographic studies revealed that the majority of cotton-wool spots developed in areas which had poor collateral flow in the early stages following embolization. Analysis of the data suggested that at some time between 3 and 20 hours irreversible damage occurs which culminates in the formation of a cotton-wool spot even if flow is then totally restored. Leakage of fluorescein into the retina, implying breakdown of the blood-retinal barrier which is normally impermeable to this dye, occurred only when the

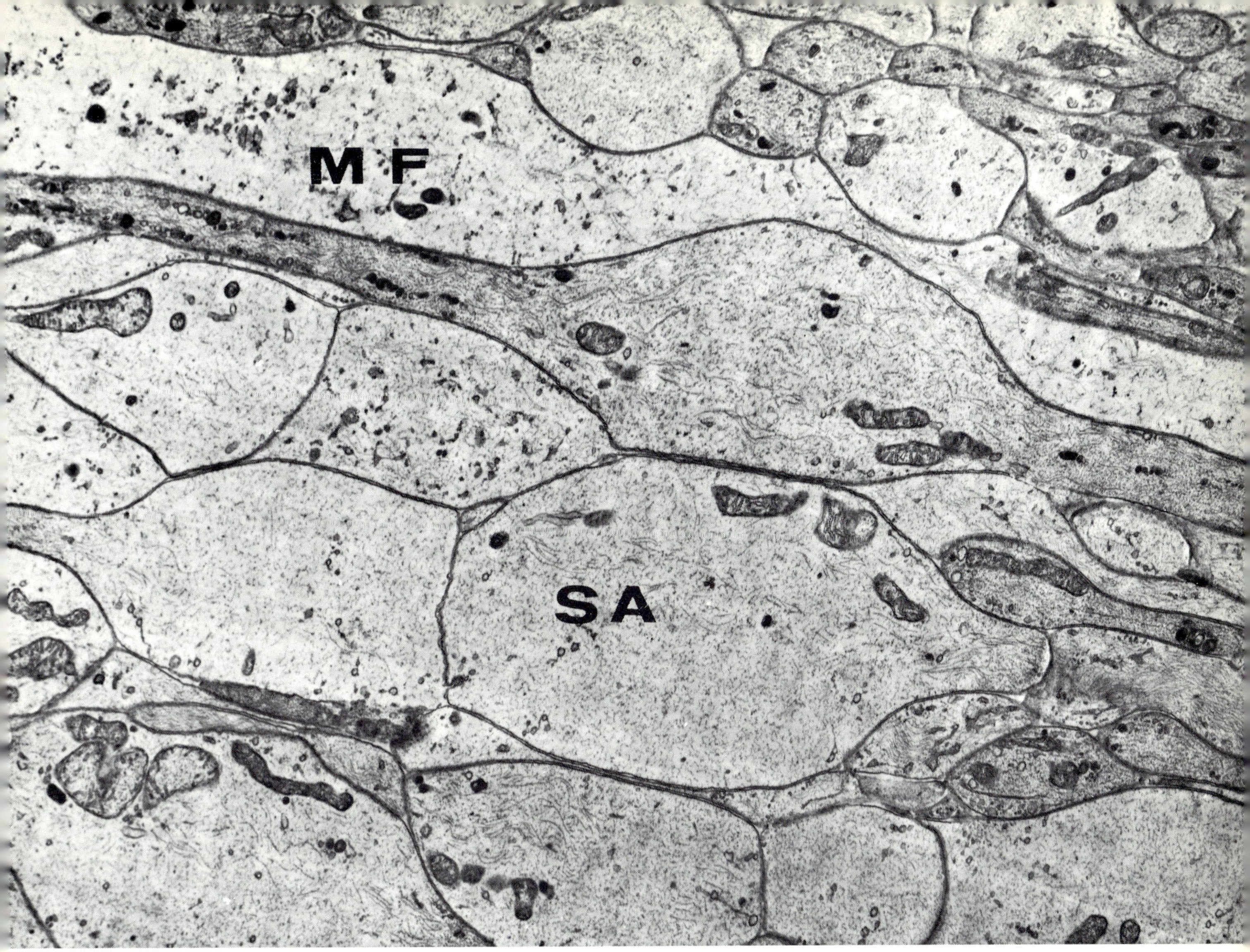

Fig. 17-14. Electron micrograph showing swollen axons **(SA)** and Müller fibers **(MF)** in the nerve fiber layer 1 hour after embolization. (From Dollery et al. *Brit. J. Ophthal. 50:*285, 1966. By permission of the Editor and Publisher.)

glass emboli injured the endothelium. It appears from the experimental evidence and from careful consideration of clinical data that most, and possibly all, cotton-wool spots result from focal retinal ischemia. From light and electron microscopic evidence, Shakib and Ashton [16] have concluded that the typical cotton-wool spot is due to intracellular swelling of the inner retinal layers, particularly of the axons, together with proliferation of axonal organelles (Fig. 17-14). The pseudonucleus of the cytoid body, long a matter of controversy as to its nature, almost certainly consists of an agglomeration of proliferating and degenerating axonal structures lying within the swollen axon, or of the cytoplasm of macrophages or astrocytes which have ingested the degenerate material (Fig. 17-15).

Hemorrhages were seen in the fundi of several cats and pigs several days after embolization. The most common were large

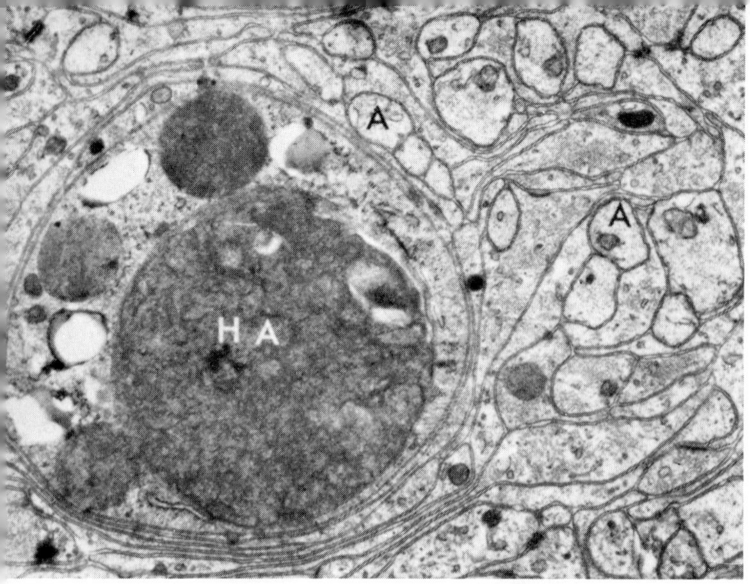

Fig. 17-15. Electron micrograph of a degenerated hypertrophic axon **(HA)** in a macrophage, 2 weeks after embolization. **A,** normal axons. (From Dollery et al. *Brit. J. Ophthal. 50*:285, 1966. By permission of the Editor and Publisher.)

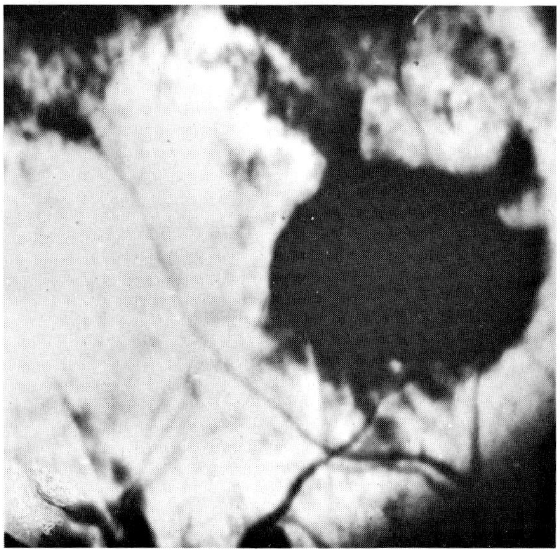

Fig. 17-16. Preretinal hemorrhage in the fundus of a cat 6 days after embolization. Blood appears to drip from the edge of the hemorrhage. (From Henkind.[8a])

Fig. 17-17. *A*, Appearance of a "blot" retinal hemorrhage 72 hours after embolization.
B, A second "blot" hemorrhage appeared to the left of the first one at 96 hours.
C, India-ink study of the same area 6 days after embolization. The hemorrhages **(arrows)** appear to come from vessels in the distribution of an embolized artery, but not from the site of the emboli themselves. (From Henkind.[8a])

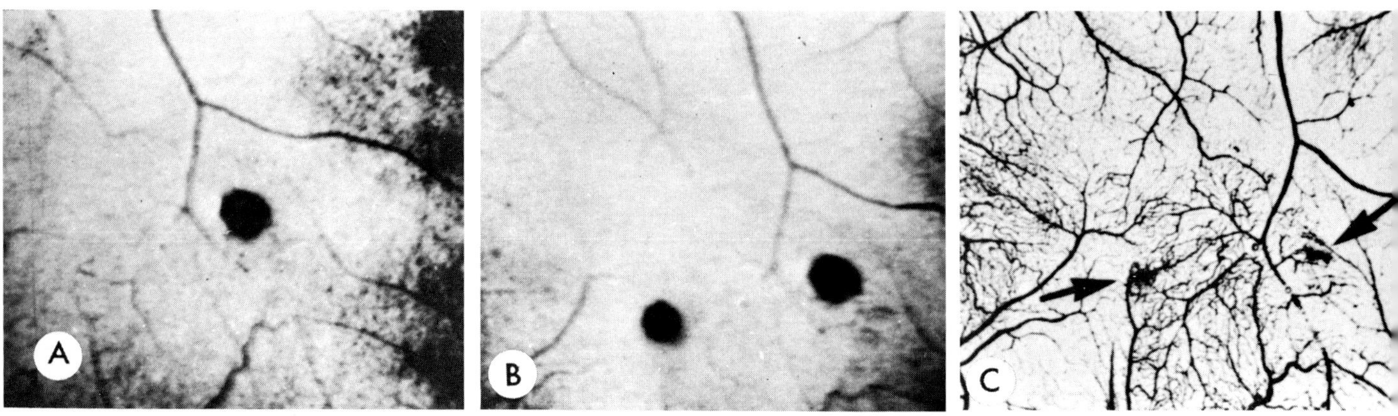

preretinal, subhyaloid extravasations of blood presumably due to the emboli disrupting a portion of the vascular wall (Fig. 17-16). Small, round intraretinal hemorrhages were seen on several occasions (Fig. 17-17). While ballotini were rarely seen in the immediate vicinity of the hemorrhages, they were generally present in neighboring arteries.

Three distinct types of retinal change have been noted clinically. The most common form, seen both in cats and pigs, was degeneration of the superficial retinal layers in the immediate area of a resolving cotton-wool spot. In these instances the retina appeared to have an irregular surface and the surface reflexes were slightly dull compared to the surrounding normal tissue. A second type of retinal atrophy was seen several times, and consisted of a deep "geographic" figure either at the equator or the retinal periphery (Fig. 17-18). Although the lesions became more prominent over a period of several days to weeks, their boundaries remained constant. This type of atrophy would appear to be related to choroidal embolism. A third type of change occurred in several animals. In these instances small cystic areas developed in the retina at the posterior pole in regions of preceding edema; in several cats a lesion developed which mimicked a human macular cyst (Fig. 17-19).

Kroll[13] has ligated the central retinal artery in squirrel monkeys (*Samiri sciurea*) and produced an experimental model which closely resembled the human condition. A "cherry-red" spot was noted at the macula. Fluorescein angiography revealed complete absence of retinal circulation, but normal filling of choroidal vessels. Swelling of neuronal mitochondria of the inner retinal layer occurred within 15 minutes of ligation, and this was followed by swelling of the endoplasmic reticulum and cell cytoplasm. Cytoplasmic membranes were found to be ruptured 3½ hours after operation, and by 16 hours there was autolysis of all cells anterior to the outer nuclear layer. Müller cells

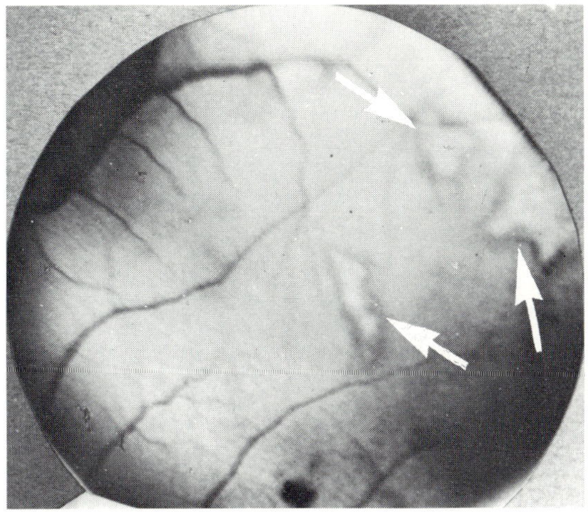

Fig. 17-18. Fundus photograph of a cat taken 10 days after embolization and showing three patches of geographic atrophy **(arrows)** of the retina. Directly below, at six o'clock, is an intraretinal blot hemorrhage. The geographic patches represent experimental Elschnig's spots. (Compare with Fig. 12-18*B*.) (From Henkind.[8a])

Fig. 17-19. Fundus photograph of a cat taken 18 days after embolization. Multiple areas of cystic retinal atrophy can be seen. The round gray lesion **(arrow)** resembles a human macular cyst. (From Henkind.[8a])

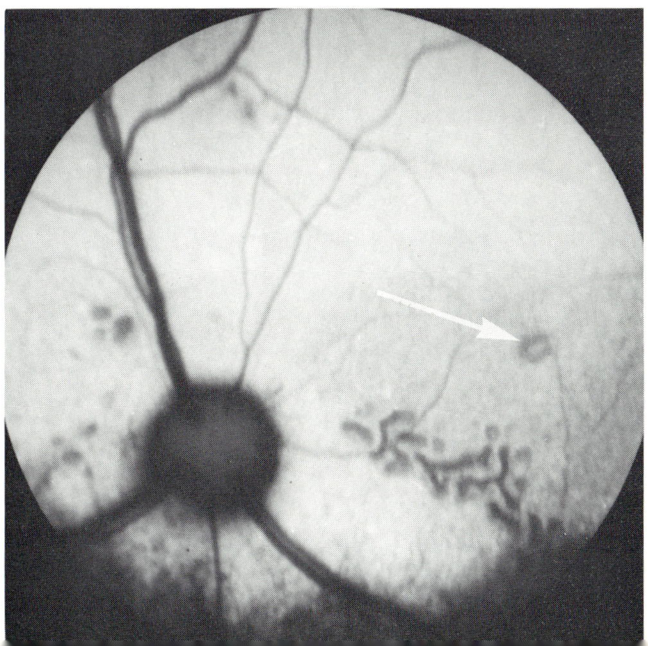

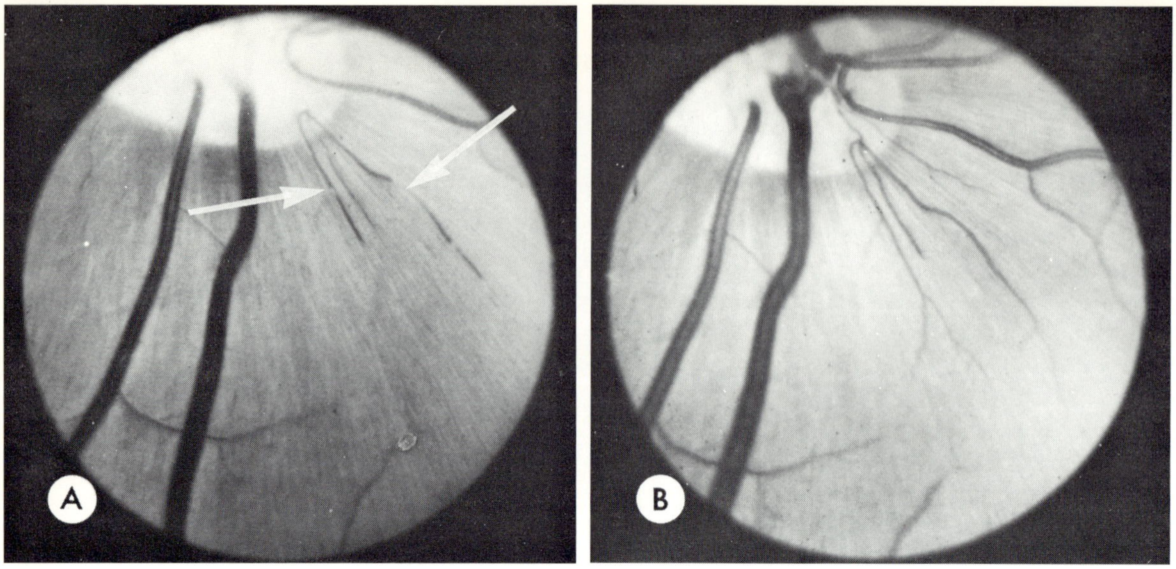

Fig. 17-20. *A*, From a color photograph taken 30 seconds after injection of platelet aggregates into the carotid artery of a pig. White bodies are plugging small arteries **(arrows).** *B*, Same area as *A* but taken 2 minutes later. The white bodies have moved on down the arteries. (From Paterson et al.[15])

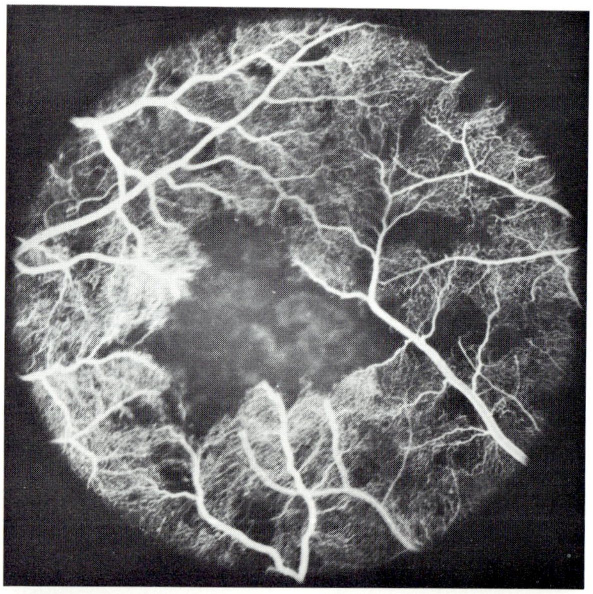

Fig. 17-21. Fluorescein angiogram after injection of platelet aggregates into the carotid artery of a pig shows multiple embolization of small arteries and nonfilling of capillaries. (From Paterson et al.[15])

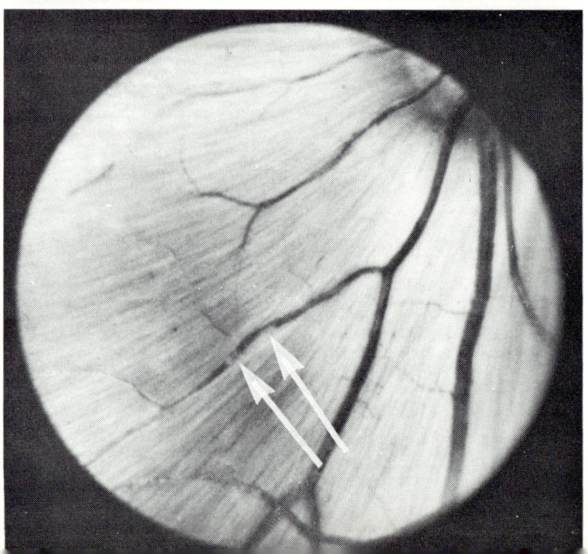

Fig. 17-22. From a color transparency of a pig fundus after intracarotid infusion of thrombin. White bodies are present in a small artery **(arrows).**

were resistant to ischemia in the early stages, but not later on. The rods and cones were undamaged.

REVERSIBLE ARTERIAL OBSTRUCTION WITH PLATELETS OR FIBRIN

Obstruction of retinal vessels with glass or latex spheres is permanent except for occasions when the embolus is dislodged to a more peripheral site. Clinically, reversible embolization of retinal arteries with "white bodies" composed of platelets or fibrin strands is of some importance. The course of these lesions has been studied experimentally in pigs by Paterson and his colleagues.[15]

Platelets clumped by adding adenosine diphosphate (ADP) to platelet-enriched plasma in vitro, or by infusing ADP into the carotid artery, appeared as opaque white emboli in the retinal arteries (Fig. 17-20). They caused a reversible obstruction of the vessels lasting from less than 1 minute up to 20 minutes (Fig. 17-21). If such emboli persisted for more than a few minutes the retina downstream became a grayish, gelatinous color but after flow was restored it returned to its normal color. After the platelet clumps had been dispersed the retinal vascular bed returned to normal.

Emboli composed of fibrin strands and platelets cause more prolonged obstruction. Infusion of thrombi into the carotid circulation of pigs causes embolization by white bodies, general slowing of flow, and later spiral strands of fibrin in the retinal arteries are seen (Fig. 17-22). Eventually the retinal circulation clots completely and flow ceases. Clot lysis occurs rapidly and many of the vessels reopened within 2 hours. Frequently large retinal and preretinal hemorrhages formed during this period while flow is being restored. These emboli consist of fibrin strands surrounded by adherent platelets.

Kulvin and David[14] have injected autologous fibrin clot into the carotid artery of owl monkeys. Some of this material entered the retinal arteries causing vascular occlusion. The fibrin clot appeared to cause endothelial damage in the arteries, for they showed a dramatic leakage of fluorescein. Accumulations of leukocytes were found in the damaged vessels.

REFERENCES

1. Ashton, N., and Henkind, P.: Experimental occlusion of retinal arterioles. *Brit. J. Ophthal. 49:*225, 1965.
2. Birch-Hirschfield, A.: Beitrag zur Kenntniss der Netzhautganglienzellen unter physiologischen und pathologischen Verhaltnissen. *Graefe. Arch. Ophthal. 50:*166, 1900.
3. Cook, C. A. G.: Role of fat emboli in diabetic retinopathy. *Brit. J. Ophthal. 41:*741, 1957.
4. Dollery, C. T., Henkind, P., Paterson, J. W., Ramalho, P. S., and Hill, D. W.: Focal retinal ischemia. *Brit. J. Ophthal. 50:*285, 1966.
5. Dollery, C. T., Ramalho, P. S., Paterson, J. W., Hill, D. W., Henkind, P., Shakib, M., and Ashton, N.: Retinal microemboli. Experimental production of "cotton-wool" spots. *Lancet 1:* 1303, 1965.
6. Gay, A. J., Goldor, H., and Smith, M.: Chorioretinal vascular occlusion with latex spheres. *Invest. Ophthal. 3:*647, 1964.
7. Goldor, H., and Gay, A. J.: Chorioretinal vascular occlusions with latex microspheres (A long-term study). Part 2. *Invest. Ophthal. 6:* 51, 1967.
8. Henkind, P.: Ballotini occlusion of retinal arteries. Collateral vessels. *Brit. J. Ophthal. 50:*482, 1966.

8a. Henkind, P.: "New Aspects of Ocular Vascularization." (Ph.D. thesis. University of London, 1965.)

9. Henkind, P., and Dollery, C. T.: Pathophysiology of the retinal vascular bed following acute embolisation. *Invest. Ophthal. 5:* 205, 1966.

10. Herrnheiser, J.: Ueber experimentelle Erzeugung von Embolien der Blutgefasse im Innern des Auges. *Klin. Mbl. Augenheilk. 33:* 315, 1895.

11. Hirose, K., and Baba, K.: A study of Takayasu-Ohnishi's (Pulseless) disease. *Amer. J. Ophthal. 55:*554, 1963.

12. Hollenhorst, R. W., Lensink, E. R., and Whisnant, J. P.: Experimental embolization of the retinal arterioles. *Trans. Amer. Ophthal. Soc. 60:*316, 1962.

13. Kroll, A. J.: Experimental central retinal artery occlusion. *Arch. Ophthal. 79:*453, 1968.

14. Kulvin, S. M., and David, N. J.: Experimental retinal embolism. Studies with high-speed fluorescein cinematography. *Arch. Ophthal. 78:*774, 1967.

15. Paterson, J. W., Dollery, C. T., Ramalho, P. S., and Kohner, E. M.: The effects of platelet aggregates on the retinal microcirculation. *Bibl. Anat. 9:*85, 1967.

16. Shakib, M., and Ashton, N.: Focal retinal ischemia. 2. Ultrastructural changes in focal retinal ischemia. *Brit. J. Ophthal. 50:* 325, 1966.

17. Shiba, S.: Experimentelle Untersuchungen uber die Embolie der Netzhaut und Aderhaut. *Graefe. Arch. Ophthal. 63:*393, 1906.

RETINAL VEIN OCCLUSION

Retinal vein occlusion is a common clinical problem and there is extensive literature on the clinical appearance and consequences of such lesions. The appearance of retinal vein occlusion in man can be duplicated in experimental animals. Such studies are beginning to clarify the circulatory and structural changes responsible for the clinical features.

Becker and Post [1] have used a diathermy probe passed across the globe and deep into the optic nerve head of cats to produce occlusion of the central retinal vein. With the electrode in the disc but touching no vessels they applied the current for 10 seconds. There was an immediate liberation of gas bubbles in the vitreous as well as constriction of arteries and marked dilatation of the veins. Fifteen to 20 hours later, hemorrhages and exudates were noted beginning in the periphery. These increased in number and after 2 or 3 days the fundus showed relatively normal arteries, dilated tortuous veins, exudates, and large hemorrhages. The retina was edematous and capillary aneurysms had formed. Flat preparations of these retinas showed numerous capillary aneurysms, distortion of capillary architecture, and newly formed vessels.

Campbell [2] has used the Zeiss photocoagulator to occlude branch retinal veins in cats. The occluded veins became dark and dilated and often showed reversal of flow and pulsation of the venous blood column. The retinal arteries showed little change initially unless involved in the coagulation, in which case they narrowed temporarily but quickly returned to normal. Several different types of hemorrhages were seen within the territory of the blocked vein. There were small flame-shaped hemorrhages along the course of the major retinal veins, small blots in the external retinal layers, and larger preretinal hemorrhages. Some of the latter resembled the classic clinical appearance with the "Napoleon's hat" configuration. Within 48 hours collateral vessels appeared and these were well developed by 7 to 10 days after occlusion. There was always some retinal detachment at the burn site and a flat separation was often evident in the territory of the blocked vein.

Mutlu[7] has used the diathermy electrode technique to occlude multiple retinal veins in rabbits. He noted that veins dilated within 5 minutes, the retina became edematous within 2 hours, and hemorrhages formed within 16 hours extending to cover the entire area within 24 hours. In several animals large collaterals formed and hemorrhages reabsorbed. After a month the fundus appeared normal apart from the presence of the collateral. If collaterals did not form by the fifth day the vessels became narrowed, white, and sclerosed and the retina atrophied. Conceivably these appearances resulted from permanent occlusion of both the artery and the vein.

Linner,[6] and Voipio and Raitta[8] both have used photocoagulation to produce branch vein occlusion. Voipio and Raitta have noted that veins often reopened after photocoagulation. Hemorrhages appeared but soon dispersed as collaterals formed. They were chiefly interested in alterations in the intraocular pressure but found this unchanged even after successful venous occlusion.

One of the most important problems in these studies is the extent to which the central retinal artery is involved by the diathermy or light beam used to occlude the vein. Hayreh[4] has pointed out the importance of this consideration. He exposed the central retinal vessels of the rhesus monkey by means of a lateral orbitotomy, and then occluded by diathermy either the vein, the artery, or both vessels. Occlusion of the vein in six animals produced venous dilatation and this subsided in 16 to 36 days. Simultaneous occlusion of both the artery and vein in three animals produced a clinical picture resembling human hemorrhagic central vein occlusion. One animal in which the artery alone was occluded showed a pale fundus and disc with a static blood column in both the artery and vein. Flow returned later but the appearance resembled central artery occlusion in man and had none of the features associated with central vein occlusion. Hayreh has stressed the importance of arterial involvement in the pathogenesis of the clinical features of vein occlusion.

Fujino, Curtin, and Norton[3] have studied the circulatory dynamics and pathology of the retinal circulation following occlusion of the central retinal vein in the owl monkey. In one group of animals they occluded the central retinal vein at the disc with neoprene. These animals developed rapid ischemic and hemorrhagic infarction of the retina and obstruction of arterial inflow. In a second group the central retinal vein was ligated as the vein left the optic nerve. In these animals a temporary and reversible venous congestion developed. In this instance it was postulated that collateral venous circulation was present at and behind the disc.

Recently Kohner et al.[5] have investigated the circulatory, ophthalmoscopic, and structural changes that take place after branch retinal vein occlusion in pigs and rhesus monkeys. The animals were studied by color and fluorescein retinal photography, including cinephotography, immediately before and after vein occlusion, and for periods up to 9 weeks. In the pig, where the main superior artery and vein are well separated, it was possible to occlude the vein without involving the adjacent artery. In rhesus monkeys, where the distribution of the vessels closely resembles man, the artery was often involved.

OPHTHALMOSCOPIC APPEARANCE

The progress of photocoagulation could be observed through the viewing system of the photocoagulator. The first change was the appearance of a whitish area where the beam struck the retina. During light exposure the blood column in the vein narrowed and flow in the vessel slowed. A dull white material accumulated in the lumen adher-

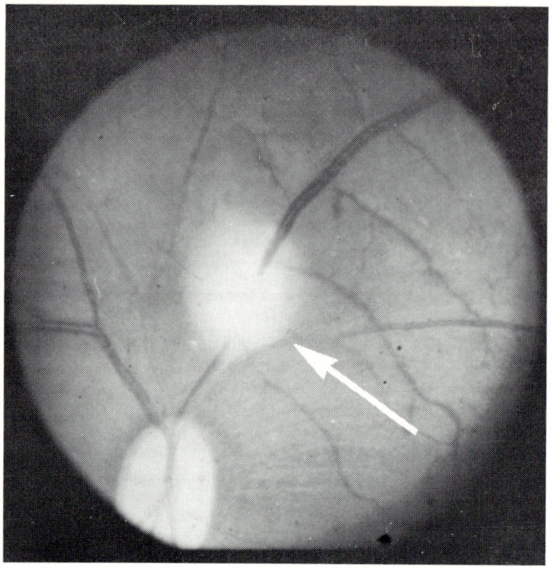

Fig. 17-23. Branch vein obstruction produced by photocoagulation in a monkey retina. The coagulated area is white **(arrow)** and the vein upstream is dark and dilated. (From Kohner et al. *Amer. J. Ophthal. 69:*778, 1970.)

ing to the wall at the site of coagulation. These "white bodies" often became detached and flow was temporarily reestablished as they shot away towards the optic disc. Once occlusion was complete the exposed segment of vein could be seen to be free of blood and the blood column immediately upstream was segmented and arrested (Fig. 17-23). Further exposure was needed to prevent the vein from reopening. Late in coagulation small hemorrhages often appeared at the edge of the burned area.

A granular, slowly moving stream of blood could be seen in the blocked vein immediately following occlusion. If a large vein had been occluded the flow in the proximal part close to the block was in the normal direction. Flow in the distal part of the blocked vein was towards the periphery. Between the two streams flowing in opposite directions in the same vessel, a section of the blood column was stationary.

Following occlusion the veins dilated by a mean of 15 per cent and also became more tortuous. The blood column was darker than normal. Arteries narrowed slightly, by an average of 10.5 per cent following occlusion of the vein draining the territory which they supplied although they had not been affected by the photocoagulator.

Shortly after occlusion the retina distal to the burn site lost its transparency. In the pig, where the nerve fibers are normally visible, the fibers became more prominent and appeared separated. The loss of transparency was rapid following occlusion of veins greater than 150 to 200 μ in diameter, but was slower to develop in the territory of small veins less than 150 μ in diameter, and sometimes did not occur at all.

Within a few minutes of a large vein obstruction multiple hemorrhages appeared within its territory. They were located predominantly around small venous twigs and began as small round blots, but quickly became larger and irregular. The same sequence was seen after occlusion of smaller veins, less than 150 μ in diameter, but it was slower to develop. It was unusual to see hemorrhages within 30 minutes of blocking a vein of that size (Fig. 17-24).

By 24 hours after occlusion of a large vein the fundic detail in the vein's drainage area was obscured by preretinal hemorrhage, retinal edema, and retinal detachment. All that could be seen were dark and tortuous large veins amid a mass of hemorrhage. Less severe hemorrhage took place in the territory of small or medium-sized veins so it was easier to observe the evolution of the changes. After several days the burn site showed a typical mottled appearance of pigment disturbance and was often surrounded by a ring of small hemorrhages.

Both in pigs and monkeys white cuffs were seen around many branch veins distal to the block. This dense sheathing sometimes persisted throughout the period of study (Fig. 17-25); arteries were rarely sheathed. In the monkey some small venous side branches disappeared during the period up to 4 weeks after vein occlusion and segments of the main vein showed irregular narrowing (Fig. 17-26).

COLLATERALS

Dilated tortuous collateral channels were first seen ophthalmoscopically at 3 days. In most experiments such vessels could be visualized by 7 days but they were often difficult to photograph because of the hemorrhage and edema. It is of interest to note that the time course of collateral development following branch vein occlusion is similar to that after arterial occlusion. Collaterals increased in size, and became fewer in number up to about 4 weeks after the vein was blocked. Side branches of adjacent patent veins which were taking the flow from developing collaterals became dilated and tortuous. When a blocked vein reopened the collaterals usually disappeared. In monkeys particularly prominent collaterals formed on either side of the fovea. No cotton-wool spots or hard fatty exudates were observed in either pig or monkey following occlusion of a vein.

CIRCULATORY CHANGES

Immediately following obstruction of the vein the arterial inflow was reduced and capillary filling with fluorescein was delayed. The velocity of flow, measured from fluorescein cineangiograms, was reduced by from 26 to 66 per cent of the control values. The capillaries in the territory of the blocked vein filled later than those of surrounding normal areas. The appearance of dye in the capillaries was often denser than in surrounding normal areas and the

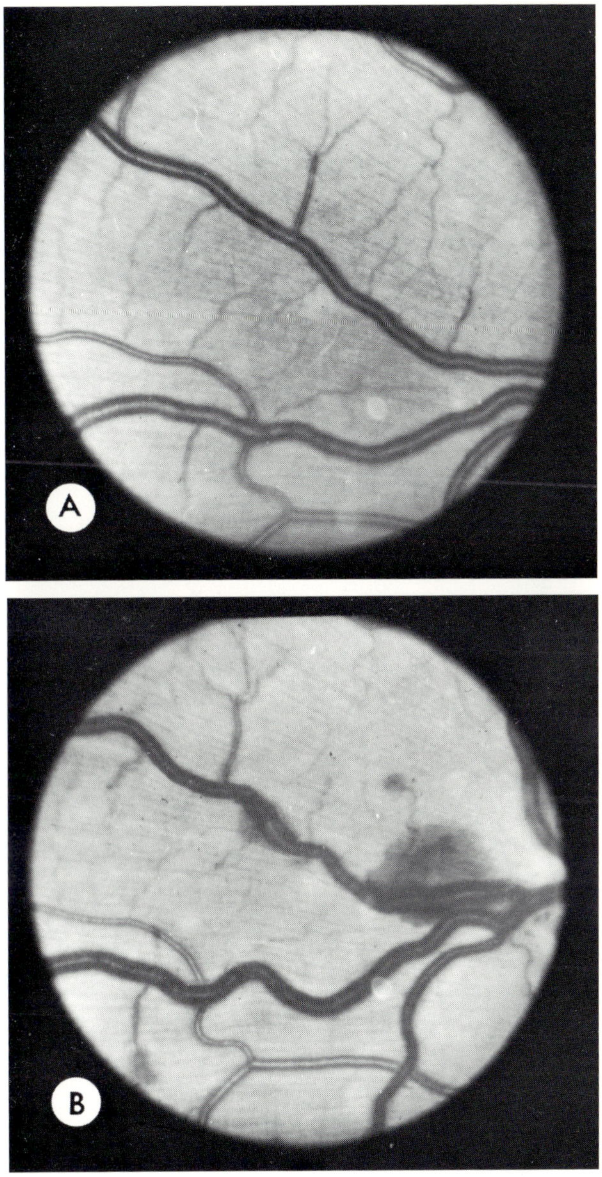

Fig. 17-24. *A*, Figure from a color transparency showing venous branches before photocoagulation in a pig. *B*, Same area as *A* but 30 minutes after photocoagulation of the vein downstream from the field (to the right). The vein is dark, dilated, and tortuous with blot hemorrhages around the main trunk and small branches. (From Kohner et al. *Amer. J. Ophthal.* *69*:778, 1970.)

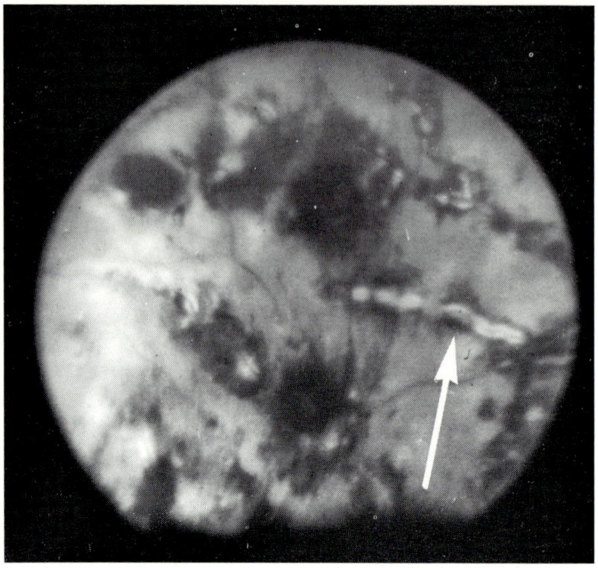

Fig. 17-25. White sheathing of branch retinal veins **(arrow)** in a rhesus monkey shown 10 days after venous occlusion. (From Kohner et al. *Amer. J. Ophthal. 69:*778, 1970.)

Fig. 17-26. Fluorescein angiogram of the right superior temporal vein in a monkey 4 weeks after obstruction. A segment of the vein remote from the site of coagulation is narrowed **(arrow).** (From Kohner et al. *Amer. J. Ophthal. 69:*778, 1970)

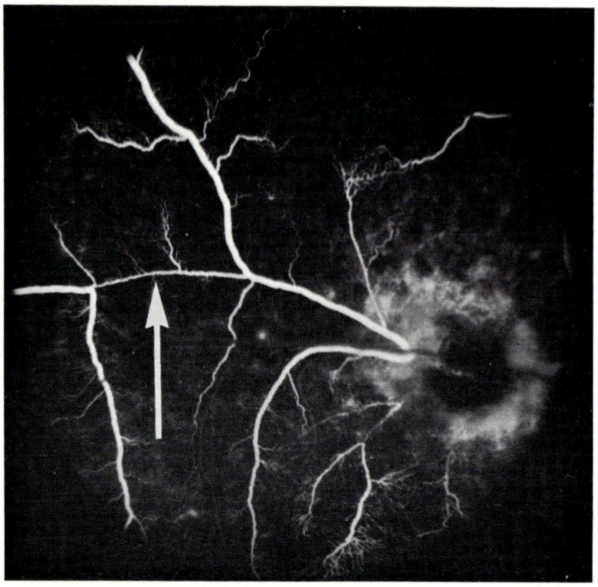

appearance suggested that the capillaries were dilated. Flow passed from the capillaries into the dilated venous branches and from them into the main trunk. Blood drained from the area through capillaries acting as collaterals (Fig. 17-27) into surrounding capillaries connected to patent veins.

LEAKAGE

Dye leaked profusely from points on capillaries and small venules. Later the area became diffusely fluorescent, particularly in the rhesus monkeys (Fig. 17-28). Leakage was no longer visible in studies carried out a week or more after obstruction but this may correspond to the development of larger collaterals reducing the venous pressure in the area.

LATE FLOW CHANGES

On fluorescein angiograms preferential channels were visible through the area of capillary collaterals as early as 24 hours following vein occlusion. These quickly dilated by 7 to 10 days following occlusion when there would be numerous tortuous collaterals whose total cross-sectional area approached or even exceeded that of the vein that had been blocked (Fig. 17-29). Despite the size of the collaterals flow was still less than before obstruction. As the resistance of a vessel varies with the inverse of the fourth power of the radius, the total resistance of these collaterals would exceed that of the original vessel although their cross-sectional area was the same. Collaterals became fewer and larger in the weeks following occlusion. There was usually a large proximal collateral circling the area of coagulation and in some instances this was the only channel present. The collaterals of largest diameter were usually shortest in

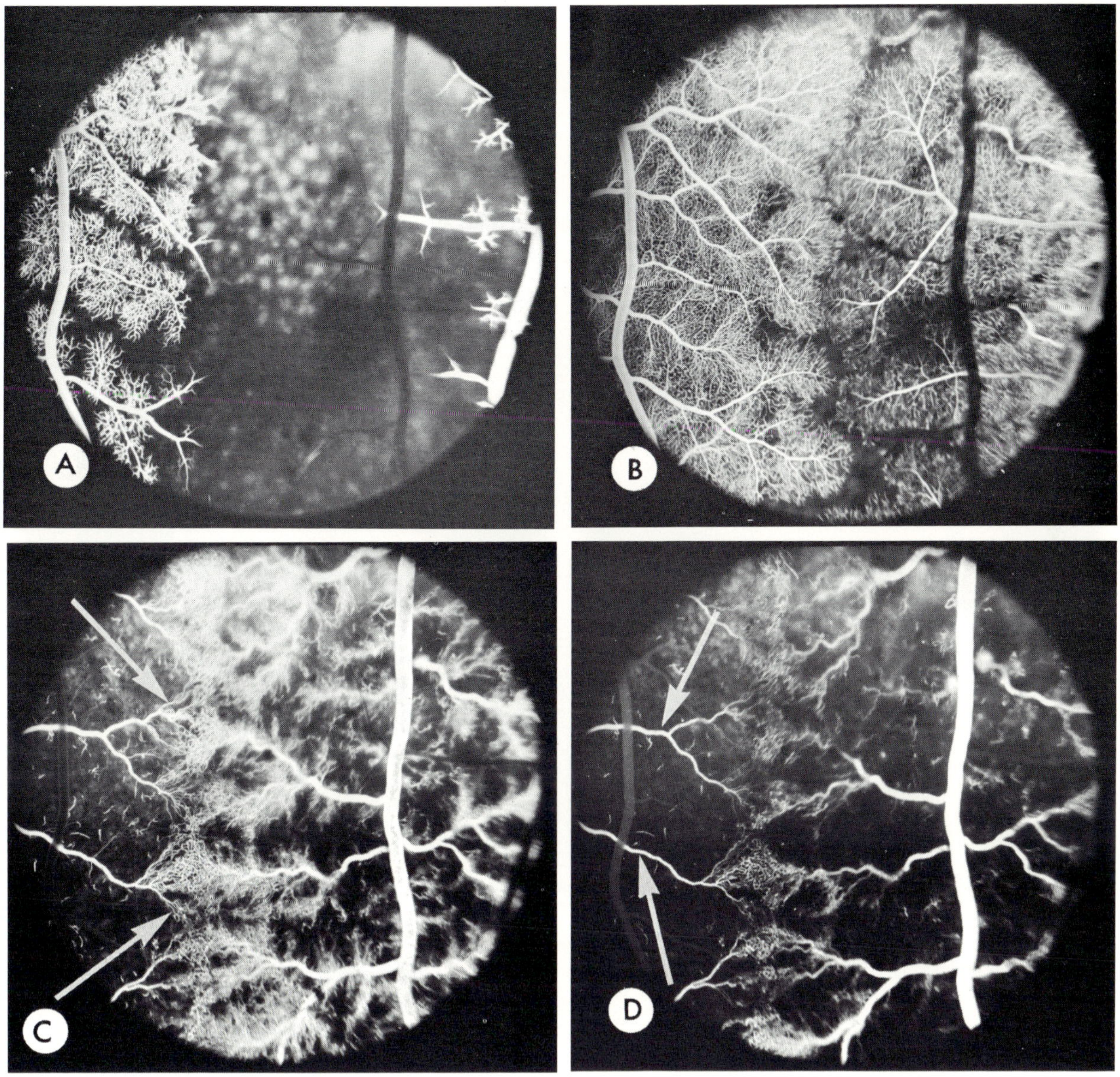

Fig. 17-27. *A*, Arterial-phase fluorescein angiogram taken immediately after branch vein obstruction in a pig. The capillary bed drained by the blocked vein has not filled at this stage. *B*, After 1.8 seconds capillary filling in the obstructed area is almost complete. *C*, Seen 3.6 seconds after *A* the main trunk of the blocked vein has filled and it is draining via capillary collaterals (**arrows**). *D*, Seen 5.4 seconds after *A* the blocked vein continues to empty into the surrounding unobstructed branches (**arrows**) via capillary collaterals. (From Kohner et al. *Amer. J. Ophthal. 69:*778, 1970.)

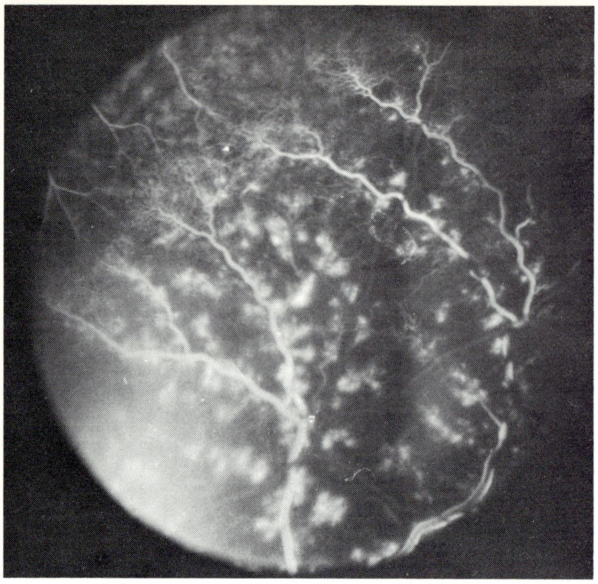

Fig. 17-28. *Left.* Fluorescein angiogram showing massive vascular leakage immediately after obstruction of a superior temporal vein in a rhesus monkey. (From Kohner et al. *Amer. J. Ophthal. 69:*778, 1970.)

Fig. 17-29. *Below.* Venous-phase fluorescein angiogram of a pig retina showing multiple collaterals 10 days after branch vein occlusion. (From Kohner et al. *Amer. J. Ophthal. 69:*778, 1970.)

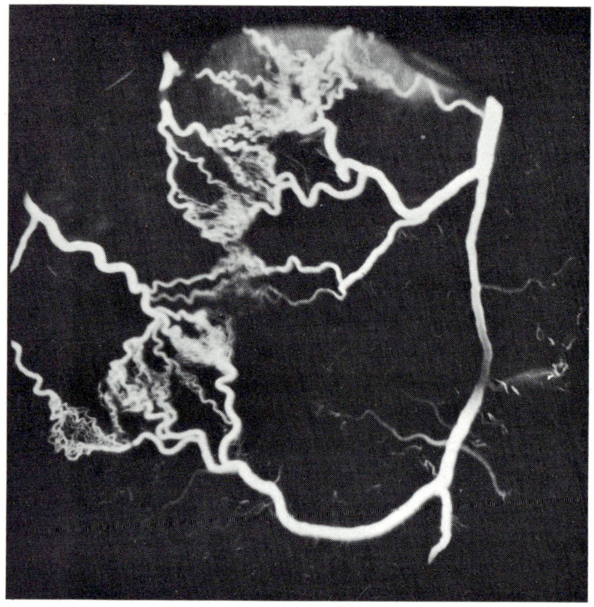

Fig. 17-30. *Below.* Large collaterals appear 3 weeks after a branch vein occlusion in a pig retina. There is no delay in filling and emptying of this area compared with surrounding unobstructed ones. (From Kohner et al. *Amer. J. Ophthal. 69:*778, 1970.)

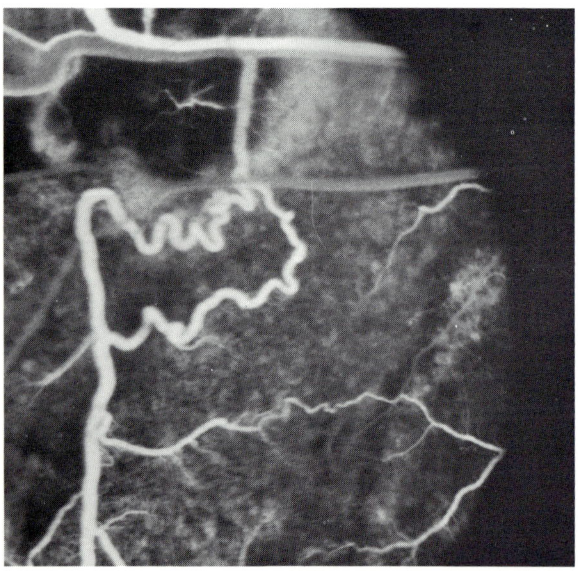

Fig. 17-31. *Below.* Capillary-phase fluorescein angiogram shows normal capillary bed **(arrow N)** drained by patent veins and a coarsening of the bed drained by an obstructed vein **(arrow C).** (From Kohner et al. *Amer. J. Ophthal. 69:*778, 1970.)

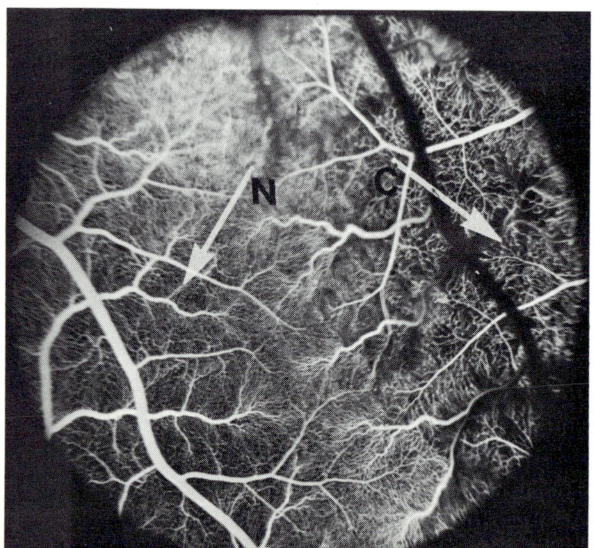

length. After 4 to 6 weeks the flow through the area with the obstructed vein had returned almost to normal (Fig. 17-30).

CAPILLARY CHANGES RELATED TO VEIN OBSTRUCTION

Immediately following vein obstruction capillary filling was delayed but essentially complete. Later capillary detail was obscured by hemorrhage in most cases. As hemorrhage cleared it was again possible to visualize the capillary bed. The most striking change was the coarsening of the capillary mesh as though some capillaries were no longer perfused and others were dilated (Fig. 17-31). Coarsening of the capillary bed persisted in pigs when the main vein reopened several days after occlusion. There were never any large areas of capillary nonperfusion in the pig. In the monkey more profound changes took place in the capillary bed. In studies 2 weeks after occlusion, large areas of the capillary bed were not perfused. The venous side-branches from these areas were not filled and appeared pruned off (Fig. 17-32). Several possible capillary microaneurysms as well as arteriovenous communications across areas of capillary closure were seen. Some veins, remote from the site of photocoagulation, showed severe caliber irregularities with some segments almost obliterated.

STRUCTURAL CHANGES

Histologic changes were noted in both the vessels and the surrounding retinal elements. Within the burn site in pigs the veins were dilated and engorged and their walls were thin (Fig. 17-33). No evidence of cellular proliferation was seen. Immediately outside the burn site there were engorged vessels, presumably veins, with hypercellularity of their intima. In digest prepara-

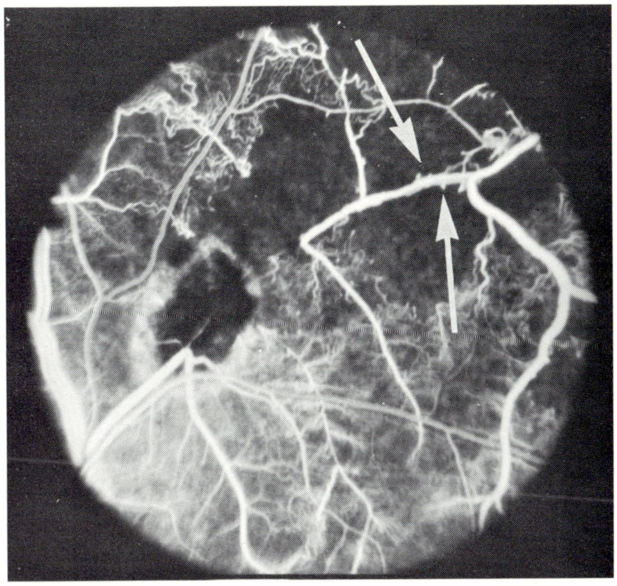

Fig. 17-32. Fluorescein angiogram of a monkey retina made 2 weeks after vein occlusion. Many capillaries are closed and venous side-branches are pruned off **(arrows).** (From Kohner et al. *Amer. J. Ophthal. 69:*778, 1970.)

Fig. 17-33. Cross section through photocoagulation site 10 days after vein occlusion in a pig. The vein is thin-walled, dilated, and engorged. There is destruction of the underlying retinal tissue as well as damage to the pigment epithelium and choroid. H & E, ×87.

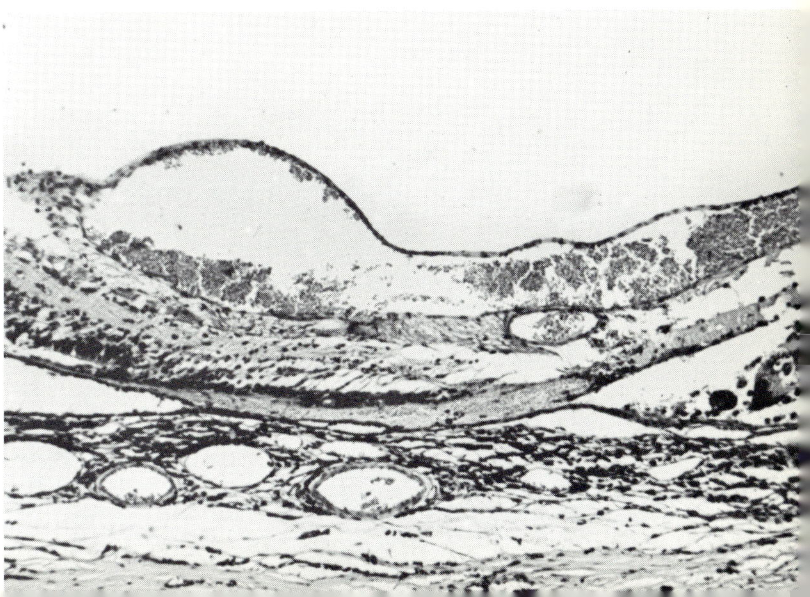

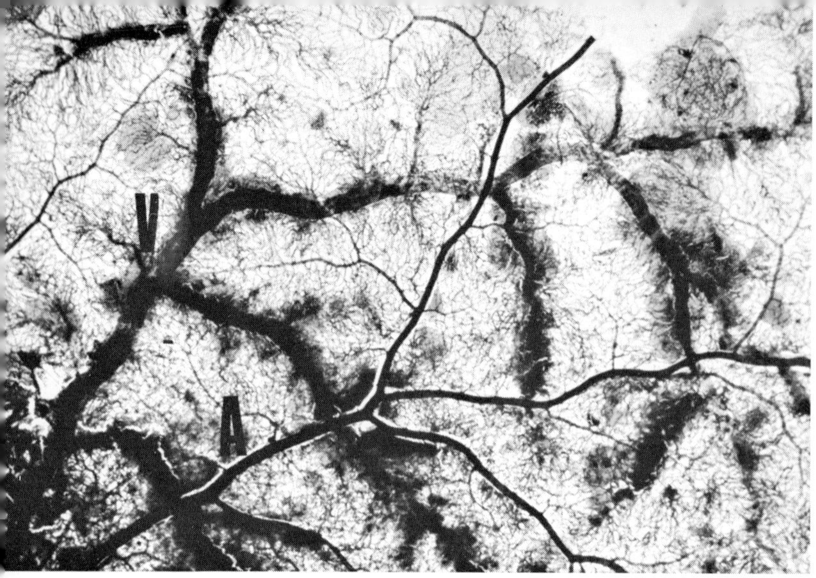

Fig. 17-34. Retinal-digest preparation from a rhesus monkey 1 day after venous occlusion. The retinal veins **(V)** are surrounded by a perivascular cuff of inflammatory cells. The arteries **(A)** lack this cellular cuff. PAS and hematoxylin, ×25.

Fig. 17-35. Retinal-digest preparation from a rhesus monkey 14 days after venous occlusion. A number of dilated, hypercellular collaterals are present. They link the occluded with patent venous channels around the macula. PAS and hematoxylin, ×87.

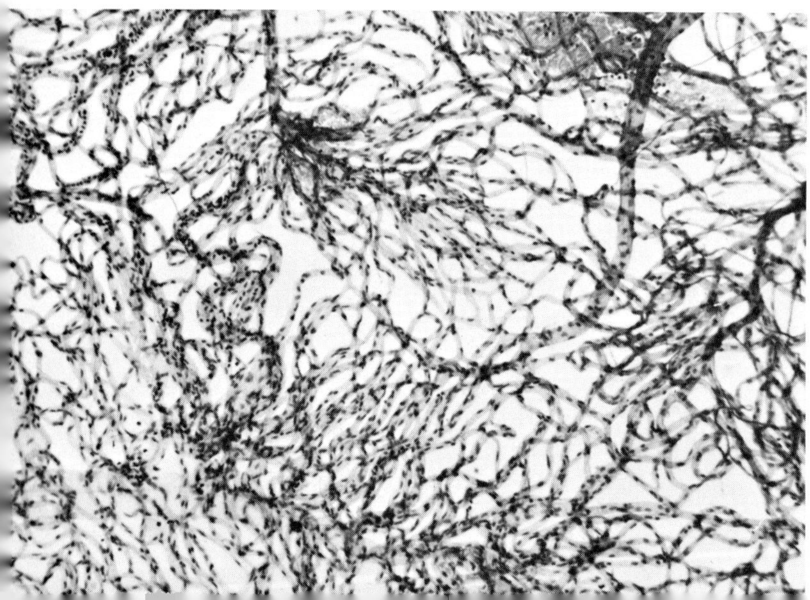

tions stained with periodic acid-Schiff (PAS) there were lumps of pinkish stained material, possibly fibrin, within the vessels. This material was mainly situated in veins or capillaries, adjacent to the obstruction. In rhesus monkeys a perivascular cuff of acute inflammatory cells was noted both on routine cross sections and in digest preparations. These cells, mainly polymorphonuclear leukocytes, were found predominantly around the venules and capillaries distal to the occlusion (Fig. 17-34). Arteries were generally spared from this process.

Edema of the nerve fiber layer and inner nuclear layer was present upstream from the occlusion, but cytoid bodies were absent except right adjacent to the burn site. The retina in the immediate area of photocoagulation was necrotic and degenerate as were the underlying choroid and inner layers of the sclera. Hemorrhage was noted around a number of vessels within the zone of obstruction, and in the inner layers of the surrounding retina.

Collateral vessels in the form of dilated capillary channels, which showed hypercellularity after several days' development, linked the blocked vein with patent venules (Fig. 17-35). In some instances the blocked vein and some of its tributaries showed degenerative changes, mainly loss of cellularity and pale staining properties, a long distance from the burn. Distal segments of these vessels were, however, normal in appearance. Microaneurysms were not a prominent feature, but several apparent ones were found in monkeys.

ULTRASTRUCTURAL CHANGES

Acute Studies

Distal to the site of occlusion the vein and its branches were dilated. The endothelium was flattened and only rarely showed the normal villous projection into the lumen. Muscle cells and endothelial cells maintained their normal electron-density, but the basement membrane was more electron-lucent and thicker than normal. Red cells, fibrin, and edematous fluid were present around the vessels.

In the nerve fiber layer most capillaries were dilated, with stretched endothelial walls and flattened nuclei. In contrast, the capillaries in the inner nuclear layer had an irregular lumen with an indented wall. These vessels were adjacent to Müller cells distended with intracellular edema.

In the nerve fiber-ganglion cell layer the intercellular spaces between the plasma membranes of adjacent Müller fibers were enlarged—in other words, extracellular edema was present. This corresponded to the edematous spaces seen on light microscopy. While bundles of nerve fibers were separated by the edematous fluid the individual ganglion cells appeared normal. Some glial cells around blood vessels were electron-lucent, suggesting intracellular edema. The inner plexiform layer seemed normal, but in the inner nuclear layer blood vessels were surrounded by swollen cells, presumably Müller cells. This intracellular swelling represented the cystic spaces which were seen by light microscopy.

Late Studies

In the pig collateral vessels were present within 3 to 7 days. They formed in the inner nuclear layer from the deep capillary meshwork. In early specimens it was difficult to differentiate them from dilated capillaries. Later their diameter was obviously larger than that of capillaries, and endothelial cell hypercellularity was seen. The cellular components of the wall of collaterals were similar to veins of comparable size, and there were no muscle cells.

In the monkey, basement membrane material surrounded by glia was all that remained of the capillaries and venous side branches not perfused on fluorescence angiograms. Macrophages were present adjacent to, or even within this basement membrane material.

By 24 hours, edema, characterized as reticulated material, was present both in enlarged extracellular spaces and in the Müller cell cytoplasm. Some Müller cells had ruptured plasma membranes. In the pig, within 1 week, the retinal architecture seemed normal with all edematous fluid disappearing from the nerve fiber ganglion cell layer. On the other hand, in a monkey studied at 7 weeks, areas that were avascular by angiography showed disappearance of the nerve fiber-ganglion cell layer and this was replaced by proliferated glia. The outer retinal layers were intact.

COMPARISONS AND CONTRASTS BETWEEN EXPERIMENTAL ARTERIAL AND VENOUS OCCLUSION

There are interesting similarities as well as important differences between the changes that take place after artery and vein occlusion. When an artery is blocked, blood enters via capillary collaterals and allows some flow to continue, while after vein occlusion it is the drainage that is impeded and blood has to find its way to adjacent veins via capillary collaterals. The most important immediate differences are the rate and the quality of the collateral blood flow. Following arterial obstruction the collateral flow is rarely more than 1 per cent of the normal forward flow. After vein occlusion the arterial inflow is 30 to 60 per cent of the normal value. Furthermore, the blood entering the blocked artery via capillary collaterals has already passed through capillaries in a relatively ischemic area and so given up most of its oxygen. Following vein obstruction the arterial blood is of normal composition. At first sight it is not obvious why there should be such a great difference in blood flow between the two situations. Both depend upon the presence of capillary links at the edge of the vascular territory and in both cases the arterial pressure drives the flow. In the case of arterial obstruction the pressure head comes from the surrounding patent arteries, via junctions in the capillary bed and in the case of vein obstruction the pressure in the blocked vein must approach the arterial level. There are two differences. Firstly, the arterial inflow pressure cannot be higher than the pressure at the junction in the capillary bed from which the flow is derived. In practice it may be much lower as the low resistance of the obstructed arterial circulation draining blood flow will tend to drop the pressure at the capillary junctions feeding it (Fig. 17-36). Secondly, the capillaries at the venous end of the circulation are likely to be of larger diameter than those nearer to the artery. Thus, following arterial obstruction the driving pressure may be less than 20 mmHg through a fairly high resistance capillary channel while following vein obstruction the driving pressure may be 80 mmHg through a lower resistance bed.

The time course of collateral development after artery and vein obstruction is similar. The first channels larger than capillaries took 1 to 3 days to appear and fully effective collaterals developed in 2 to 6 weeks. However, channels formed after vein occlusion were of much larger diameter than after artery occlusion.

The retinal changes consequent upon vascular obstruction were completely different but largely explicable upon the basis of the observed changes in blood flow and intravascular pressure. Arterial obstruction caused very severe ischemia. Retinal elements supplied by the retinal capillaries suffered cloudy swelling and ischemic necrosis with subsequent development of cotton-wool spots. Following vein obstruction the degree of ischemia was much less severe but the high venous pressure caused leakage, hemorrhage, edema and detachment.

One important and inexplicable finding following vein obstruction was coarsening of the capillary bed in pigs and large zones of capillary obliteration in rhesus monkeys. Although temporary capillary occlusion might occur as a result of the high tissue pressure following leakage and hemorrhage this should be reversible as the collaterals form. In fact capillary damage persisted even when the vein reopened only a few days after occlusion. The explanation of this phenomenon would be of the greatest significance because it might throw light on the pathogenesis of capillary closure in other conditions, particularly diabetes.

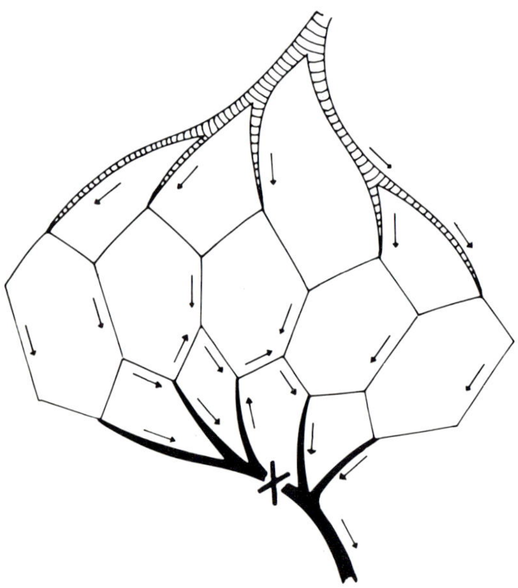

Fig. 17-36. Schematic diagram of the retinal microcirculation following branch vein occlusion **(X)**. Pressure in capillaries rises to near arterial level. Collateral flow takes place via capillary connections between patent and blocked veins at the venous end of the capillary bed **(arrows)**.

REFERENCES

1. Becker, B., and Post, L. T.: Retinal vein occlusion. Clinical and experimental observations. *Amer. J. Ophthal. 34:*677, 1951.
2. Campbell, F. P.: Retinal vein occlusion. An experimental study. *Arch. Ophthal. 65:*2, 1961.
3. Fujino, T., Curtin, V. T., and Norton, E. W. D.: Experimental central retinal vein occlusion. *Arch. Ophthal. 81:*395, 1969.
4. Hayreh, S. S.: Occlusion of the central retinal vessels. *Brit. J. Ophthal. 49:*626, 1965.
5. Kohner, E. M., Dollery, C. T., Shakib, M., Henkind, P., Paterson, J. W., de Oliveira, L. N. F., and Bulpitt, C. J.: Experimental retinal vein occlusion. *Amer. J. Ophthal. 69:* 778, 1970.
6. Linner, E.: Occlusion of the retinal veins in rabbits induced by light coagulation. *Acta Ophthal. 39:*739, 1961.
7. Mutlu, F.: Experimental retinal vein occlusion and treatment with fibrinolysin. *Amer. J. Ophthal. 62:*282, 1966.
8. Voipio, H., and Raitta, C.: Branch vein occlusion by photocoagulation in the rabbit eye. *Acta Ophthal. 42:*544, 1964.

EFFECT OF ALTERED INTRAOCULAR PRESSURE ON RETINAL CIRCULATION

There have been few studies of the effect of altered intraocular pressure on the retinal vascular system.

Elevated intraocular pressure, induced with a limbal suction cup, slowed retinal blood flow in pigs.[4] The no-flow point depended upon both the level of intraocular pressure and the mean systemic blood pressure; the higher the mean arterial pressure of the animal, the higher the intraocular pressure necessary to halt retinal blood flow (Fig. 17-37). Sinuous pulsation of the retinal arterioles became more prominent (Fig. 17-38) as intraocular tension increased, but there was little measurable change in the caliber of either arteries or veins. Increased intraocular pressure, with a constant mean arterial systemic pressure, slowed capillary filling and exaggerated time differences between filling of different portions of the retinal capillary bed. Analysis of high-definition fluorescein angiograms revealed that virtually all retinal capillaries of the posterior pole appeared to be perfused even when flow was slowed to less than 10 per

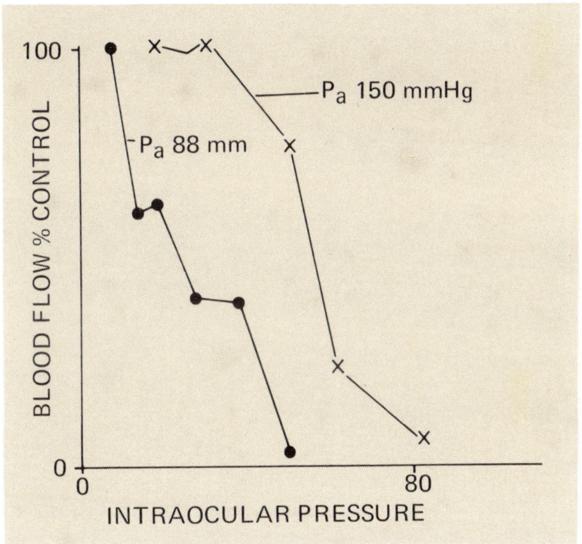

Fig. 17-37. Plot of percentage change (from control) in mean velocity flow in the axial stream of two large arteries in two different pigs as the intraocular pressure was increased. One pig had a mean systemic arterial pressure of 88 mmHg and blood flow ceased at an intraocular pressure just above 50 mmHg, while the other had a systemic arterial pressure of 150 mmHg and flow did not cease until the intraocular pressure exceeded 80 mmHg. (From Dollery et al.[4])

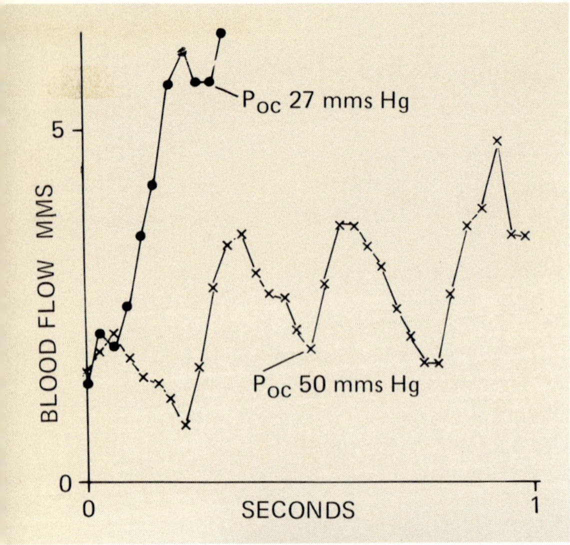

Fig. 17-38. Movement of the dye front in millimeters from the reference points on the optic disc in a retinal artery 160 μ in diameter at two levels of intraocular pressure, 27 mmHg (**x – x**) and 50 mmHg (●—●). Flow is pulsatile at both levels of intraocular pressure but the mean forward flow is much lower, and the back flow in diastole much greater, at the higher level of intraocular pressure. (From Dollery et al.[4])

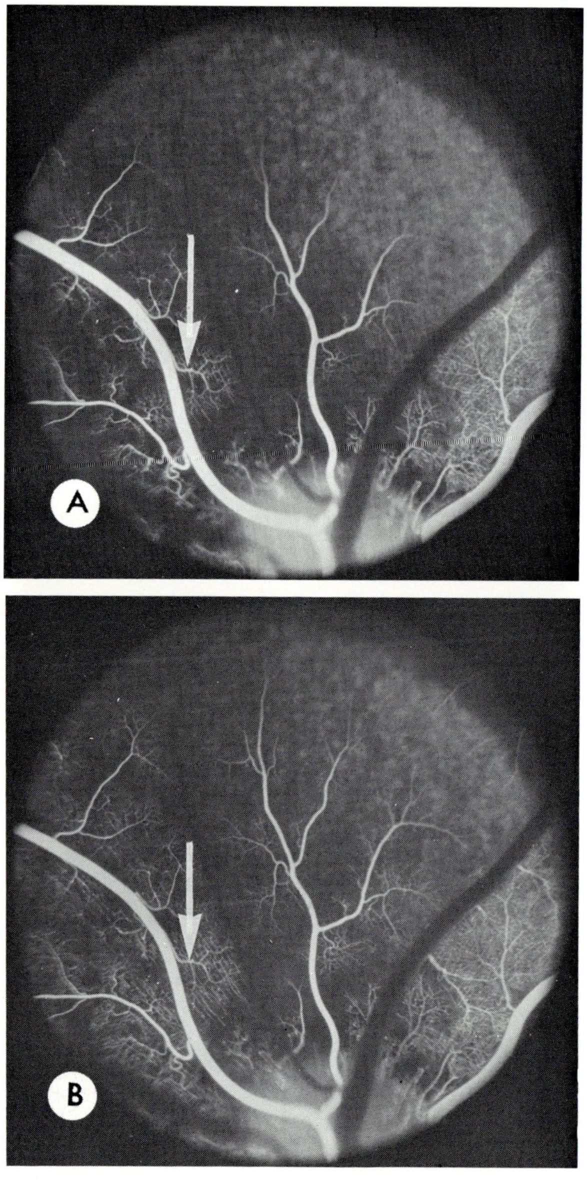

Fig. 17-39. *A*, Arterial-phase fluorescein angiogram at an intraocular pressure of 36 mmHg. Early filling of radial peripapillary capillaries is taking place from a small intraretinal arterial branch **(arrow).** *B*, One second later, radial capillaries continue to fill from intraretinal arterial branches **(arrow).** (From Dollery et al.[4])

cent of control values. Furthermore, there was no evidence of selective perfusion of any preferential channels. These studies confirmed the fact that the radial peripapillary capillaries, at least in the pig, derive from intraretinal arterioles, and not from arterioles of the disc head (Fig. 17-39). Elevated intraocular pressure slowed flow in some of the radial capillaries, but this was not a constant finding. A further observation was that the vascular supply of the optic nerve head, at least the arterial portion, is distinct from that of the surrounding retina. The disc fluoresces at the same time as the choroid, and prior to retinal vessel infilling. This observation of the dichotomy between nerve head and retinal vascular supply has also been demonstrated in human studies.

These studies illustrate the importance of recording both the intraocular and arterial pressures in clinical and experimental investigations of the retinal circulation.

Perfusion of the eye in experimental glaucoma has also been studied using india ink injected into the carotid artery. In owl monkeys with elevated intraocular pressure caused by injection of alpha-chymotrypsin, dental moulding cement, or talcum powder, ink only entered the larger retinal vessels.[5] Ink studies in cats with acute unilateral elevation of intraocular pressure to 30 to 50 mmHg and a mean arterial pressure of about 120 mmHg showed underfilling of the capillaries at the posterior pole particularly the radial peripapillary bed.[2]

The effect of severe retinal ischemia caused by elevating the intraocular pressure to very high levels has been studied in cats and rats. Reinecke and his colleagues[6] have raised the intraocular pressure of cats to approximately 155 mmHg for periods ranging from 1 to 45 days. Histologic studies showed destruction of the retina if ischemia was maintained for more than 1½ hours. Retinal vessels showed an early proliferation of endothelial cells. More prolonged ischemia caused death of these cells and finally destruction of the intramural pericytes. Agrawal,[1] using rats, has found irreversible retinal vascular damage after only 3 minutes of total ischemia induced by elevating intraocular pressure to 80 mmHg. Cunha-Vaz[3] has caused retinal ischemia in rats by elevating the intraocular pressure to from 110 mm to 160 mmHg. He studied the breakdown of the blood-retinal barrier by injecting carbon particles. Initially leakage was more marked in the terminal arterioles but later the whole arterial tree was involved and after 24 hours the veins were the most severely affected vessels.

REFERENCES

1. Agrawal, P. K.: The effect of experimental ischaemia on the retinal vessels of the cat. *Orient. Arch. Ophthal. 3:*184, 1965.
2. Alterman, M., and Henkind, P.: Radial peripapillary capillaries. 2: Possible role in Bjerrum scotoma. *Brit. J. Ophthal. 52:*26, 1968.
3. Cunha-Vaz, J. G.: Studies on the permeability of the blood-retinal barrier. 3. Breakdown of the blood-retinal barrier by circulatory disturbances. *Brit. J. Ophthal. 50:*505, 1966.
4. Dollery, C. T., Henkind, P., Kohner, E., and Paterson, J. W.: Effect of raised intraocular pressure on the retinal and choroidal circulation. *Invest. Ophthal. 7:*191, 1968.
5. Kalvin, N. H., Hamasaki, D. I., and Gass, J. D. M.: Experimental glaucoma in monkeys. 2. Studies of intraocular vascularity during glaucoma. *Arch. Ophthal. 76:*94, 1966.
6. Reinecke, R. D., Kuwabara, T., Cogan, D. G., and Weis, D. R.: Retinal vascular patterns. Part 5. Experimental ischemia of the cat eye. *Arch. Ophthal. 67:*470, 1962.

EXPOSURE TO LIGHT

The retina is readily damaged by exposure to intense light sources. Eclipse burns and accidental observation of atomic fireballs, or clinical use of lasers or xenon arc photocoagulators can produce sufficient thermal energy in the retina to coagulate and destroy it.[2,8,12,13] Recent work has shown that less intense light sources, which do not produce an immediately visible lesion in the retina, may cause sufficient damage for a lesion to appear, over hours or days and evolve into complete retinal necrosis.[5] Exposures of several days' duration to much less intense light sources can produce severe damage and eventually complete destruction of the photoreceptors.[10]

Intense light causes severe damage to the pigment epithelium and the immediately adjacent photoreceptors. However, very high intensities or prolonged exposures can damage the retinal blood vessels.[7,9,11,13] The xenon arc photocoagulator is widely used to destroy abnormal vascular structures such as angiomas or patches of neovascularization. For experimental purposes it has been used to obstruct large branch veins in cats, pigs, and monkeys. Caution is necessary with the photocoagulator in both clinical and experimental use. Too prolonged exposure may cause immediate rupture of blood vessels with massive hemorrhages or extensive late retinal scarring. It is best to use a number of brief exposures often spaced over a period of time rather than a large single dose to destroy or occlude a vascular structure.

PHOTOCOAGULATION

Photocoagulation was introduced by Meyer-Schwickerath[8] and is now widely used in therapy. Several instruments are available. The Carl Zeiss (Oberkochen) instrument makes use of a xenon arc lamp and the duration and intensity of exposure can be varied at will. The Carl Zeiss (Jena) instrument has improved viewing optics and uses a xenon flash tube as the coagulating source. The intense and short duration pulse is suitable for occluding smaller vessels but not large veins. The ruby laser was first used in the eye experimentally by Zaret and his colleagues[13] and it is used clinically when a small-diameter, brief, and intense coagulation is required.

A number of workers have used these devices to produce experimental retinal burns in animals and they have also been used to cause experimental obstruction of large retinal veins.

Okun and Collins[11] have noted hypercellularity of retinal veins in dogs following their photocoagulation with the xenon arc. Microaneurysmal formations were found distal to the experimental branch vein occlusions. Their attempts at photocoagulation of retinal arteries were unsuccessful. Miles and Ruiz[9] have photocoagulated the larger retinal vessels of rabbits. They found loss of normal nuclei in the vessel walls and lumens filled with polymorphonuclear leukocytes to occur within 1 day. After 3 days, the walls of both arteries and veins were thickened and invaded by round cells and the lumens of the coagulated veins were patent. By 7 days there was fibrosis of the outer layers of the vessels, and the smaller branching vessels were partially or completely occluded. Sections made 12 weeks after coagulation showed distortion and shrinkage of the lumen both of the arteries and veins.

Ham and his colleagues[4] have used a searchlight to produce retinal burns in rabbits. Exposures of 500 to 1000 msec immediately produced a dense white retinal lesion. In globes enucleated and fixed immediately after exposure there was moderate swelling of the nerve fiber layer and pyknosis of the nuclei of the inner and outer nuclear layers. The structure of the rods and cones was lost or modified in the burn area. In eyes enucleated 3 or 4 days later the changes were similar but there was also choroidal hyperemia and damage to the sclera. Some pigment cells at the edge of the lesion had begun to proliferate.

These authors have noted that the thermal energy required to produce a visible lesion varied inversely with its size. For an image size of 0.4 mm on the retinal surface the critical dose to produce almost immediate whitening of the retina was 5.6 cal/cm^2 while for a 1.1-mm diameter lesion it was 3.6 cal/cm^2

Kohner and her colleagues[5] have shown that a xenon light source that gave a retinal irradiance of 0.25 cals/cm^2 sec caused severe retinal damage if exposure was prolonged. The lamp illuminated an area of retina approximately 8 mm in diameter. Exposures of up to 30 seconds caused no retinal lesions either immediately or later. Forty- to 60-second exposures caused no clinically visible change within the first hour although fluorescein studies showed deep leakage from the pigment epithelium (Fig. 17-40). Eighty- to 180-second burns of the retina became an opalescent white color within a few minutes of exposure. Later there were pigmentary changes and extensive hemorrhage. After 3 weeks hemorrhage reabsorbed leaving a scarred retina with tortuous, abnormal vessels and loss of capillaries (Fig. 17-41). In one animal a large artery that appeared undamaged at the conclusion of a 120-second exposure to light became occluded 5 days later (Fig. 17-42).

Ruby lasers can be used to produce retinal lesions [13] in both experimental animals and man.[2,15] The intense, narrow, red beam of coherent radiation produces a small, sharply demarcated area of retinal coagulation. The technique is used for sealing leaking points in central serous retinopathy and other retinal conditions but it is not, because of its wavelength, very useful in the treatment of retinal vascular lesions or in the production of experimental vascular occlusion.

L'Esperance [7] was among the first to examine the response of the retinal vasculature to laser radiation. He has studied cross sections of rabbit and monkey retinas whose vessels were subjected to ruby laser radiation (wavelength 6, 943 Å; energy 0.03–0.27 J). The retinal blood vessels of rabbits were unaffected by even intensive laser irradiation. Monkey eyes enucleated within 2 weeks after their last treatment showed slight edema of the intramural pericytes. The edema was more pronounced in the vessel walls that lay in close approximation to the pigment layers. More intense irradiation led to decreased intramural cell population and thickening and disruption of the vessel wall. Wood and Watzke [13] have compared the response of retinal vessels of dogs to xenon arc and ruby laser coagulation. They used light intensities similar to those given for the treatment of human retinal disease. Digest preparations showed that laser radiation caused an early minimal inflammatory response in the venules and a delayed atrophy of retinal capillaries. Minimal laser coagulation caused no damage to the retinal arterioles. Light coagulation produced a moderate venous inflammatory response

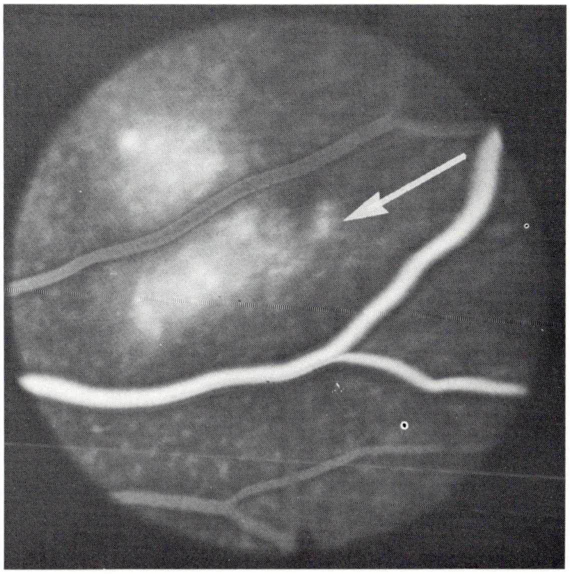

Fig. 17-40. Venous-phase fluorescein angiogram made 1 hour after exposure of the pig retina to high-intensity light for 40 seconds. There is a diffused area of deep leakage **(arrow).** (From Kohner et al. *Amer. J. Ophthal. 63:*1793, 1967.)

Fig. 17-41. Fluorescein angiogram shows the edge of a burned area 3 weeks after an 80-second exposure. The capillary bed in the burned area has been replaced by tortuous dilated new vessels **(arrow).** (From Kohner et al. *Amer. J. Ophthal. 63:*1793, 1967.)

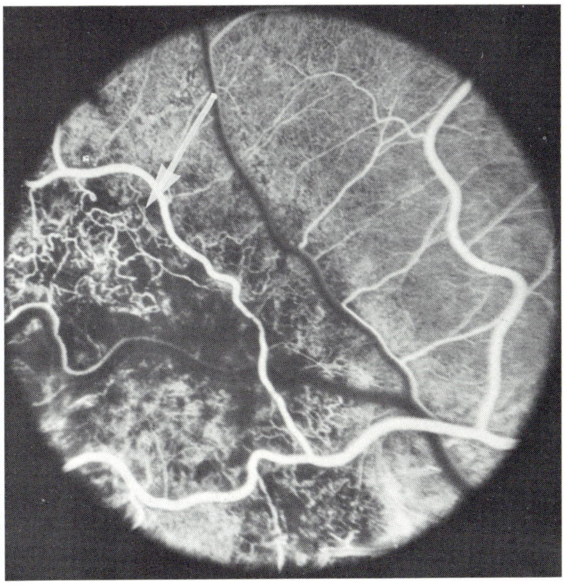

and early capillary necrosis. Arterioles exhibited loss of cellular architecture and hypocellularity 4 weeks after treatment. Repeated applications of light coagulation caused more severe retinal vascular damage than single doses.

The development of the argon laser, with its wavelength more suitable for vessel coagulation, should add a new dimension to the field of retinal vessel photocoagulation.

Fig. 17-42. Fluorescein angiogram made 5 days after 120-second exposure. A blocked artery is filling retrogradely from the collateral (**arrow**). A ring of dilated capillaries surrounds the central zone of hemorrhages. (From Kohner et al. *Amer. J. Ophthal. 63:*1793, 1967.)

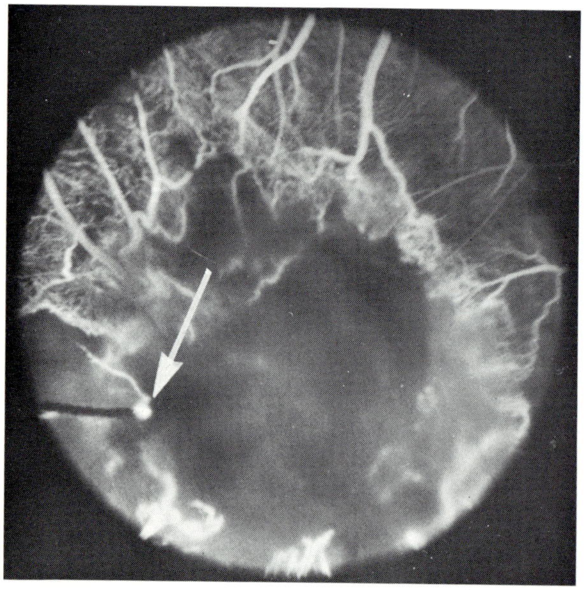

PHOTORECEPTOR DAMAGE

In 1966 Noell[10] observed that rats in open cages exposed to ordinary fluorescent lighting for long periods developed irreversible damage to their photoreceptors.

Kuwabara and Gorn[6] have studied changes in the ultrastructure of the photoreceptors in albino rats exposed to light at a brightness of 750 fc for periods from an hour to several weeks. After an hour a few layers of the myelin discs of the outermost tips of the photoreceptors became thinner and showed separation of the disc membranes. After 24-hours' exposure the membranes had lost their regular lamellar structure and were separated and vacuolated. Three days of exposure converted the whole outer segment into tubular structures and at 5 days it consisted of round and pear-shaped masses filled with tubular material. Up to this stage the changes were reversible and the normal myelin membranes could be slowly reformed. When light exposure was continued for more than a week the retina was irreversibly damaged and all the photoreceptor cells disappeared. The same authors have correlated different periods of light exposure with electroretinogram (ERG) changes.[3]

Damage to retinal vessels has not been reported in these studies.

EFFECT OF LIGHT ON RETINAL CIRCULATION

Morris, Bellhorn, and Henkind[9a] have examined benzidine-stained, retinal flatmount preparations of rats and cats whose eyes were exposed to various levels of illumination. There was no apparent difference in distribution of red cells in retinal vessels of light-adapted versus dark-adapted eyes. Intense light and flicker did not seem to cause any alteration in the number or distribution of red cells within the vessels.

REFERENCES

1. Campbell, C. J., Rittler, M. C., Koester, C. J.: The optical laser as a retinal coagulator. An evaluation. *Trans. Amer. Acad. Ophthal. 67:*58, 1963.
2. Flynn, J. A. F.: Eclipse blindness, prevention is better than cure. *Trans. Ophthal. Soc. Austr. 12:*7, 1952.
3. Gorn, R. A., and Kuwabara, T.: Retinal damage by visible light. A physiologic study. *Arch. Ophthal. 77:*115, 1967.
4. Ham, W. T., Weisinger, H., Guerry, D., Schmidt, M. S., Williams, R. C., Ruffins, R. S., and Shaffer, M. C.: Experimental production of flash burns in the rabbit retina. *Amer. J. Ophthal. 43:*711, 1957.
5. Kohner, E. M., Dollery, C. T., Henkind, P., Paterson, J. W., and Ramalho, P. S.: Retinal vascular changes following exposure to high-intensity light. *Amer. J. Ophthal. 63:* 1793, 1967.
6. Kuwabara, T., and Gorn, R. A.: Retinal damage by visible light. *Arch. Ophthal. 79:*69, 1968.
7. L'Esperance, F. A., Jr.: The effect of laser radiation on the retinal vasculature. *Arch. Ophthal. 74:*752, 1965.
8. Meyer-Schwickerath, G.: Lichtkoagulation: Eine Methode zur Behandlung und Verhutung der Netzhautablosung. *Graefe. Arch. Ophthal. 156:*2, 1954.
9. Miles, D. R., and Ruiz, R. S.: The effects of photocoagulation on the large retinal vessels of the rabbit eye. *Amer. J. Ophthal. 64:*1098, 1967.

9a. Morris, D., Bellhorn, R., and Henkind, P.: Study of the retinal circulation: 1. Effect of light. *Brit. J. Ophthal. 54:*99, 1970.

10. Noell, W. K.: Retinal damage by light in rats. *Invest. Ophthal. 5:*450, 1966.
11. Okun, E., and Collins, E. M.: Histopathology of experimental photocoagulation in the dog: 3. Microaneurysm-like formations following branch vein occlusion. *Amer. J. Ophthal. 56:*40, 1963.
12. Rose, H. W., Brown, D. V. L., Brynes, V. A., and Cibis, P. A.: Human chorioretinal burns from atomic fireballs. *Arch. Ophthal. 55:*205, 1956.
13. Wood, L. W., and Watzke, R. C.: The effects of photo- and laser coagulation on the retinal vasculature. A comparative study. *Arch. Ophthal. 82:*499, 1969.
14. Zaret, M. M., Ripps, H., Siegel, I. M., and Breinin, G. M.: Laser photocoagulation of the eye. *Arch. Ophthal. 69:*97, 1963.
15. Zweng, H. E., Flocks, M., Kapany, N. S., Silbertrust, N., and Peppers, N. A.: Experimental laser photocoagulation. *Amer. J. Ophthal. 58:*353, 1964.

EFFECT OF OXYGEN ON IMMATURE RETINAL VESSELS

The recognition that the epidemic of retrolental fibroplasia in the later 1940s and 1950s [10,11,21] was due to treatment with oxygen stimulated a great deal of experimental work on the effects of oxygen on immature retinal vessels. Indeed, the proof that oxygen was the causative agent came in large part from the experimental work.[8,12,20]

Gyllensten and Hellström [12] had exposed newborn mice to 100% oxygen intermittently for periods of up to 16 days. The results of intermittent exposure were relatively slight on the retina itself. There were some hemorrhages, retinal folding, and fibrovascular cellular proliferation from the retina into the vitreous. There was marked persistence, proliferation, and dilatation of the hyaloid vessels. Continuous administration of oxygen for up to 5 days retarded formation of the retinal vessels and, when the animals were returned to air, the retinal vessels proliferated and capillaries invaded the vitreous. In later papers [13,14] these same authors have compared the effect of exposure to oxygen in newborn mice and animals that

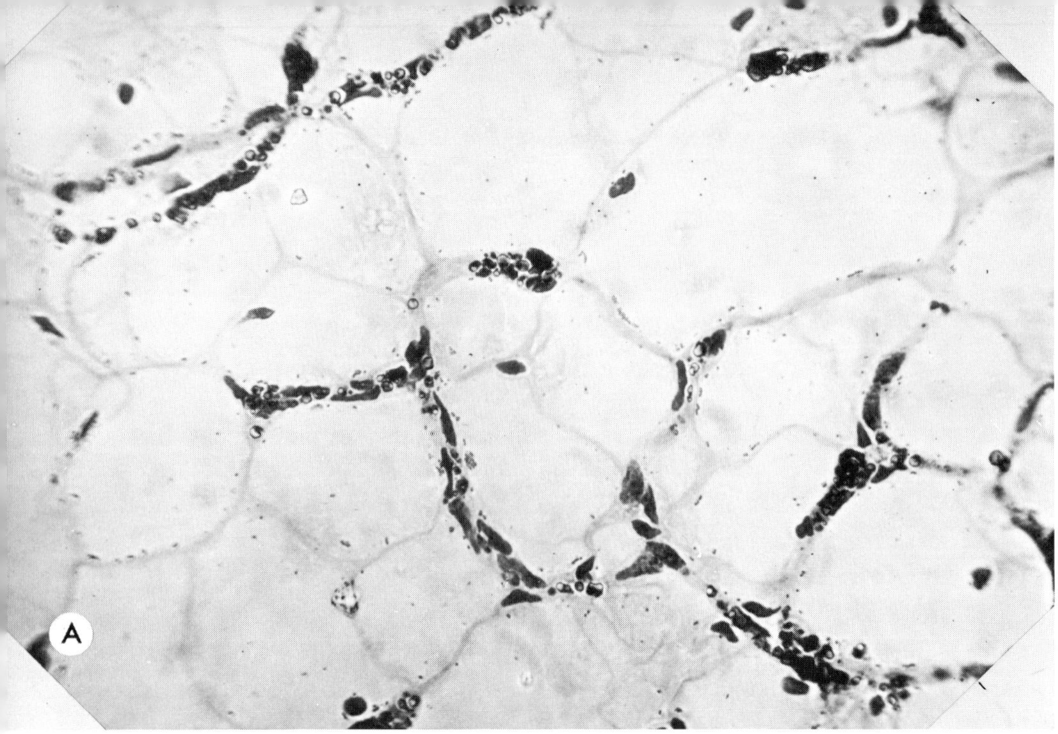

Fig. 17-43. *A*, Retinal-digest preparation giving general picture of the process of oxygen vaso-obliteration in kitten retina. Degenerating endothelial cells are withdrawing into isolated capillary islands, while the capillary network is represented only by delicate threadlike strands. Digest preparation. H & E, ×440. *B*, Digest preparation of retinal vessels of a premature infant subjected to oxygen for 90 hours. Note that the obliterative process is identical to that in the kitten, being an exaggeration of the normal process of retraction and migration. PAS and hematoxylin, ×390.
(*A* and *B* from Ashton. *Amer. J. Ophthal.* *62*:412, 1966.)

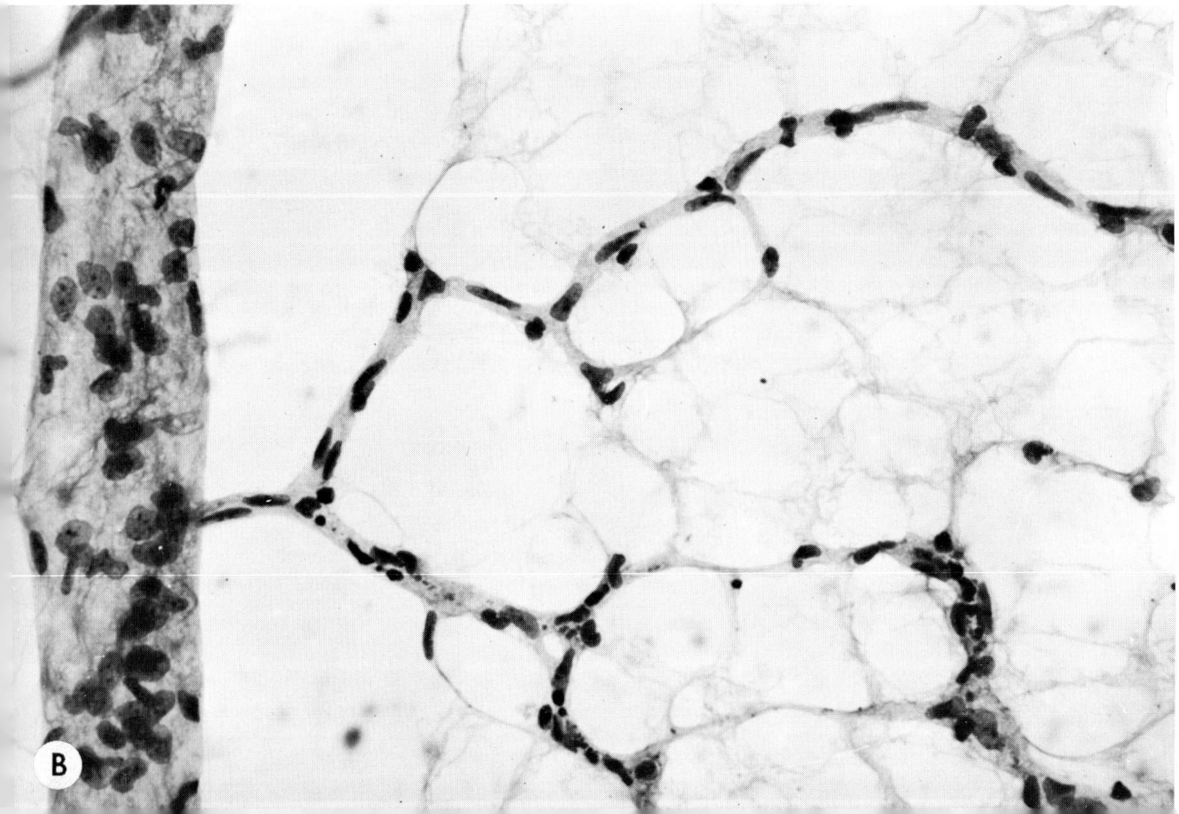

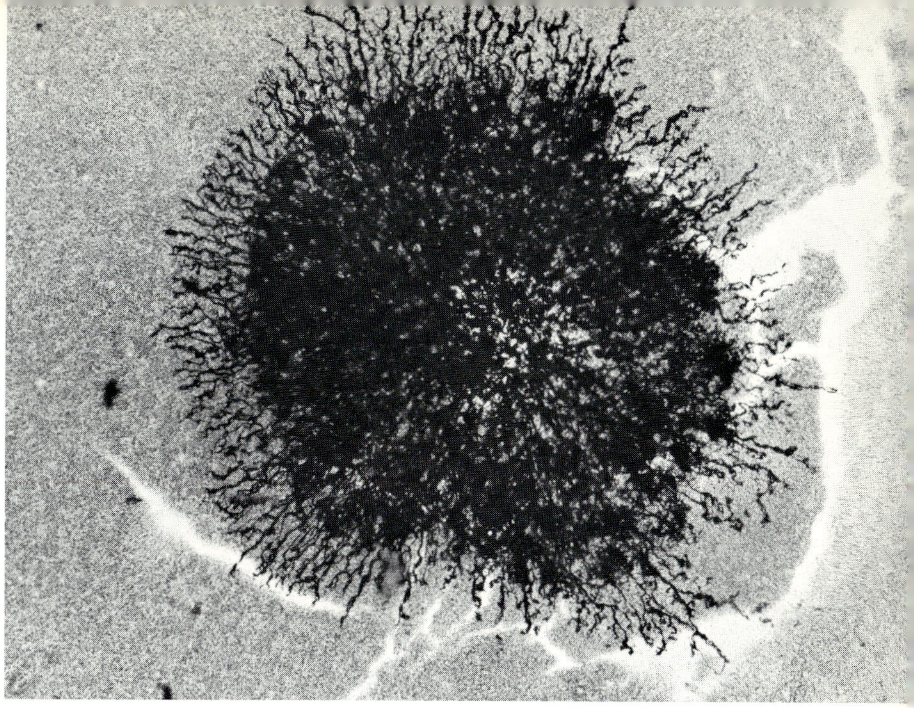

Fig. 17-44. India-ink injected, flat retinal preparation from a 21-day-old kitten raised in 80% oxygen for 6 days, then in room air for 15 days; note the abnormal vascularization which extends only a short distance from the disc. (From Patz.[19])

were aged 5 to 10 days. In newborn mice the vascular changes were concentrated around the optic disc and in the older ones it was more peripheral. Ocular hemorrhages and irregular vasoproliferation of the retinal vessels were more conspicuous in the younger mice. The vasoproliferative changes closely resembled the early stages of human retrolental fibroplasia.

Patz and co-workers[20] had exposed newborn opposums, rats, mice, kittens, and puppies to continuous 70 to 80% oxygen. Changes were noted mainly in the mouse and kitten. The abnormalities seen in the mouse included intraocular hemorrhage, abnormal persistence and proliferation of the tunica vasculosa lentis, vitreous changes, retinal edema, and nodules of endothelial or glial cells in the retina. The tabulated results in this paper suggested that exposure to oxygen for 21 days produced greater changes than exposure for 7 to 14 days. This led to the conclusion that continuous exposure to oxygen may lead to proliferative retinopathy. Patz recognized that proliferative retinopathy could occur if animals were removed abruptly from oxygen to air, but his experimental evidence was in favor of the changes being produced by continuous administration of oxygen.

Ashton, Ward, and Serpell[8] have shown that continuous exposure of newborn kittens to 60 to 70% oxygen at atmospheric pressure caused vasoconstriction of the growing retinal vessels. If oxygen was administered continuously for 4 to 6 days complete obliteration of the vessels occurred. If the kittens exposed to oxygen were removed into air, retinal vascular proliferation with tufts of vessels invading the vitreous, and retinal detachment took place. Ashton and his colleagues have shown that the severity of the constriction and subsequent obliteration of the vessels varied inversely with their maturity. Although mature retinal vessels exposed to oxygen constricted they could not be obliterated. The concentration of oxygen was also of crucial importance and this effect could not be produced by less than 35% concentration.

This research has demonstrated the crucial importance of the biphasic response, first vaso-obliteration and second vasoproliferation.

Retinal digest and ink-injected preparations of man and animals exposed to continuous oxygen demonstrate capillary retraction, narrowing and eventually obliteration (Figs. 17-43 and 17-44). Endothelial cells migrate into the remaining part of the bed

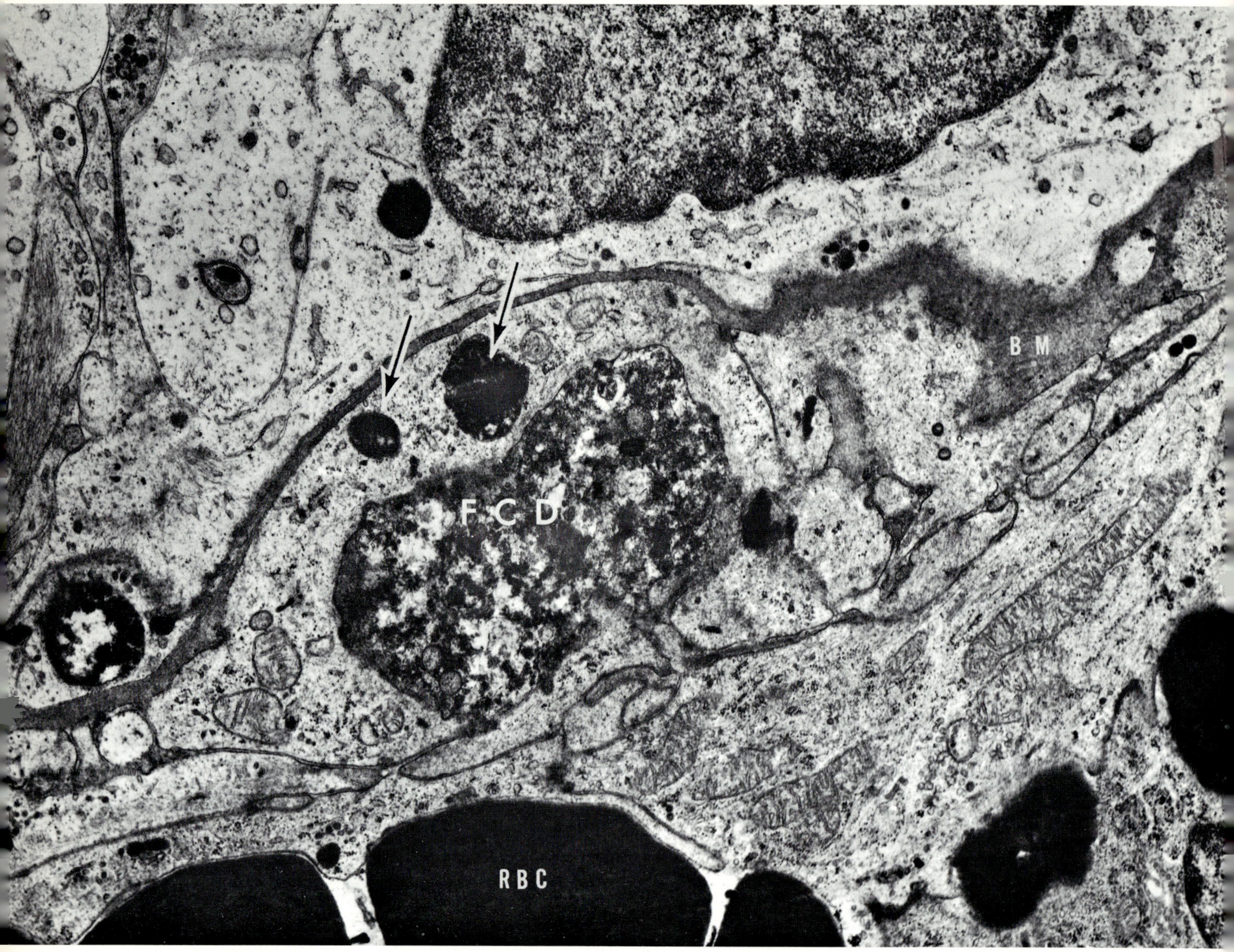

Fig. 17-45. Electron micrograph of the retina of a 10-day-old kitten subjected to 80 to 90% oxygen for 2 days shows a large intracellular vesicle of focal cytoplasmic degeneration **(FCD)** in the wall of a small vessel cut longitudinally. The dense bodies **(arrows)** probably also represent advanced focal cytoplasmic degeneration. Red cells **(RBC)**; basement membrane **(BM)**. Uranyl acetate-lead citrate. Araldite-embedded, ×18,000. (From Ashton. *Brit. J. Ophthal. 52:*505, 1968. By permission of the Editor and Publisher.)

but they eventually become necrotic until all that remains is a delicate network made up of the basement membrane of the obliterated capillaries.[1,2] Electron microscopic studies show that oxygen has a remarkably selective effect upon the blood vessels. The constricted and disintegrating vessels lie among apparently normal retinal tissue.[7,18,19] The transition from a normal endothelial cell to complete disintegration is signalled by dense granular bodies in the cytoplasm (Fig. 17-45). Intramural pericytes either degenerate in situ or are shed into the lumen of the capillary along with endothelial cell debris.

Attempts to produce vasodilatation during exposure to oxygen by use of carbon dioxide, sympathectomy, or vasodilator drugs have been unsuccessful.[8,17] Although vitamin E has been claimed to protect against the vascular obliteration,[19] Ashton[2] found that doses of 500 mg per kilogram per day had no protective action in kittens. Anticoagulants have been claimed to prevent vaso-obliteration induced by oxygen;[9] however, this observation has not been followed up. Patz and co-workers have recently used the fluorescein angiographic technique to study flow changes during the obliterative phase. The vessels were studied by direct observation through a limbal window and intraocular pressure was maintained manometrically. In five kittens exposed to 80% oxygen for 72 hours complete cessation of retinal blood flow resulted (Fig. 17-46).[19]

Following their removal to room air there was marked dilatation and tortuosity of the larger retinal vessels. Delicate tufts of neovascularization appeared and broke through the internal limiting membrane to form capillaries in the adjacent vitreous.[20] These vessels soon had an adult structure with a basement membrane and pericytes and they became surrounded by collagen (Fig. 17-47). The proliferating vessels leaked fluorescein (Fig. 17-48).[19]

The site and extent of the proliferative change depends upon the extent of the original obliterative changes. If obliteration is complete, proliferation begins from the optic disc; otherwise, it begins from the edge of the obliterated zone. There are species differ-

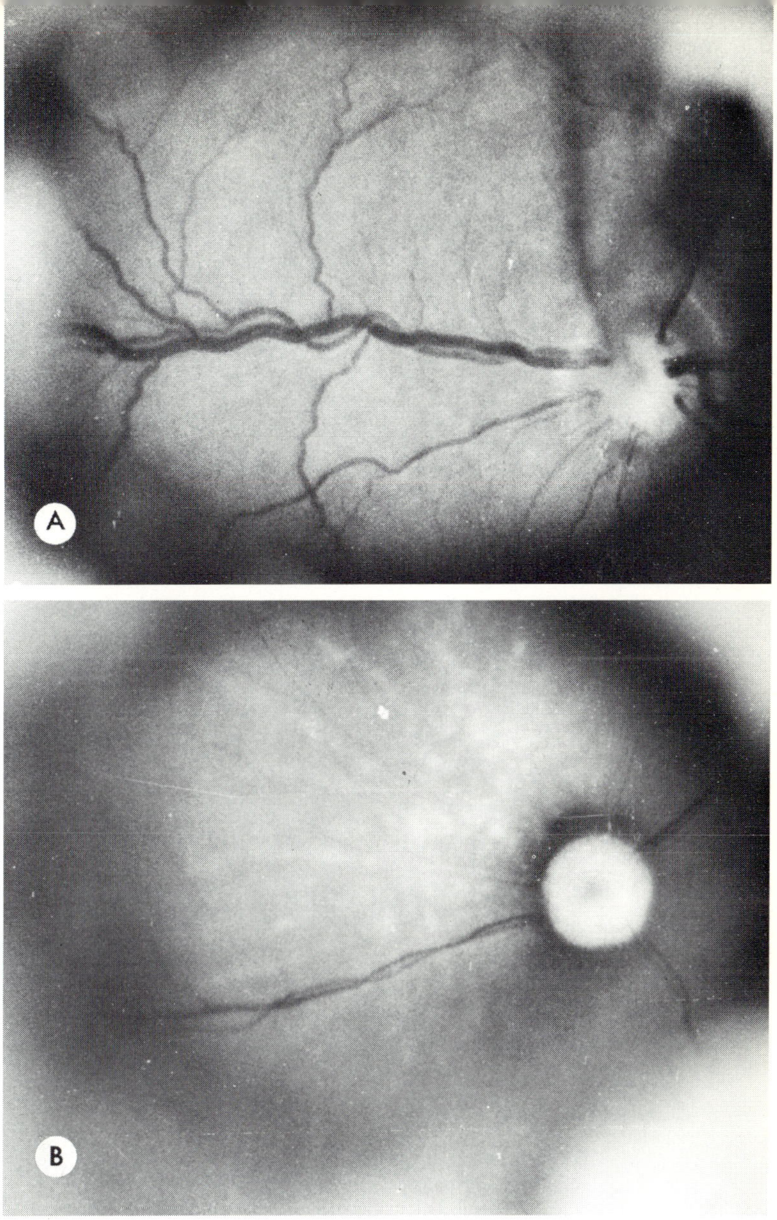

Fig. 17-46. *A*, Retinal vessels seen through artificial anterior chamber in normal 14-day-old kitten. ×25. *B*, Litter mate to animal in *A* shows extreme degree of vasoconstriction of major vessels and obliteration of capillary bed and smaller branch vessels after being subjected to 80% oxygen for 24 hours. (From Patz.[19])

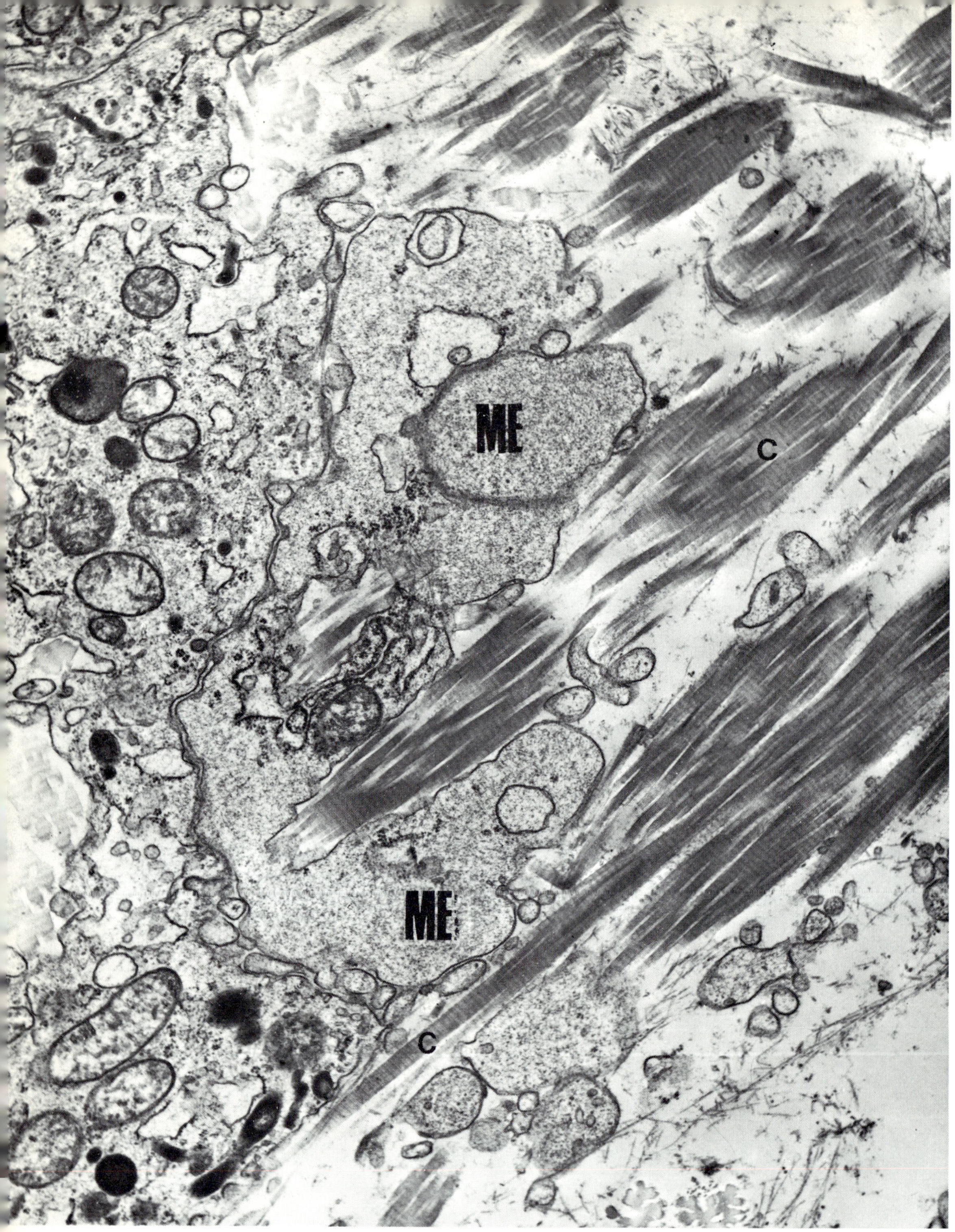

Fig. 17-47. Electron micrograph showing collagen fibers **(c)** in intimate relation with proliferating cells in the vitreous of a kitten which was subjected for 3 days to 80 to 90% oxygen at 10 days of age. Later kitten was removed to 38 days of air. Mesenchymal cell **(ME)**. Uranyl acetate-lead citrate. Epon embedded, ×22,000. (From Ashton, *Brit. J. Ophthal. 52:*505, 1968. By permission of the Editor and Publisher.)

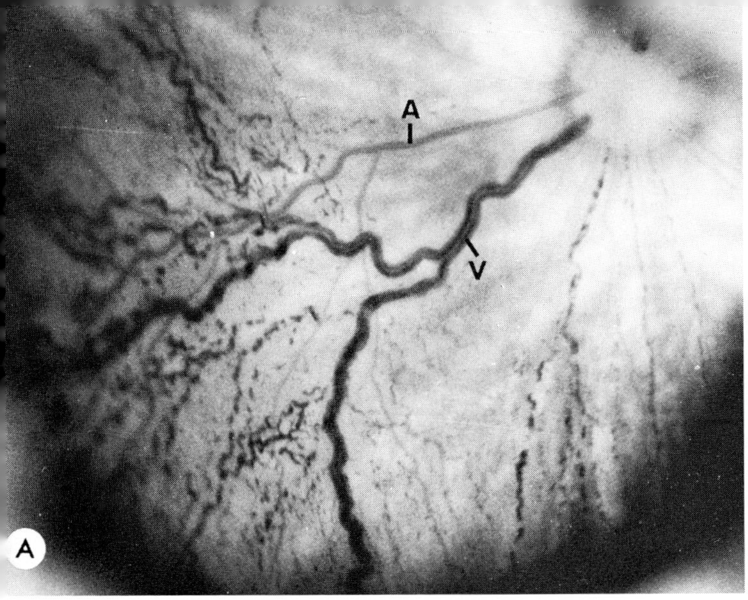

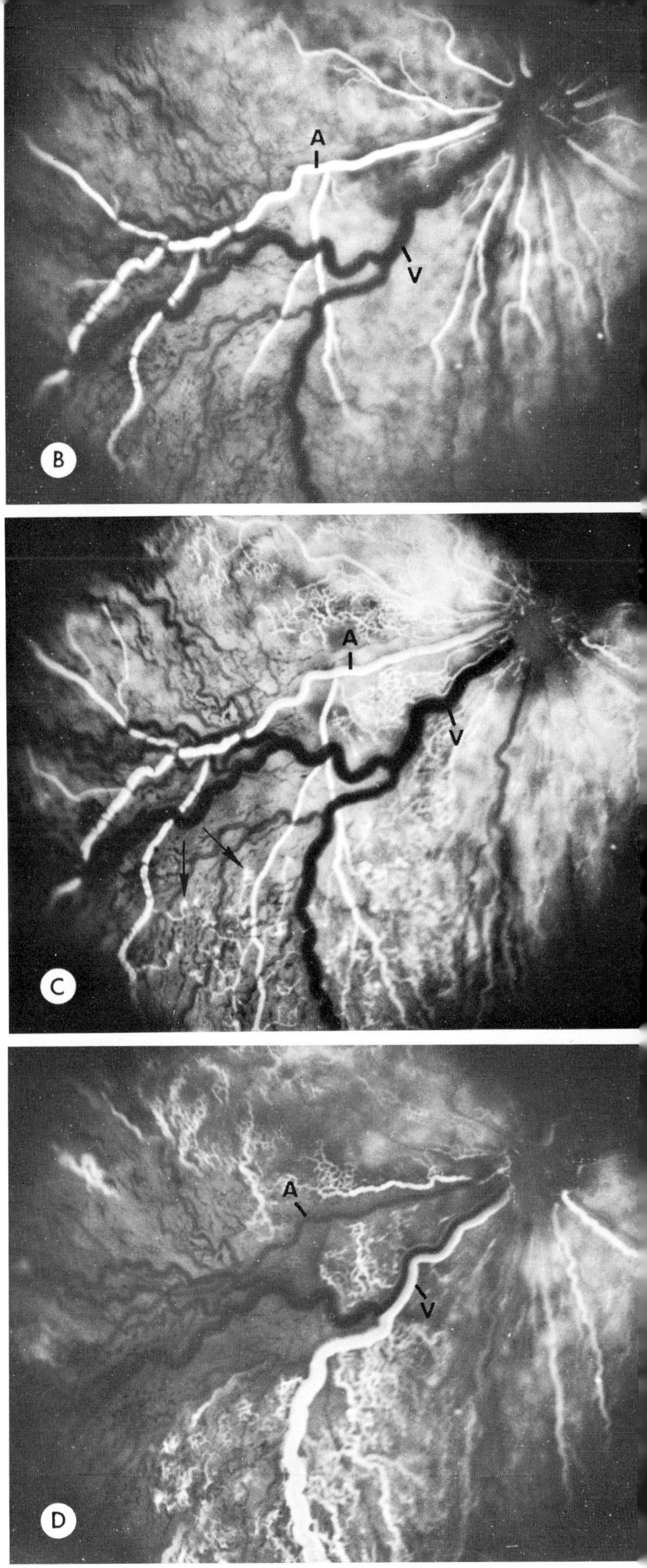

Fig. 17-48. *A*, Retinal vessels of kitten treated from tenth to twelfth day of age in 80% oxygen and removed to room air for 7 days; note the marked dilatation and tortuosity of larger retinal vessels and abnormality of capillary bed: **A,** artery, **V,** vein.

B, Same animal as in *A* showing arterial phase of fluorescein-filling retinal vessels.

C, Eight seconds after *B*; **arrows** point to delicate tufts of neovascularization.

D, One second after *C* shows filling of the venous side of the capillary bed. The neovascular tufts appear to be leaking fluorescein.

(From Patz.[19])

ences in the proliferative response which is best seen in the kitten and man and occurs to a much smaller extent in the rabbit, rat, mouse, and dog.[2,3,16]

In addition to the above-mentioned in vivo studies, Ashton has performed in vitro experiments which demonstrate the toxic effect of oxygen on developing vessels.[2]

While oxygen has been incriminated as the inciting agent in retrolental fibroplasia, Imre[15] has suggested, on the basis of some experimental work, that lactic acid may induce retinal neovascularization. He injected lactic acid in varying concentration into 7- to 9-day-old kittens, and found that a 0.1% solution caused retinal neovascularization.

REFERENCES

1. Ashton, N.: Oxygen and the growth and development of retinal vessels. In vivo and in vitro studies. *Amer. J. Ophthal. 62:*412, 1966.
2. Ashton, N.: Some aspects of the comparative pathology of oxygen toxicity in the retina. *Brit. J. Ophthal. 52:*505, 1968.
3. Ashton, N., and Blach, R.: Studies on developing retinal vessels. 8. Effect of oxygen on the retinal vessels of the ratling. *Brit. J. Ophthal. 45:*321, 1961.
4. Ashton, N., and Cook, C.: Direct observation of the effect of oxygen on developing vessels. Preliminary report. *Brit. J. Ophthal. 38:* 433, 1954.
5. Ashton, N., and Cook, C.: Studies on developing retinal vessels. 1. Influence of retinal detachment. *Brit. J. Ophthal. 39:*449, 1955.
6. Ashton, N., and Cook, C.: Studies on developing retinal vessels. 2. Influence of retinal detachment on oxygen vaso-obliteration. *Brit. J. Ophthal. 39:*457, 1955.
7. Ashton, N., and Pedler, C.: Studies on developing retinal vessels. 9. Reaction of endothelial cells to oxygen. *Brit. J. Ophthal. 46:* 257, 1962.
8. Ashton, N., Ward, B., and Serpell, G.: Role of oxygen in the genesis of retrolental fibroplasia. A preliminary report. *Brit. J. Ophthal. 37:*513, 1953.
9. Ashton, N., Ward, B., and Serpell, G.: Effect of oxygen on developing retinal vessels with particular reference to the problem of retrolental fibroplasia. *Brit. J. Ophthal. 38:*397, 1954.
10. Campbell, K.: Intensive oxygen therapy as a possible cause of retrolental fibroplasia: A clinical approach. *Med. J. Austr. 2:*48, 1951.
11. Crosse, V. M., and Evans, P. J.: Prevention of retrolental fibroplasia. *Arch. Ophthal. 48:* 83, 1952.
12. Gyllensten, L. J., and Hellström, B. E.: Retrolental fibroplasia animal experiments. The effect of intermittingly administered oxygen on the postnatal development of the eyes of fullterm mice. A preliminary report. *Acta Paediat. Scand. 41:*577, 1952.
13. Gyllensten, L. J., and Hellström, B. E.: Experimental approach to the pathogenesis of retrolental fibroplasia. 1. Changes of the eye induced by exposure of newborn mice to concentrated oxygen. *Acta Paediat. 43* (Suppl.100): 1954.
14. Gyllensten, L. J., and Hellström, B. E.: Experimental approach to the pathogenesis of retrolental fibroplasia. 2. The influence of the developmental maturity on oxygen induced changes in the mouse eye. *Amer. J. Ophthal. 39:*475, 1955.
15. Imre, G.: Studies on the mechanism of retinal neovascularization. Role of lactic acid. *Brit. J. Ophthal. 48:*75, 1964.
16. Patz, A.: Oxygen studies in retrolental fibroplasia. 4. Clinical and experimental observations. *Amer. J. Ophthal. 38:*291, 1954.
17. Patz, A.: Experimental studies. *Amer. J. Ophthal. 40:*174, 1955.
18. Patz, A.: The effect of oxygen on immature retinal vessels. *Invest. Ophthal. 4:*988, 1965.
19. Patz, A.: The role of oxygen in retrolental fibroplasia. *Trans. Amer. Ophthal. Soc. 66:* 940, 1968.
20. Patz, A., Eastham, A., Higginbotham, D. H., and Kleh, T.: Oxygen studies in retrolental fibroplasia. 2. The production of the microscopic changes of retrolental fibroplasia in experimental animals. *Amer. J. Ophthal. 36:* 1511, 1953.
21. Patz, A., Hoeck, L. E., and DeLaCruz, E.: Studies on the effect of high oxygen administration in retrolental fibroplasia. 1. Nursery observations. *Amer. J. Ophthal. 35:*1248, 1952.

EFFECT OF VISUAL CELL DEGENERATION ON RETINAL VESSELS

Gerstein and Dantzker,[1] using a strain of rats with hereditary visual cell degeneration, have shown that there is a close temporal relationship between progressive degeneration and thinning of the outer retinal layers and degeneration of retinal capillaries. Studying retinal digest preparations, they noted the loss both of endothelial cell and intramural pericyte nuclei. In addition, they found irregularity of the capillary wall outline progressing through diminution in capillary width to a stage of anuclear fibrous strands. They feel that the degeneration and consequent thinning of the outer retinal layers brings the retinal vascular network into closer proximity to the choroid. This, plus the lessened tissue mass to metabolize oxygen, leads to increased oxygen tension in the outer retina. Presumably this combination of factors has a vasoconstrictive and degenerative effect on the retinal capillaries. These authors have further studied the problem by inducing damage to the outer retinal layers of rats with high-intensity light exposure, and by damaging the outer retinal layers in cats with intravenous iodoacetate.[2] Retinal capillary damage was induced in both instances and was considered secondary to the visual cell loss. According to Dantzker and Gerstein the capillary degeneration is not primarily related to either the state of the inner nuclear layer or the pigment epithelium. Interestingly, Henkind has noted that the retinal capillaries appear to maintain their integrity after loss of the inner retinal layers, for example, following optic nerve or chiasmal lesions.

REFERENCES

1. Gerstein, D. D., and Dantzker, D. R.: Retinal vascular changes in hereditary visual cell degeneration. *Arch. Ophthal.* *81*:99, 1969.

2. Dantzker, D. R., and Gerstein, D. D.: Retinal vascular changes following toxic effects on visual cells and pigment epithelium. *Arch. Ophthal.* *81*:106, 1969.

EFFECT OF CRYOPEXY ON RETINAL VESSELS

Cryogenic surgery is commonly used in retinal detachment operations. Wood and Watzke[1] have studied the effect of cryopexy upon the retinal vascular system of the dog. They used a temperature of −30° to −40° C for 1 to 3 seconds. This produced capillary damage which was first noted on retinal digest preparations 3 days after operation. There was a notable decrease in endothelial and intramural pericyte nuclei. In addition round cells were found in the walls of venules in the involved area. Later the capillaries became acellular and the venules became sheathed with pigment which had migrated from the retinal pigment epithelium. Little damage was found in the arterial portion of the retinal vascular tree.

REFERENCE

1. Wood, L. W., and Watzke, R. C.: Effects of cryopexy upon the retinal vasculature. *Arch. Ophthal.* *81*:254, 1969.

Index

PAGE NUMBERS IN *italics* REFER TO ILLUSTRATIONS.
FOOTNOTES ARE INDICATED BY *n* FOLLOWING THE PAGE NUMBER.
REFERENCES TO CONTINUING DISCUSSIONS ARE INDICATED BY *ff* FOLLOWING THE PAGE NUMBER.

Text and cover designed by M. S. Karkucinski
Composition in Century Schoolbook, linofilm, by Quinn & Boden Company, Inc.
Printed by Quinn & Boden Company, Inc.
HARPER & ROW, PUBLISHERS

71 72 73 74 75 9 8 7 6 5 4 3 2 1